Biopsy Pathology in Colorectal Disease

Biopsy Pathology in Colorectal Disease

SECOND EDITION

Ian Talbot
Consulting Pathologist at St Mark's and Northwick
Park Hospitals and Professor of Histopathology at
Imperial College Faculty of Medicine

Ashley Price
Consulting Pathologist at Northwick Park
and St Mark's Hospitals and Professor of
Gastrointestinal Pathology at Imperial College
Faculty of Medicine

Manuel Salto-Tellez
Associate Professor at the Department of Pathology,
Yong Loo Lin School of Medicine, National University
of Singapore and Senior Consultant Pathologist at
the National University Hospital in Singapore

Hodder Arnold

A MEMBER OF THE HODDER HEADLINE GROUP

First published in Great Britain in 1987
This second edition published in 2006 by
Hodder Arnold, an imprint of Hodder Education and a member of the Hodder Headline Group,
338 Euston Road, London NW1 3BH

http://www.hoddereducation.com

Distributed in the United States of America by
Oxford University Press Inc.,
198 Madison Avenue, New York, NY10016
Oxford is a registered trademark of Oxford University Press

Whilst the advice and information in this book are believed to be true and accurate at the date of going to
press, neither the author[s] nor the publisher can accept any legal responsibility or liability for any errors or
omissions that may be made. In particular (but without limiting the generality of the preceding disclaimer)
every effort has been made to check drug dosages; however it is still possible that errors have been missed.
Furthermore, dosage schedules are constantly being revised and new side-effects recognized. For these reasons
the reader is strongly urged to consult the drug companies' printed instructions before administering any of the
drugs recommended in this book.

British Library Cataloguing in Publication Data
A catalogue record for this book is available from the British Library

Library of Congress Cataloging-in-Publication Data
A catalog record for this book is available from the Library of Congress

ISBN-10   0 340 759 224
ISBN-13   978 0 340 759 226

1 2 3 4 5 6 7 8 9 10

Commissioning Editor: Philip Shaw
Project Editor: Heather Fyfe
Production Controller: Karen Tate
Cover Designer: Tim Pattinson
Indexer: Lawrence Errington

Typeset in 9.5/12 RotisSerif by Charon Tec Ltd (A Macmillan Company), Chennai, India
www.charontec.com
Printed and bound in Italy

What do you think about this book? Or any other Hodder Arnold title?
Please visit our website at www.hoddereducation.com

CONTENTS

Preface   xi
Acknowledgements   xiii

1   Introduction   1
     1.1   The clinician's role   1
     1.2   The pathologist's report   2
     1.3   Research and development   3
            References   3

2   Normal features   5
     2.1   Normal mucosal architecture   5
     2.2   The normal epithelium   5
     2.3   The lamina propria   9
     2.4   The muscularis mucosae   10
     2.5   The submucosa   11
            References   11

3   Assessment of abnormalities: diagnostic signposts   14
     3.1   Introduction   15
     3.2   The lumen   15
     3.3   Surface epithelium   16
     3.4   Intercryptal erosion   18
     3.5   Subepithelial zone   18
     3.6   Mucosal crypt architecture   19
     3.7   Crypt epithelium   29
     3.8   Lamina propria – cells   33
     3.9   Lamina propria – matrix   44
     3.10   Muscularis mucosae   49
     3.11   Submucosa   50
     3.12   Vasculature   52
     3.13   Nerves   53
     3.14   Pigment deposition   53
            References   53

4   Infective colitis   56
     4.1   Introduction   56
     4.2.   Acute bacterial diarrhoeas/infective colitis and proctitis   57

4.3	Enterocolitic syndromes	65
4.4	Sexually transmitted diseases	66
4.5	Intestinal spirochaetosis	69
4.6	Viral causes of colitis	70
4.7	Protozoal infection	74
4.8	Helminths	77
4.9	Nematodes	79
4.10	Fungal infection	82
	References	82

5   Ulcerative colitis   90

5.1	Introduction	90
5.2	The biopsy for diagnosis	91
5.3	The equivocal biopsy	101
5.4	Sequential biopsies	101
5.5	Colonoscopic biopsy	102
5.6	Inflammatory polyps ('pseudopolyps')	106
5.7	Fulminant acute colitis (toxic dilatation)	106
5.8	Follicular proctitis	107
5.9	Conclusions	107
	References	107

6   Crohn's disease   113

6.1	Introduction	113
6.2	Making the diagnosis	113
6.3	Histopathology	114
6.4	Differential diagnosis	118
6.5	Disease activity	119
6.6	Indicators of prognosis	120
6.7	Colonoscopic biopsy in Crohn's disease	120
6.8	Complications	121
6.9	Conclusions	121
	References	121

7   Ileoanal pouch pathology   124

7.1	Introduction: clinical indications for pouch surgery	124
7.2	Normal adaptive changes: ileal mucosa vs. residual rectal cuff mucosa	124
7.3	Inflammation and pouchitis	125
7.4	Risk factors for pouchitis	126
7.5	Pre-pouch ileitis	128
7.6	Differential diagnosis of pouchitis	128
7.7	Neoplasia	130
	References	131

8   Pseudomembranous colitis   133

8.1	Introduction: pseudomembranous colitis, antibiotic-associated colitis and diarrhoea	133
8.2	The biopsy diagnosis	134
8.3	Problems in the differential diagnosis	140
8.4	*Clostridium difficile* and its toxin	140

8.5   The pathologist's role in the diagnosis of pseudomembranous colitis   142
8.6   Conclusions   142
     References   142

9   Microscopic colitis – collagenous colitis, lymphocytic colitis and their variants   146
9.1   Introduction   146
9.2   Terminology   147
9.3   The biopsy diagnosis   148
9.4   Aetiology and pathogenesis   161
9.5   Course and therapy   162
9.6   Conclusions   163
     References   163

10   Ischaemic colitis   168
10.1   Introduction   168
10.2   Anatomical considerations   168
10.3   Precipitating causes   169
10.4   Natural history of ischaemic bowel disease   171
10.5   Endoscopic features   171
10.6   Biopsy appearances   172
10.7   Difficulties with diagnosis   175
10.8   Vasculitis   176
10.9   Necrotizing colitis syndromes   177
     References   177

11   Iatrogenic disease   182
11.1   Radiation colitis   182
11.2   Barium granuloma   184
11.3   Oleogranuloma   184
11.4   Drug-associated colitis   185
11.5   Diversion proctocolitis   191
11.6   Graft-versus-host disease   192
11.7   Neutropenic colitis   194
11.8   Colitis caused by bowel preparation and instrumentation   194
11.9   Anastomotic ulceration   195
11.10   Melanosis coli and laxative abuse   195
     References   196

12   The differential diagnosis of inflammatory bowel disease   202
12.1   General principles   203
12.2   Significance of the normal biopsy   203
12.3   Minor abnormalities   204
12.4   Major disease entities: ulcerative colitis vs. Crohn's disease vs. infection   209
12.5   Other forms of colitis   212
12.6   The terminal ileal biopsy   219
12.7   Backwash ileitis and ileal complications of ulcerative colitis   224
12.8   Ileal nodular lymphoid hyperplasia   225
12.9   Conclusions   226
     References   226

13   Disorders of motility   233
      13.1   Introduction   233
      13.2   The normal innervation   233
      13.3   Congenital megacolon: neuronal dysplasias, including Hirschsprung's disease   235
      13.4   Idiopathic megacolon of childhood   242
      13.5   Acquired megacolon   242
      13.6   Features associated with megacolon   244
              References   246

14   Neoplasia in the colon and rectum and its classification   248
      14.1   Definitions   248
              References   250

15   Polyps   251
      15.1   Definition   251
      15.2   Handling   251
      15.3   Classification   252
      15.4   Aberrant crypt foci   252
      15.5   Adenomatous polyps   253
      15.6   Serrated polyps   260
      15.7   Juvenile polyps   264
      15.8   Peutz–Jeghers polyps   266
      15.9   Inflammatory polyps   268
      15.10   Mucosal prolapse syndrome, including inflammatory cap polyp and
              inflammatory myoglandular polyp   271
      15.11   The Cronkhite–Canada syndrome   275
      15.12   Problems in the diagnosis of mucosal polyps: differential diagnosis   275
      15.13   Lymphoid polyps   276
      15.14   Leiomyomatous polyps   277
      15.15   Lipomatous polyps   278
      15.16   Vascular hamartoma   279
      15.17   Neurofibroma   279
      15.18   Ganglioneuroma   279
      15.19   Cowden's (multiple hamartoma) syndrome   282
      15.20   Granular cell tumour   282
      15.21   Heterotopic gastric mucosa   282
      15.22   Colonoscopic polypectomy   284
      15.23   The reporting of polyps   285
              References   286

16   The diagnosis of malignancy   292
      16.1   Introduction   292
      16.2   Overdiagnosis of malignancy   293
      16.3   The stroma of invasive adenocarcinoma   293
      16.4   Focal carcinoma in adenomatous polyps ('malignant polyps')   295
      16.5   Decisions when reporting biopsies of neoplastic tissue   298
              References   300

17   Dysplasia in inflammatory bowel disease   301
        17.1   Introduction   301
        17.2   Definitions   302
        17.3   Patients at risk and cancer incidence   303
        17.4   The reliability of dysplasia in cancer surveillance   305
        17.5   The macroscopic lesion in dysplasia   306
        17.6   Histological recognition and classification of dysplasia   307
        17.7   Observer variation   316
        17.8   Other stains and methodologies   316
        17.9   Molecular investigations   317
        17.10   Implication of the pathologist's report   317
        17.11   The sporadic adenoma and dysplasia-associated lesion or mass in ulcerative colitis   319
        17.12   Failure to find a lesion following recommendation for surgery   323
                References   323

18   Malignant tumours   330
        18.1   Carcinoma   330
        18.2   Endocrine cell (carcinoid) tumours   337
        18.3   Lymphoma and leukaemia   340
        18.4   Mesenchymal tumours   342
        18.5   Metastatic tumours   345
                References   347

19   Anal biopsy   351
        19.1   Introduction   351
        19.2   Inflammatory lesions   352
        19.3   Tumours of the anal canal   361
        19.4   Lesions of perianal skin   368
                References   374

20   Miscellaneous conditions   377
        20.1   Angiodysplasia and other primary vascular lesions   377
        20.2   Cystic pneumatosis (pneumatosis cystoides intestinalis, pneumatosis coli)   380
        20.3   Malakoplakia   380
        20.4   Chronic granulomatous disease of childhood   381
        20.5   Whipple's disease   382
        20.6   Sarcoidosis   382
        20.7   Ceroid lipofuscinosis (including Batten's disease)   383
        20.8   Amyloidosis   383
        20.9   Cronkhite–Canada syndrome   385
        20.10   Mucoviscidosis (cystic fibrosis)   386
        20.11   Colitis cystica profunda   386
        20.12   Endometriosis   387
        20.13   Primary immunodeficiency syndromes   387
        20.14   Irritable bowel syndrome   388
        20.15   Brown bowel syndrome   389
                References   389

Index   395

The sections illustrated in the figures have been stained with haematoxylin and eosin unless otherwise stated.

PREFACE

Mucosal biopsies of the colon, rectum and anus are some of the most frequently encountered specimens in hospital histopathology departments. This revised and updated edition of *Biopsy Pathology of Colorectal Disease*, builds on the popular first edition. Almost all of the figures are now in colour and the chapters are re-arranged. The book should continue to provide practising pathologists and those in allied disciplines with a thorough guide to the diagnosis of colorectal conditions, both common and rare, and offer expert guidance in the handling of biopsy specimens.

The most valuable information for diagnostic interpretation of the various types of inflammatory disease is presented clearly and succinctly, avoiding the use of non-diagnostic terms such as 'non-specific colitis'. Optimal ways of handling and examining polyps as well as biopsies, the assessment of biopsies in motility disorders and the interpretation of biopsies of anal lesions are described. A rational classification and practical approach to dysplasia is presented.

The early chapters describe how to recognize the many different features, both normal and abnormal, which can be regarded as *signposts* to diagnosis. The significance of these diagnostic signposts is briefly described and cross referenced to later chapters. In these the relevant signposts are amalgamated to describe the histological features of the specific diseases in greater depth. Some of the views expressed are personal opinions.

This book is for hospital pathologists and postgraduate students of histopathology, whether novices or experts. Its size is suitable for use close to the microscope during reporting. It is also a unique source of information for physicians and surgeons with an interest in gastroenterology and proctology; perhaps their compendium for a greater appreciation of the multidisciplinary team biopsy meetings that are now part and parcel of so many gastroenterology departments.

Ian Talbot
Ashley Price
Manuel Salto-Tellez
June 2006

ACKNOWLEDGEMENTS

This book would not have been written without the inspiration we have received from Dr Basil Morson, who set us on our way through the pageant of Gastrointestinal Pathology. We are indebted to our staff in the Northwick Park and St Mark's Hospitals Department of Histopathology for their technical assistance, particularly Paul Dunscombe. We also thank our colleagues in pathology at other departments who have provided slides of elusive material, specifically acknowledged throughout the book. Last but not least, we thank our respective wives and families for their forbearance in allowing us to steal so much time from them.

CHAPTER 1

INTRODUCTION

1.1 The clinician's role   1   1.3 Research and development   3
1.2 The pathologist's report   2   References   3

Colorectal biopsies form a significant proportion of the work of most departments of diagnostic histopathology. Colorectal diseases are common, carcinoma of the large bowel, for example, being the second most frequent malignant neoplasm to cause death in developed countries (Office of Population, Censuses and Surveys, 2003; World Health Organization, 1995). Rectal biopsy has always been a highly cost-effective and non-invasive investigation, but since the introduction of flexible fibre-optic colonoscopy and sigmoidoscopy and subsequent digital and other technologies (Saunders, 2005; Brown and Saunders, 2005) the scope of biopsy diagnosis of large bowel diseases has greatly increased. It is now a routine matter to examine and biopsy the terminal ileum. This has led to an acceleration in the rate of advance in our understanding of these diseases and the development of new forms of treatment. The range of diagnostic material now presented to the pathologist reflects these developments and demands a wide knowledge of the tissue changes in interpreting ever-smaller biopsy samples. These changes are described and illustrated in subsequent chapters, but in their interpretation the clinician and pathologist must appreciate each other's roles.

1.1 THE CLINICIAN'S ROLE

In all branches of diagnostic pathology accurate reporting depends on the clinical input, especially in inflammatory bowel disease, when the radiological and gross appearance of the colonic mucosa can be as important as the appearance under microscopy. The endoscopist's description of the colon, giving the distribution and pattern of the pathology is equivalent to the gross examination of the surgical specimen. Thus, one may appreciate such features as 'skip' areas in the case of Crohn's disease or the diffuse left-sided disease of typical ulcerative colitis. These may be diagnostic appearances even when the histological features are not. No clinical gastroenterologist can expect a helpful report if the relevant clinical data are not documented on the pathology request form. At all times the clinician should be aware that normal endoscopy does not necessarily mean normal histology and a biopsy should usually accompany an endoscopic examination. It is important that biopsies are not crushed or damaged by diathermy wires and that the tissue is not left exposed to air for more than a few minutes, as the tissue will dry out and histological examination will be unsatisfactory.

When taking a colonoscopic series of biopsies it is important that the sites from which the various biopsies are taken are identifiable. Many endoscopists achieve this by using a separate container for each biopsy, resulting in numerous 'pots' for each series of biopsies. We avoid this by mounting the biopsies along a straight line on a single strip of cellulose nitrate filter material (Catalogue no. 11404-50-N; Sartorius AG, Goetingen, Germany) (Sheffield and Talbot, 1992; Villanacci et al., 1993) (Fig. 1.1). The tissue fragments remain adherent to the strip during processing (Fig. 1.2) and all are easily sectioned together with the cellulose strip, so that the biopsies remain in correct sequence on the slide (Fig. 1.3). Up to eight biopsies can be comfortably accommodated on a single 2-cm long strip. By noting on the request form the order in which the biopsy sites are represented on the strip and using an identifier for the proximal end of the strip, such as cutting off a corner, all of the biopsies can be incorporated in one or two wax blocks instead of 8–16 blocks. This significantly reduces the laboratory work and reduces the number of slides for the reporting pathologist. An additional advantage is that, provided that the biopsy is mounted the correct way up, the tissue will be properly orientated.

Improvements in the methods of treatment of Hirschsprung's disease and related motility problems, with the adoption of surgical techniques such as the 'pull-through' operations of Duhamel and others (Nixon, 1978), have demanded special techniques in the diagnostic laboratory (see Chapter 13) and clinicians need to be aware of what can be done and how to make best use of the facilities of histochemistry.

Therapeutic polypectomy (Williams *et al.*, 1974), and the local excision of tumours (Wolff and Shinya, 1975), including submucosal resection (developed in Japan as the 'strip biopsy' technique) (Karita *et al.*, 1991) are developments which require the closest collaboration between clinician and pathologist if the endoscopist is to make the most of diagnostic and therapeutic opportunities (Whiteway *et al.*, 1985).

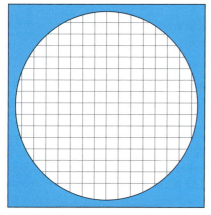

Figure 1.1 Disc of cellulose nitrate filter, material (Sartorius AG, Goetingen, Germany). Note the 3 mm grid pre-printed on the material. The whole disc measures 5 cm in diameter.

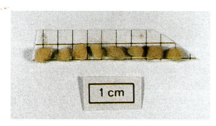

Figure 1.2 Strip of cellulose nitrate bearing a series of colonoscopic biopsies, complete with mounting strip, 2-cm long. The most proximal biopsy is situated at the end with the corner cut away. To obtain sections in the same plane, the embedded strip will need to be trimmed until the sections cut through the equator of the majority of the biopsies.

1.2 THE PATHOLOGIST'S REPORT

The construction of the pathologist's report is the art form of histopathology. It should fulfil two roles: first, to provide a basic description of the stained slide and second, to translate this description into a conclusion. An attempt should be made to interpret the features in diagnostic terms. It is, for example, inadequate to conclude a report, 'this is non-specific proctitis or colitis' (see Section 12.3.3c). The chances

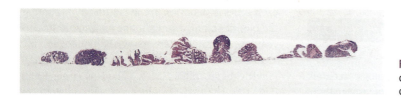

Figure 1.3 Section of a colonoscopic series of biopsies, complete with mounting strip.

are that the clinician knew this at the time of the examination. With polyps and neoplastic conditions it is essential that the report is adequate to indicate to the endoscopist what further course of action is most appropriate. This entails, in addition to precise diagnosis, an assessment of whether excision is complete and a comment on the likely behaviour of any tumour. Diagnoses apart, a biopsy may be undertaken to assess:

• the extent of the disease;
• the effect of therapy;
• the cause of the disease;
• the detection of complications.

When a biopsy is taken for any of these reasons the report should provide the answer to the specific clinical question asked.

The first part of the surgical report usually details the main 'physical signs' present in the biopsy or colonoscopic series. In practice, clinicians leap directly to the report's conclusions and the pathologist's descriptive prose may seldom be read. However, the main distinguishing attributes should be described in sufficient detail to provide, on any subsequent review, a justification of the conclusion drawn.

When several biopsies are taken at different levels or when reporting a colonoscopic series, ideally, each biopsy needs a separate descriptive paragraph, the site of each being clinically identified. If all are similar, then a collective description, simply documenting the differences between sites, is adequate. For example, 'the biopsies from 10 cm, 20 cm, and 40 cm are similar and show ..., only the biopsy from 40 cm is actively inflamed, with polymorphs infiltrating, ... etc.'

1.3 RESEARCH AND DEVELOPMENT

A regular biopsy review or multidisciplinary team meeting, attended by clinicians, is a useful way of improving the diagnostic interplay. It allows the discussion of ideas too subtle to be conveyed in writing, either on the request form or on the report. It is our experience that regular seminars provide an invaluable forum for communication of information about the handling of biopsy specimens that leads to improvements in the quality and orientation of biopsy material. They facilitate the training of junior staff and raise the standards of diagnosis. They also provide a 'second look', reducing the risk of an erroneous diagnosis, a phenomenon no pathologist should be too proud to recognize.

In the context of research a more detailed descriptive section is justified on a report. It is from meticulous documentation that 'new histological signs' may emerge to improve the diagnostic distinction between the varieties of inflammatory bowel disease, to identify improved markers for pre-cancer, to relate the features of polypoid lesions to other diseases and to help with our understanding of motility disorders.

Every department should have a system of disease classification and retrieval. It is not within the remit of this book to discuss the relative merits of particular systems. But whatever system is used every report should be indexed. This provides a simple database for further study, whether in a large university department or in a smaller district general hospital.

REFERENCES

Brown, G.J., Saunders, B.P. (2005) Advances in colonic imaging: technical improvements in colonoscopy. *Eur. J. Gastroenterol. Hepatol.*, 17, 785–92.

Karita, M., Tada, M., Okita, K., Kodama, T. (1991) Endoscopic therapy for early colon cancer: the strip biopsy resection technique. *Gastrointest. Endosc.*, 37, 128–32.

Nixon, H.H. (1978) *Surgical conditions in paediatrics*. London, Boston, Sydney, Wellington, Durban and Toronto: Butterworths, pp. 228–42.

Office of Population Censuses and Surveys (2003) DH2 No. 30, *Mortality statistics, review of the Registrar General on deaths by cause, sex and age in England and Wales*. London: Office for National Statistics, HMSO.

Saunders, B.P. (2005) Colonoscopy techniques. *Gastrointest. Endosc. Clin. N. Am.*, 15(4), xii–xiv.

Sheffield, J.P., Talbot, I.C. (1992) ACP Broadsheet 132. Gross examination of the large intestine. *J. Clin. Pathol.*, 45, 751–5.

Villanacci, F., Baroncelli, C., Ravelli, P., Missale, G., Williams, C., Talbot, I.C., Cestari, R. (1993). Orientamento delle biopsie endoscopiche del tratto gastroenterico mediante l'impiego di filtri Millipore di acetato di cellulose: aspetti endoscopici e anatomo patologici. *G. Ital. Endoscop. Dig.*, 16, 213–17.

Whiteway, J.E., Nicholls, R.J., Morson, B.C. (1985) The role of surgical local excision in the treatment of rectal cancer. *Br. J. Surg.*, 72, 694–7.

Williams, C.B., Hunt, R.H., Loose, H., Riddell, R.H., Sakai, Y., Swarbrick, E.T. (1974) Colonoscopy in the management of colon polyps. *Br. J. Surg.*, 61, 673–82.

Wolff, W.I., Shinya, H. (1975) Definitive treatment of malignant polyps of the colon. *Ann. Surg.*, 182, 516–25.

World Health Organization (1995) *World health statistics annual.* Geneva: World Health Organization.

CHAPTER 2

NORMAL FEATURES

2.1	**Normal mucosal architecture**	5	2.2.5	Lymphoid follicle-associated epithelium	8
2.2	**The normal epithelium**	5	2.3	**The lamina propria**	9
	2.2.1 Goblet cells	6	2.4	**The muscularis mucosae**	10
	2.2.2 Tall columnar cells	7	2.5	**The submucosa**	11
	2.2.3 Endocrine cells	7		**References**	11
	2.2.4 Stem cells	8			

It is not always easy to be sure that an intestinal biopsy is normal. Allowances have to be made for the mechanical effects of colonoscopy or sigmoidoscopy – congestion (Section 3.9.5), haemorrhage (Section 3.9.6), exudation of small numbers of neutrophils (Section 3.8.2) – and for the effects of enemas and purgatives used in preparation for the endoscopy – slight mucin depletion (Section 3.7.1) and minor regenerative features (Section 3.7.2). The following are the features to be found in a normal biopsy, the pathologist having taken account of the variation mentioned above.

2.1 NORMAL MUCOSAL ARCHITECTURE

The large intestinal mucosa increases in thickness gradually from 500 µm in the caecum to 1000 µm in the rectum. The crypts, which extend vertically from immediately above the muscularis mucosae, to open on the surface, are therefore deeper in the rectum and sigmoid colon than in the more proximal large bowel. The crypts are parallel-sided, straight, narrow, unbranched tubes. They lie close together and occupy most of the volume of the

mucosa, being only separated from each other by a thin rim of lamina propria when examined in 5 µm histological sections (Fig. 2.1).

2.2 THE NORMAL EPITHELIUM

Depending on the location in the colon and rectum, there are 500 to 2000 epithelial cells in each crypt (Potten *et al.*, 1992), with the maximum numbers appearing distally. The large intestinal epithelium is made up of three differentiated cell types: goblet cells, tall columnar cells and endocrine cells. Paneth cells are normally present only in the caecum, and even then in small numbers confined to the crypt bases. The cells in the lower third of the crypt (the proliferative compartment) are mitotically active. Within this basal third of the crypt the columnar cells (differentiating cells) are immature with increased nucleo-cytoplasmic ratio and pale finely vacuolated cytoplasm (Fig. 2.2) (Laorenssonn and Trier, 1968). The epithelial stem cells lie in the base of the proliferative compartment (vide infra).

A thin, barely visible, basal lamina extends, in continuity, beneath the epithelium of both the crypts and the luminal surface (Fig. 2.3).

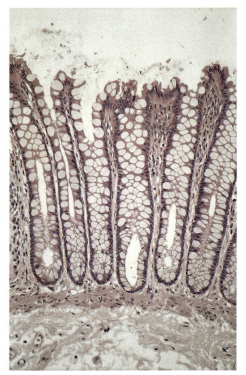

Figure 2.1 Normal rectal mucosal biopsy. The straight, parallel crypts extend down to the muscularis mucosae. They lie close together.

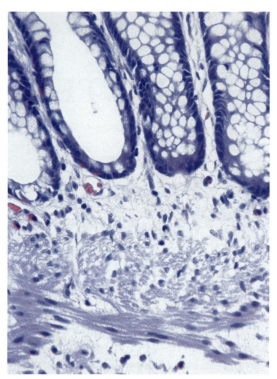

Figure 2.2 Basal portions of rectal mucosa with normal crypts. The immature goblet cells have relatively large, vesicular nuclei and multivesicular mucus. Between the goblet cells are the slimmer columnar cells, with dark elongated nuclei and inconspicuous cytoplasm. Endocrine cells with intensely eosinophilic cytoplasm, are present. Stem cells are not identifiable. The two layers of the muscularis mucosae (inner circular and outer longitudinal) can be seen.

Changes in the activity and numbers of epithelial cell types are responsible for many of the morphological features useful in biopsy interpretation.

2.2.1 Goblet cells

These account for the largest proportion, by volume, of the crypt epithelium but, numerically, they are outnumbered by the tall columnar cells in a ratio of 4 to 1 (Neutra and Padykula, 1984). There are subtle differences between the goblet cells in the rectum and distal colon and those in the proximal colon (Shamsuddin *et al.*, 1982). The mucin vacuoles in the mature goblet cells of the rectum and distal colon are larger and are inconspicuously subdivided into smaller globules. In the caecum and ascending colon, and in the lower parts of the crypts of the more distal colon and rectum, in addition to being smaller, the mucin goblets are more

obviously subdivided by refractile septa into numerous small vacuoles (Fig. 2.2). Chemical differences in goblet cell mucin parallel these morphological differences. In the distal large bowel the mucin is strongly acidic and stains blue or purple with alcian blue/periodic acid–Schiff (PAS) stain, whereas the mucin in the proximal colon is less acidic and is stained magenta or purple by this method. The reason for these differences is that the acid mucin of the left side of the colon and rectum is mostly sulphated but in the right side of the colon and caecum the proportion of sulphated mucin is less. The goblet cell mucin throughout the colon and rectum is sialylated which inhibits staining with PAS. Goblet cell staining by PAS is weak in the left colon but is stronger in the right colon because of a higher ratio of neutral sugars (fucose) to sialic acid in the proximal colon. However, in alcian blue/PAS stained sections, this is masked by the acidic sulphated mucosubstance in the more proximal colon taking up alcian blue (Jass and Roberton, 1994). The mucin types are best demonstrated by the high iron diamine/alcian blue technique; sialomucins stain blue and sulphomucins brown. Changes in their expression within the crypts may be of some diagnostic use. There is also goblet cell sialomucin heterogeneity within the general population (Sugihara and Jass, 1986) and between Sino-Japanese and Caucasians (Campbell *et al.*, 1994). In 9 per cent of Caucasians and in a much higher proportion of Asians, goblet cells are more strongly stained with PAS. This is because of a congenital inactivity of both alleles of the *O*-acetyl transferase (OAT) gene (the trait is recessive). In 42 per cent of Caucasians there is focal strong PAS staining of scattered isolated crypts caused by somatic loss of heterozygosity of the inactive OAT gene brought about by non-disjunction at stem cell division (Jass and Roberton, 1994).

As the goblet cells approach the necks of the crypts they begin to discharge their mucus, with the result that, by the time the surface epithelium is reached, only a few goblet cells remain identifiable (Fig. 2.3).

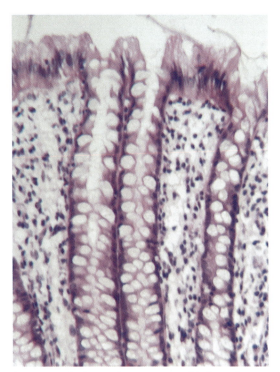

Figure 2.3 Surface and upper crypt epithelium of normal rectal mucosa. The goblet cells are most prominent in the crypts, those on the luminal surface having partly discharged their mucin. Note the thin subepithelial collagen plate and the inconspicuous, small blood vessels immediately beneath it.

2.2.2 Tall columnar cells

These slender cells, with a brush border of microvilli, appear on light microscopy to lack mucin vacuoles. However, Neutra *et al.* (1977) demonstrated by autoradiography that columnar cells are more active than goblet cells in synthesizing and secreting glycoproteins and, by electron microscopy, vesicles are seen in the apex of each columnar cell (Shamsuddin *et al.*, 1982). The vesicles become smaller, more uniform and more electron-dense towards the caecum. Columnar cell mucin is membrane-bound and, unlike goblet cell mucin, is not secreted. Furthermore, the protein core expresses MUC1 and MUC3 (non-secretory, membrane-associated glycoproteins), rather than MUC2, a glycoprotein of goblet cell mucin (Jass and Roberton, 1994). Staining with

PAS reveals finely granular, diastase-resistant material in the vesicles, indicating a neutral mucin secretory product. The relationship between this material and the role that these cells are believed to have in absorption of water, lipid and solutes is still uncertain.

After discharging mucin, goblet cells gain microvilli and resemble tall columnar cells (Shamsuddin and Trump, 1981) (Fig. 2.3). However, although no doubt both are derived from the same crypt stem cells, the two cell types represent different lineages (Jass and Roberton, 1994).

2.2.3 Endocrine cells

These cells, being small and few, tend to be inconspicuous in routine sections stained with

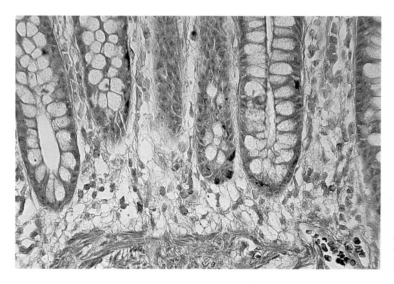

Figure 2.4 Biopsy of normal rectal mucosa, showing distribution of enterochromaffin cells, located towards the crypt bases (lead haematoxylin).

haematoxylin and eosin (H and E). Cristina *et al.* (1978) showed, by electron microscopy, that although 69 per cent of endocrine cells in the caecum were of enterochromaffin type and therefore likely to be argentaffin, this proportion fell to 42 per cent in the rectum. This means that less than half the endocrine cells in the rectal mucosa will stain with Masson–Fontana. The remainder are argyrophil rather than argentaffin and therefore fall into the category of 'enterochromaffin-like' cells.

Endocrine cells are sparsely scattered along the bowel among the other epithelial cells (Fig. 2.4), an average of four to each crypt in paraffin sections (Gledhill *et al.*, 1986). They are pyramidal, with a narrow apex which presents a small luminal surface covered with microvilli (Neutra and Padykula, 1984). The argyrophil granules are basally situated beneath the nucleus and are visible, owing to their intense eosinophilia, in routine H and E stained sections. The granules stain by immunohistochemical methods for chromogranin. Some contain serotonin, whereas others react with antisera to a number of polypeptide hormones, including substance P (Sokolski and Lechago, 1984), pancreatic polypeptide, glucagon and somatostatin (O'Briain *et al.*, 1982). The non-granular antigen, neurone-specific enolase, can be used as a non-specific marker for all of these cells but, in our experience, is less reliable and sensitive as an immunohistochemical marker than chromogranin (Carlei *et al.*, 1985).

2.2.4 Stem cells

At the base of the proliferative compartment in the lower third of the crypt is a group of four to six stem cells (Potten, 1998) clustered in a niche. These cells show no morphologically distinguishing features (Shamsuddin *et al.*, 1982) but can be investigated by studying crypt cell phylogeny with respect to methylation of CpG islands within isolated crypt epithelial cell DNA (Kim and Shibata, 2002). These latter authors estimate that each crypt is populated by a single clone of stem cells which is renewed every 8 years. It is normal to find mitoses in, or immediately above, the proliferative compartment.

2.2.5 Lymphoid follicle-associated epithelium

It is normal for crypt epithelial cells adjacent to lymphoid follicles to be more fusiform and compactly arranged than ordinary columnar cells (Fig. 2.5) (Laorenssonn and Trier, 1968). The surface epithelium overlying lymphoid follicles (dome epithelium) is also of this type and functions as a semipermeable gateway through which antigenic material can gain access to antigen-presenting cells in the lamina propria (O'Leary and Sweeney, 1986), prior to antigen processing (Sarsfield *et al.*, 1996). It is important not to mistake these for dysplastic cells in ulcerative colitis.

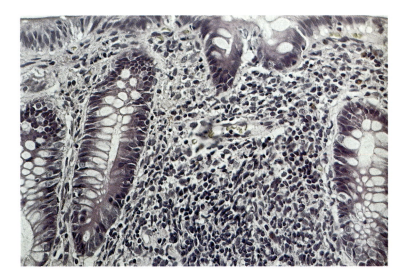

Figure 2.5 Crypt epithelium adjacent to lymphoid follicle, showing a more compact arrangement, with densely eosinophilic cells lacking mucin goblets.

2.3 THE LAMINA PROPRIA

The normally small amount of connective tissue between the large intestinal mucosal crypts is of areolar type and consists of sparsely arranged fibroblasts and reticulin fibres separated by poorly staining ground substance (Fig. 2.6). There is a layer of collagen up to 3 μm thick immediately beneath the basement membrane of the surface epithelium (Gledhill and Cole, 1984) (Fig. 2.6) but this is not evident in relation to the crypt basement membrane, a feature that has been confirmed by electron microscopy (Donnellan, 1965). Thin smooth muscle fibres pass up from the muscularis mucosae to be attached to this superficial collagen layer and fibroblasts are embedded in it (Donnellan, 1965; Kaye *et al.*, 1968).

Immediately beneath the collagen layer underlying the basement membrane of the surface epithelium there are sparsely scattered PAS-positive cells (Fig. 2.7). Some of these cells may be muciphages, as described by Azzopardi and Evans (1966) (Section 3.8.9, Fig 3.37) but others are antigen-presenting cells ('veiled' cells or dendritic reticulum cells) (Sarsfield *et al.*, 1996).

The gut-associated lymphoid tissue (Parrott, 1976) comprises singly scattered lymphocytes which are mostly T cells and B lymphocytes arranged in lymphoid follicles (Fig. 2.8). The follicles are most numerous in the caecum and rectum (Langman and

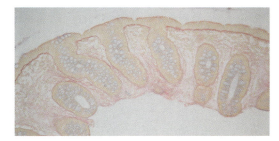

Figure 2.6 Normal rectal mucosal connective tissue. There are only fine collagen fibres in the lamina propria and a thin subepithelial collagen plate. The 'spaces' between the fibres are occupied by blood capillaries and vertically orientated smooth muscle cells (van Gieson, ×170).

Rowland, 1986). They frequently extend through the muscularis mucosae into the upper submucosa. In children and adolescents they have pale germinal centres, such as are seen in lymph nodes, owing to the presence of large lymphoblastic cells. However, no more than 1 per cent of follicles should contain such germinal centres in normal adults, unless there is inflammation (O'Leary and Sweeney, 1986). Also scattered throughout the colorectal mucosal lamina propria are plasma cells, mainly immunoglobulin A (IgA)-containing, with small numbers of immunoglobulin G (IgG)- and immunoglobulin M (IgM)-producing cells (Bjerke *et al.*, 1986). Plasma cells and lymphocytes are scanty in infancy and the lymphoid cells of the large intestine do not reach their maximum numbers until the age of 3–5 years.

At points where the muscularis mucosae is breached by lymphoid follicles, mucosal crypts may also extend into the submucosa, forming 'lymphoid–glandular complexes' (Kealy, 1976) (Section 3.11.4). O'Leary and Sweeney (1986) found approximately one such complex in each 3-mm length of colonic mucosa and double this number in the rectum. They observed antigen-processing M cells in the overlying surface epithelium by electron microscopy, analogous to the situation in the small intestine.

The blood vessels of the mucosa are small, capillary-sized, thin-walled, low-pressure vessels and are concentrated beneath the surface collagen layer, with their feeder vessels of similar size passing vertically between the crypts (Fig. 2.6). Knowledge of this arrangement helps in the appreciation of artefactual haemorrhage (Section 3.9.6) and the histogenesis of ischaemic damage (Section 10.6) and angiodysplasia (Section 20.1.1).

Sparse, fine, non-myelinated nerve fibres lie vertically in the lamina propria between the crypts, together with occasional ganglion cells. They are detectable only by special techniques such as immunocytochemistry for CD56 (N-CAM) antigen. Cholinesterase staining is more sensitive, but requires frozen sections of unfixed tissue (Fig. 13.2). Assessment of the number and nature of neuronal processes is useful in cases of Hirschsprung's disease and other neuronal dysplasias (Chapter 13).

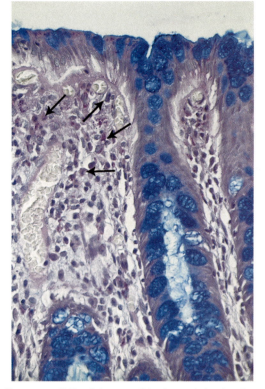

Figure 2.7 Cells of the normal lamina propria, showing macrophages and probable dendritic reticulum, antigen-processing cells (Alcian blue/periodic acid–Schiff)

2.4 THE MUSCULARIS MUCOSAE

This consists of elastic fibres and an inner circular and outer longitudinal layer of smooth muscle,

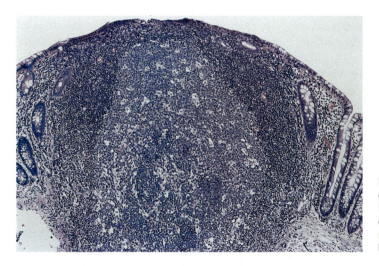

Figure 2.8 Lymphoid follicle in biopsy of normal rectum. This hyperplastic lymphoid follicle contains a germinal centre and extends through the muscularis mucosae, which appears to be interrupted.

30–40 μm in total thickness (Fig. 2.2). The muscularis mucosae is innervated by single parasympathetic nerve fibres, which can be identified like those in the mucosa (Fig. 13.2), and their assessment is important when considering Hirschsprung's disease and other neuronal dysplasias.

2.5 THE SUBMUCOSA

Similar to the lamina propria mucosae, this consists of areolar connective tissue with loosely arranged collagen fibres and scanty elastic fibres (Fig. 2.9) which allow a considerable degree of elasticity, a property of some importance to the technical procedure of mucosal biopsy. Plexuses of veins and small arteries are present.

Meissner's plexus of autonomic nerve fibres, with associated ganglion cells lies in the submucosa (Fig. 2.10).

A detailed knowledge of the normal innervation of the submucosa is required for interpretation of biopsies taken for motility disorders (Hirschsprung's disease, etc., Section 13.3).

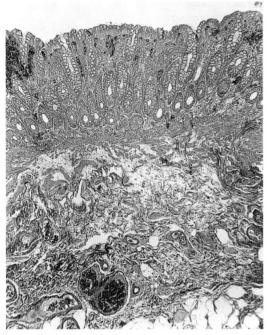

Figure 2.9 Normal submucosal collagen and elastic fibres (elastic–van Gieson).

REFERENCES

Azzopardi, J.G., Evans, D.J. (1966) Mucoprotein containing histiocytes (muciphages) in the rectum. *J. Clin. Pathol.*, 19, 368–74.

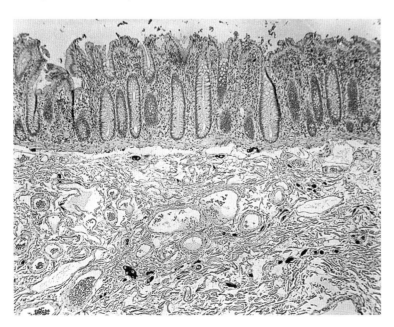

Figure 2.10 Normal submucosal nerves, stained for S-100 by immunoperoxidase, showing Schwann cells. The superficial (Meissner plexus) and deep submucosal ganglia are evident.

Bjerke, K., Brandtzaeg, P., Rognum, T.O. (1986). Distribution of immunoglobulin producing cells is different in normal human appendix and colon mucosa. *Gut*, 27, 667–74.

Campbell, F., Appleton, M.A., Fuller, C.E. *et al.* (1994) Racial variation in the *O*-acetylation phenotype of human colonic mucosa. *J. Pathol.*, 174, 169–74.

Carlei, F., Bishop, A.E., Bonamico, M. *et al.* (1985) Gut endocrine cells in coeliac disease estimated by immunocytochemistry using monoclonal antibody to chromogranin. *J. Pathol.*, 145, 116A (Abstract).

Cristina, M.L., Lehy, C.R., Zeitoun, P., Dufougeray, F. (1978) Fine structural classification and comparative distribution of endocrine cells in normal human large intestine. *Gastroenterology*, 75, 20–8.

Donnellan, W.L. (1965) The structure of the colonic mucosa. *Gastroenterology*, 49, 496–514.

Filipe, M.L., Branfoot, C.A. (1976) Mucin histochemistry of the colon. In: Morson, B.C. (ed.) *Pathology of the gastrointestinal tract, current topics in pathology*, vol. 63. Berlin: Springer-Verlag, pp. 143–78.

Gledhill, A., Cole, F.M. (1984) Significance of basement membrane thickening in the human colon. *Gut* 25, 1085–8.

Gledhill, A., Hall, P.A., Cruse, J.P., Pollock, D.J. (1986) Enteroendocrine cell hyperplasia, carcinoid tumours and adenocarcinoma in long-standing ulcerative colitis. *Histopathology*, 10, 501–8.

Jass, J.R., Roberton, A.M. (1994) Colorectal mucin histochemistry in health and disease: a critical review. *Pathol. Int.*, 44, 487–504.

Kaye, G.I., Lane, N., Pascal, R.R. (1968) Colonic pericryptal fibroblast sheath: replication, migration and cytodifferentiation of a mesenchymal cell system in adult tissue. *Gastroenterology*, 54, 835–51.

Kealy, W.F. (1976) Colonic lymphoid-glandular complex (microbursa) nature and morphology. *J. Clin. Pathol.*, 29, 241–4.

Kim, K.M., Shibata D. (2002) Methylation reveals a niche: stem cell succession in human colon crypts. *Oncogene*, 21, 5441–9.

Langman, J.M., Rowland R. (1986) The number and distribution of lymphoid follicles in the human large intestine. *J. Anat.*, 149, 189–94.

Laorenssonn, V., Trier, J.S. (1968) The fine structure of human rectal mucosa. *Gastroenterology*, 55, 88–101.

Neutra, M.R., Padykula, H.A. (1984) The gastrointestinal tract. In: Weiss, L. (ed.) *Modern concepts of gastrointestinal histology.* New York, Amsterdam and Oxford: Elsevier, pp. 696–706.

Neutra, M.R., Grand, R.J., Trier, J.S. (1977) Glycoprotein synthesis, transport and secretion by epithelial cells of human rectal mucosa: normal and cystic fibrosis. *Lab. Invest.*, 36, 535–46.

O'Briain, D.S., Dayal, Y., Delellis, R.A. *et al.* (1982) Rectal carcinoids as tumors of the hind-gut endocrine cells: a morphological and immunohistochemical analysis. *Am. J. Surg. Pathol.*, 6, 131–42.

O'Leary, A.D., Sweeney, E.C. (1986) Lympho-glandular complexes of the colon: structure and distribution. *Histopathology*, 10, 267–83.

Parrott, D.M.V. (1976) The gut as a lymphoid organ. *Clin. Gastroenterol.*, 5, 211–28.

Potten, C.S. (1998) Stem cells in the gastrointestinal epithelium: numbers, characteristics and death. *Phil. Trans. R. Soc. Biol. Sci.*, 353, 821–30.

Potten, C.S., Kellett, M., Roberts, S.A., Rew, D.A., Wilson, G.D. (1992) Measurement of *in vivo* proliferation in human colorectal mucosa using bromodeoxyuridine. *Gut*, 33, 71–8.

Sarsfield, P., Rinne, A., Jones, D.B., Johnson, P., Wright, D.H. (1996). Accessory cells in physiological lymphoid tissue from the intestine: an immunohistochemical study. *Histopathology*, 28, 205–11.

Shamsuddin, A.K.M., Trump B.F. (1981) Colon epithelium 1. Light microscopic, histochemical and ultrastructural features of normal colon epithelium of male Fischer 344 rats. *J. Nat. Cancer Inst.*, 66, 375–88.

Shamsuddin, A.M., Phelps, P.C., Trump, B.F. (1982) Human large intestinal epithelium: light microscopy, histochemistry and ultrastructure. *Hum. Pathol.*, 13, 790–803.

Sokolski, K.N., Lechago, J. (1984) Human colonic substance P-producing cells are a separate population from the serotonin-producing enterochromaffin cells. *J. Histochem. Cytochem.*, 32, 1066–74.

Sugihara, K., Jass, J.R. (1986) Colorectal goblet cell sialomucin heterogeneity: its relation to malignant disease. *J. Clin. Pathol.*, 39, 1088–95.

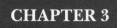

CHAPTER 3

ASSESSMENT OF ABNORMALITIES: DIAGNOSTIC SIGNPOSTS

3.1	Introduction	15
3.2	The lumen	15
3.3	Surface epithelium	16
3.4	Intercryptal erosion	18
3.5	Subepithelial zone	18
3.6	Mucosal crypt architecture	19
	3.6.1 Crypt branching	19
	3.6.2 Crypt atrophy	21
	3.6.3 Crypt degeneration	21
	3.6.4 Crypt serration	24
	3.6.5 Crypt dilatation	25
	3.6.6 Crypt enlargement – transitional mucosa	26
	3.6.7 The crypt abscess	27
	3.6.8 Incipient crypt abscess (cryptitis)	28
	3.6.9 Misplaced crypts	29
3.7	Crypt epithelium	29
	3.7.1 Mucin depletion	29
	3.7.2 Regenerative hyperplasia	29
	3.7.3 Dysplastic epithelium	30
	3.7.4 Paneth cells	32
	3.7.5 Endocrine cells	33
3.8	Lamina propria – cells	33
	3.8.1 Inflammatory cells	33
	3.8.2 Neutrophil exudate	34
	3.8.3 Plasma cells	34
	3.8.4 Lymphocytes	35
	3.8.5 Eosinophils	35
	3.8.6 Mast cells	36
	3.8.7 Proportions of inflammatory cells	36
	3.8.8 Distribution of inflammatory cells	36
	3.8.9 Histiocytes	37
	3.8.10 Giant cells	37
	3.8.11 Granulomas	38
	3.8.12 Pseudolipomatosis	41
	3.8.13 Microorganisms	42
3.9	Lamina propria – matrix	44
	3.9.1 Fibrosis	44
	3.9.2 Hyalinization	46
	3.9.3 Oedema	46
	3.9.4 Muscle fibres	47
	3.9.5 Vasculature	48
	3.9.6 Haemorrhage	48
	3.9.7 Granulation tissue	48
3.10	Muscularis mucosae	49
3.11	Submucosa	50
	3.11.1 Submucosal oedema	50
	3.11.2 Inflammation	50
	3.11.3 Submucosal fat	51
	3.11.4 Misplaced epithelium	51
	3.11.5 Pseudocarcinomatous invasion (pseudoinvasion)	52
3.12	Vasculature	52
3.13	Nerves	53
	3.13.1 Ganglia	53
	3.13.2 Nerve bundles	53
3.14	Pigment deposition	53
References		53

3.1 INTRODUCTION

In this chapter individual lesions are described and illustrated and the diagnostic significance of each is evaluated. However, a single abnormal feature is rarely of specific significance on its own and our purpose is to provide a series of diagnostic signposts – the parts that go to make up the whole. Subsequent chapters are more conventional in style and deal with the specific disease entities which can be considered the sum of the individual changes described in this chapter.

It cannot be overemphasized that the individual signs are not diagnostic but merely building bricks. The bricks from any one building look much the same, yet each building viewed as a whole is entirely different. This chapter, therefore, is very much a dictionary, to be used in conjunction with later, specific disease descriptions.

3.2 THE LUMEN

It is easy to omit inspection of the debris covering the mucosa. Often it has become detached and is seen lying a few millimetres from the main biopsy (Fig. 3.1a). The debris reflects the luminal contents and is worth careful inspection. Sloughed epithelial cells, collections of neutrophil polymorphs and/or eosinophils are common cellular constituents.

In practice 'pus' in the lumen is a frequent finding, even when the mucosa of the biopsy is not inflamed. It raises the question of pathology nearby and is an indication to cut deeper levels, perhaps to expose focal disease. In pseudomembranous colitis the luminal polymorphs may have an unusual linear

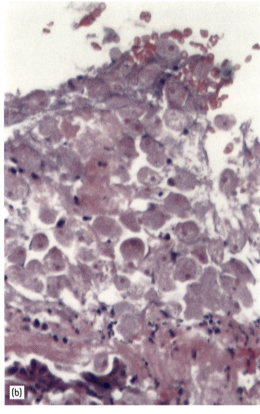

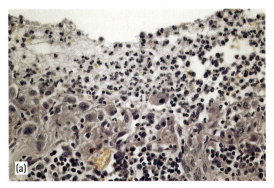

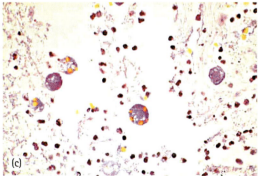

Figure 3.1 Luminal debris and cells. (a) Vacuolated macrophages, degenerate epithelial cells and inflammatory cells overlying a non-specific ulcer. (b) and (c) Amoebae, containing partly digested red blood cells, apart from being larger, are better preserved and their cytoplasmic structures better defined than the macrophages in (a). ((b) Haematoxylin and eosin; (c) periodic acid–Schiff/Martius yellow.)

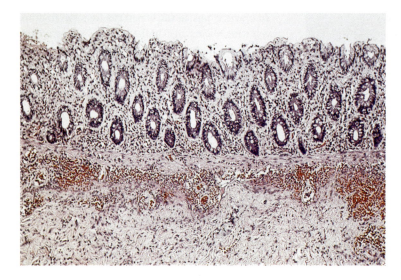

Figure 3.2 Surface epithelial degeneration in a patient with ischaemic colitis. There is a mild inflammatory reaction in the lamina propria.

arrangement (Fig. 8.3), again not a diagnostic feature but a pointer to the need for further levels and perhaps clinical discussion (Section 8.2.1a).

Amoebiasis is an important diagnosis to be made from inspection of the surface debris but care is necessary to distinguish the organisms from sloughed epithelial cells and macrophages (Fig. 4.20). It is useful to remember that the nuclei of amoebae are pale and indistinct in comparison with those of histiocytes (Fig. 3.1b). The periodic acid–Schiff (PAS) reaction also helps in this distinction (Section 4.7.1) (Fig. 3.1c). As well as amoebae, *Candida* and other organisms, such as cryptosporidia and spirochaetes, may be noted, though they are usually intimately associated with the surface epithelium (Section 3.8.13).

3.3 SURFACE EPITHELIUM

The epithelium between the crypts may be absent, degenerate, infiltrated by inflammatory cells, serrated or show an irregular 'tufted' growth pattern. It is the site to search for cryptosporidia and spirochaetes (Section 3.8.13). Although strictly part of the lamina propria, the collagen plate immediately beneath the surface epithelial basement membrane is also usually assessed along with the epithelium (Section 3.5).

Trauma at the time of biopsy, or subsequently, may simply remove the surface. Viable cells may then be obvious in the luminal debris and the exposed lamina propria will not show any signs of inflammation. Free blood cells usually cover the denuded mucosa.

Degeneration of the surface epithelium in the absence of accompanying inflammation is uncommon. It may represent poor tissue fixation or be the result of enthusiastic bowel preparation. In the latter case a few inflammatory cells are often present.

Surface degeneration accompanied by an acute inflammatory cell infiltrate is a common and non-specific feature of any of the causes of coloproctitis (Chapter 12) and usually occurs in conjunction with other changes in the lamina propria (Fig. 3.2). In isolation, as a sign, it suggests an irritative enema or some form of iatrogenic or self-induced trauma. It should always initiate a request for deeper levels. Diarrhoea in itself, however, is not a cause of surface inflammation (Mandal *et al.*, 1982).

Close scrutiny of the surface epithelium will often reveal nuclear dust apparently within and between the columnar cells (Fig. 3.3). This is not a specific diagnostic feature, but is seen in many cases of resolving acute inflammation, particularly in the later stages of infective colitis. It can also be seen in microscopic colitis and can be the result of administration of a phosphate enema as part of bowel preparation for colonoscopy (Driman and Preiksaitis, 1998). The surface epithelium is constantly being shed, with loss of cells by apoptosis, but apoptotic bodies are usually inconspicuous. Conspicuous apoptotic bodies in the surface

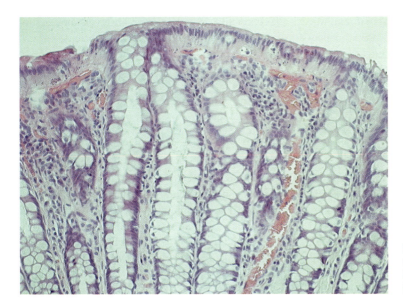

Figure 3.3 Nuclear dust within surface epithelial layer. Rectal biopsy from patient with resolving infective proctocolitis.

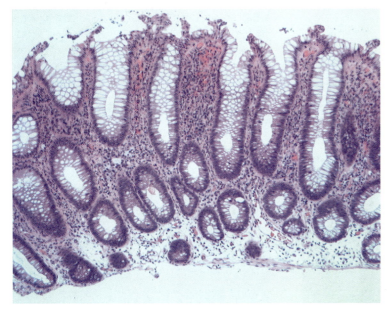

Figure 3.4 Tufting of degenerate surface epithelium, suggesting a toxic effect (seen in some cases of antibiotic-associated colitis).

epithelium are markers of increased epithelial cell destruction. They can result from virus infection and various luminal influences, including disturbances of short chain fatty acids and surfactant loss (Strater *et al.*, 2002).

The surface epithelial cells may occasionally be grouped into protruding tufts (Fig. 3.4). These are usually associated with some inflammatory cells. Although we would not claim this as a specific sign, it does appear to be more common in infective

colitis and antibiotic-associated diarrhoea than other causes of colitis (Sections 4.2.1, 8.2.1 and 8.2.2). It may be used as a prompt to search for other features of these diseases.

In spirochaetosis the luminal surface of the epithelial cells appears thickened and 'fuzzy' (see Figs 3.49b and 4.11). The PAS reagent, or better still a Warthin–Starry stain, emphasizes this thick line and the 'tails' of the spirochaetes can be seen (Section 4.5).

Cryptosporidia are seen as tiny haematoxyphilic dots on the surface (see Figs 3.49d, 4.22a), easily confused with stain deposits or nuclear debris (Section 4.7.4).

3.4 INTERCRYPTAL EROSION

A particularly striking abnormality may be termed the intercryptal erosion. Here the surface epithelium is lost and replaced by a spray of fibrin, mucus and inflammatory cells (Fig. 3.5). In the correct setting (Section 8.2.1a) it is a diagnostic lesion of pseudomembranous colitis. However, careful interpretation is needed, as it is also typically seen in mucosal prolapse (solitary ulcer syndrome; Section 15.10), can be found in ischaemic colitis

(Section 10.6.2) and we have observed similar surface erosion in many unrelated conditions.

3.5 SUBEPITHELIAL ZONE

When observing the surface, attention should also focus on the basal lamina and acellular collagen band beneath. It should be noted that the nuclei of the surface epithelial cells are not always basally located and are often displaced upwards. This results in a thick eosinophilic band of basal cytoplasm (Fig. 3.6a). The significance of this nuclear shift is uncertain but it is probably an artefact of fixation and contraction of the biopsy, with concertina-like

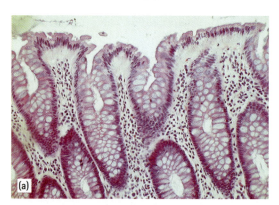

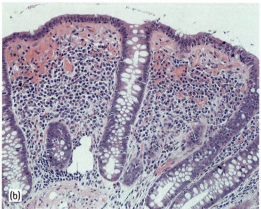

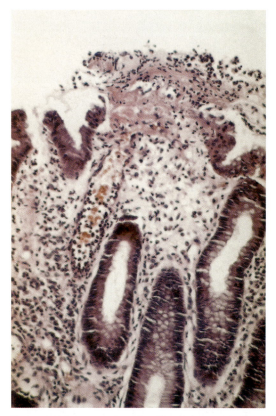

Figure 3.5 Intercryptal erosion. The surface epithelium is lost and replaced by fibrino-purulent exudate in this typical lesion of pseudomembranous colitis, also seen at lower magnification in Fig. 8.3b on page 135.

Figure 3.6 (a) Subepithelial zone. Upward shift of nuclei of surface epithelial cells, with superficial resemblance to thickened basement membrane. This artefact may be due to foreshortening of the biopsy on fixation. (b) Minimal thickening (10 μm) of subepithelial collagen zone. Blood capillaries are embedded in the collagen layer. The lamina propria is diffusely infiltrated by plasma cells.

foreshortening of the surface. Its importance is to avoid mistaking it for the thickened collagen zone of collagenous colitis.

The normal thickness of the subepithelial collagen is between 3 μm and 6.9 μm (Bogomoletz *et al.*, 1980; Gledhill and Cole, 1984). This must be remembered before labelling a biopsy as abnormal (Fig. 3.6b). Any thickening can be patchy within one biopsy and at different levels. The presence of a thickened band at one point does not warrant the immediate diagnosis of collagenous colitis (the interpretation of real or apparent thickening is more fully covered in Chapter 9). Other situations in which the collagen band can be thickened are ischaemia, radiation injury and metaplastic polyps.

3.6 MUCOSAL CRYPT ARCHITECTURE

Inspection of the crypt architecture initially at low power may reveal either circumscribed non-inflammatory abnormalities affecting a group of crypts, as in polyps (Fig. 3.7), or inflammatory abnormalities affecting the crypts along the length of mucosa, as in the various forms of colitis.

3.6.1 Crypt branching

The colonic mucosa has regular natural undulations and the crypts situated astride these areas (at the innominate grooves) may be branched (Fig. 3.8). Apart from this situation, crypt branching is an abnormal sign, implying prior mucosal damage. The crypts may be bifid (Fig. 3.9) or, after severe damage, even run parallel to the surface (Fig. 3.10). This can be seen in a variety of serrated adenoma, when it has a different connotation (Section 15.6.2). In a well-orientated biopsy the failure to cut any crypts along their length, with the majority being cross-cut, is also a sign of crypt branching and irregularity (Fig. 3.11).

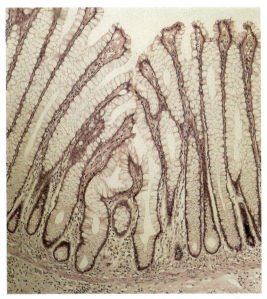

Figure 3.8 Normal mucosa: crypt branching at the junctions of mucosal undulations (innominate grooves)

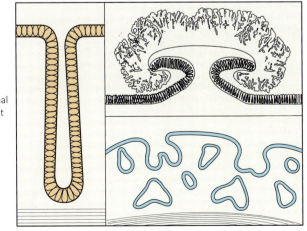

Normal crypt

Polyp

Deformed crypts

Figure 3.7 Patterns of crypt architecture: a polyp is a circumscribed focal abnormality, whereas in established colitis the glandular irregularity is diffuse (lower right).

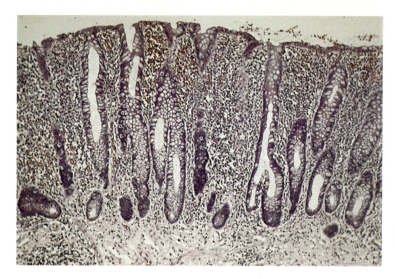

Figure 3.9 Crypt bifurcation following damage in ulcerative colitis.

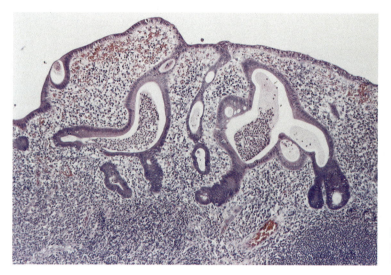

Figure 3.10 Severe deformity, with crypts parallel to luminal surface, in longstanding ulcerative colitis.

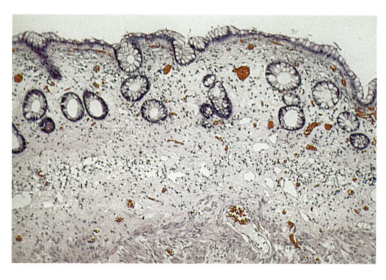

Figure 3.11 Unavoidable cross-cutting of distorted crypts in ulcerative colitis.

Small numbers of irregular crypts have no specific diagnostic significance, apart from the implication of previous damage, but when irregularity dominates the biopsy it is a strong pointer towards the diagnosis of ulcerative colitis (Section 5.2.1a). It may also be seen in healing mucosa after any bout of severe ulceration, for example, in ischaemia (Section 10.6.3). The interpretation must take account of this and, hence, of the clinical story, and endoscopic findings are needed to evaluate the problem. In infective colitis and Crohn's disease the basic crypt alignment is usually maintained.

3.6.2 Crypt atrophy

A reduction in the number of crypts seen in a biopsy represents crypt atrophy. When fully established, it is an attribute most commonly in favour of the diagnosis of ulcerative colitis. As with branching, it may be the end result of healing after severe acute ulceration. As well as showing lateral separation, the crypts are generally shorter, with an obvious gap between their bases and the muscularis mucosae (Fig. 3.12). The individual mucous cells lining the crypts are usually intact and may even appear larger than normal (Fig. 5.9).

Crypt atrophy is found in chronic disease states, particularly chronic ulcerative colitis (Section 5.2.3),

healed ischaemic colitis (Section 10.6.4), radiation damage (Section 11.1) and graft-versus-host disease (Section 11.6). A helpful marker of atrophy caused by chronic disease is the finding of Paneth cells in the shortened crypts (Section 3.7.4).

Situations that mimic crypt atrophy are thickening of the lamina propria owing to oedema (Section 3.9.3) and, conversely, thinning of the mucosa caused by stretching in an over-zealous attempt at orientation, when the crypts become separated from each other (Fig. 3.13). It is normal for the crypts to appear attenuated in the rectal mucosa close to the anal canal and in the relatively thin mucosa of the caecum (Fig. 3.14). Failure to recognize these artefacts and variants can lead to a mistaken diagnosis of atrophy and possibly quiescent ulcerative colitis.

3.6.3 Crypt degeneration

This may involve the whole crypt or the superficial half of the crypt.

Damage to the superficial half of the crypt is a useful pointer to ischaemia and pseudomembranous colitis (Fig. 3.15). The bases frequently survive and the remaining epithelial cells appear hyperchromatic and basophilic. Pseudomembranous colitis is fully discussed in Chapter 8 and ischaemia in Chapter 10.

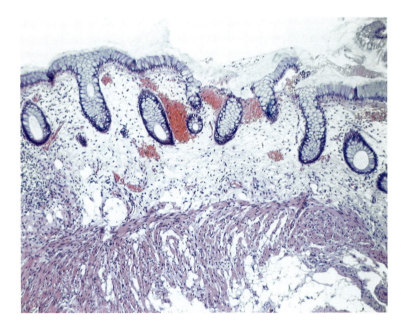

Figure 3.12 Crypt atrophy in long-standing ulcerative colitis. The crypts are widely spaced and short, the crypt bases lying well above the muscularis mucosae. The lamina propria contains few lymphocytes.

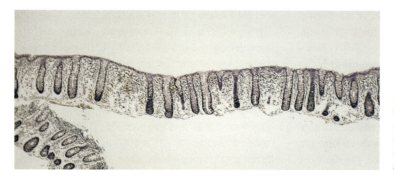

Figure 3.13 Overstretched rectal biopsy, with separation of crypts mimicking atrophy. The lack of muscularis mucosae in this biopsy may have contributed to this artefact.

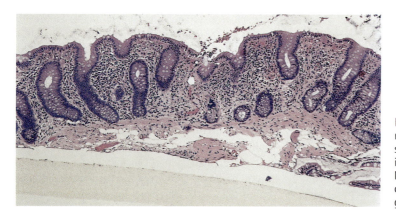

Figure 3.14 Normal thin caecal mucosa. Similar appearances, with short, spaced-out crypts, are normal in the lower rectum and upper anus. Note that in the caecum and right colon the lamina propria shows greater cellularity.

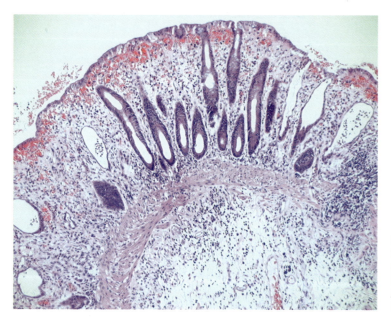

Figure 3.15 Crypt degeneration. Superficial crypt damage and dilatation, with preservation of crypt bases in acute ischaemic colitis. A similar picture can occur in infection.

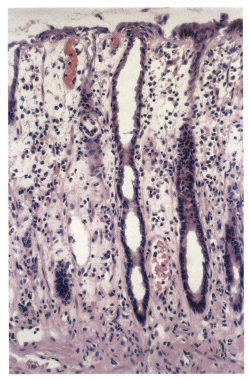

Figure 3.16 Withering of crypts caused by reduction in bulk of epithelial cells following mucin discharge in infective proctocolitis. The crypt bases are characteristically pointed.

Degenerative changes throughout the length of the crypts may occur in either ischaemic disease or infective proctocolitis. In ischaemia the appearances are mainly of cell death but in infection the affected crypt cells appear small, lose their mucin and have pyknotic nuclei. Some may appear flattened (Fig. 3.16). The crypts therefore look thinner than normal or 'withered' with an uneven lumen, giving a 'beaded' appearance. The crypt base is no longer blunt and rounded, but sharply pointed. If only single crypts show this latter change no diagnosis is possible, but when it is a prominent feature it is usual to see the other changes of infective proctocolitis (Section 4.2.1). Ischaemia, as mentioned, may produce a similar pattern of damage but the accompanying mucosal morphological signs will be different (Section 10.6.2).

Another form of crypt degeneration is seen in graft-versus-host disease (Section 11.6). This has been termed the 'exploding crypt'. Here, individual crypt epithelial cells are seen to be necrotic and surrounded by lymphocytes and plasma cells (Fig. 3.17). Much nuclear apoptotic debris is noted. A characteristic is individual foci of cellular necrosis rather than complete degeneration of crypts. Apoptosis of crypt cells with individual cell change may also be seen in biopsies from patients with the acquired immunodeficiency syndrome (AIDS)

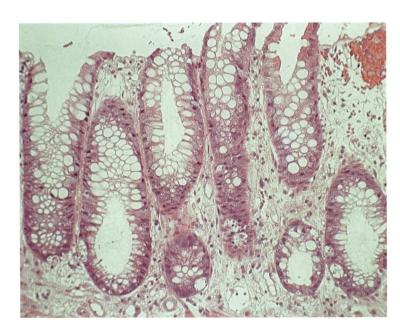

Figure 3.17 Multifocal crypt base cell apoptosis in graft-versus-host disease. The crypts have a 'moth-eaten' appearance.

(Section 4.4.4) and is a signpost for drug-induced lesions (Section 11.4.3), especially non-steroidal anti-inflammatory drugs (NSAIDs) (Section 11.4.4).

3.6.4 Crypt serration

This abnormality is the basis of the architecture of the commonest polyp occurring in the colon, the metaplastic polyp (Section 15.6.1). The crypts have a serrated outline, with abundant absorptive cells in the luminal half and hyperplastic columnar cells occupying the base (Fig. 3.18a). The usual problem is to see a star-shaped crypt in a poorly orientated biopsy cut in cross-section (Fig. 3.18b). When large numbers of crypts like this are seen the diagnosis is obvious but, on many occasions, there may be only one or two affected crypts, which can be easily missed.

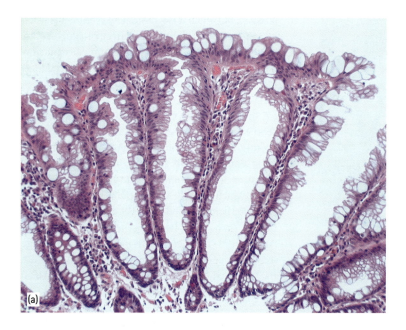

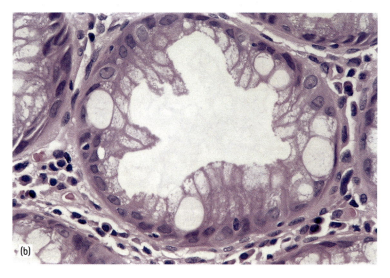

Figure 3.18 Crypt serration in metaplastic polyps: (a) vertical section. (b) transverse section. The crowding and tufting is caused by an accumulation of excess numbers of tall columnar cells.

Serrated crypt epithelium is also frequently seen in quiescent ulcerative colitis, especially when the disease is of long standing (Fig. 5.11).

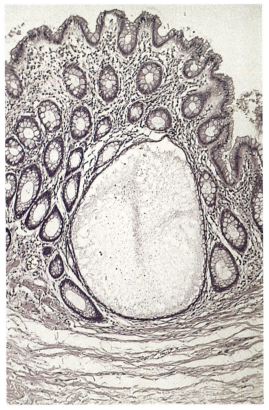

Figure 3.19 Isolated cystically dilated crypt, containing a few polymorphs and debris from a patient with diverticular disease.

3.6.5 Crypt dilatation

The isolated cystic crypt is not uncommon in what may otherwise be a normal biopsy. Such crypts contain small numbers of polymorphs (Fig. 3.19). The pathogenesis is uncertain but it is most likely caused by obstruction of the mouth of the crypt by mucus. We are not aware that, in its own right, this is a helpful sign but it is an indication to examine deeper levels for other pathology. Two or three such crypts in a biopsy should provoke consideration of the category of focal active colitis as described by Greenson *et al.* (1997) (Sections 3.6.7 and 12.3.3a).

Groups of dilated crypts with flattened epithelial cells, expanded by mucin and containing inflammatory debris (Fig. 8.6a) are a useful sign for pseudomembranous colitis and the related antibiotic-associated colitis (Chapter 8). The mucous cells may be shed from the luminal half of the crypts, giving the appearance of superficial crypt necrosis. Some may come to resemble signet ring cells and be mistaken for malignancy, a pattern occasionally seen in pseudomembranous colitis (Section 8.2.1b) An important feature is that the dilatation and disarray of cells is contained within the overall configuration of the normal mucosal architecture. Groups of cystic crypts that disrupt the mucosal pattern are present in colitis cystica superficialis (Fig. 3.20). This is an uncommon finding, associated with vitamin deficiencies and, occasionally, *Shigella* dysenteries. If cystic dilatation is of a degree that produces polypoid lesions, then juvenile polyps, inflammatory polyps and the Cronkhite–Canada syndrome need to be considered (Chapter 15).

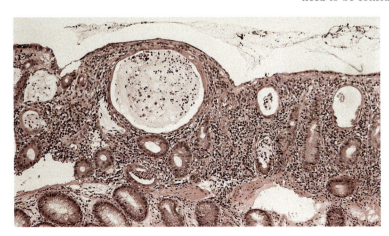

Figure 3.20 Cystically dilated crypts *en masse*, in a biopsy from a patient with an acute infective colitis due to *Campylobacter jejuni*; the picture is that of colitis cystica superficialis.

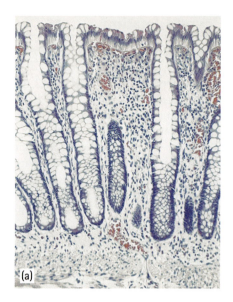

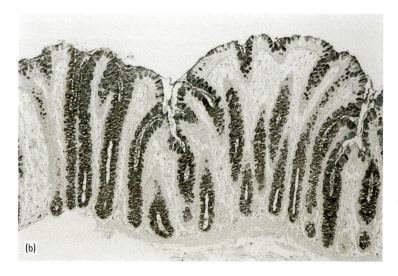

Figure 3.21 Crypt enlargement – transitional mucosa: (a) normal rectal mucosa. (b) High iron-diamine–Alcian green (HID–AG) showing normal dark brown staining of sulphomucin.

Diffuse distension of crypts by unusually eosino-philic mucus, with only slight accompanying inflammation, is the picture seen in mucoviscidosis (Section 20.10).

3.6.6 Crypt enlargement – transitional mucosa

In some biopsies it will be observed that the crypts, though regular, seem longer and lined by taller mucus-secreting cells. Such an epithelial pattern has been termed 'transitional' (Fig. 3.21). The tall epithelial cells are filled with mucin, and are pale when stained with haematoxylin and eosin (H and E), but differ from goblet cells both morpho-logically and histochemically (Fig. 3.21c). Staining with the combined high iron diamine and alcian blue method (Totty, 2002) shows that, in contrast to normal goblet cells, these cells contain acid sialomucin but do not stain for sulphated mucin

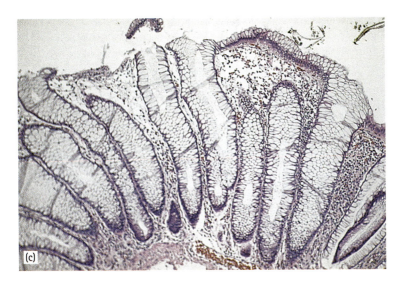

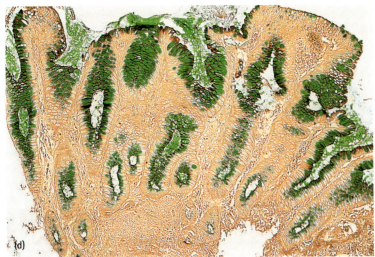

Figure 3.21 (c) elongated crypts, lined by tall epithelium–transitional mucosa adjacent to rectal carcinoma (haematoxlin and eosin); (d) HID–AG showing pale green sialomucins rather than sulphated mucins.

(Figs 3.21b,d), and are analogous to small intestinal epithelium (Robey-Caffney *et al.*, 1990).

Transitional mucosa is found adjacent to, or overlying tumours of any type, including adenocarcinoma, large adenomas, mucosal prolapse syndrome (Section 15.10), endometriosis and colostomies. It is therefore likely that the morphological and mucin changes in transitional epithelium are the result of proximity to such lesions, rather than being histogenetically implicated in neoplasia. Nevertheless, transitional mucosa may be useful as a marker for a nearby tumour, when a biopsy has failed to include diagnostic tissue (Williams, 1985).

3.6.7 The crypt abscess

The presence of polymorphs within the lumen of the crypt constitutes a crypt abscess. There may be only a few inflammatory cells or the crypt may be expanded by voluminous cellular exudate and the lining cells flattened. The numbers of crypts involved and the accompanying mucosal signs obviously determine the specific diagnosis. However, as a working rule, more than two crypts involved in any one biopsy constitute active inflammation and additional abnormalities are then commonly present (Fig. 3.22). When only one or two are seen and

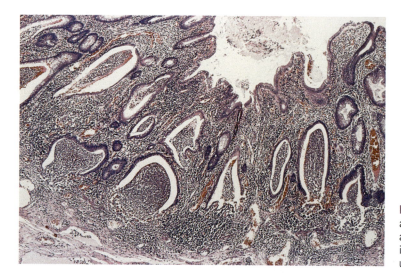

Figure 3.22 Multiple crypt abscesses – active colitis. The architectural distortion and diffuse inflammation support a diagnosis of ulcerative colitis.

when these contain only small numbers of inflammatory cells in the absence of other signs, the term focal active colitis has been used (Greenson *et al.*, 1997). Greenson *et al.* found an association with infection, antibiotic use or immunosuppression (see Section 12.3.3a). Excessive instrumentation, laxative abuse or energetic enemas can produce such minor abnormalities. It is still advisable to cut levels into the biopsy, as infective and antibiotic-associated colitis can be focal and these few crypt abnormalities may simply be marking convincing, deeper, inflammation.

Although crypt abscesses are common in ulcerative colitis they are certainly not diagnostic of that condition and are seen in colitis of any cause. The crypt abscess classifies the biopsy as inflamed and justifies the label of 'colitis' but it is from the other features that a diagnosis is derived. However, when crypt abscesses dominate the picture, ulcerative colitis has to be the histologist's first diagnosis. Crohn's disease and bacterial diarrhoeas can produce this picture but in these it is less conspicuous (Section 4.2.1).

3.6.8 Incipient crypt abscess (cryptitis)

In contrast to the established crypt abscess, here the polymorphs lie between the crypt cells, with only a few within the lumen (Fig. 3.23). When this

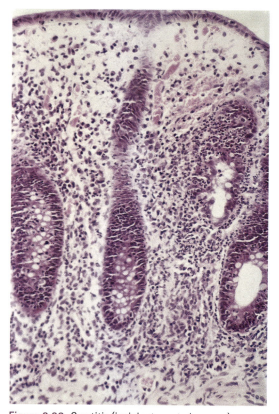

Figure 3.23 Cryptitis (incipient crypt abscesses). The neutrophil polymorphs lie between crypt epithelial cells. Biopsy from a patient with bacterial dysentery.

pattern of crypt disease predominates it is a most useful indicator of a bacterial colitis (Section 4.2.1). However, when seen only in single crypts or in the company of large numbers of developed crypt abscesses it is unhelpful.

The dynamic relationship between cryptitis and crypt abscesses has not been studied. It is not simply one of time, as patients with bacterial colitis will not go on to develop a picture dominated by crypt abscesses, neither do patients with ulcerative colitis have an initial inflammatory pattern largely composed of incipient crypt abscesses.

3.6.9 Misplaced crypts

Cryptal epithelium may be found misplaced within or beneath the muscularis mucosae (Fig. 3.24) in:

(a) Mucosal prolapse syndrome, as in solitary ulcer of the rectum (Section 15.10).

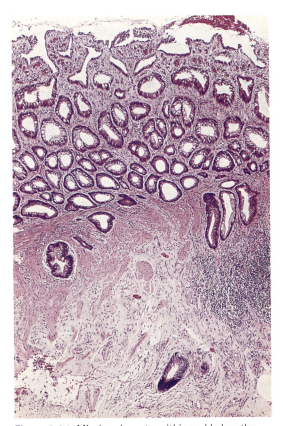

Figure 3.24 Misplaced crypts, within and below the muscularis mucosae, in this instance caused by mucosal prolapse (solitary ulcer syndrome).

(b) In association with any polypoid lesion in which there has been localized mucosal damage from torsion or ischaemic infarction ('pseudo-carcinomatous invasion'; Section 16.2.2).

(c) Colitis cystica profunda (Section 20.11).

(d) Healed fissuring ulcers, as in Crohn's disease and amoebiasis (Sections 6.3.5 and 4.7.1).

(e) In association with lymphoid follicles which extend into the submucosa (lymphoid–glandular complexes; Section 3.11.4).

In a woman, the possibility that misplaced glands represent endometriosis should be considered (Section 20.12).

3.7 CRYPT EPITHELIUM

3.7.1 Mucin depletion

This is the result of discharge and exhaustion of goblet cells, which become morphologically indistinguishable from absorptive columnar cells. Goblet cell discharge occurs commonly and can simply be a response to the irritant effect of enema fluid, such as is used before colonoscopy (Leriche *et al.*, 1978), when the mucin depletion, although diffuse, is mild (Fig. 3.25a). Diffuse loss of goblet cells, ranging in severity through mild, moderate and severe (Fig. 3.25) is seen in infective and ulcerative colitis, ischaemia and radiation colitis. Mucin depletion also occurs in Crohn's disease, but is usually focal and less conspicuous. This is a useful attribute in discriminating between ulcerative colitis and Crohn's disease (Section 12.4.1), though, outside this context, it is of limited value.

3.7.2 Regenerative hyperplasia

Goblet cells are also reduced in numbers when there is regenerative hyperplasia of immature differentiating cells. This is the result of increased surface epithelial cell loss, accompanied by a progressive reduction in numbers of differentiated cells in the crypt lining. There is a compensatory increase in the proportion of undifferentiated crypt base cells. The nuclei of the undifferentiated epithelial cells are

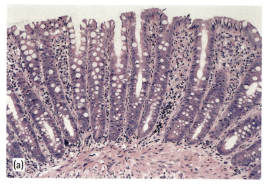 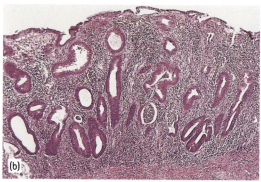

Figure 3.25 Mucin depletion: (a) mild, with loss of a few goblet cells – can be caused by enemas or low grade colitis; (b) severe, with almost complete absence of goblet cells – an indicator of active disease, in this case ulcerative colitis.

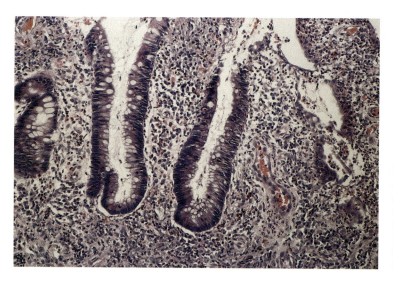

Figure 3.26 Actively regenerating epithelium. The cells are immature columnar cells and goblet cells with only apical mucin vacuoles. There is a heavy plasma cell and lymphocytic infiltrate and foci of neutrophils are present. Rectal biopsy in active ulcerative colitis.

large, the cytoplasm is deeply stained and there is an increase in the nucleo-cytoplasmic ratio, with mitotic figures often present high up, away from their normal situation in the crypt base (Fig. 3.26).

Regenerative hyperplasia of crypt epithelium occurs after any ulcerative process. It can be particularly prominent in active ulcerative colitis (Section 5.2.1a) and care is then needed to avoid confusion with epithelial dysplasia (Sections 3.7.3 and 7.7.2). It is also important to remember that, even in quiescent ulcerative colitis, if there is mucosal atrophy, there can be paradoxical hyperplasia of the epithelium of the reduced number of crypts. This is the result of the compensatory effort to maintain the integrity of the surface epithelium from a smaller reserve of epithelial stem cells. An excess of mitotic figures,

above their normal position in the crypt base, is often seen in otherwise normal mucosa, the result of enemas and mechanical trauma related to colonoscopy, but is of relatively minor degree.

3.7.3 Dysplastic epithelium

Dysplasia of crypt epithelium may be evident at both the cytological level and the architectural level. At the cytological level the cells show 'atypia' (Fig. 3.27), with nuclear hyperchromatism, enlargement and pleomorphism. The most significant abnormality is, however, loss of polarity. This is manifested in columnar cells as stratification of nuclei and varies in severity from mild, when the majority of the nuclei remain in the basal half of

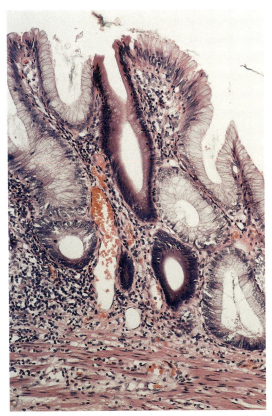

Figure 3.27 Dysplasia, low grade. A single crypt shows hyperchromasia of epithelial cell nuclei and cytoplasm. Nuclear enlargement and stratification are relatively mild. Goblet cells are disturbed. (From a patient with a long history of extensive ulcerative colitis.)

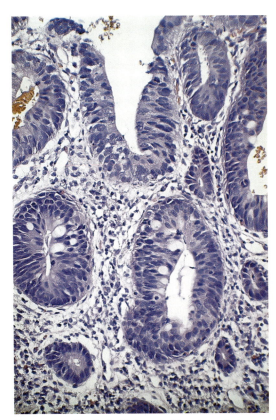

Figure 3.28 Dysplasia, high grade. There is marked nuclear enlargement and stratification as well as hyperchromasia. Goblet cells are greatly reduced. From a patient with a long history of extensive ulcerative colitis.

the epithelium (Fig. 3.27), to severe, when the nuclei are randomly situated (Fig. 3.28). Loss of polarity also affects goblet cells, which fail to discharge their mucin and become rounded off and enlarged, their nuclei often being eccentrically positioned and even inverted (Fig. 17.17). This leads to the appearance described as 'upside-down' or dystrophic goblet cells (Riddell *et al.*, 1983). Sometimes, there is alteration of mucin to non-sulphated, small intestinal type or there may be mucin depletion. The architectural changes involve crypt branching, budding, bridging or transformation of the mucosal surface to a villous configuration (Fig. 17.4).

Before a firm opinion can be expressed about dysplasia it is essential to ensure that the histological material under consideration is of adequate quality. Crushing artefact, particularly at the edge of a

biopsy, can make the epithelium of damaged crypts appear disorderly and hyperchromatic (Fig. 3.29).

Dysplasia is invariably present in adenomatous mucosa (Section 15.5) and is sometimes found in the flat mucosa of patients who have had active ulcerative colitis for several years (Chapter 17). In both situations the histological features are similar and in both situations the grade of severity varies.

The dysplasia, in adenomas and in ulcerative colitis, must be regarded as a pre-cancerous change, analogous to intraepithelial neoplasia of the uterine cervix. However, in the flat mucosa from an ulcerative colitic, dysplasia can closely resemble the regenerative hyperplasia that is always found in active ulcerative colitis. A firm diagnosis of dysplasia is difficult in the presence of active disease (i.e. the presence of large numbers of polymorphs in

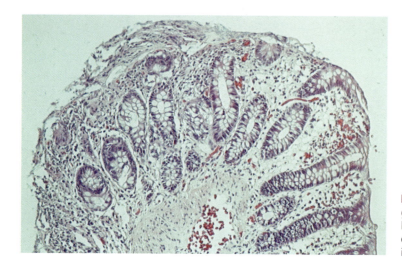

Figure 3.29 Crushing artefact, giving a disorderly and hyperchromatic appearance to crypt epithelium which may, on casual inspection, resemble dysplasia.

the lamina propria and crypts; Figs 3.26 and 3.22). The assessment of such cases is discussed more fully in Chapter 17.

3.7.4 Paneth cells

Cells with the characteristic features of Paneth cells are normally confined to the caecum and proximal right colon but may, in certain disease states, be found scattered among the other cells of the epithelium in the colon or rectum, most frequently at the crypt base.

These cells can be easily recognized in H and E sections by their large, round, highly refractile eosinophilic granules, rich in lysozyme, concentrated at the apices of the cells (Fig. 3.30). Paneth cells may arise by divergent differentiation, a process termed Paneth cell metaplasia by Watson and Roy (1960).

Paneth cells are typically found in chronic ulcerative colitis, but, away from the caecum can be regarded as markers of any long-standing inflammatory state in which there is epithelial regeneration.

Paneth cells are equipped for antibacterial functions, containing natural antibiotics (defensins) (Porter *et al.*, 1997; Elphick and Mahida, 2005), lysozyme (Erlandsen *et al.*, 1974), immunoglobulin A (IgA) and immunoglobulin G (IgG) (Rodning *et al.*, 1976), as well as being highly cationic. Paneth cell metaplasia therefore might be a homeostatic

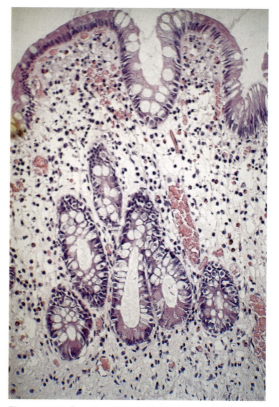

Figure 3.30 Paneth cell metaplasia. Paneth cells at the base of crypts. Rectal biopsy from a patient with ulcerative colitis, in remission. Note the branched crypts and the relatively 'empty' lamina propria.

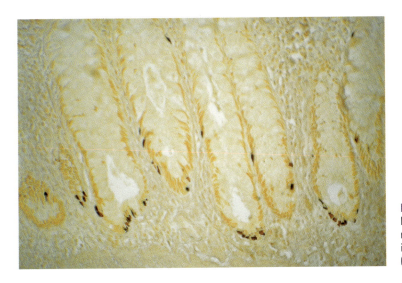

Figure 3.31 Endocrine cells in long-standing ulcerative colitis. The number of these cells in each crypt is increased (compare with Fig. 2.4). (Grimelius).

mechanism concerned with regulation of the flora of the gut lumen (Elmes *et al.*, 1984).

3.7.5 Endocrine cells

Although there is no recognized primary condition of diffuse endocrine cell hyperplasia in the large intestine, the proportion of argyrophilic endocrine cells (Section 2.2.3) in each crypt is increased in inflammatory disease of long standing, particularly ulcerative colitis (Fig. 3.31) (Gledhill *et al.*, 1986a,b). It has been suggested by Lampert *et al.* (1985) that, at least in graft-versus-host disease, the observed preservation of endocrine cells results from their relative resistance to the harmful stimulus which is damaging the remainder of the crypt epithelium (Section 11.6).

3.8 LAMINA PROPRIA – CELLS

The stroma of the lamina propria consists of a normal inflammatory cell component and a connective tissue matrix. In the normal mucosa lymphocytes and plasma cells show a characteristic gradient from superficial to deep, with the majority in the upper one-third of the lamina propria. There are more of these cells in the proximal right colon (Fig. 3.14) and care should be taken that this is not mistaken

for proximal inflammation when seen in contrast to the left side.

3.8.1 Inflammatory cells

The clearest evidence of inflammation is an increase in cellularity of the lamina propria and loss of the above gradient. The excess cells may be neutrophil polymorphs, lymphocytes, plasma cells or eosinophils in varying proportions. It is an excess of neutrophil polymorphs which is the essential marker of active versus inactive chronic inflammation. It is important to recognize that the intensity of any cellular infiltrate may be masked by accompanying oedema. This is particularly the case in infective colitis.

A reduction in the number of inflammatory cells may lead to an apparently 'empty' lamina propria (Fig. 3.12). This is a picture seen, though as yet unexplained, in chronic ulcerative colitis (Section 5.2.3b) and, when there is stromal obliteration by smooth muscle or collagen, in the mucosal prolapse syndrome (Section 15.10) or chronic ischaemia (Section 10.6.4). In chronic ulcerative colitis some of this effect may be related to steroid therapy.

It is quite common to see foamy histiocytes or fat-like vacuoles in the lamina propria in otherwise normal mucosa. These elements will be considered separately.

3.8.2 Neutrophil exudate

This is a manifestation of the classical pattern of acute inflammation, with dilatation of mucosal capillaries and venules, margination of neutrophils in these vessels and exudation of fluid and polymorphs into the surrounding lamina propria (Fig. 3.32). The polymorphs are often seen migrating through the glandular epithelium (cryptitis) and may accumulate in the crypt lumina, to form crypt abscesses (Sections 3.6.7 and 3.6.8).

The presence of neutrophil polymorphs is not a specific marker of any particular disease; indeed, small numbers are often seen in normal mucosa, as a result of the preparation for, or trauma of, colonoscopy (Chapter 2). However, more than a few polymorphs indicate that an active inflammatory process is present. Different aetiologies produce differing intensities and patterns of neutrophil exudate. Neutrophils can be reduced in numbers or absent, even in the presence of clinically fulminant colitis, in patients with neutropenia (neutropenic colitis, Section 11.7).

The most florid acute inflammatory exudate is manifested by crypt abscesses (Fig. 3.7), with or without purulent exudate on the luminal surface of the mucosa. This picture is typical of the active phases of ulcerative colitis (Section 5.2.1b) but can occur in Crohn's disease (Section 6.3.2), amoebiasis (Section 4.7.1) and acute infective colitis (Section 4.2.1).

A neutrophil exudate in the lamina propria, extending into, but not through, crypt epithelium (Section 3.6.8), as shown in Figure 3.32, often with prominent vascular margination and unaccompanied by other inflammatory cells, is typical of infective colitis caused, for example, by *Campylobacter* or *Salmonella* infection (Section 4.2.1).

3.8.3 Plasma cells

Plasma cells are normal constituents of the lamina propria and increase to varying degrees in all forms of colitis (Fig. 3.6b). They are, therefore, a non-specific marker of inflammation, although the proportion in relation to the numbers of polymorphs present has some diagnostic implications

(Section 3.8.7). In the absence of any other diagnostic signs one can do little more than record 'chronic inflammation' of a particular severity. As the acute phase of the various forms of colitis wanes, so the ratio of plasma cells to polymorphs increases, though in mild infection, for example, the numbers involved may be small. In inflammatory conditions of any type, the proportion of IgA-producing plasma cells falls in proportion to the increased number of other types of plasma cell but no unequivocal pattern of immunoglobulin-producing cells has yet been shown to relate to any particular type of inflammatory disease (Day *et al.*, 2003).

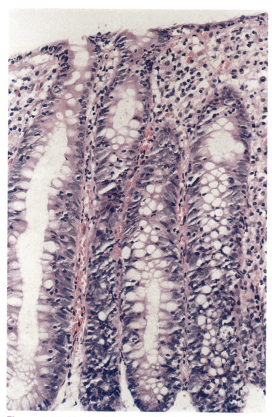

Figure 3.32 Neutrophils. As well as being scattered throughout the lamina propria, neutrophil polymorphs are present within the epithelium of the surface and crypts. Rectal biopsy from a patient with infective colitis.

In hypogammaglobulinaemic patients plasma cells are frequently absent (Section 20.13).

3.8.4 Lymphocytes

Since lymphocytes are numerous in the lamina propria of normal mucosa, an increase in numbers is difficult to assess and only a large increase is of diagnostic significance. Excluding lymphomas, such an excess is rarely homogeneous, and usually takes the form of hyperplasia of the normal rectal mucosal lymphoid follicles (Fig. 3.33), a picture referred to as follicular proctitis or colitis (Section 5.8). The other pattern is of aggregated clusters of lymphocytes, adjacent to the bases of crypts or in the submucosa (Fig. 3.34).

Follicular proctitis is commonly, though not exclusively, associated with ulcerative colitis and usually indicates chronic disease. The alternative picture of lymphoid aggregates is associated with Crohn's disease, and should be an indication to seek other signs of this condition (Chapter 6).

Increased numbers of intraepithelial lymphocytes should raise the suspicion of microscopic colitis – lymphocytic variety (Section 9.3.2) or lymphoma (Section 18.3). In the latter, the lymphocytes tend to destroy the crypts but this is not seen in lymphocytic colitis.

3.8.5 Eosinophils

Eosinophils are normally scanty in the large intestinal lamina propria, comprising less than 2.7 per cent of the inflammatory cells of the rectal mucosa (Binder, 1970). Eosinophils are increased in inflammatory bowel disease (Bischoff *et al.*, 1996) may

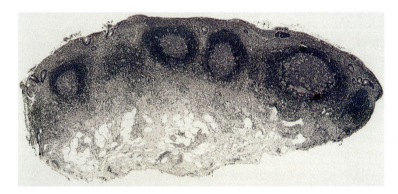

Figure 3.33 Hyperplasia of lymphoid follicles (follicular proctitis) and crypt atrophy, in a patient with ulcerative colitis.

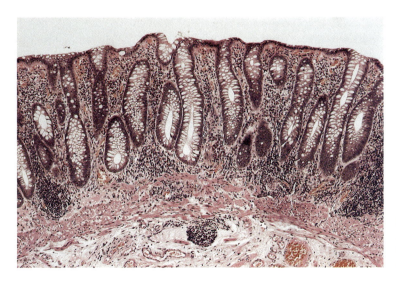

Figure 3.34 Irregularly arranged dense aggregates of lymphocytes, with extension into submucosa in a patient with Crohn's disease.

be numerous in ulcerative colitis (Section 5.2.1b), and are prominent in schistosomiasis (Section 4.8.1) or as part of a systemic reaction in atopic disease such as asthma. They are also seen in Crohn's disease (Section 6.3.2) (Al-Haddad and Riddell, 2005). They may be a feature of polyarteritis nodosa and can accompany lymphomas. Inflammatory fibroid polyps contain large numbers of eosinophils but these are excessively rare in the colon. Eosinophil infiltration of the rectal mucosa has also been described in the acute phase of irradiation proctitis (Gelfand et al., 1968), although this is unusual in our experience. As with eosinophils in any tissue, they are probably a sequel of acute inflammation and do not indicate any specific disease. Frustratingly, it is our experience, in biopsy work, that an increase in numbers is often seen without any obvious explanation.

3.8.6 Mast cells

Mast cells are inconspicuous in routinely stained sections, but can be found in increased numbers in inflamed tissue on immunocytochemical staining for CD117 (Arber, 1998) or when traditional stains such as toluidine blue or Csaba's modification of alcian blue (Bancroft, 2002) are used. Changes in the mast cell granules have also been noted in ultrastructural studies of large intestinal biopsies in inflammatory bowel disease (Dvorak, 1979; Heatley and James, 1979). Spuriously low mast cell counts may be caused by degranulation (Bischoff et al., 1996).

Although, along with eosinophils, mast cells are often considered to be specifically concerned with type I hypersensitivity (allergic) reactions, they are known to be activated by complement components C3a and C5a and a variety of non-immunological stimuli (Wasserman, 1979). Mast cells evidently participate in many acute inflammatory reactions and are not specific markers for any particular pathogenetic mechanism.

No diagnostic or prognostic role has been established for the observation of increased numbers of mast cells in inflammatory bowel disease. Large numbers are characteristically found in the large intestinal mucosa and in many tissues, in systemic mastocytosis.

3.8.7 Proportions of inflammatory cells

The number of neutrophil polymorphs probably reflects the degree of epithelial damage that is taking place. Neutrophils are therefore predominant in acute colitis (Fig. 3.32), particularly when caused by bacteria (Campylobacter, Shigella, Salmonella, etc., Chapter 4), and in the active phases of ulcerative colitis, however long the history (Chapter 5). They are less numerous in ischaemic colitis (Section 10.6.2).

A variable or patchy concentration of neutrophils is found in diseases in which there are focal ulcers, such as amoebiasis, Crohn's disease and varieties of vasculitis. The ulcers of amoebic infection (Section 4.7.1) which are characteristically lined by granulation tissue have a polymorph exudate, forming a pyogenic membrane-like structure. The fissuring ulcers of Crohn's disease (Section 6.3.5) are lined by similar elements, but are associated with chronic inflammation and dense lymphoid aggregates in the surrounding tissue.

The number of neutrophils is reduced in relation to other cells as acute colitis goes into remission or responds to treatment (Fig. 5.13). In neutropenic colitis they are depleted from the outset (Section 11.7).

3.8.8 Distribution of inflammatory cells

Inflammation may be diffuse, patchy or focal. The diseases associated with the various patterns of distribution of inflammatory cells are shown in Figure 3.35.

Diffusely distributed inflammatory cells throughout the mucosa indicate a disease process affecting the surface and crypt epithelium uniformly. Lymphoid follicles, rather than focal lymphoid aggregates, may be present. Ulcerative colitis is a typical example.

Variation in the intensity of inflammation from one part of the mucosa to another (i.e. 'patchy' inflammation) can occur in a wide variety of diseases, but is not always evident in a biopsy because of the small area available for examination. Meaningful interpretation of patchy inflammation is not possible without taking account of

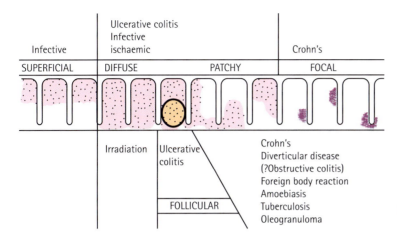

Infective | Ulcerative colitis / Infective / ischaemic | Crohn's

SUPERFICIAL | DIFFUSE | PATCHY | FOCAL

Irradiation | Ulcerative colitis

FOLLICULAR

Crohn's
Diverticular disease
(?Obstructive colitis)
Foreign body reaction
Amoebiasis
Tuberculosis
Oleogranuloma

Figure 3.35 Diagram of patterns of inflammation.

other features, such as crypt architecture, state of the epithelium and the nature of the lamina propria and submucosa. Diffuse patterns of inflammation become patchy as remission occurs.

Focal mucosal inflammation, with a background of normal mucosa is typically seen in Crohn's disease (Section 6.3.2), but is not in itself specific and may represent the last residues of infective colitis (Section 4.2.2c). It can also be found in diverticular disease and obstructive colitis (Section 13.6.2).

3.8.9 Histiocytes

Histiocytes with phagocytic function are identified in the mucosa by the material which they have ingested and may be inconspicuous unless PAS-stained sections are examined (Fig. 3.36). Small collections of such cells, containing mucin (muciphages) are found in the lamina propria in 50 per cent of normal subjects and are rarely of diagnostic value (Azzopardi and Evans, 1966). They may be a response to crypt damage (Salto-Tellez and Price, 2000) during which there has been disruption of goblet cells, with passage of mucin through the basement membrane.

Disease states associated with PAS-positive histiocytes are: melanosis coli (Sections 11.0 and 13.6.1); Whipple's disease (Section 20.5); malakoplakia (Section 20.3); lipid storage diseases and histoplasmosis (Section 4.10).

Confluent sheets of mononuclear phagocytes form in relation to extravasated barium and such a lesion is conventionally termed 'barium granuloma'

(Fig. 11.4). The barium can be visualized as finely divided grey, unstained, refractile granular material which is variably birefringent in polarized light (Section 11.2).

Sheets of finely vacuolated lipid-containing histiocytes in the superficial lamina propria constitute a xanthoma (Fig. 3.37). This is a feature of uncertain clinical significance which can develop in the absence of any other histological abnormality.

Brown pigment within macrophages can indicate haemosiderin (Section 3.14) but is usually a manifestation of melanosis coli. Large cells, with granular golden-brown cytoplasm, stand out in the superficial lamina propria (Fig. 3.38). Melanosis coli is often of no significance but does have a tendency to develop in patients with chronic motility disorders, particularly when they have habitually taken laxatives (Section 13.5).

3.8.10 Giant cells

Giant cells, not part of epithelioid granulomas, may be seen both in the mucosa and in the submucosa. They should not be confused with ganglion cells (Fig. 3.39). This mistake is easily made in a poorly orientated and prepared biopsy.

3.8.10a Mucosal giant cells

It is of critical importance to distinguish granulomas from the giant cells which form in response to crypt destruction in order to avoid an erroneous diagnosis of Crohn's disease (Fig. 3.40). It is unwise to base a diagnosis of Crohn's disease solely on giant cells or granulomas related to such damaged crypts (granulomatous crypt abscesses) (Lee *et al.*, 1997). These can occur in infective colitis (Section 4.2.4c) and ulcerative colitis (Section 5.2.1d) (Mahadeva *et al.* 2002). In difficult cases immunostaining for cytokeratin may highlight surviving crypt cells. We have seen isolated giant cells in the mucosa, occasionally with ingested foreign debris, faecal material (Fig. 3.41) or barium. Finding such a cell in the absence of foreign material calls for examination of multiple levels through the block, to exclude a true granuloma.

3.8.10b Submucosal giant cells

Giant cells are frequently seen in and around fistulae (Section 19.2.2). Obviously, Crohn's disease is the first diagnosis to exclude (Chapter 6), but low rectal fistulae are commonly biopsied and by no means all are caused by Crohn's disease. There must be a careful search for foreign material in such circumstances.

Giant cells will also occur around any injected material, particularly the oil used to treat haemorrhoids (Section 11.3), and around the gas cysts of pneumatosis (see Fig. 3.58 and Section 20.2). A giant cell in the submucosa may also be the first indication that there is pathology in deeper sections. Schistosomiasis must be thought of, as it may excite a giant cell response (Section 4.8.1). Furthermore, the eggs may be mistaken for giant cells.

3.8.11 Granulomas

A granuloma is defined as a collection of inflammatory cells which includes epithelioid histiocytes

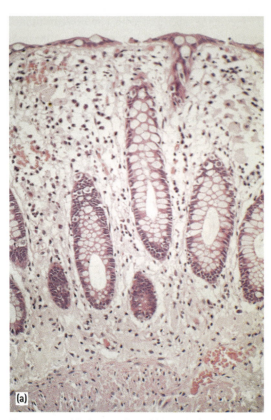
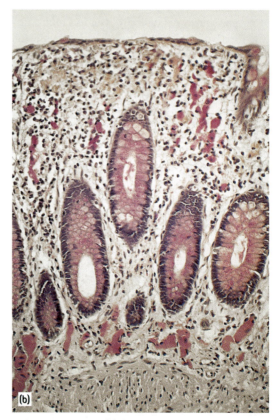

Figure 3.36 Histiocytes. Rectal biopsy taken during the investigation of diarrhoea. (a) Routine haematoxylin and eosin staining shows only mucosal oedema. (b) Staining of a parallel section with periodic acid–Schiff after diastase treatment reveals groups of histiocytes (macrophages) in both the superficial and the deep lamina propria.

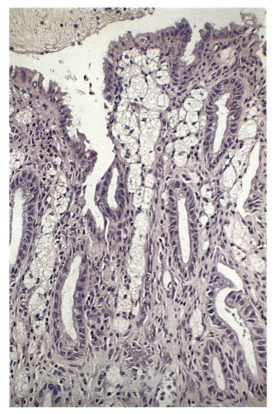

Figure 3.37 Mucosal xanthoma. Sheets of finely vacuolated, lipid-containing histiocytes in the superficial lamina propria are occasionally found incidental to other disease. They can appear as sessile polyps at endoscopy.

(Figs 3.42 and 3.43). Multinucleate giant cells may or may not be present. Within this definition there is considerable scope for variation, but, as mentioned above (Section 3.8.10a), isolated multinucleate giant cells, sometimes found in relation to the base of a damaged crypt (Fig. 3.40) or in response to foreign material in the submucosa should not be confused with granulomas (Mahadeva *et al.*, 2002). Also to be distinguished from granulomas are small blood vessels lined by swollen endothelial cells (Fig. 3.44) and the pericrypt fibroblasts, which, when they are seen in a tangential plane of section, passing close to the basement membrane of a crypt, take on the appearance of epithelioid cells (Fig. 3.45).

Tiny collections of epithelioid cells, less than 50 μm across, may be ill-defined and are easily overlooked (Fig. 3.42). Small, genuine, granulomas of this kind constitute good evidence of Crohn's disease (Section 6.3.3). Small granulomas found incidentally in the absence of overt intestinal disease, in rare cases, may be markers for sarcoidosis (Section 20.6). Ribbons of serial sections from multiple levels should be searched to avoid missing such lesions in the relevant clinical case.

Larger, well-defined granulomas with or without necrosis (Fig. 3.43), imply Crohn's disease, but it should not be forgotten that they may be signs of intestinal tuberculosis, particularly in certain ethnic groups of patients. Caseation need not necessarily

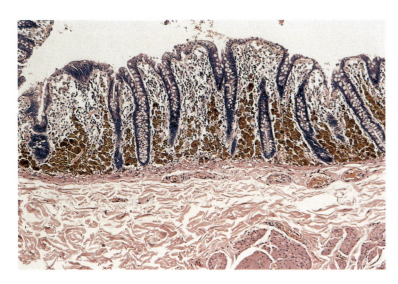

Figure 3.38 Melanosis coli. Collections of brown pigment-laden macrophages in the lamina propria, usually a sign of laxative abuse.

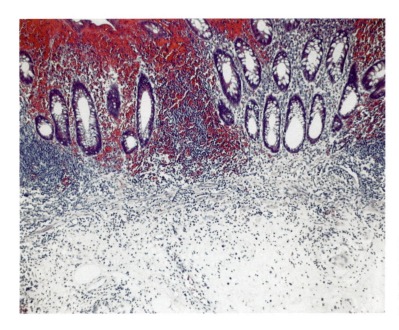

Figure 3.39 Submucosal ganglia. In this biopsy, from a patient with Crohn's disease, conspicuous ganglia in the presence of oedema should not be confused with multinucleate giant cells.

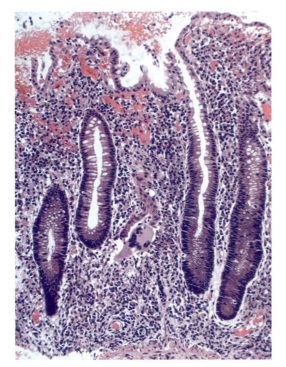

Figure 3.40 Giant cell response to crypt damage. Foreign body-type giant cells sometimes develop in relation to damaged crypt epithelium. They are markers of active epithelial destruction. This is an example in ulcerative colitis but they can equally be found in infective colitis.

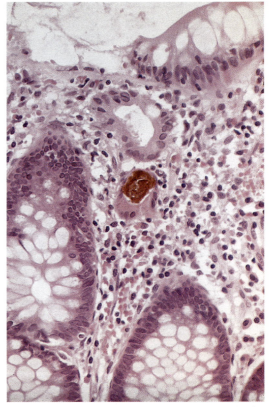

Figure 3.41 Foreign body giant cell reaction to faecal material.

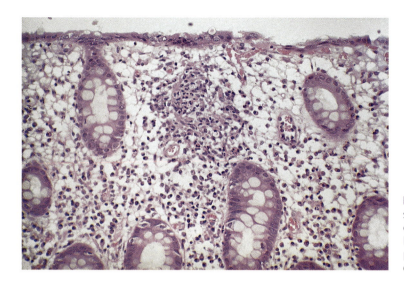

Figure 3.42 Microgranuloma. A small collection of inflammatory cells, including epithelioid histiocytes, in the upper lamina propria, in a patient with Crohn's disease.

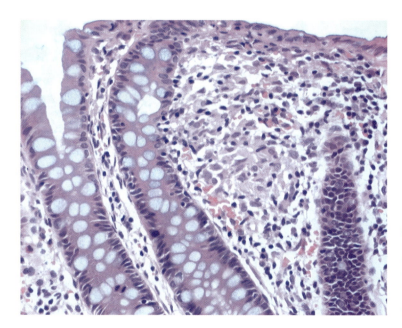

Figure 3.43 Well-defined granulomas in Crohn's disease. Florid granulomas in both the mucosa and submucosa, with focal dense lymphocytic infiltration, can also be seen in tuberculosis, despite the lack of caseation.

be present. Large granulomas, with confluent sheets of histiocytes, are found in chronic granulomatous disease of childhood (Section 20.4) and in overwhelming infection with *Mycobacterium avium-intracellulare* in patients with AIDS (Section 4.4.4).

Discrete granulomas are sometimes found around ova in chronic schistosomiasis (Fig. 3.46) and occasionally, related to lymphatics, in the vicinity of tumours such as adenocarcinoma.

3.8.12 Pseudolipomatosis

Focal groups of small vacuoles, similar in appearance to the cells of mature adipose tissue are not uncommon in the lamina propria of the large intestinal mucosa (Fig. 3.47). Snover *et al.* (1985) have shown, by histochemistry and electron microscopy that these are not fat cells as previously thought, but appear to be extracellular collections of gas.

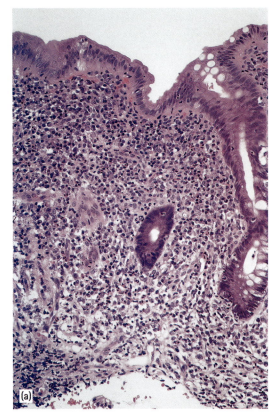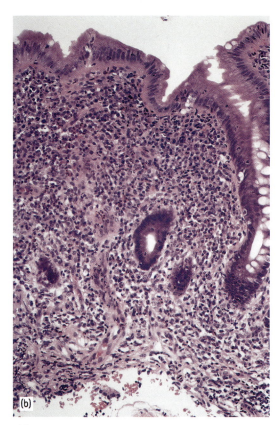

Figure 3.44 Small mucosal blood vessel mimicking granuloma. (a) The swollen endothelial cells of a small blood vessel resemble epithelioid cells in this section but the vascular nature of these cells is revealed in a deeper section (b).

They are most frequent in quiescent long-standing ulcerative colitis but can be seen in other diseases, particularly pneumatosis coli (Gagliardi *et al.*, 1996) or even in normal mucosa. They appear to be the result of gas passing from the colonic lumen through tiny defects in the surface epithelium and can be a complication of the air-insufflation which accompanies colonoscopy (Waring *et al.*, 1989) or the result of insufficient rinsing of hydrogen peroxide used for cleaning the endoscope (Ryan and Potter, 1995) They tend to be located at sites previously occupied by lymphocytes (Whitehead, 1985) and may be related to lymphatics. This latter hypothesis is supported by the occasional finding of such cysts in submucosal lymphoid follicles (Fig. 3.48).

3.8.13 Microorganisms

Bacteria are normally present in the lumen of the large intestine. It is not practicable to identify them in histological sections. Spirochaetes are also sometimes found, forming a blue layer on the surface epithelium in haematoxylin and eosin-stained sections; they are not necessarily indicative of disease (Section 4.5).

The following other organisms may be found in a mucosal biopsy in disease (Fig. 3.49):

1. Protozoa: Amoebae (Section 4.7.1), *Balantidium* (Section 4.7.3), cryptosporidia (Section 4.7.4), schistosomal ova (Section 4.8.1)
2. Bacteria: *Actinomyces*
3. Viruses: Cytomegalovirus (Section 4.6.1), Herpes simplex (Section 4.6.2)

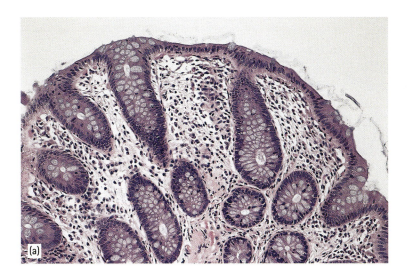

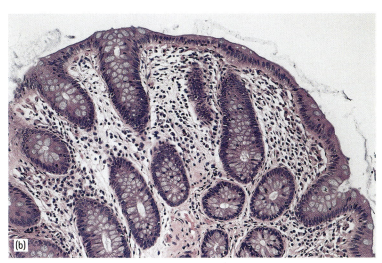

Figure 3.45 (a) Pericrypt sheath cells mimicking a granuloma.(b) The parallel section reveals that the ill-defined collection of epithelioid cells is, in fact, the pericrypt sheath of myofibroblasts.

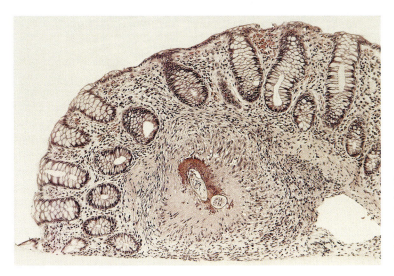

Figure 3.46 Schistosomiasis. A circumscribed granuloma in an otherwise normal, or oedematous mucosa is typical of schistosomiasis. If ova, such as those seen here, are not evident, multiple serial sections may reveal the diagnosis.

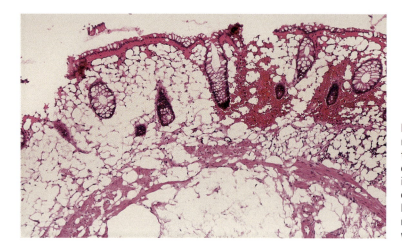

Figure 3.47 Pseudolipomatosis of rectal mucosa. Vacuoles resembling the cells of adipose tissue have collected in the lamina propria. This is probably a iatrogenic artefact caused by gas under pressure in the lumen finding its way into the mucosa. Vacuoles can be seen within the surface epithelium.

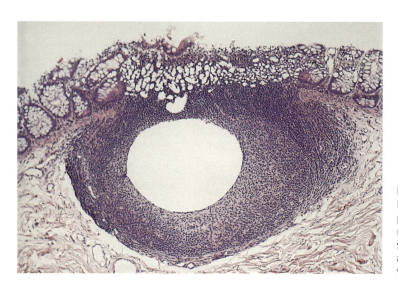

Figure 3.48 Cyst in submucosal lymphoid follicle, associated with pseudolipomatosis of overlying mucosa. Biopsy of otherwise normal sigmoid mucosa, proximal to aganglionic segment in an infant with Hirschsprung's disease.

Of these, amoebae are easily missed, lying as they do, camouflaged in granulation tissue or surface slough and cryptosporidia, too, can be mistaken for surface debris.

3.9 LAMINA PROPRIA – MATRIX

3.9.1 Fibrosis

The normal lamina propria in routine sections appears clear or slightly eosinophilic apart from a normal complement of cells (Section 2.3). In obvious fibrosis the lamina propria is densely eosinophilic, the crypt architecture is distorted and the cellular background frequently appears diminished. Small blood vessels may be unusually prominent (Fig. 3.50). Minor degrees of fibrosis are not so readily appreciated. In doubtful cases connective tissue stains, such as van Gieson or Masson's trichrome, confirm the fibrous replacement of the lamina propria. This is the end stage of the reparative process in ischaemia. Imperfect regeneration of the crypts, together with iron-containing macrophages in the lamina propria provide additional clues to the

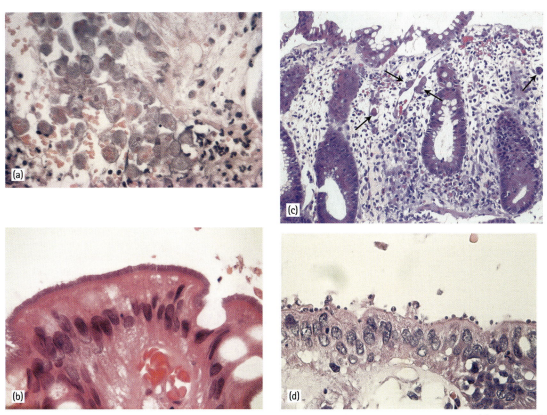

Figure 3.49 Microorganisms which may infect the large intestine and which can be easily overlooked: (a) amoebae; (b) spirochaetes; (c) cytomegalovirus; (d) cryoptosporidia.

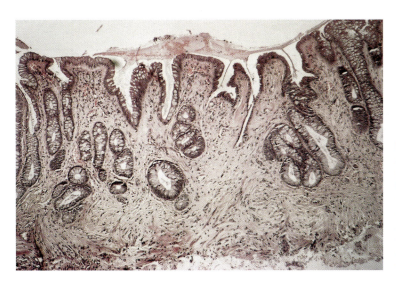

Figure 3.50 Fibrosis of the lamina propria. The cellularity of the lamina propria is reduced and the normally loose areolar tissue is replaced by solid fibrous tissue containing numerous blood capillaries. This picture may result from chronic ischaemia and, particularly in the rectum, mucosal prolapse (solitary rectal ulcer), as in this case.

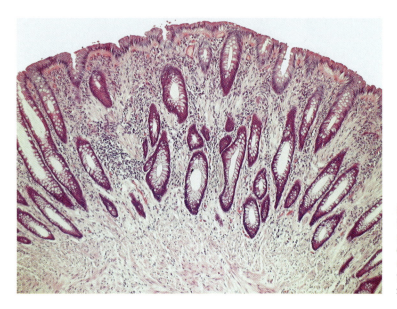

Figure 3.51 Smooth muscle fibres in the lamina propria in mucosal prolapse. Hypertrophic myocyte, in continuity with the muscularis mucosae, pass upwards between the crypts to be inserted in the subepithelial collagen plate.

aetiology of the changes (Alschibaja and Morson, 1977). The presence of atypical glandular epithelium in association with fibrous tissue is a sign of adenocarcinoma (Section 16.3). This is referred to as desmoplasia.

Fibrosis of the lamina propria accompanies the solitary ulcer syndrome (Section 15.10), which is also believed to have an ischaemic pathogenesis, produced by mucosal prolapse. In this syndrome it is helpful to note the strands of muscle from the muscularis mucosae, which also contribute to the obliteration of the lamina propria (Fig. 3.51). Fibrosis and elastosis of the lamina propria associated with angulation of the crypt bases are features of solitary ulcer syndrome/mucosal prolapse (Section 15.10) (Warren et al., 1990).

Fibrosis must be evaluated with the knowledge that it will occur at the edge of any ulcerated area along with some cryptal distortion as part of the healing process. Following radiation damage, fibrosis is accompanied by other changes in the matrix (Sections 3.9.2 and 11.1).

3.9.2 Hyalinization

This pattern of degenerative change appears as an even, glass-like eosinophilia of the connective tissue of the lamina propria (Fig. 3.52). It is diagnostic of chronic radiation damage and is accompanied by other signs of this condition (Section 11.1). Similar change can be seen in the submucosal connective tissue and in the walls of vessels. The glass-like quality of hyalinization plus the distribution in the lamina propria is different from that of the collagen band in collagenous colitis and amyloid disease, with which it could be confused (Sections 9.3.1 and 20.8).

An increased eosinophilic density of the lamina propria is often seen in early ischaemic damage and is a useful sign, the exact nature of which is unclear.

3.9.3 Oedema

Oedematous mucosa appears thicker than normal. The crypts fail to reach the muscularis mucosae and the space between them is increased (Fig. 3.53). In other respects the crypts remain normal. Oedema is best appreciated when inflammation is absent or mild, when the lamina propria appears empty or focally depleted of cells. The oedematous connective tissue may take on a mild eosinophilia – not to be confused with the denser staining and texture of hyalinization (Section 3.9.2).

It can be difficult to distinguish the appearances produced by oedema from those of mild atrophy. The crypts and other mucosal features must be carefully inspected for other signs of chronic damage that would favour atrophy (Section 3.6.2).

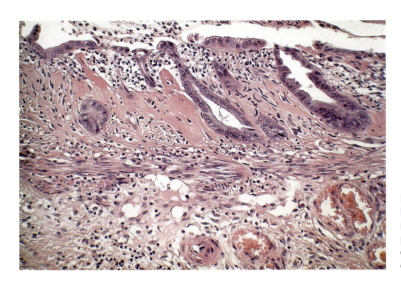

Figure 3.52 Hyalinization of lamina propria in a patient with radiation proctitis. The lamina propria is empty of inflammatory cells and the matrix is hyaline and eosinophilic.

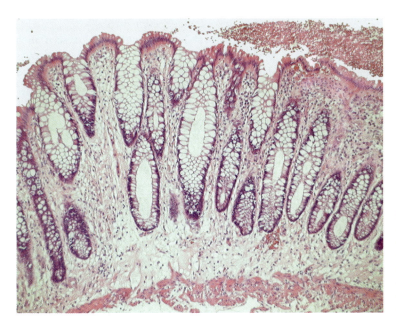

Figure 3.53 Oedema. Biopsy from close to a rectal carcinoma. The mucosa is slightly thickened and the crypt bases lie above the muscularis mucosae. The lamina propria appears empty of cells. The oedema may have been caused by lymphatic obstruction.

Oedema is often the only abnormality in a biopsy but its usefulness as a diagnostic sign is limited. It is usual to report it as an observation without comment. There is no evidence that it is a response to diarrhoea.

When seen together with other changes suggestive of infective colitis, oedema is a helpful sign (Section 4.2.1). In severe active ulcerative colitis and Crohn's disease the heavy infiltrate of inflammatory cells in the mucosa usually obscures the fact that it is also oedematous.

3.9.4 Muscle fibres

Individual fibres extend up from the muscularis mucosae into the lamina propria in the normal biopsy but in certain conditions this becomes more extensive, owing to hypertrophy of myocytes

(Fig. 3.51). It is most obvious in the solitary ulcer syndrome (Section 15.10) but can be seen in polyps of any description (Section 15.10). Polyps probably suffer mechanical stresses similar to the 'prolapsing mucosa' of the solitary ulcer syndrome and they may, indeed, develop as a result of prolapse of a mucosal fold (inflammatory 'cap' polyps; Section 15.9.2). In polyps of the Peutz–Jeghers syndrome the muscle seen in the lamina propria surrounding the crypts, although considered part of the hamartomatous malformation, may also result from mucosal prolapse (Section 15.8).

Like many of the abnormalities described in this section, a derangement of muscle fibres, with splaying into the lamina propria, may accompany healing of ulceration which has originated from any cause.

3.9.5 Vasculature

Mucosal capillary congestion is a common finding and has little discriminating potential on its own. Vigorous instrumentation before biopsy may produce congestion. It also accompanies most of the major forms of colitis and is especially prominent in acute ulcerative colitis (Section 5.2.1b). In infective proctocolitis there is margination of polymorphs within dilated capillaries (Section 4.2.1). Ectasia of capillaries within the mucosa accompanies other more specific changes in mucosal prolapse (Section 15.10 and Fig. 3.54) and radiation damage (Section 11.1). Abnormal numbers of large capillaries, closely grouped, suggest the possible diagnosis of a vascular abnormality. The problems of vascular hamartomas and angiodysplasia are considered in Sections 15.16 and 20.1.1, respectively.

3.9.6 Haemorrhage

Free blood is frequently seen in the mucosa and may even occupy most of the lamina propria (Fig. 3.55). It is commonly an artefact, a product of zealous instrumentation. On such occasions other mucosal elements are all seen to be normal. It may, however, be a helpful sign in acute ischaemic colitis. It is then seen alongside congested capillaries and degenerative changes in the superficial half of the mucosa (Section 10.6.2).

Discrete focal haemorrhage may be seen in a biopsy and it is our impression that this pattern is a pointer to infective colitis when interpreted with other signs (Section 4.2.1) (Fig. 3.55).

3.9.7 Granulation tissue

Granulation tissue can be found in any healing ulcer, but is especially seen in relation to ischaemia. Within exuberant granulation tissue highly atypical

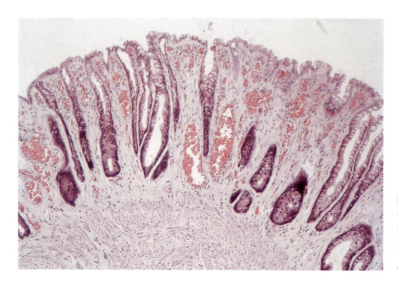

Figure 3.54 Ectasia of mucosal capillaries. This is a feature accompanying ischaemia and may result from solitary rectal ulcer, as in this case, or from radiation damage.

large cells may sometimes be noted (Fig. 3.56). These have pleomorphic nuclei, prominent nucleoli and often abundant cytoplasm. Many may be swollen endothelial cells, as suggested by Isaacson (1982) but others seem unrelated to vessels and may be of fibroblastic or myofibroblastic origin (Shekitka and Helwig, 1991). These cells should not be mistaken for a malignant infiltrate. They do not appear to be related to any particular condition.

Their precise histogenesis is unknown. Following immunocytochemistry, they are vimentin-positive (Shekitka and Helwig, 1991) but do not express factor VIII antigen or any other differentiation marker. Some of the cells may display features resembling an infection by cytomegalovirus. There is generally an overlying layer of fibrino-purulent exudate.

3.10 MUSCULARIS MUCOSAE

The muscularis mucosae is not a source of useful diagnostic information. A few abnormal patterns are recognized, namely thickening, fibrosis and splaying of fibres into the mucosa.

It is difficult to recognize thickening of the muscularis mucosae in a biopsy. Indeed, artefactual contraction and curling up of the muscle may lead to misinterpretation. True thickening is seen in the vicinity of obstructive lesions of whatever cause (e.g. carcinoma or Hirschsprung's disease). Thus, its appreciation, in the absence of other mucosal abnormalities may be a clue to a lesion nearby. There can also be thickening of the muscularis mucosae in chronic ulcerative colitis, but as a useful sign it is over-shadowed by other features (Section 5.2.3b).

Splaying of muscle fibres upwards into the lamina propria is the commonest anomaly (Section 3.9.4), prompting consideration of the 'mucosal

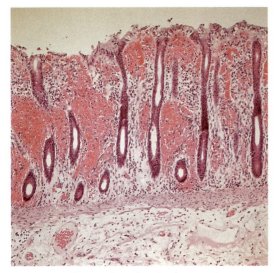

Figure 3.55 Haemorrhage into lamina propria. Although an artefact, this is often the result of rupturing of congested capillaries in ischaemia or, as in this case, infective colitis.

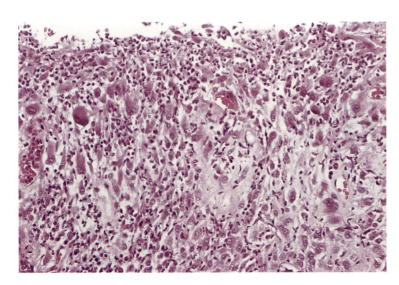

Figure 3.56 Granulation tissue from a patient with ulcerative colitis containing, beneath surface exudate, bizarre primitive cells of possible endothelial or fibroblastic lineage.

prolapse syndrome' (Section 15.10), healing ulceration, Peutz–Jeghers polyps and polyps suffering
torsion or trauma (Sections 15.8 and 15.10).

In non-malignant strictures fibres of the muscularis mucosae are often intermingled with fibrous
tissue and this arrangement can replace the loose
connective tissue of the submucosa. This is not a
feature specific to any particular underlying disease, but does occur in Crohn's disease and may
occasionally be detected along the deep margin of
well-taken biopsies.

3.11 SUBMUCOSA

Submucosal signposts depend entirely on the size of
the biopsy, for only in deep biopsies will submucosa
be present. The significance of 'connective tissue
changes' and any inflammatory infiltrate in general is the same as described for the mucosa but
certain features are worth emphasizing.

3.11.1 Submucosal oedema

Submucosal oedema accounts for the radiological sign of 'thumbprinting' and is a marker for
ischaemia. Microscopically, attention is often drawn
to the large amount of submucosa in the biopsy, the
oedematous submucosa having been easily picked
up by the biopsy forceps. It is also a feature that can
be recognized in pseudomembranous colitis and
antibiotic-associated colitis (Chapter 4).

3.11.2 Inflammation

An inflammatory cell infiltrate in the submucosa is
sometimes in excess of that observed in the overlying mucosa (Fig. 3.57). This has been designated
disproportionate inflammation and is most often a
sign of Crohn's disease (Section 6.3.6).

The inflammation may seem to bear no relation
to an almost normal mucosa above, in which case
a lesion close by is the most likely. An undermin-
ing ulcer, a deep, 'flask-shaped' ulcer of amoebiasis (Section 4.7.1), the edge of a fissure, inflammation adjacent to a diverticulum or abscess and

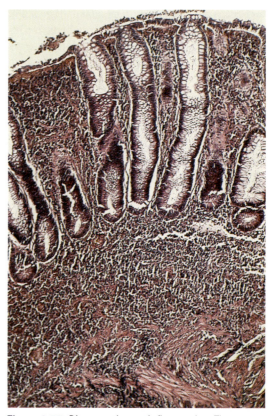

Figure 3.57 Disproportionate inflammation. The
inflammatory cell infiltrate in the submucosa is denser
than in the mucosa. Rectal biopsy, Crohn's disease.

tuberculosis (Section 4.2.7b) are the main possibilities to be considered and other evidence sought.
However, inflammation may extend into the submucosa beneath severe ulceration of any cause,
even in ulcerative colitis.

Eosinophilic colitis can have a predominantly
submucosal distribution (Section 12.5.10).

Collections of foamy histiocytes in the submucosa, often with large foreign body-type multinucleate giant cells, are seen surrounding submucosal
gas cysts (cystic pneumatosis; Fig. 3.58 and
Section 20.2). The cysts themselves are not always
evident in biopsies. A similar picture, but with multiple round vacuoles, rather than large irregular
cysts, is presented by oleogranuloma (Section 11.3).
Discrete granulomas in the submucosa are, on their
own, highly suggestive of Crohn's disease (Section
6.3.3) but it is important to beware of mistaking

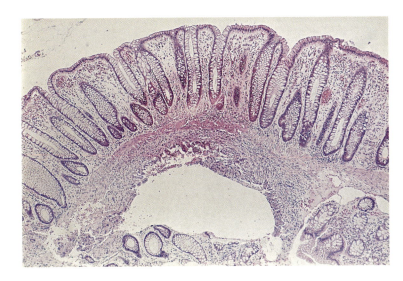

Figure 3.58 Cystic pneumatosis. Submucosal gas cyst, lined by plump, foreign body-type giant cells.

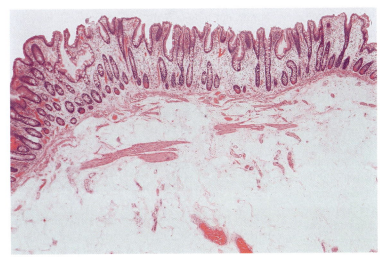

Figure 3.59 Fat in submucosa. Submucosal adipose tissue can be a manifestation of atrophy, as in ulcerative colitis. This is a biopsy from a focus of caecal lipohyperplasia.

submucosal ganglia in inflamed bowel for granulomas (Fig. 3.39).

Inconspicuous groups of brown-tinged histiocytes in the submucosa, shown by Perl's stain to contain haemosiderin, are markers of previous ischaemic damage (Sections 10.6.3 and 10.6.4).

3.11.3 Submucosal fat

Fat cells are normally present in small numbers in the submucosa but submucosal adipose tissue becomes conspicuous in some cases of bowel atrophy, as in ulcerative colitis of long duration, especially when there has been a defunctioning colostomy or ileostomy. It is found in the idiopathic condition of lipohyperplasia (Fig. 3.59).

3.11.4 Misplaced epithelium

It is within the normal spectrum to find occasional misplaced glands beneath the muscularis mucosae in relation to lymphoid follicles, so-called lymphoid–glandular complexes (Kealy, 1976; Section 2.2.5). The epithelium looks normal or reflects the features of the overlying mucosa (Fig. 3.60). Submucosal glandular misplacement is more frequently seen in cases of long-standing inflammatory bowel disease than in normal mucosa and, if the epithelium is

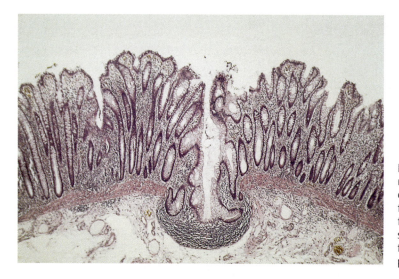

Figure 3.60 Misplaced colonic mucosa: lymphoid–glandular complexes (herniation). It is normal for occasional transmural lymphoid follicles to extend into the submucosa, accompanied by crypts from the overlying mucosa. From a patient with infective colitis.

dysplastic, can resemble invasive adenocarcinoma (Allen and Biggart, 1986). The presence of lamina propria around the misplaced glands excludes malignancy (Section 16.2.2).

Irregular clusters of glands occur within the muscularis mucosae and in the submucosa in colitis cystica profunda (Fig. 20.6). These have been referred to as mucous retention cysts (Goodall and Sinclair, 1957; Stolar and Silver, 1969). There is usually an accompanying architectural disturbance in the mucosa and the muscularis mucosae is often splayed out. In the rectum, the derangement is believed to be a complication of mucosal prolapse, a combination of ulceration and prolapse preventing normal healing. It is part of the picture of the solitary ulcer (Section 15.10). The epithelium is not dysplastic and is surrounded by normal or slightly inflamed submucosa. A more diffuse form of colitis cystica profunda may develop in the sigmoid or more proximal colon following severe ulceration caused by ulcerative colitis or bacterial dysentery (Tedesco *et al.*, 1976).

3.11.5 Pseudocarcinomatous invasion (pseudoinvasion)

'Misplaced' glands can be seen within the muscularis mucosae and in the submucosa in relation to adenomatous polyps (Section 15.12.1). The glands may be dysplastic, as in the head of the adenoma,

but do not have a malignant cytological or architectural pattern. The most helpful sign in distinguishing this potentially worrying picture from carcinoma is the presence of lamina propria around the glands, often containing haemosiderin-laden macrophages (Fig. 16.2). In contrast, malignant epithelium in the submucosa excites a desmoplastic response (Section 16.3).

3.12 VASCULATURE

Within the submucosa there are veins and small muscular arterioles. Rectal biopsy is a useful diagnostic tool in the detection of amyloid (Section 20.8) and systemic vasculitis (Section 10.8). It is essential to examine step sections as the vasculitis may not only be patchy, but vessels may be tortuous and not appear throughout the biopsy. Amyloid is also easily missed and a Congo red-stained section should always be examined by polarized light in a suspected case, even if at first inspection of the H and E section the vessels appear normal.

The size and distribution of vessels in the submucosa may also give a clue to the diagnosis of angiodysplasia and other vascular anomalies, even though the mucosa above may not seem overtly abnormal. Large venous channels especially, or a clustered arrangement are typical features (Section 20.1.1).

3.13 NERVES

3.13.1 Ganglia

Submucosal nerve ganglia are occasionally unusually prominent. This feature is not in itself of significance, but may be associated with thickening of the bowel wall, as in diverticular disease or Crohn's disease (Dvorak *et al.*, 1980), when there is usually accompanying inflammation. Absence of submucosal ganglia is not diagnostic of Hirschsprung's disease, but their presence excludes it (Section 13.3).

Perhaps the most frequent cause of absent or reduced density of submucosal ganglia in biopsy material is the overstretching of the bowel which occurs in constipation or pseudo-obstruction. Assessment of submucosal ganglia in endoscopic biopsies therefore lacks reliability. Ganglia may be genuinely reduced in absolute number (hypoganglionosis) in rare instances of neuronal dysplasia associated with constipation (Section 13.3.4) or increased and extend through the muscularis mucosae into the mucosa in hyperganglionic neuronal dysplasia. This is an occasional cause of a clinical picture resembling Hirschsprung's disease (Section 13.3.5).

3.13.2 Nerve bundles

Abnormal, thick and irregular nerve bundles are present in the submucosa in large numbers in Hirschsprung's disease. These may be inconspicuous in routine haematoxylin and eosin-stained sections, but are easily seen in cryostat sections of unfixed biopsy tissue stained for nonspecific esterase, or more specifically for acetylcholinesterase. Submucosal neural hypertrophy can also be a conspicuous feature of Crohn's disease (Section 6.3.6).

3.14 PIGMENT DEPOSITION

The commonest reason to find brown pigment within macrophages in the lamina propria is melanosis coli, in which lipofuscin accumulates because of epithelial cell destruction by anthroquinone laxative administration (Section 13.6.1). Lipofuscin deposition in ganglia and nerves, as well as the muscularis mucosae, is characteristic of Batten's disease (Section 20.7).

Small, inconspicuous groups of brown, pigment-containing cells in the deeper lamina propria or, more typically, in the submucosa, are likely to contain haemosiderin, which can be confirmed by Perl's stain. This is a marker of previous ulceration, particularly that caused by ischaemia (Sections 10.6.2 and 10.6.3).

REFERENCES

Al-Haddad, S., Riddell, R.H. (2005) The role of eosinophils in inflammatory bowel disease. *Gut*, 54, 1674–5.

Allen, D.C., Biggart, J.D. (1986) Misplaced epithelium in ulcerative colitis and Crohn's disease of the colon and its relationship to malignant mucosal changes. *Histopathology*, 10, 37–52.

Alschibaja, T., Morson, B.C. (1977) Ischaemic bowel disease. *J. Clin. Pathol.* 11, (Suppl. 30), 68–77.

Arber, D.A., Tamayo, R., Weiss, L.M. (1998) Paraffin section detection of the *c*-kit gene product (CD117) in human tissues: value in the diagnosis of mast cell disorders. *Hum. Pathol.*, 29, 498–504.

Azzopardi, J.G., Evans D.J. (1966) Mucoprotein-containing histiocytes (muciphages) in the rectum. *J. Clin. Pathol.*, 19, 368–74.

Bancroft, J.D. (2002) Paraffin section detection of the *c*-kit gene product (CD117) in human tissues: value in the diagnosis of mast cell disorders. Mast Cells. In: Bancroft J. D., Gamble M. (eds.) *Theory and practice of histological techniques*, 5th edn. London, Edinburgh, New York, St Louis, Philadelphia, Sydney, Toronto: Churchill Livingstone, pp. 346–7.

Binder, V. (1970) The content of eosinophil granulocytes in the colonic mucosa in ulcerative colitis. *Scand. J. Gastroenterol.*, 5, 707–12.

Bischoff, S.C., Wedemeyer, J., Hermann, A. *et al.* (1996) Quantitative assessment of intestinal eosinophils and mast cells in inflammatory bowel disease. *Histopathology*, 28, 1–13.

Bogomoletz, W.V., Adnet, L.J., Birembaut, P., Feydy, P., Dupont, P. (1980) Collagenous colitis: an unrecognized entity. *Gut*, 21, 164–8.

Day, D.W., Jass, J.R., Price A.B. *et al.* (2003) *Morson and Dawson's gastrointestinal pathology*, 4th edn. Oxford: Blackwell, p. 489.

Driman, D.K., Preiksaitis, H.G. (1998) Colorectal inflammation and increased cell proliferation associated with oral sodium phosphate bowel preparation solution. *Hum. Pathol.*, 29, 972–8.

Dvorak, A.M. (1979) Mast-cell hyperplasia and degranulation in Crohn's disease. In: Pepys, J., Edwards, A.M. (eds) *The mast cell*. London: Pitman, pp. 657–62.

Dvorak, A.M., Osage, J.E., Monahan, R.A., Dickersin, G.R. (1980) Crohn's disease. Transmission electron microscopic studies. III Target tissues. Proliferation of and injury to smooth muscle and the autonomic nervous system. *Hum. Pathol.*, 11, 620–34.

Elmes, M.E., Stanton, M.R., Howells, C.H.L., Lowe, G.H. (1984) Relation between the mucosal flora and Paneth cell population of human jejunum and ileum. *J. Clin. Pathol.*, 37, 1268–71.

Elphick, D.A., Mahida, Y.R. (2005) Paneth cells: their role in innate immunity and inflammatory disease. *Gut*, 54,1802–9.

Erlandsen, S.L., Parsons J.A., Taylor T.D. (1974) Ultrastructural immunocytochemical localization of lysozyme in the Paneth cells of man. *J. Histochem. Cytochem.*, 22, 401–13.

Gagliardi, G., Thompson, I.W., Hershman, M.J. *et al.* (1996) *Pneumatosis coli*: a proposed pathogenesis based on study of 25 cases and review of the literature. *Int. J. Colorectal Dis.*, 11, 111–8.

Gelfand, M.D., Tepper, M., Katz, L.A. *et al.* (1968) Acute irradiation proctitis in man. Development of eosinophilic crypt abscesses. *Gastroenterology*, 54, 401–11.

Gledhill, A., Cole, F.M. (1984) Significance of basement membrane thickening in the human colon. *Gut*, 25, 1085–8.

Gledhill, A., Enticott, M.E., Howe, S. (1986a) Variation in the argyrophil cell population of the rectum in ulcerative colitis and adenocarcinoma. *J. Pathol.*, 149, 287–91.

Gledhill, A., Hall, P.A., Cruse, J.P., Pollock, D.J. (1986b) Enteroendocrine cell hyperplasia, carcinoid tumours and adenocarcinoma in long-standing ulcerative colitis. *Histopathology*, 10, 501–8.

Goodall, H.B., Sinclair, L.S. (1957) Colitis cystica profunda. *J. Pathol. Bacteriol.*, 73, 33–42.

Greenson, J.H., Stern, R.A., Carpenter, S.L., Barnett, J. (1997) The clinical significance of focal active colitis. *Hum. Pathol.*, 28, 729–33.

Heatley, R.V., James, P.D. (1979) Eosinophils in the rectal mucosa. *Gut*, 20, 787–91.

Isaacson, P.G. (1982) Biopsy appearances easily mistaken for malignancy in gastrointestinal endoscopy. *Histopathology*, 6, 377–89.

Kealy, W.F. (1976) Colonic lymphoid–glandular complex (microbursa) nature and morphology. *J. Clin. Pathol.*, 29, 241–4.

Lampert, I.A., Thorpe, P., van Noorden, S. *et al.* (1985) Selective sparing of enterochromaffin cells in graft versus host disease affecting the colonic mucosa. *Histopathology*, 9, 875–86.

Lee, F.D., Maguire, C., Obeidat, W., Russell, R.J. (1997) Importance of cryptolytic lesions and pericryptal granulomas in inflammatory bowel disease. *J. Clin. Pathol.*, 50, 148–52.

Leriche, M., Devroede, G., Sanchez, G. (1978) Changes in the rectal mucosa induced by hypertonic enemas. *Dis. Colon Rectum*, 21, 227–36.

Mahadeva, U., Martin, J.P., Patel, N.K., Price, A.B. (2002) Granulomatous ulcerative colitis: a re-appraisal of the mucosal granuloma in the distinction of Crohn's disease from ulcerative colitis. *Histopathology*, 41, 50–5.

Mandal, B.K., Schofield, P.F., Morson, B.C. (1982) A clinicopathological study of acute colitis: the dilemma of transient colitis syndrome. *Scand. J. Gastroenterol.*, 17, 865–9.

Porter, E.M., Liu, L. Oren, A., Anton, P.A., Ganz, T. (1997) Localization of human intestinal defensin 5 in Paneth cell granules. *Infect. Immun.*, 65, 2389–95.

Riddell, R.H., Goldman, H., Ransohoff, D.F. *et al.* (1983) Dysplasia in inflammatory bowel disease: standardized classification with provisional clinical applications. *Hum. Pathol.*, 14, 931–68.

Robey-Cafferty, S.S., Ro, J.Y., Ordonez, N.G., Cleary, K.R. (1990) Transitional mucosa of colon. A morphological, histochemical, and immunohistochemical study. *Arch. Pathol. Lab. Med.*, 114, 72–5.

Rodning, C.B., Wilson, I.D., Erlandson, S.L. (1976) Immunoglobulins within small intestinal Paneth cells. *Lancet*, i, 984.

Ryan, C.K., Potter, G.D. (1995) Disinfectant colitis. Rinse as well as you wash. *J. Clin. Gastroenterol.*, 21, 6–9.

Salto-Tellez, M., Price, A.B. (2000) What is the significance of muciphages in colorectal biopsies? The significance of muciphages in otherwise normal colorectal biopsies. *Histopathology*, 36, 556–9.

Shekitka, K.M., Helwig, E.B. (1991) Deceptive bizarre stromal cells in polyps and ulcers of the gastrointestinal tract. *Cancer*, 67, 2111–17.

Snover, D., Sandstad, J., Hutton, S. (1985) Mucosal pseudolipomatosis of the colon. *Am. J. Clin. Pathol.*, 84, 575–80.

Stolar J., Silver, H. (1969) Differentiation of pseudo-inflammatory colloid carcinoma from colitis cystica profunda. *Dis. Colon Rectum*, 12, 63–6.

Strater, J., Walczak, H., Pukrop, T., von Muller *et al.* (2002) TRAIL and its receptors in the colonic epithelium: a putative role in the defense of viral infections. *Gastroenterology*, 122, 659–66.

Tedesco, F.J., Sumner, H.W., Kassens, W.D. (1976) Colitis cystica profunda. *Am. J. Gastroenterol.*, 65, 339–43.

Totty, B.A. (2002) Mucins. In: Bancroft, J.D., Gamble, M. (eds) *Theory and practice of histological techniques*, 5th edn. London, Edinburgh, New York, Philadelphia, St Louis, Sydney, Toronto: Churchill Livingstone, pp. 188–9.

Waring, J.P., Manne, R.K., Wadas, D.D., Sanowski, R.A. (1989) Mucosal pseudolipomatosis: an air pressure-related colonoscopy complication. *Gastrointest. Endosc.*, 35, 93–4.

Warren, B.F., Dankwa, E.K., Davies, J.D. (1990) 'Diamond-shaped' crypts and mucosal elastin: helpful diagnostic features in biopsies of rectal prolapse. *Histopathology*, 17, 129–34.

Wasserman, S.L. (1979) The mast cell and the inflammatory response. In: Pepys, J., Edwards, A.M. (eds) *The mast cell.* London: Pitman, pp. 9–20.

Watson, A.J., Roy, A.D. (1960) Paneth cells in the large intestine in ulcerative colitis. *J. Pathol. Bacteriol.*, 80, 309–16.

Whitehead, R.H. (1985) *Mucosal biopsy of the gastrointestinal tract. Major problems in pathology 3*, 3rd edn. Philadelphia, London, Toronto, Mexico City, Rio de Janiero, Sydney, Tokyo: Saunders, p. 299.

Williams, G.T. (1985) Commentary: transitional mucosa of the large intestine. *Histopathology*, 9, 1237–43.

CHAPTER 4

INFECTIVE COLITIS

4.1	Introduction	56
4.2	Acute bacterial diarrhoeas/ infective colitis and proctitis	57
	4.2.1 The typical biopsy in invasive infection	57
	4.2.2 Other patterns	60
	4.2.3 Resolution	61
	4.2.4 Specific bacteria	61
	4.2.5 Distinguishing infectious colitis (acute self-limiting colitis) from chronic inflammatory bowel disease	62
	4.2.6 Non-invasive infections	63
	4.2.7 Miscellaneous infections	63
4.3	Enterocolitic syndromes	65
4.4	Sexually transmitted diseases	66
	4.4.1 Gonorrhoea	66
	4.4.2 *Treponema pallidum*	66
	4.4.3 *Chlamydia trachomatis*	67
	4.4.4 Colitis in acquired immuno-deficiency syndrome (AIDS)	67
4.5	Intestinal spirochaetosis	69
4.6	Viral causes of colitis	70
	4.6.1 Cytomegalovirus infection	70
	4.6.2 Herpes simplex	73
	4.6.3 Adenovirus	73
4.7	Protozoal infection	74
	4.7.1 Amoebiasis	74
	4.7.2 Giardiasis	76
	4.7.3 *Balantidium*	77
	4.7.4 Coccidia (*Cryptosporidium*)	77
4.8	Helminths	77
	4.8.1 *Schistosoma mansoni* and *Schistosoma japonicum*	79
4.9	Nematodes	79
	4.9.1 Strongyloidiasis	79
	4.9.2 Trichuriasis	79
	4.9.3 Oxyuriasis	81
4.10	Fungal infection	82
	References	82

4.1 INTRODUCTION

Biopsy in intestinal infection may occasionally result in the direct identification of an organism or, more usually, permit a presumptive diagnosis from the pattern of inflammation (e.g. tuberculosis in the presence of caseating granulomas). Perhaps the commonest biopsy dilemma in routine practice is to distinguish infective colitis from the first attack of chronic inflammatory bowel disease (CIBD), that is Crohn's disease or ulcerative colitis (Section 4.2.5). In North America the former is generally referred to as acute self-limiting colitis (ASLC). The standard classifica.tion of infective colitis is aetiological, namely viral, bacterial, protozoal, fungal infections and infestations by helminths. In Western countries it is the bacterial diarrhoeas which form the large majority of the diagnostic problems.

A particular clinical problem is 'Traveller's diarrhoea'. This has a polymicrobial aetiology and patients seldom come to biopsy. On the rare occasions when a biopsy is taken, the histology reflects the aetiological agent at that point in its natural history (Taylor *et al.*, 1985; Arduino and DuPont, 1993).

4.2 ACUTE BACTERIAL DIARRHOEAS/INFECTIVE COLITIS AND PROCTITIS

A pertinent first question is, why bother with a biopsy to solve an apparently microbiological problem? There are two reasons. First, the majority of cases of bacterial infective diarrhoeas in routine practice are culture-negative (Thomas and Tillett, 1975; Dickinson *et al.*, 1979; Koplan *et al.*, 1980; Nostrant *et al.*, 1987; Schumacher *et al.*, 1991) and if the characteristic histological picture of infective proctocolitis is present the biopsy is of diagnostic help. Matsumoto *et al.* (1994) found that culture of biopsies was more sensitive than culturing faeces (50 per cent vs. 20 per cent). Second, it is important that pathologists are familiar with these histological features (Dickinson *et al.*, 1979; Jewkes *et al.*, 1981) so that patients with a relatively minor self-limiting infectious disease are not mislabelled Crohn's disease or ulcerative colitis, both of which carry long-term medical and social implications.

A useful subclassification of the infective diarrhoeas, based partly on symptomatology and partly on pathogenesis is shown in Table 4.1. It is the inflammatory/invasive group (Table 4.1, column 2) that is the most important, for it is infections in this group which can be mistaken for CIBD. *Salmonella* species, *Shigella* species, enteroinvasive *Escherichia coli* and *Campylobacter* species account for the large majority of the culture-positive cases (Loosli *et al.*, 1985). Typically, all produce similar histology, with an 'infective' biopsy pattern (Price *et al.*, 1979).

4.2.1 The typical biopsy in invasive infection

The initial impression at low magnification is of a thick mucosa widened by oedema. The oedema separates the crypts both from each other and from the muscularis mucosae. It also diminishes the apparent intensity of the inflammatory cell infiltrate, which has the look of 'sprinkled salt grains' across an otherwise clear lamina propria (Fig. 4.1). Focal clusters of polymorphs are present throughout the biopsy, often adjacent to dilated capillaries or alongside the crypts. Their margination within capillaries is prominent. A characteristic strongly suggestive of infectious proctocolitis is the presence of polymorphs caught up between the lining cells of the

Table 4.1 Infective causes of diarrhoea

1. Non-inflammatory/non-invasive	2. Inflammatory/invasive	3. Miscellaneous

Enteric viruses
  e.g. Coxsackie AB, Norwalk types
  and rotavirus
Vibrio cholera
Bacillus cereus
Staphylococcus aureus
Vibrio parahaemolyticus
Enterotoxic *Escherichia coli*
Clostridium perfringens
	Salmonella spp. (typhoid and
	  non-typhoid types
	Shigella spp.
	Campylobacter spp.
	Enteroinvasive *Escherichia coli*
	Clostridium *difficile*
	Staphylococcus aureus
		Mycobacterium tuberculosis
		Yersinia spp.
		Cytomegalovirus
		Venereal infections
		Neisseria gonorrhoea
		Treponema pallidum
		Herpes simplex virus
		Chlamydia spp.
		Enterocolitic syndromes
		Pseudomembranous and
		  antibiotic associated colitis
		Neonatal necrotizing enterocolitis
		Intestinal spirochaetosis

crypts but not in great numbers within the crypt lumen (Figs 3.23, 4.2 and 4.3). This appearance, 'the incipient crypt abscess' or 'cryptitis' (Price *et al.*, 1979) contrasts with the true crypt abscess, which often occurs in infection but does not dominate the picture as it does in active ulcerative colitis and Crohn's disease (Anand *et al.*, 1986) (Fig. 3.22). Similar clusters of polymorphs infiltrate between the cells of the surface epithelium. The latter may be degenerate or may be gathered into small projecting tufts between individual crypts (Figs 3.4 and 8.10). The absolute numbers of plasma cells and lymphocytes within the lamina propria may well be increased but this is often masked by the oedema. It is the prominence of polymorphonuclear neutrophils compared with the plasma cell infiltrate that is of key diagnostic importance when making the distinction between infection and other causes of proctocolitis coupled with the inflammatory cell balance in favour of cryptitis versus crypt abscesses (Figs 4.2, 4.3 and 5.6). Furthermore, the distribution of inflammation across the biopsy is patchy. The crypt pattern remains regular but the superficial crypt epithelium shows reactive and degenerative changes along with numerous neutrophils (Kumar *et al.*, 1982; Surawicz and Belic, 1984). There is mucin depletion and individual epithelial cells appear flat or attenuated, leading to dilatation of the luminal half of many of the crypts. In some crypts this area may degenerate completely (Fig. 4.4). The overall crypt abnormalities form a conspicuous feature at the initial examination of a biopsy at low magnification. The term crypt 'withering' has been suggested (Fig. 4.5) for this pattern of abnormalities or, when superficial, the 'string of pearls' sign

(Surawicz and Belic, 1984) (Fig. 4.6). This manifests as apparent bridging of degenerate lining cells across the crypt lumen in conjunction with an infiltrate of neutrophil polymorphs. A degree of crypt dilatation

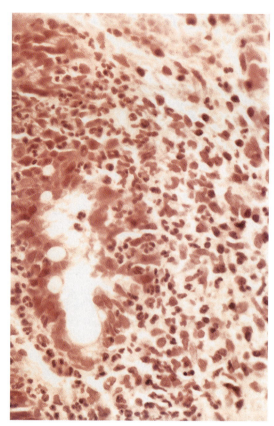

Figure 4.2 Acute infective colitis. Typical cryptitis in which neutrophil polymorphs predominate in intraepithelial and pericryptal positions rather than in the crypt lumen as crypt abscesses. The latter is more a feature of ulcerative colitis and Crohn's disease.

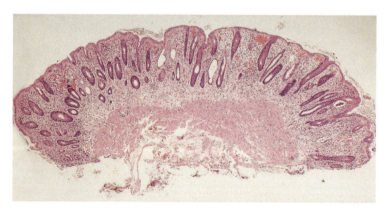

Figure 4.1 Acute infective colitis. The mucosa appears thickened due to oedema. The inflammatory cells in the lamina propria are dispersed, giving the so-called 'sprinkled salt' appearance. The crypts show degenerative features resulting in dilatation and crypt withering. Their alignment remains intact.

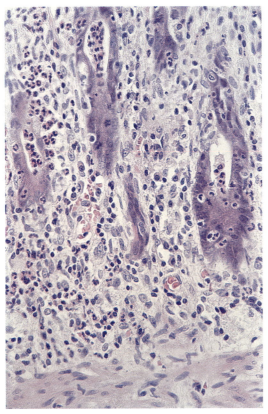

Figure 4.3 A case of *Salmonella* colitis showing cryptitis and pericryptitis but also with some lumenal neutrophils. There is crypt cell degeneration (withering) and oedema with a loose even sprinkling of inflammatory cells across the lamina propria.

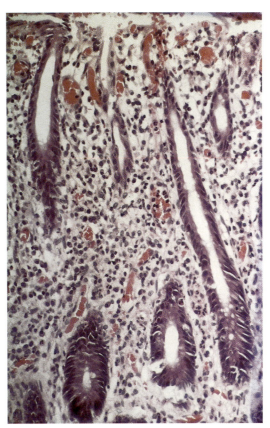

Figure 4.5 Acute infective colitis. There is superficial crypt withering with preservation of the perpendicular crypt alignment against an oedematous background of evenly distributed inflammatory cells.

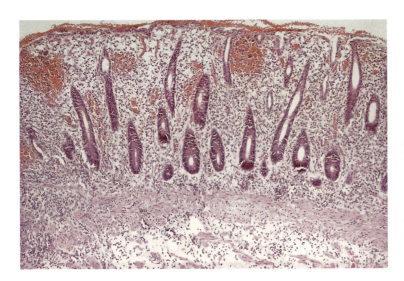

Figure 4.4 Acute infectious colitis. This shows the preservation of architecture along with crypt withering. The latter is most obvious superficially resulting in apparent luminal crypt dilatation. The oedema accentuates foci of haemorrhage, which while entirely non-specific, may contribute to the overall diagnostic picture.

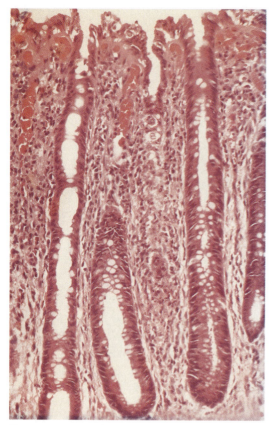

Figure 4.6 Acute infective colitis. In this pattern of crypt withering there is degenerative bridging of the epithelium across the crypt lumen giving a 'string of pearls' appearance. Neutrophil polymorphs are often seen within the individual 'pearls'.

and branching, sufficient to cause some confusion with ulcerative colitis, may be seen in *Shigella* infections (Anand *et al.*, 1986).

The other abnormalities present are less specific. Luminal pus is frequent and margination of polymorphs is prominent within congested capillaries. Capillary microthrombi have been described (Mathan and Mathan, 1985), which may account for the focal haemorrhage in the lamina propria (Choudari *et al.*, 1985). The changes, though usually seen throughout the biopsy, are patchy and occasionally restricted to one focus. The above description represents the characteristic pattern and is most common in patients biopsied at the onset of their symptoms or within the first 7 days (Kumar *et al.*, 1982). As far as is known at present, there is no histological difference between culture-positive cases and cases that are clinically infective but culture-negative. The umbrella term to cover both situations is that of ASLC. Surawicz and Belic (1984) looked at the reliability of histological signs in ASLC and could only identify three. These were: invariably regular crypt architecture, superficial giant cells and superficial crypt abscesses. The frequency of the last two was only 16 per cent. Indeed, they have rarely been features of our own material.

4.2.2 Other patterns

Not all biopsies in infectious diarrhoea show the above typical features (Dickinson *et al.*, 1979; Nostrant *et al.*, 1987). Unfortunately, no other patterns permit a diagnostic statement.

4.2.2a Normal or oedematous

Unaccountably, even in the face of positive cultures some biopsies remain normal or show only mild oedema.

4.2.2b Mild acute non-specific proctitis

This is dealt with more fully in Section 12.3.1. There is a definite minor increase in plasma cells usually limited to the superficial mucosa. A few polymorphs are present, including some infiltrating the cryptal or surface epithelium. The goblet cell population is slightly reduced and the cells can show signs of degeneration and vacuolation.

No diagnosis is possible, but this pattern is most likely in biopsies taken early in the second week of disease, as resolution occurs (Kumar *et al.*, 1982). It is likely that this is the commonest picture seen by pathologists because of the time lag from onset of symptoms to hospital referral and biopsy.

4.2.2c Chronic inflammation

In this pattern, described and illustrated in Section 12.3.2, the only abnormality is the plasma cell infiltrate in the lamina propria. This can be diffuse but, more often, is focal and light. Lymphoid aggregates can be present, and should not be overinterpreted as suggesting Crohn's disease. Without a suitable clinical story infection is only part of a large differential. In the natural history of infectious diarrhoea this pattern also represents part of the spectrum of resolution seen from the second week onwards (Kumar *et al.*, 1982). However, in a biopsy taken during a first attack of colitis the presence of chronic inflammation, in particular plasma cells in the lower fifth of the lamina propria, is considered a strong pointer towards CIBD. We have seen these appearances persist for many weeks. What determines the rate of resolution is unknown.

4.2.3 Resolution

In the typical case full resolution of the changes occurs within 2–3 weeks, and virtually always within 3 months (Dickinson *et al.*, 1979; Schumacher *et al.*, 1991). A follow-up biopsy is therefore an important part of the diagnostic procedure, especially in culture-negative cases.

4.2.4 Specific bacteria

In general, it is not possible from biopsy appearances to distinguish between the main causes of bacterial colitis.

4.2.4a *Escherichia coli* species

There is only limited documentation of the biopsy pathology of diarrhoea caused by *E. coli*. However the bacteria are the most prevalent aerobic organisms in the gut and five main variants exist that are believed to be responsible for diarrhoeal illnesses (Echeverria *et al.*, 1993): enterotoxigenic species, which account for approximately 30 per cent of traveller's diarrhoea (Taylor *et al.*, 1985; Arduino and DuPont, 1993); enteroinvasive species, closely related to *Shigella,* which do cause a colitis and damage the mucosa; enteropathogenic species that are responsible for outbreaks of diarrhoea in childhood, demonstrate plasma-mediated adherence to the microvilli of the intestinal mucosa and have been shown to produce a mild coloproctitis (Candy and McNeish, 1984); enterohaemorrhagic species; and enteroadherent species. The first group includes 0157:H7 which produces a verocytotoxin and causes a haemorrhagic colitis described as similar to ischaemic colitis (Pai *et al.*, 1984; Morandi *et al.*, 2003). It may also precipitate the haemolytic-uraemic syndrome (Smith *et al.*, 1987; Murray and Patterson, 2000) and even appendicitis (Rosen *et al.*, 2005). The enteroadherent species play a role in travellers diarrhoea and an enteroaggregative subgroup can cause chronic diarrhoea (Echeverria *et al.*, 1993).

4.2.4b *Aeromonas* species

These organisms produce an array of virulence factors and are now an accepted cause of gastroenteritis, especially in young children (George *et al.*, 1985; Chopra and Houston, 1999). Chronic symptoms have also been documented (Lee and Surawicz, 2001).

4.2.4c *Campylobacter* species

These organisms now rank with *Salmonella* species as the commonest cause of infective diarrhoea in Western countries (Weir, 1985) and were first isolated from faecal specimens by Dekeyser *et al.* in 1972. *Campylobacter jejuni* is the most important species. The biopsy is usually typical of infectious proctocolitis (Section 4.2.1) (Price *et al.*, 1979) and organisms have been seen in the lamina propria at electron microscopy (van Spreeuwel *et al.*, 1985). Giant cells and occasional granulomas have also been described. As with the other organisms a small number of biopsies remain normal, non-specific or, it is claimed, even resemble ulcerative colitis (Lambert *et al.*, 1979). Toxic megacolon has been reported (Anderson *et al.*, 1986) consequent to infection as has appendicitis. The Guillain–Barré syndrome may also complicate infection with a quoted incidence of 1 per 1000 cases (Butzler, 2004).

4.2.4d *Shigella* species

The biopsy picture is similar to that produced by the other enteroinvasive bacteria (Speelman *et al.*, 1984; Sachdev *et al.*, 1993), though slight differences may point towards shigellosis. Crypt dilatation and branching are frequent and neutrophils are less dominant. Indeed, confusion with chronic inflammatory bowel disease is more likely (Anand *et al.*, 1986). Multiple cystic crypts may result in colitis cystica superficialis (Fig. 3.20 on page 25). In *Shigella* infection only 10–100 organisms are required as the infecting dose (DuPont *et al.*, 1989).

4.2.4e *Salmonella* species

These divide into the typhoid and non-typhoid organisms. Classical typhoid fever due to S. *typhi* is an ileal disease and mostly beyond the range of endoscopic instruments.

Non-typhoid salmonellosis involves the colon as well as the small bowel (Mandal and Mani, 1976). Together with *Campylobacter* species it is one of the commonest causes of infectious diarrhoea. At sigmoidoscopy it appears much like the other bacterial infections, with a wide range of appearances, including mild oedema, areas of petechial haemorrhage and, in severe cases, friability and ulceration (McGovern and Slavutin, 1979).

The biopsy is indistinguishable from the preceding causes (Day *et al.*, 1978; Sachdev *et al.*, 1993) but it is interesting to note the prominence of polymorphs for, in *Salmonella typhi* infection polymorphs are scant, the picture being dominated by mononuclear cells. As with the other major bacterial causes of diarrhoea occasionally toxic megacolon can occur (Bellary and Isaacs, 1990).

4.2.4f *Clostridium difficile*

This organism is considered in conjunction with pseudomembranous colitis in Chapter 8.

4.2.4g *Staphylococcus aureus*

Between 15 and 20 per cent of normal adults carry coagulase-positive *Staphylococcus aureus* in the stool (Hinton *et al.*, 1960) and it is disputed whether a true staphylococcal enterocolitis exists that is independent of the mechanism in staphylococcal food poisoning. Suppression of the normal flora by antibiotics, akin to the pathogenesis of pseudomembranous colitis, is claimed to be responsible (Cook, 1993). In two case reports the biopsies were said to show typical infective proctocolitis but in neither case were cultures for *Clostridium difficile* or *Campylobacter* species set up (Dickinson *et al.*, 1980). The organism probably only has importance if seen in large numbers in the direct stool smear and if it is grown on non-selective culture media (Hinton *et al.*, 1960).

4.2.5 Distinguishing infectious colitis (acute self-limiting colitis) from chronic inflammatory bowel disease

This is an important issue with what can be life-long implications for the patient. The reliability of the histological features on which the diagnosis depends have been addressed by several groups of authors for not all biopsies will conform to the typical picture described earlier (Section 4.2.1) (Surawicz and Belic, 1984; Allison *et al.*, 1987; Nostrant *et al.*, 1987; Surawicz, 1988; Schumacher *et al.*, 1991; Dundas *et al.*, 1997; Jenkins *et al.*, 1997).

Seven features were selected by Surawicz and Belic (1984) in favour of CIBD: distorted crypt architecture; increased lamina propria cellularity that included plasma cells, lymphocytes and neutrophils; a villous mucosal surface; crypt atrophy; basal lymphoid aggregates; basal isolated giant cells; and epithelioid granulomas. Only three were considered to favour ASLC: preserved normal architecture (Figs 4.1 and 4.4), superficial isolated giant cells and superficial crypt abscesses. However, as previously stated (Section 4.2.1), these last two had a frequency of only 16 per cent. Surawicz and Belic (1984) concluded that the diagnosis of ASLC is based more on an absence of criteria for CIBD than on positive attributes for ASLC. Of the seven features favouring CIBD their frequency varied from 13 per cent for basal giant cells to 48 per cent for distorted crypt architecture but one or more was present in 79 per cent of cases and the predictive probability for any one was in the region of 90 per cent or above.

The other papers mentioned above focus on evaluating features selected by Surawicz and Belic (1984) as the most likely to help distinguish first attacks of CIBD from infectious colitis (ASLC) since it is the interpretation of a biopsy taken during the first attack that is perhaps the most difficult for the diagnostic pathologist. There was consistent agreement among them that crypt architectural distortion and increased numbers of plasma cells, lymphocytes and neutrophils in the lamina propria were the most reliable pointers to CIBD. The variation expressed in predictive probability, sensitivity and specificity for several of the parameters has been ascribed to the differing timing of biopsies relative to the onset of symptoms and by differing definitions of the terms used. For example, if architectural distortion is defined as requiring only one branched gland, rather than two or more, its specificity and sensitivity as a distinguishing attribute change from 100 per cent and 24 per cent respectively to 87 per cent and 58 per cent (Schumacher *et al.*, 1991; Dundas *et al.*, 1997). Nostrant *et al.* (1987) point out that branching of crypts can be seen within 3–4 weeks of the onset of symptoms (or perhaps sooner) for CIBD is likely to have had a subclinical period with evolving mucosal damage prior to the patient's first clinical presentation. This contrasts with the sudden acute onset of ASLC which is usually both rapidly evolving and resolving. The recognition of the diagnostic features, as mentioned earlier, is generally limited to the first week of the attack (Price *et al.*, 1979; Nostrant *et al.*, 1987). Biopsy beyond this time produces a variable picture accounting for a broad morphological complex, blurring the ability to discriminate between CIBD and ASLC. The distinction must be based on a cluster of histological criteria, not on any single one (Nostrant *et al.*, 1987; Schumacher *et al.*, 1991). An approach that is applicable to the whole area of diagnostic colorectal biopsy practice.

The presence of chronic inflammation favoured CIBD, as would be expected, but it is most reliable when increased numbers of plasma cells are to be found in the lower fifth of the mucosa (Nostrant *et al.*, 1987; Schumacher *et al.*, 1991; Jenkins *et al.*, 1997). However, in their discussion of the problem of CIBD versus ASLC at the time of the first attack of colitis Allison *et al.* (1987), while confirming the discriminative value of crypt distortion and chronic inflammation for CIBD, point out that 30 per cent of their cases of ASLC had one or both of these features. The analysis of Dundas *et al.* (1997) was restricted to rectal biopsies and not solely first-attack biopsies. They found a positive predictive value of 100 per cent in favour of CIBD if there was villous mucosal architecture and Paneth cell metaplasia. However, the respective sensitivities were but 26 per cent and 15 per cent.

Undoubtedly, in first attacks, distorted crypt architecture and a transmucosal predominantly chronic inflammatory cell infiltrate are the commonest and most reliable attributes on which to base a diagnosis of CIBD over ASLC. Such a diagnosis will be strengthened when there is a villous mucosal surface and Paneth cell metaplasia. The typical crypt and inflammatory features of ASLC depend on examining a biopsy in the first week of the attack, otherwise the diagnosis is mainly one of inference based on an absence of those features favouring CIBD. However Therkilsden *et al.* (1989), Schumacher *et al.* (1991) and Dundas *et al.* (1997), from their follow-up data, point out that a first biopsy is not always predictive and care must be taken before attaching an irreversible diagnostic label. Furthermore Dundas *et al.* (1997) quote a figure of 1:17 for the chances of a biopsy diagnosis of ASLC evolving into CIBD in time. Both of these points are important caveats for clinicians to appreciate and emphasize the need for the diagnosis to take account of all the available clinical information. This might have to include a follow-up period and further biopsies to strengthen diagnostic confidence.

4.2.6 Non-invasive infections

The organisms broadly categorized as non-invasive and non-inflammatory are those mostly responsible for food poisoning (excluding *Salmonella* species; see Table 4.1, column 1). Biopsy has no role in the diagnosis. *Clostridium perfringens* has been implicated as a cause of infective colitis via its *theta* toxin (Borriello *et al.*, 1984) and is at least in part responsible for necrotizing enteritis (Section 4.3).

The biopsy data are scant, with a few minor abnormalities entirely within the designation of non-specific.

4.2.7 Miscellaneous infections

4.2.7a *Yersinia* species

Yersinia enterocolitica and *Yersinia pseudotuberculosis* are Gram-negative aerobic cocco-bacilli. *Y. pseudotuberculosis* may cause a colitis but generally produces a terminal ileitis and mesenteric adenitis with granulomas and micro-abscesses (El-Maraghi and Mair, 1979). *Yersinia enterocolitica,* however, is a well-documented cause of an acute colitis (Editorial, 1984), though there are few endoscopic studies of colonic disease (Vantrappen *et al.,* 1977; Simmonds *et al.,* 1987; Matsumoto *et al.,* 1990) and additional data are from autopsy series (Bradford *et al.,* 1974) or surgical resections (Gleason and Patterson, 1982). The mucosa is often erythematous and friable and shows tiny yellow-white ulcers. Large ulcers up to 5 cm, have been described. Generally, biopsies are not diagnostic and the pattern of inflammation does not have the typical characteristics of the other common bacterial infections. Simmonds *et al.* (1987) in their analysis of patients with positive faecal cultures for *Y. enterocolitica* found that the majority had normal colonoscopies and biopsies. Extrapolating to biopsies from the features described in the surgical resections documented by Gleason and Patterson (1982) one might expect to see prominent lymphoid follicles, possibly with microabscesses (Fig. 4.7) and clumps of bacteria. Granulomas are not seen in *Y. enterocolitica* infection though there may be clusters of histiocytes.

An association between yersiniosis and collagenous colitis has been proposed (Makinen *et al.,* 1998; Bohr *et al.,* 2002). On occasions *Yersinia* may also cause an apparent diffuse colitis in which case background ulcerative colitis should be considered (Simmonds *et al.,* 1987). About 2 per cent are associated with a reactive arthritis (Griffiths and Gorbach, 1993).

4.2.7b Mycobacterium tuberculosis

Tuberculosis involving the colon is uncommon away from endemic areas. The ileocaecal area is the commonest site to be involved and it occurs with decreasing frequency distal to this region. It has been an uncommon biopsy diagnosis in the West but this is tending to change because of the current patterns of global migration. Because of the contrasting therapies, namely antituberculous therapy versus possible steroid use, it is essential to distinguish it from Crohn's disease and, indeed, in the case of an isolated mass lesion, from carcinoma. The former is a well documented mistake

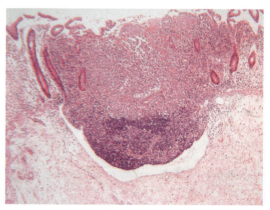

Figure 4.7 *Yersinia* enterocolitica infection. This illustrates microabscess formation centred on a mucosal lymphoid follicle with overlying ulceration. The inflammatory cell infiltrate in the lamina propria to either side is mild.

(Arnold *et al.,* 1998; Chatzicostas *et al.,* 2002) and Patel *et al.* (2004), studying the gastrointestinal profile of 260 cases with an initial diagnosis of gastrointestinal tuberculosis which had warranted commencing antituberculous therapy, found 3.9 per cent of cases had a final diagnosis of Crohn's disease. Colonoscopic distinction can be difficult and there are a wide range of appearances described. Typically, ulceration is in the transverse axis as opposed to the linear serpiginous pattern commonly seen in Crohn's disease. There can be segmental involvement, short strictures and hypertrophic polypoid masses (Singh *et al.,* 1996). Aphthoid ulceration has also been described (Shah *et al.,* 1992). When a diagnosis of tuberculosis is suspected the diagnostic yield is increased by taking multiple biopsies of which some should be sent for culture and multiple levels cut on those routinely processed (Franklin *et al.,* 1979; Shah *et al.,* 1992). The highest positive yield for the detection of acid-fast bacilli is from an ulcer, especially if part of an ulcerated mass (Patel *et al.,* 2004). The biopsy characteristics that favour tuberculosis over Crohn's disease are well documented in the papers of Pulimood *et al.* (1999, 2005). Granulomas in tuberculosis are much larger than in Crohn's disease with 90 per cent being over 200 μm in Pulimood *et al.'s* studies, compared with an average of 95 μm in their Crohn's diseases cases. The

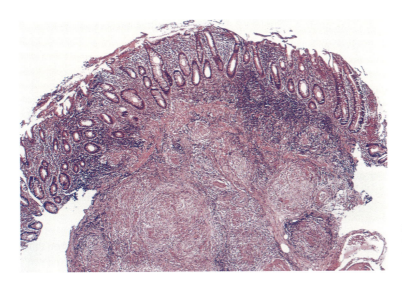

Figure 4.8 A single granuloma or small number encompasses a wide differential diagnosis but confluent granulomas, as seen in this biopsy, favour a diagnosis of tuberculosis.

granulomas are frequently confluent (Fig. 4.8) and caseation is common. If the biopsy is deep enough granulomas can be observed in the submucosa. Finding a band of epithelioid histiocytes in the base of any ulcers present is also a useful sign in favour of tuberculosis (Pulimood *et al.*, 2005; Kirsch *et al.*, 2006). By contrast, in Crohn's disease, it is rare to see more than single granulomas in a biopsy with no caseation, although foci of necrosis can occur. Microgranulomas are a feature of Crohn's disease but not seen in tuberculosis. Moreover while it is a feature of Crohn's disease to see focal acute and chronic inflammation in endoscopically normal mucosa this is infrequent in tuberculosis. Being able to demonstrate acid-fast bacilli is the diagnostic gold standard for tuberculosis. From a survey of the literature Marshall (1993) quoted figures of between 35 per cent and 60 per cent for cases in which there can be a rapid diagnosis by the finding of large caseating granulomas and/or acid-fast bacilli. However some sizeable published studies fail to identify any organisms (Shah *et al.*, 1992) while for Patel *et al.* (2004) tuberculosis remained a presumed diagnosis in 29.5 per cent of their series; this presumption is based on the response to anti-tuberculous therapy. Hopefully, the more frequent use of the polymerase chain reaction to establish a diagnosis should ease the diagnostic difficulty (Anand *et al.* 1994).

4.3 ENTEROCOLITIC SYNDROMES

Pseudomembranous colitis and antibiotic-associated colitis are dealt with separately (Chapter 8). Necrotizing enterocolitis (pigbel, PB) and neonatal necrotizing enterocolitis must be mentioned as part of the spectrum of infectious disease of the intestinal tract (Price, 1985), although neither really impinges on biopsy practice, as their main impact is in the small intestine. Necrotizing enterocolitis (PB) is believed to be caused by the toxin of *C. perfringens*, type C and primarily involves the jejunum and ileum. Only a few sporadic cases have been reported outside New Guinea (Murrell *et al.*, 1966; Murrell and Walker, 1991) with such reports usually confined to severely malnourished children or elderly diabetics (Gui *et al.*, 2002). *Clostridium perfringens* type C can also cause bloody watery diarrhoea unassociated with necrotizing enteritis (van Loon *et al.*, 1990). *Clostridium perfringens* type A has been identified as the likely pathogen in a few cases of necrotizing enteritis occurring in healthy adults (Sobel *et al.*, 2005).

Neonatal necrotizing enterocolitis (Kafetzis *et al.*, 2003) can involve the large bowel and is the major gastrointestinal complication of preterm neonates (Guthrie *et al.*, 2003) though it may rarely be seen in full term infants (Maayan-Metzger *et al.*, 2004).

Biopsy evidence of colitis has been documented following the use of an auroscope for proctoscopic examination in infants (Fenton *et al.*, 1981). *Clostridium* species, *E. coli* species, *Klebsiella* species and *Pseudomonas* species have all been incriminated (Kliegman, 1979) in conjunction with ischaemia, hypoxia and mucosal immaturity (Kafetzis *et al.*, 2003; Fell, 2005).

4.4 SEXUALLY TRANSMITTED DISEASES

Proctitis is common in homosexual men and an infective cause can be proven in many (McMillan *et al.*, 1983; Surawicz *et al.*, 1986; Laughon *et al.*, 1988). The 'gay' bowel syndrome (Weller, 1985) is merely diarrhoea in a homosexual patient due to one (or more) of the causative agents listed in Table 4.2. It is probably no longer an appropriate term (Scarce, 1997). The most frequent infections are with *Neisseria gonorrhoeae*, *Treponema pallidum*, *Chlamydia* and *Herpes simplex* virus (Quinn *et al.*, 1983) and the symptoms are usually mild. However, enteric infections with *Shigella*, *Campylobacter* (Quinn *et al.*, 1984), *Giardia* and amoebae can also be transmitted by sexual contact (Weller, 1985; Laughon *et al.*, 1988). Studying a cohort of 388 homosexual or bisexual men, Laughon *et al.* (1988) found 68 per cent of those with proctitis or diarrhoea harboured a pathogen as did 12 per cent of the asymptomatic group. Half of those with a pathogen proved to be human immunodeficiency virus (HIV)-positive compared with 25 per cent without.

4.4.1 Gonorrhoea

Anorectal gonorrhoea is one of the most common infections in women and homosexual men (Klein *et al.*, 1977; Klausner *et al.*, 2004). The symptoms, if present, vary from pruritus to severe proctitis and diarrhoea.

The biopsy appearances are variable but include the typical florid picture of infective proctocolitis. Gonorrhoea is, therefore, very much part of the differential diagnosis of the histological pattern of acute proctitis. Abnormalities are, however, always limited to the rectum (McMillan *et al.*, 1983). It is

Table 4.2 Sexually transmitted infective agents

Salmonella and *Shigella* species
Campylobacter species
Neisseria species
Treponema pallidum
Chlamydia species
Giardia lamblia
Entamoeba histolytica
Herpes simplex virus type II
Cytomegalovirus
Enterobius vermicularis
Pthrirus pubis
Candida and *Cryptosporidium* (in AIDS patients)

commoner to find either a normal biopsy or mild but acute inflammatory changes in the lamina propria (Surawicz *et al.*, 1986). It is claimed that, in some cases, intracellular diplococci may be recognized if a Gram stain of the biopsy is carefully scrutinized.

In the study by McMillan *et al.* (1983) of homosexuals with rectal gonorrhoea, although over 50 per cent had normal biopsies a significant number showed a non-specific inflammatory response compared with a control, uninfected, homosexual group. Only 3 per cent had a classical infective picture.

4.4.2 *Treponema pallidum*

The anus and anorectal margin is a recognized site for a primary chancre but the lesion may occasionally be seen on the rectal mucosa. However, it is not widely appreciated that a proctitis and an abnormal rectal biopsy occur in secondary syphilis (Klausner *et al.*, 2004). McMillan and Lee (1981) looked at rectal biopsies in ten cases of syphilis. Out of seven which were abnormal, three showed marked inflammatory changes resembling an infectious picture and, in two of these, both with secondary syphilis, small granulomas with giant cells were present. In the remaining four, there was only an increase in plasma cells within the lamina propria. Five out of the 10 patients had secondary syphilis and, overall, the mucosal changes were more florid than in the same authors' cases of gonorrhoeal proctitis. In the study of rectal biopsies in symptomatic homosexual men by Surawicz *et al.* (1986) the presence of *Treponema pallidum* was associated with both chronic inflammation as well as acute inflammatory changes and, in one case, a granuloma.

4.4.3 *Chlamydia trachomatis*

Chlamydia are obligate intracellular bacteria which may be classified into (a) lymphogranuloma venereum immunotypes and (b) non-lymphogranuloma venereum immunotypes. They rank among the commonest cause of sexually transmitted clinical proctitis (Laughon *et al.*, 1988; Klausner *et al.*, 2004).

4.4.3a Lymphogranuloma venereum

Like the other venereal infections this seldom causes acute symptoms but may cause mild or chronic diarrhoea, owing to proctitis. In long-standing cases rectal strictures occur and subsequently a carcinoma may develop (Levin *et al.*, 1964; Day *et al.*, 2003; Papagrigoriadis and Rennie, 1998).

In the acute case the rectal mucosa is infiltrated by neutrophils, plasma cells, and lymphocytes. There can be mild crypt irregularities. Giant cell granulomas occur and are usually seen in relation to disrupted crypts. The problem is to distinguish lymphogranuloma venereum from Crohn's disease (Quinn *et al.*, 1981). The relationship of the giant cells to disrupted crypts is of some value; in Crohn's disease at least some of the granulomas are unrelated to crypt disruption. The distinction seldom poses a clinical problem, but to help an immunofluorescent method of identifying the lymphogranuloma venereum *Chlamydia* in tissue sections, using a monoclonal antibody, has been described by Klotz *et al.* (1983).

In the rectum the disease is mostly transmural, becoming more superficial proximally; again, a difference from Crohn's disease but difficult to appreciate in a biopsy series. There may be marked rectal lymphoid hyperplasia, giving a pattern of follicular proctitis which can cause some confusion with ulcerative colitis (de la Monte and Hutchins, 1985).

4.4.3b Non-lymphogranuloma venereum immunotypes

These organisms are also responsible for a proctitis, though generally milder than that caused by the previous group. Biopsies are rarely carried out but, when performed, have in some cases shown definite minor inflammatory changes. Focal collections of neutrophils were seen within the lamina propria (Quinn *et al.*, 1981) and isolated giant cells with some chronic inflammation have also been reported (Surawicz *et al.*, 1986). There is no diagnostic picture but one to be interpreted in its clinical setting (Munday *et al.*, 1981).

4.4.4 Colitis in acquired immunodeficiency syndrome (AIDS)

The interpretation of colorectal biopsies in AIDS is primarily focused on the recognition of the opportunistic infections that are an integral part of the syndrome. Blanshard *et al.* (1996) identified a pathogen in 83 per cent of the AIDS cohort of 155 patients with chronic diarrhoea but the whole gut was examined as well as stool culture being done. The most frequent organisms are *Candida*, atypical *Mycobacteria*, *Cryptosporidium*, *Herpes simplex* virus and cytomegalovirus (Francis *et al.*, 1989) of which the last three are commonly associated with the large bowel and dealt with in their relevant sections. However, there are case reports implicating a much wider range of infective agents that include *Microsporidia*, *Toxoplasma* (Pauwels *et al.*, 1992), *Histoplasma* (Clarkston *et al.*, 1991) and even *Pneumocystis* (Bellomo *et al.*, 1992). All biopsies from AIDS patients should also be carefully inspected for more than one pathogen. The one most easily overlooked is adenovirus (Maddox *et al.*, 1992) (Section 4.6.3). In the 'look-back' study of Orenstein and Dieterich (2001) of AIDS patients with chronic bowel symptoms the virus had been totally overlooked and subsequently identified in 12 per cent of the study material. They point out, however, that with a negative stool culture and restricting the investigations to merely examining colonoscopic biopsies, in contrast to the wider investigative approach of Blanshard *et al.* (1996), 60–70 per cent of cases will fail to provide a specific diagnosis.

At the time of seroconversion from HIV negative to positive there is often an infectious mononucleosis-like illness with gastrointestinal symptoms, including diarrhoea. The latter may occur in the absence of a demonstrable pathogen. Kotler *et al.* (1984, 1986) describe changes in the rectal mucosa in such cases emphasizing the prominence of apoptosis in the base of crypts and increased mast cells with a picture not unlike graft-versus-host disease (Section 11.6), In patients with chronic diarrhoea and proven HIV infection but not yet fulfilling the criteria for AIDS Hing *et al.* (1992) observed a proctocolitis with superficial ulceration. The biopsies showed diffuse mucosal infiltration by mixed inflammatory cells but an intact crypt architecture. Tubuloreticular structures can be found in the lamina propria, epithelial cells, monocytes and macrophages that are thought to be a product of α- or β-interferon production. Their significance is unclear for they are found in certain other diseases but there is a suggestion they are related to disease progression (Kostianovsky *et al.*, 1987).

It does seem that chronic diarrhoea with biopsy evidence of inflammation in the colorectal mucosa occurs not only as a consequence of a range of opportunistic infective agents but is caused by HIV infection itself prior to the onset of AIDS. While it is important to look for more than one pathogen (Francis *et al.*, 1989) a substantial number of cases will still remain negative and non-diagnostic (Boylston *et al.*, 1987; Orenstein and Dieterich, 2001). This has been estimated as between 15 and 51 per cent (Maddox *et al.,* 1992), the range reflecting many factors relating to the scope of the investigative procedures.

A picture resembling Whipple's disease has been reported in a few patients with AIDS and immuno-suppressed non-HIV individuals. This is due to infection with *Mycobacterium avium-intracellulare* (Roth *et al.*, 1985; Nguyen *et al.*, 1999). Large foamy macrophages can be seen in the rectal mucosa (Wolke *et al.*, 1984). These cells are periodic acid–Schiff (PAS)-positive. Ziehl–Nielsen stain will demonstrate the acid-fast organisms of *M. avium* (Fig. 4.9) and distinguishes the macrophages of this condition from those seen in Whipple's disease. However, only 24 per cent of biopsies yield organisms and the majority show mild non-specific inflammatory features (Boylstun *et al.*, 1987). There is also a report of a genuine case of Whipples disease mimicking AIDS enteropathy (Maliha *et al.*, 1991).

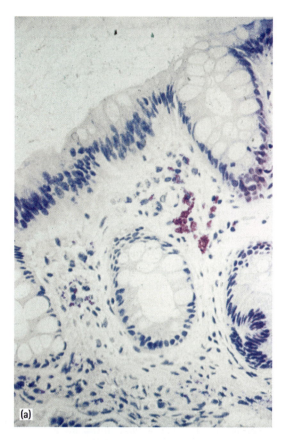

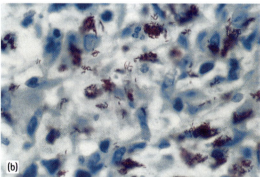

Figure 4.9 (a) Seen here are a small cluster of macrophages containing *Mycobacterium avium-intracellulare* organisms. The background lamina propria is only minimally inflamed highlighting how easily the condition may be overlooked if special stains are not requested in what might at first seem a non-diagnostic biopsy. (b) The organisms are seen more clearly using the oil-immersion lens in this biopsy from another case of Mycobacterium avium-intercellulare infection. (Haematoxylin and Ziehl–Nielsen) (Courtesy Dr N. Francis)

4.5 INTESTINAL SPIROCHAETOSIS

A small number of colonic and rectal biopsies may show a haematoxyphilic blurred margin, approximately 3 μm thick, on the luminal aspect of the surface epithelial cells (Figs 3.49b and 4.10). It is easily overlooked. The PAS or Warthin–Starry method (Fig. 4.11) emphasizes the abnormality but only scanning or transmission electron microscopy (Antonakopoulas *et al.*, 1982) reveals that the appearance results from rows of spiral organisms embedded in the epithelial cell border. The organisms can have a variable distribution around the colon with occasionally the rectum uninvolved and colonization restricted to the right colon (Prior *et al.*, 1987; Lo *et al.*, 1994; van Mook *et al.*, 2004). The taxonomy of the organism has been disputed, but the spirochaetes are now accepted as genus *Brachyspira* with *B. aalborgi* and *B. pilosicoli* being the two species found in humans (Hovind-Hougen *et al.*, 1982; Mikosza and Hampson, 2001). These organisms lie between and parallel to the microvilli and do not usually penetrate the cell, although Antonakopoulos *et al.* (1982) and Padmanabhan *et al.* (1996) report invasion of epithelial cells, macrophages and even Schwann cells by the spirochaetes. Numerous partly degranulated mast

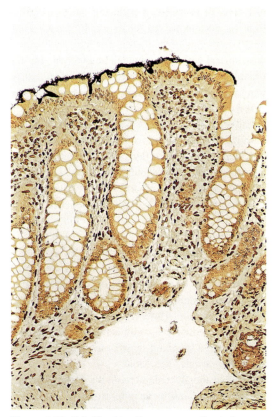

Figure 4.11 This Warthin–Starry preparation is the optimal stain for demonstrating the surface covering of spirochaetes. Individual hair-like organisms can be appreciated even at low magnifications.

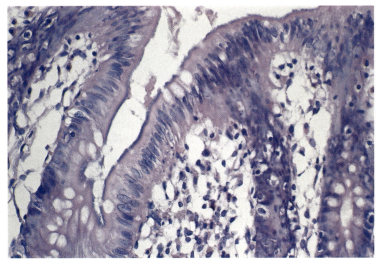

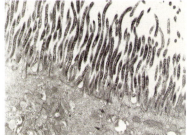

Figure 4.10 Intestinal spirochaetosis. The blurred and haematoxyphilic margin on the surface epithelial cells is clearly seen. It is formed by the spirochaetes embedded in the surface but not penetrating the cytoplasm. This effect is shown in the adjacent electron micrograph.

cells have been observed within the surface epithelium in relation to spirochaetosis (Gebbers et al., 1987). In the majority of cases the mucosa is otherwise normal with on-going debate over whether the organism is of clinical significance (Christie, 2003; van Mook et al., 2004). However, McMillan and Lee (1981) found accompanying mild inflammatory changes in 32 per cent of biopsies from a group of homosexuals in whom spirochaetosis was the only abnormality identified. Mild inflammation was also documented by Padmanabhan et al. (1996) and Kostman et al. (1995) reported a more severe colitis in a patient with advanced immunodeficiency in which invasive spirochaetes were the only putative pathogens identified. Gebbers et al. (1987) also describe an excess of IgE plasma cells within the lamina propria in spirochaetosis. This decreased after treatment with metronidazole, suggesting that an unusual immunological response may be elicited by the infestation. However marked inflammatory changes in a biopsy showing spirochaetosis should suggest that a second disease process is more likely to be responsible. van Mook et al. (2004) propose that while mostly commensal, the organisms can become pathogens in an opportunistic fashion in patients with the appropriate profile of diminished immunocompetence and this includes children (Christie, 2003).

Clinically, most authors feel that the presence of spirochaetosis has no proven clinical importance and its elimination does not affect symptoms (Nielsen et al., 1983; Christie, 2003; van Mook et al., 2004). Nevertheless, there are a few reports of patients with diarrhoea in whom spirochaetosis was the only abnormal finding and in whom a course of antibiotics eliminated the organisms and cured the diarrhoea (Douglas and Crucioli, 1981; Gebbers et al., 1987; Rodgers et al., 1986; Lo et al., 1994). When identified in a biopsy taken during the course of a screening colonoscopy for cancer, or as part of the routine follow-up of polyps, clinicians usually adopt a wait and see policy. Interestingly, some adenomas identified in such instances may show a conspicuous absence of colonization of the neoplastic epithelium in contrast to the adjacent heavily colonized non-neoplastic epithelium (Coyne et al., 1995).

The prevalence of intestinal spirochaetosis in rectal biopsies is quoted as between 2 and 7 per cent in the West in patients with diverse gastrointestinal conditions (Lee et al., 1971; Nielson et al., 1983; van Mook et al., 2004) but is much higher in the less developed parts of the world with figures in the range 11–34 per cent (van Mook et al., 2004). The highest prevalence is in homosexual men and HIV-infected subjects with prevalence rates of up to 54 per cent (McMillan and Lee, 1981; Surawicz et al., 1986; Trivett-Moore et al., 1998).

4.6 VIRAL CAUSES OF COLITIS

Viral causes of gastroenteritis were mainly unknown much before 1970. The main viral groups now responsible are rotavirus, enteric adenovirus, calicivirus (Norwalk and Norwalk-like) and astrovirus (Schwab and Shaw, 1993). The emergence of AIDS has made cytomegalovirus (CMV) more common. In biopsy work CMV, adenovirus and herpes simplex virus are the only ones likely to be seen in routine preparations and are considered here.

4.6.1 Cytomegalovirus infection

This is a herpes group virus and is common throughout the human population. Infection is usually subclinical and overt disease is mostly confined to patients who are immunologically suppressed, in particular, patients with AIDS (Meiselman et al., 1985; Francis et al., 1989). However, it can occur in immunocompetent patients (Galiatsatos et al., 2005) when there is usually some comorbidity. In the meta-analysis by these authors infected patients under 55 years generally did well while in those over 55 years negative factors influencing survival were surgical intervention, immune modulating comorbidity and male gender. Gastrointestinal disease is one of the rarer presentations and of 190 patients with HIV-1 or AIDS Francis et al. (1989) found gastrointestinal tract CMV in 7.7 per cent and 13 per cent respectively. Any site in the gut can be involved but colorectal involvement was the commonest of the gastrointestinal sites in that study.

Ulceration is a prominent feature and one of three basic patterns are seen at colonoscopy (Wilcox et al.,

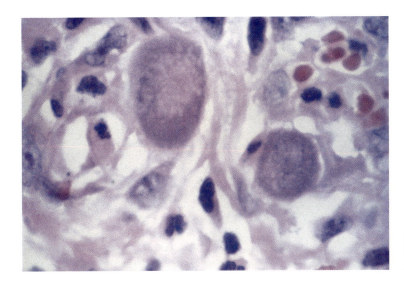

Figure 4.12 Intranuclear cytomegalovirus inclusions in macrophages in the lamina propria.

1998), ulcers, ulcers and colitis or purely a colitis. As far as obtaining biopsy evidence is concerned it is worth noting that in four of their 31 cases the changes were restricted to the proximal half of the colon. There has been some debate whether CMV initiates ulceration (Foucar *et al.*, 1981) or merely represents a superinfection that simply prevents established ulcers from healing (Goodman *et al.*, 1979; Hommes *et al.*, 2004). In established secondary infection CMV is commoner in patients with ulcerative colitis than Crohn's disease (Cooper *et al.*, 1977; Kaufman *et al.*, 1999) and because it may be a reason for resistance to medical therapy (Kamhan *et al.*, 2004) special care is required with such a history to search for inclusions.. Primary disease probably does occur (Galiatsatos *et al.*, 2005), and it can be shown that in some instances the virus is causing a vasculitis (Meiselman *et al.*, 1985; Muldoon *et al.*, 1996).

Diagnosis depends on demonstrating the characteristic intranuclear inclusions within macrophages in the lamina propria (Fig. 4.12). Although easily visible on light microscopy they are often overlooked, as this condition is infrequently met in routine biopsy practice (Figs 3.49c and 4.13). This is especially problematic in severely ulcerated areas with florid granulation tissue in which there are often atypical stromal cells present that can mimic the appearances of CMV (Serra and Chetty, 2005)

(Fig. 3.56). Capillary endothelial cells are the other site to search for inclusions (Figs 3.49c and 4.13) but epithelial cells are rarely involved (Fig. 4.14). The intensity of the accompanying inflammatory infiltrate within the mucosa is related to ulceration and this can occasionally mimic chronic inflammatory bowel disease (Roskell *et al.*, 1995). The typical infected cells show nuclear and cytoplasmic enlargement with a single, dark amphophilic nuclear 'owl's eye' inclusion that is pinkish-red with Geimsa stain. However, often the infected cells are elongated and have indistinct smudged haematoxyphilic nuclei (Francis *et al.*, 1989). The cytoplasm of the involved cells can show granular inclusions or be foamy. Electron microscopy of the inclusions reveals capsids with both dense and empty cores and it is possible to distinguish the morphology of CMV from that of other herpes viruses (Freeman *et al.*, 1977).

As mentioned above CMV should be thought of when confronted with the interpretation of atypical cells in the granulation tissue of intensely inflamed and ulcerated biopsies (Section 3.9.7). In such circumstances immunohistochemistry should be carried out as a routine (Fig. 4.15); this will also allow unusual morphological variants of the infected cells to be appreciated (Francis *et al.*, 1989). In particular, it will allow identification of positive staining in infected cells where the nucleus is not

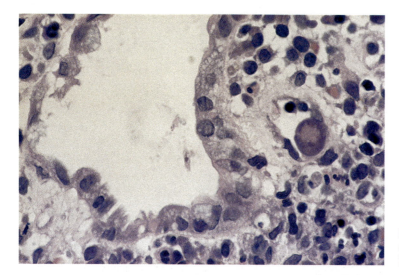

Figure 4.13 A capillary endothelial cell which contains a cytomegalovirus inclusion body.

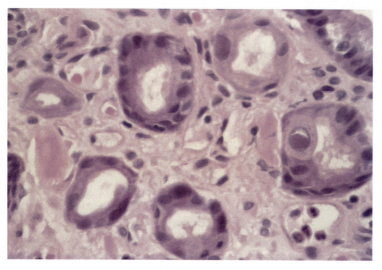

Figure 4.14 It is uncommon to observe cytomegalovirus, as seen here, within glandular epithelial cells.

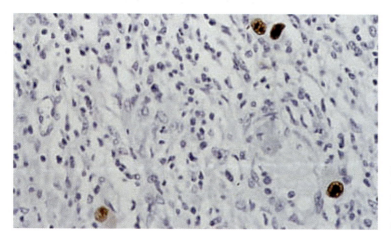

Figure 4.15 As an aid to diagnosis immunocytochemistry with antibody to cytomegalovirus helps identify virus-containing macrophages, which can be overlooked on routine staining. (Immunoperoxidase.)

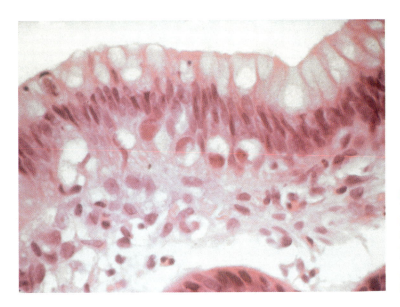

Figure 4.16 Adenovirus infection. The infected surface epithelial cells have irregular basal amphophilic nuclei associated with mucin-containing vacuolated cytoplasm. The nuclei can be shown to contain variably sized inclusions. (Courtesy Dr N. Francis)

in the plane of the section and they would not otherwise be recognized. In look-back studies Kamham *et al.* (2004) showed that immunohistochemistry for CMV increased the number of positive cases from 5 per cent to 25 per cent and Orenstein and Dieterich (2001), in a similar exercise, increased their yield of positive cases by 14 per cent. Safe practice is to be aware of the clinical situations in which CMV is likely, looking carefully on the routine haematoxylin and eosin preparation for inclusions in macrophages, capillary endothelial cells and in any granulation tissue. If negative or suspicious, have a low threshold for undertaking immunohistochemistry.

4.6.2 Herpes simplex

This virus is a common cause of proctitis in homosexuals and a common opportunist in AIDS or in any other immunosuppressed patient (Goodell *et al.*, 1983; Surawicz *et al.*, 1986; Laughon *et al.*, 1988). Anorectal ulceration occurs with giant cells at the margin. These can be shown to contain virions by electron microscopy. The inflammatory infiltrate is non-specific but most often includes acute inflammatory cells in the lamina propria and more rarely chronic inflammation is present (Surawicz *et al.*, 1986). These authors reported the

rectal biopsy findings in 12 proven cases of which the biopsy was normal in five and oddly, none of the twelve showed inclusions. In two there was perivascular cuffing. Occasionally, widespread ulceration can occur with a severe acute colitis (Leprince *et al.*, 1993).

4.6.3 Adenovirus

This is an accepted cause of diarrhoea in children and has now been recognized in HIV patients. Janoff *et al.* (1991) identified the virus in just over 7 per cent of a group of sixty-seven HIV-positive homosexual men with diarrhoea of whom only one had a potential second enteric pathogen. They suggested it may therefore have a role in the aetiology of the diarrhoea. There is still, however, some uncertainty about the pathogenic role of the virus (Cunningham *et al.*, 1988) for HIV itself can be associated with diarrhoea (Hing *et al.*, 1992) and Maddox *et al.* (1992) found eight of their 10 reported cases with the virus had an alternative enteric pathogen present. However as the viral cytoplasmic changes can be recognized in a biopsy and, in some patients, they are accompanied by a mild to moderate chronic inflammatory cell infiltrate plus occasional neutrophils (Janoff *et al.*, 1991; Maddox *et al.*, 1992) it behoves the pathologist to report their presence.

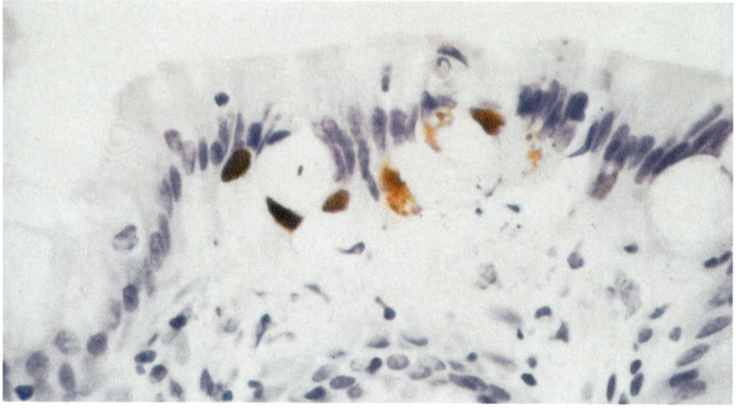

Figure 4.17 Adenovirus infection. Immunocytochemistry using antibody to adenovirus identifies the virus containing nuclei within the cytoplasmic vacuoles of the surface epithelial cells. (Immunoperoxidase.) (Courtesy Dr N. Francis.)

A good description of the features is that of Maddox *et al.* (1992). Infected epithelial cells are usually found on or close to the surface. The cells are vacuolated (Fig. 4.16), contain mucin and the range of changes in the amphophilic nuclei is from crescentic to moderately enlarged with an irregular outline. Small intranuclear inclusions are visible at high power. The vacuoles are sialomucin positive and the presence of the virus can be confirmed by immunocytochemistry (Fig. 4.17) with commercially available antibodies.

The vacuolar appearance and nuclear shape allows recognition at low power since the infected cells appear as goblet cells lying below the level of the nuclei of adjacent uninfected cells.

As with all HIV-positive cases, having identified involved cells a careful search should be made for other pathogens, in particular CMV (Thomas *et al.*, 1999). Where adenovirus and a colitis was identified these latter authors found a significant association with chronic diarrhoea.

4.7 PROTOZOAL INFECTION

The common human pathogens belong to four main classes: the Rhizopoda (*Amoebae*), the Mastigophora (*Giardia*), the Ciliata (*Balantidium*), and the Sporozoa (*Coccidia–Cryptosporidium*). Diagnosis depends on identifying the protozoa and this is best done by examination of fresh stool. There is no characteristic histological pattern on biopsy and the organisms are easily overlooked in sections unless a careful inspection is made. Because of this, it is important for the clinician to draw attention to any unusual clinical details.

4.7.1 Amoebiasis

The organism responsible (*Entamoeba histolytica*) is found in all climates of the world but is commonest in areas of poor sanitation. In industrialized societies a history of foreign travel is common but not invariable, as demonstrated by sexually transmitted cases (McMillan *et al.*, 1984). Infection is via faecal contamination and ingestion of cysts. Liberated protozoa colonize the large bowel. The clinical spectrum of disease is wide. At one extreme some patients are symptomless, at the other some develop toxic megacolon and may perforate (Juniper, 1978; Abbas *et al.*, 2000). The range in symptomatology is, in part, explained by the existence of as many as 22 different variants (zymodenes) of *E. histolytica*, only some of which are pathogenic (types 2, 6, 7 and 12) (Sargeaunt and Williams, 1979).

In the homosexual population with proctitis there is dispute as to whether amoebae play a role. McMillan *et al.* (1984) suggest the organism is responsible for a proctitis, while our own experience was at variance with this (Goldmeier *et al.*, 1986) and they were not found in either of the large series of Surawicz *et al.* (1986) and Laughon *et al.* (1988).

It is important to remember that antidiarrhoeal preparations can destroy the amoebae and such medications should be avoided prior to biopsy. The organism may reside in the debris over the biopsy and all material must be carefully processed with levels cut. This is especially important in endemic areas. Prathap and Gilman (1970) describe several stages prior to the development of the classical flask-shaped ulcer. Initially, there is a mild non-specific proctitis, with neutrophils in small groups in the lamina propria, within the lumen of capillaries and adjacent to the surface epithelium. This is accompanied by oedema, making the mucosa appear thickened. The only amoebae present are on the surface, usually in an overlying exudate (Fig. 3.1b and c). Confirmation of their presence is essential for diagnosis.

In a well-orientated biopsy it is possible to recognize the next stage. A small depressed area of mucosa is accentuated by the thickened mucosa on either side (Fig. 4.18). In this area there is goblet cell depletion and usually micro-ulceration of the epithelium. A basophilic exudate covers the denuded lamina propria and contains the organisms, which are not found within the mucosa at this stage. Overall, there are increased numbers of polymorphs in the lamina propria but crypt abscesses are not conspicuous.

Tissue necrosis is the hallmark of the most severe changes and ulceration occurs down to the level of the submucosa (Fig. 4.19). In routine haematoxylin and eosin sections the mucosa is replaced by a thick amorphous grey/blue exudate separated from underlying viable tissue by a 'fibrinoid' band. With any exudate there are only occasional inflammatory cells but at this stage, the organisms are abundant. Intact mucosa on either side is congested and infiltrated by neutrophils as in the earlier phases. An increase in plasma cells and eosinophils may also be present. At all stages the amoebae are best demonstrated in the amorphous exudate on the mucosal surface or covering an ulcer and, although invasion of the mucosa occurs, it is limited. When only a few organisms are present they are easily confused with sloughed-off epithelial cells or macrophages (Figs 3.1 and 4.20). The PAS reaction

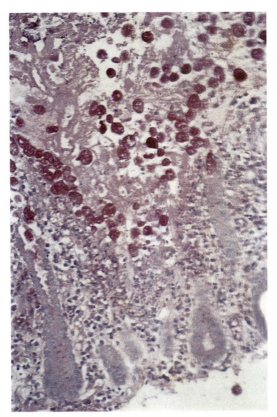

Figure 4.18 Early amoebic colitis. Ulceration is superficial but large numbers of organisms are seen in the surface debris and their recognition facilitated by use of the periodic acid–Schiff reagent.

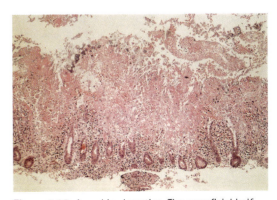

Figure 4.19 Amoebic ulceration. The superficial half of the mucosa has been destroyed and replaced by amorphous debris in which there are numerous amoebae but relatively few inflammatory cells. (Haematoxylin and eosin.)

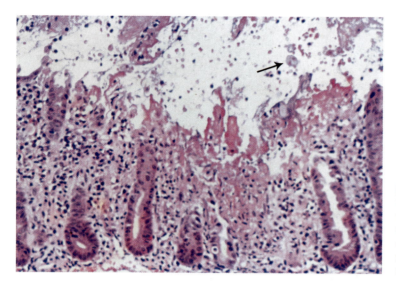

Figure 4.20 Amoebic colitis. There is degeneration and sloughing of the surface epithelium intermingled with macrophages but only an occasional amoeba (arrow), here seen having ingested a red blood cell.

aids the recognition of the amoebae, especially when counterstained with Martius yellow (Fig. 3.1c). In active disease the organisms are about 60 μm in diameter, with ingested red blood cells frequently visible in the cytoplasm. There is a small nucleus containing one or several deeply-stained karyosomes.

4.7.1a Differential diagnosis

In addition to positive identification of the organisms the inflammatory profile of amoebiasis should be distinguishable from ulcerative colitis by its focal nature and from Crohn's disease by the absence of lymphoid aggregates and granulomas. However, there are many accounts of amoebic colitis closely mimicking chronic inflammatory disease, co-existing with it and exacerbating attacks, especially of ulcerative colitis (Radhakrishnan *et al.*, 1986; Chan *et al.*, 1995). It is found to be a commoner accompaniment of ulcerative colitis than Crohn's disease (Ustun *et al.*, 2003). A mistaken diagnosis of chronic inflammatory bowel disease can have serious consequences, for inappropriate therapy with steroids may lead to perforation (Abbas *et al.*, 2000). Examination of the stools and serology can be negative, in which case the diagnosis hinges on careful inspection of the biopsy (Larsson *et al.*, 1991) and its levels. Rarely and unfortunately it may be only after colonic resection

that the true diagnosis is made (Lysy *et al.*, 1991; Abbas *et al.*, 2000). In the correct clinical setting a diagnosis might be considered on seeing a thick cellular basophilic ulcer slough alongside mucosa containing a few crypt abscesses. Levels through the tissue should be cut, looking for organisms. Prior to this stage the picture most resembles that seen in the acute bacterial diarrhoeas and care is required when examining biopsies with these appearances so that amoebiasis is not overlooked. Occasionally, amoebiasis may follow a prolonged course, with persisting ulceration and even stricture formation (Powell and Wilmot, 1966). This post-dysenteric colitis syndrome is extremely difficult to distinguish from ulcerative colitis.

4.7.2 Giardiasis

Giardia lamblia, a flagellate protozoa of the class Mastigophora, causes malabsorption, together with chronic and, occasionally, acute diarrhoea. Although examination of the stool for protozoa and cysts is part of the diagnostic procedure the organism resides in the small bowel and rectal or colonic biopsy is not normally undertaken (Allison *et al.*, 1988). Cases of colonic infection are documented (Kacker, 1973) in sexually transmitted giardiasis following anal intercourse but biopsy appearances have not yet been described.

4.7.3 *Balantidium*

Balantidium coli (Class Ciliata) is a ciliate proto-zoan which can rarely cause human dysentery. The main hosts from which man becomes infected are the pig and rat. Infection usually occurs in conditions of poor personal hygiene and, in insti-tutions, may reach epidemic proportions. Patients present with acute diarrhoea, fulminant colitis and perforation, or with chronic intermittent diarrhoea (Ladas *et al.*, 1989). Asymptomatic carriers are also recognized.

Following ingestion of cysts of *B. coli* the liber-ated trophozoites reside predominantly in the colon. The gross lesions are similar to amoebiasis (Fig. 4.21).

Diagnosis depends on demonstrating the organism (Baskerville, 1970), which is best done by examin-ation of fresh stool, as there is no characteristic histological pattern on biopsy.

4.7.4 Coccidia (*Cryptosporidium*)

Coccidia is the collective name for the sub-order Eimerinia, which includes the other human pathogens *Isospora*, *Sarcocystis* and *Toxoplasma* (Knight, 1978). Their diagnoses along with the coccidian microsporidia, also intracellular organ-isms, are not usually in the realm of colorectal biopsy practice and they are not considered further.

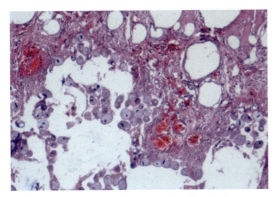

Figure 4.21 *Balantidium coli* trophozoites in the submucosa. These protozoa have maximum dimensions of between 55 μm and 80 μm and are approximately twice the size of amoebae. They have a characteristic macronucleus and are ciliate.

Cryptosporidium, however, belongs to a different genus (Bird and Smith, 1980) and is a diagnostic biopsy challenge.

The first case of human cryptosporidiosis appears to have occurred in a previously healthy infant (Nime *et al.*, 1976) and, since then, infection has been reported in both immunocompromised (Soave *et al.*, 1984) and normal subjects (Fletcher *et al.*, 1982; Isaacs *et al.*, 1985). In the former it may pro-duce severe diarrhoea, in the latter self-limiting 'flu-like gastroenteritis. It is a common opportunist in patients with AIDS, when it is often in associa-tion with other micro-organisms (Section 4.4.4) and one case of toxic megacolon has been documented in such a patient infected with cryptosporidia (Connolly and Gazzard, 1987). It has also been recognized as a cause of traveller's diarrhoea (Jokipii *et al.*, 1983). The pattern of inflammation in the biopsy is not characteristic. Often it is minimal, with oedema and a few plasma cells and eosinophils in the lam-ina propria. Occasionally, ulceration occurs. Cryp-tosporidial organisms are seen as groups of tiny haematoxyphilic dots on the epithelial cell surface or within crypts (Figs 3.49d and 4.22) it is easy to mistake their appearance for stain deposit or nuclear debris. The latter is a special problem when signif-icant inflammation and karyorrhexis is present. A PAS reaction or Grocott silver impregnation shows up the cyst walls and the Geimsa stain is helpful. Scanning and transmission electron microscopy (Fig. 4.22c) reveal the characteristic cytological details of the life cycle, the organism apparently lying embedded in the surface but not within the cytoplasm of the epithelial cells.

The organisms involve the small as well as the large intestine and the diagnosis must be con-sidered in any case of malabsorption in which the common aetiologies have been excluded. Varying degrees of villous atrophy accompany infection in the jejunal mucosa.

4.8 HELMINTHS

Infection by helminths is not a significant diagnos-tic problem in the temperate climates of developed Western countries, though it is a major cause of

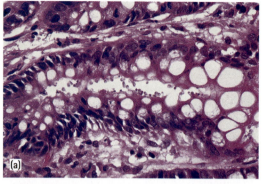

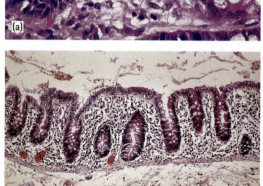

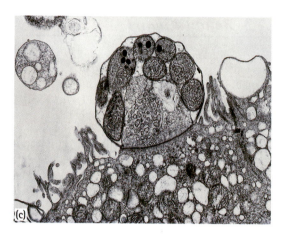

Figure 4.22 Cryptosporidiosis. Numerous tiny protozoa lie in close contact with the epithelium of the crypts (a). The lamina propria of the mucosa may appear normal and the organisms easily overlooked when initially screening a biopsy (b). (c) Electron micrograph shows a schizont with developing merozoites attached to the free surface of a caecal epithelial cell.

Table 4.3 Common human helminths

Trematodes (flukes)	Nematodes (roundworms)	Cestodes (tapeworms)
Schistosoma spp.	*Ascaris lumbricoides*	* *Taenia* spp.
	* Hookworms	* *Diphyllobothrium* spp.
	Strongyloides spp.	* *Sparganum* spp.
* (*Fasciola* spp.)	*Trichuris trichura*	* (*Echinococcus* spp.)
* (*Clonorchis* spp.)	*Enterobius vermicularis*	* Hydatid disease
* (*Paragonimus* spp.)	*Oesophagostomum* spp.	
	* *Trichinella spiralis*	
	* (Filarial diseases)	

*Denotes colon not involved. ( ), Denotes other important members of the class but not primary gut pathogens.

disease in the tropics and in societies with poor standards of hygiene. Human infection is produced by the three main classes of worm (Table 4.3) but only in schistosomiasis do colonic and rectal biopsy have any role. This is because most worms inhabit the small intestine and the examination of stools for stages in the life cycles of these worms is the preferred method of diagnosis. For those worms that spend part of their life cycle in the colon a specific diagnosis from a biopsy can only be made

when the parasite, its eggs or larval forms are seen. In the absence of the parasite, but in the correct clinical setting, infestation should be considered if an isolated granuloma is present or there is a focal inflammatory mucosal lesion in which eosinophils predominate. In old burnt-out parasitic lesions there may be fibrosis and calcification, which can produce mucosal and submucosal nodules. The biopsy may then show an apparently unexplained focus of scarring and calcification.

4.8.1 *Schistosoma mansoni* and *Schistosoma japonicum*

These are the two common trematode worms that affect the large bowel (Prata, 1978; Warren, 1978). *Schistosoma haematobium* is found in the bladder and only rarely involves the intestine. Disease is caused by the reaction to the eggs. Adults reside in the superior mesenteric or inferior mesenteric veins. The severity of the reaction depends on host immunity and the infecting dose, and varies from no reaction to acute inflammation and mucosal necrosis. In countries with endemic schistomiasis the whole length of the large bowel may become fibrotic, shortened and studded with polyps and ulcers. The picture may also resemble Crohn's disease.

The rectum is a good site for the identification of *S. mansoni* eggs, which can easily be seen in the mucosa and submucosa (Fig. 3.46). The eggs of *S. japonicum* are generally in the right colon and colonoscopic biopsies are required. The eggs are oval and have a haematoxyphilic shell which may be calcified, enclosing the remnants of miracidia. The presence of preserved miracidial nuclei indicates live, mature and active schistosomes. It is possible to identify the species of schistomes by the subterminal spines of the eggs of *S. mansoni,* in contrast to the terminal spines of *S. haematobium* ova. The eggs of *S. japonicum* have ill-defined subterminal knobs, are smaller and more rounded than the other species and tend to be present in larger numbers. In some cases the eggs may be surrounded by an eosinophilic zone of fibrinoid material, representing an antigen–antibody complex (Fig. 3.46). Beyond this, a variable cellular infiltrate is found. It is rare to see florid acute inflammation (Fig. 4.23a) and more commonly a granulomatous picture is present. In the mucosa or submucosa the eggs can be surrounded by lymphocytes, macrophages, giant cells and eosinophils. However, in many instances, particularly with old, effete ova, no reaction is present at all and the calcified shell is simply surrounded by a thin rim of collagen (Fig 4.23b,c). It is important to examine multiple levels through any biopsy from patients in whom schistosomiasis is suspected, be it from the history, from an initial finding of a granuloma, from an ill-defined focus of chronic inflammatory cells or a collection of eosinophils and macrophages. Deeper levels may reveal disintegrating shells of schistosome eggs. A Ziehl–Neelsen stain is useful, as *S. mansoni* eggs are positive (Fig 4.23d). Without the identification of an egg the diagnosis of schistosomiasis cannot be made, but it must be included in the differential diagnosis of isolated mucosal or submucosal granulomas in biopsy material (Section 3.8.11).

There is an increased incidence of carcinoma of the large bowel in patients with chronic infection (Ming-Chai *et al.*, 1981). It is believed that mucosal epithelial dysplasia precedes the development of carcinoma in a fashion similar to that in long-standing ulcerative colitis. In patients at risk, biopsies should be carefully examined for evidence of dysplasia. Inflammatory polyps are an occasional presenting feature of schistosomiasis.

4.9 NEMATODES

4.9.1 Strongyloidiasis

Like the other major nematode infestations, *Strongyloides stercoralis* is usually restricted to the small intestine. However, the migratory larvae which develop during passage through the colon are capable of burrowing into the colonic mucosa, causing auto-infection. This is most likely to occur if there is any cause for intestinal delay such as megacolon and in massive infections associated with immunological suppression (AIDS) (Boram *et al.*, 1981; Lemos *et al.*, 2003). Adult worms may also be found in the colon in such circumstances. The crypts and superficial mucosa are usually the sites to find the parasites. A florid transmural eosinophilic granulomatous inflammation can occur in small numbers of patients, a reaction believed to destroy most of the larvae. This is in contrast to their rapid passage through the colonic wall in the usual pattern of hyperinfection syndrome (Gutierrez *et al.*, 1996),

4.9.2 Trichuriasis

Trichuris trichura is the whipworm, which preferentially infests the caecum, sometimes in large numbers (Neafie and Connor, 1976). The anterior

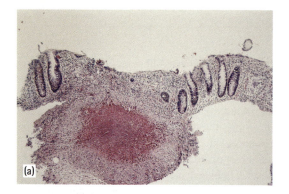

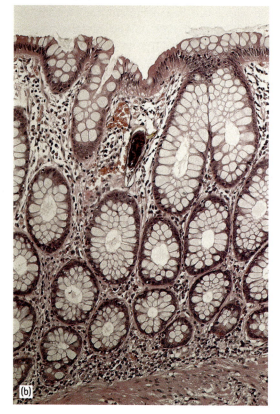

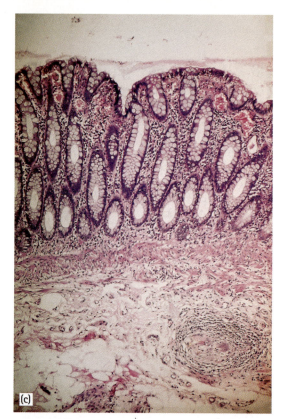

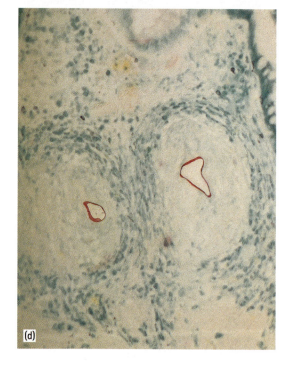

Figure 4.23 The uncommon necrotizing response to schistosomal eggs is present in the deep mucosa and submucosa of (a). However it is more common to see old effete eggs and no surrounding reaction (b) or a minor granulomatous response as in the submucosa in (c). A Ziehl–Neelsen stain is useful for identifying *Schistosoma mansoni* at the centre of a granulomatous response (d).

end is inserted into the mucosa and the bulk of the worm is visible on the surface. Penetration reaches the submucosa. An intense focal infiltrate of eosinophils may mark the worm track but focal inflammation may also occur up to 20 cm beyond such sites (Kaur *et al.*, 2002). Theoretically, colonoscopic biopsy is capable of demonstrating part of this track.

4.9.3 Oxyuriasis

Oxyuris or *Enterobius vermicularis is* the pinworm or threadworm (Neafie *et al.*, 1976). It is perhaps the most prevalent of the parasitic worms in Europe and the USA. The adults attach themselves to the caecal mucosa but, in routine histopathology, the parasite is most commonly seen in the lumen of appendicectomy specimens. Its role as a primary cause of appendicitis is disputed. The main symptomatology results from the nocturnal migration of the adult female, which lays eggs on the perianal skin. This causes intense pruritis. Scratching may result in abrasion and the parasite may become embedded in the submucosa (Fig 4.24). The inflammatory reaction may then produce a presenting polyp or even a mass mistaken for carcinoma (Lee *et al.*, 2002).

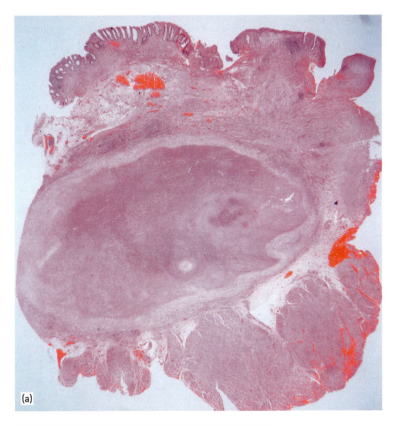
(a)

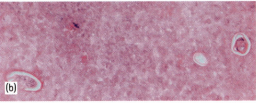
(b)

Figure 4.24 (a, b) Invasive *Enterobius vermicularis.* This was a polyp at the anorectal junction caused by the inflammatory reaction induced by the threadworm which had become implanted into the submucosa. Although the worm is dead the ova (b) may have been viable.

4.10 FUNGAL INFECTION

Fungal infections of the gastrointestinal tract, and the large bowel, in particular, are rare (Smith, 1969). In European countries they are usually opportunistic infections in immunologically compromised hosts, though in regions of North and South America histoplasmosis, coccidioidomycosis and paracoccidioidomycosis are endemic. Histoplasma is the organism most likely to involve the gut (Collins, 1956). The diagnostic challenge is clinical and the histological diagnosis depends solely on recognizing the fungus in the biopsy material. This is best done with the aid of the PAS reaction or a Grocott silver impregnation. Gram's stain is also effective. The fungi may be in either yeast or mycelial forms rarely forming a mass which should not to be misinterpreted as a carcinoma (Khalil *et al.*, 1989).

REFERENCES

Abbas, M.A., Mulligan, D.C., Ramzan, N.N. *et al.* (2000) Colonic perforation in unsuspected amebic colitis. *Dig. Dis. Sci.*, 45, 1836–41.

Allison, M.C., Hamiton-Dutoit, S.J., Dhillon, A.P., Pounder, R.E. (1987) The value of rectal biopsy in distinguishing self-limiting colitis from early inflammatory bowel disease. *Q. J. Med.*, 65, 985–95.

Allison, M.C., Green, E.L., Bhattacharya, D.N., Smith, A., Pounder, R.E (1988) A microscopic and immunodiagnostic search for giardiasis in patients with gastrointestinal disorders. *Scand. J. Gastroenterol.*, 23, 209–12.

Anand, B.S., Malhotra, V., Bhattacharya, S.K. *et al.* (1986) Rectal histology in acute bacillary dysentery. *Gastroenterology,* 90, 654–60.

Anand, B.S., Schneider, F.E., El-Zaatari, F.A., Shawar, R.M., Clarridge, J.E., Graham, D.Y. (1994) Diagnosis of intestinal tuberculosis by polymerase chain reaction on endoscopic biopsy specimens. *Am. J. Gastroenterol.*, 89, 2248–9.

Anderson, J.B., Tanner, A.H., Brodribb, A.J.M. (1986) Toxic megacolon due to *Campylobacter* colitis. *Int. J. Colorectal Dis.*, 1, 58–9.

Antonakopoulas, G., Newman, J., Wilkinson, M. (1982) Intestinal spirochaetosis: an electron microscopic study in an unusual case. *Histopathology*, 6, 477–88.

Arduino, R.C., DuPont, H.L. (1993) Travellers' diarrhoea. *Baillieres Clin. Gastroenterol.*, 7(2), 365–85.

Arnold, C., Moradpour, D. Blum, H.E (1998) Tuberculous colitis mimicking Crohn's disease. *Am. J. Gastroenterol.*, 93, 2294–6.

Baskerville, L. (1970) Balantidium colitis. Report of a case. *Am. J. Dig. Dis.*, 15, 727–31.

Bellary, S.V., Isaacs, P. (1990) Toxic megacolon (TM) due to salmonella. *J. Clin. Gastroenterol.*, 12, 605–7.

Bellomo, A.R., Perlman, D.C., Kaminsky, D.L., Brettholtz, E.M., Sarlin, J.G. (1992) Pneumocystis colitis in a patient with the acquired immunodeficiency syndrome. *Am. J. Gastroenterol.*, 87, 759–61.

Bird, R.G., Smith, M.D. (1980) Cryptosporidiosis in man: parasite life cycle and fine structural pathology. *J. Pathology*, 132, 217–33.

Blanshard, C., Francis, N., Gazzard, B.G. (1996) Investigation of chronic diarrhoea in acquired immunodeficiency syndrome. A prospective study of 155 patients. *Gut*, 39, 824–32.

Bohr, J., Nordfelth, R., Jarnerot J., Tysk, C. (2002) Yersinia species in collagenous colitis: a serologic study. *Scand. J. Gastroenterol.*, 37, 711–14.

Boram, L.H., Keller, K.F., Justus, P.E., Collins, J.P. (1981) Strongyloidiasis in immunosuppressed patients. *Am. J. Clin. Pathol.*, 76, 778–81.

Borriello, S.P., Larson, H.E., Welch, A.R., Barclay, F., Stringer, M.F. (1984) Enterotoxigenic *Clostridium perfringens*: a possible cause of antibiotic-associated diarrhoea. *Lancet*, i, 305–7.

Boylston, A.W., Cook, H.T., Francis, N.D., Goldin, R.D. (1987) Biopsy pathology of acquired immunodeficiency syndrome (AIDS) *J. Clin. Pathol.*, 40, 1–8.

Bradford, W.D., Noce, P.S., Cutman, L.T., Durham, N.C. (1974) Pathologic features of enteric infection with *Yersinia enterocolitica*. *Arch. Pathol.*, 98, 17–22.

Butzler, J.P. (2004) *Campylobacter*, from obscurity to celebrity. *Clin. Microbiol. Infect.*, 10, 868–76.

Candy, D.C.A., McNeish, A.S. (1984) Human *Escherichia coli* diarrhoea. *Arch. Dis. Child.*, 59, 395–6.

Chan, K.L., Sung, J.Y., Hsu, R., Liew, C.T. (1995) The association of amoebic colitis and chronic ulcerative colitis. *Singapore Med. J.*, 36, 303–5.

Chatzicostas, C., Koutroubakis, I.E., Tzardi, M., Roussomoustakaki, M., Prassapoulos, P., Kouroumalis, E.A. (2002) Colonic tuberculosis mimicking Crohn's disease: case report. *BMC Gastroenterol.*, 2, 10.

Chopra, A.K., Houston, C.W. (1999) Enterotoxins in *Aeromonas*-associated gastroenteritis. *Microbes Infect.*, 1, 1129–37.

Choudari, C.P., Mathan, M., Rajan, D.P., Raghavan, R., Mathan, V.L. (1985) A correlative study of etiology, clinical features and rectal mucosal pathology in adults with acute infectious diarrhoea in Southern India. *Pathology*, 17, 443–50.

Christie, J.D. (2003) Intestinal spirochaetosis; an organism in search of a disease. *Am. J. Clin. Pathol.*, 120, 820–21.

Clarkston, W.K., Bonacini, M., Peterson, I. (1991) Colitis due to *Histoplasma capsulatum* in the acquired immunodeficiency syndrome. *Am. J. Gastroenterol.*, 86, 913–16.

Collins, D. (1956) Histoplasmosis and the coloproctologist. *Am. J. Proctol.*, 7, 379–91.

Connolly, G.M., Gazzard, B.G. (1987) Toxic megacolon in cryptosporidiosis. *Postgrad. Med. J.*, 63, 1103–4.

Cook, G.C. (1993) Diagnostic procedures in the investigation of infectious diarrhoea. *Baillieres Clin. Gastroenterol.*, 7(2), 421–49.

Cooper, H.S., Raffenberger, E.C., Jones, L. (1977) Cytomegalovirus inclusions in patients with ulcerative colitis and toxic dilatation requiring colonic resection. *Gastroenterology*, 72, 1253–6.

Coyne, J.D., Curry, A., Purnell, P., Haboubi, N.Y. (1995) Colonic tubular adenomas and spirochaetosis: an incompatible association. *Histopathology*, 27, 377–9.

Cunningham, A.L., Grohman, G.S., Harkness, J., Law, C., Marriott, D., Tindal, B., Cooper, D.A. (1988) Gastrointestinal infections in homosexual men who were symptomatic and seropositive for human immunodeficiency virus. *J. Infect. Dis.*, 158, 386–91.

Day, D.W., Mandal, B.K., Morson, B.C. (1978) The rectal biopsy appearances in *Salmonella* colitis. *Histopathology*, 2, 117–31.

Day, D.W., Jass, J.R., Price, A.B. *et al.* (2003) *Morson and Dawson's Gastrointestinal Pathology*, 4th edn. Oxford: Blackwell, Ch. 36.

Dekeyser, P., Cassvin-Detrain, M., Butzler, J.P., Sternon, J. (1972) Acute enteritis due to related *Vibrio*: first positive stool culture. *J. Infect. Dis.*, 125, 390–2.

Dickinson, R.J., Gilmour, H.M., McClelland, D.B.L. (1979) Rectal biopsy in patients presenting to an infectious diseases unit with diarrhoeal disease. *Gut*, 20,141–8.

Dickinson, R.J., Dixon, M.F., Axon, A.T.R. (1980) Staphylococcal enterocolitis and inflammatory bowel disease. *J. Clin. Pathol.*, 33, 604–5.

Douglas, J.G., Crucioli, V. (1981) Spirochaetosis: A remediable cause of diarrhoea and rectal bleeding? *Br. Med. J.*, 283, 1362.

Dundas, S.A.C., Dutton, J., Skipworth, P. (1997) Reliability of rectal biopsy in distinguishing between chronic inflammatory bowel disease and acute self-limiting colitis. *Histopathology*, 31, 60–66.

DuPont, H.L., Levine, M.M., Hornick, R.B., Formal, S.B. (1989) Inoculum size in shigellosis and implications for expected mode of transmission. *J. Infect. Dis.*, 159, 1126–8.

Echeverria, P., Savarrino S.J., Yamamoto,T. (1993) *Escherichia coli* diarrhoea. *Baillieres Clin. Gastroenterol.*, 7(2), 243–62.

Editorial (1984) Yersiniosis today. *Lancet*, i, 84–5.

El-Maraghi, N.R.H., Mair, N.S. (1979) The histopathology of enteric infection with *Yersinia pseudotuberculosis*. *Am. J. Clin. Pathol.*, 71, 631–9.

Fell, J.M. (2005) Neonatal inflammatory intestinal diseases: necrotizing enterocolitis and allergic colitis. *Early Hum. Dev.*, 81, 117–22.

Fenton, T.R., Walker-Smith, J.A., Harvey, D.R. (1981) Proctoscopy in infancy with reference to its use in necrotizing enterocolitis. *Arch. Dis. Child.*, 56, 121–4.

Fletcher, A., Sims, T.A., Talbot, L.C. (1982) Cryptosporidial enteritis without general or selective immune deficiency. *Br. Med. J.*, 285, 22–3.

Foucar, E., Mukai, K., Sutherland, D.E., van Buren, C.T. (1981) Colon ulceration in lethal cytomegalovirus infection. *Am. J. Clin. Pathol.*, 76, 788–801.

Francis, N.D., Boylston, A.W., Roberts, A.H., Parkin, J.M., Pinching, A.S.J. (1989) Cytomegalovirus infection in gastrointestinal tracts of patients with HIV-1 or AIDS. *J. Clin. Pathol.*, 42, 1055–64.

Franklin, G., Mohapatra, M, Perillo, R.P. (1979) Colonic tuberculosis diagnosed by colonoscopic biopsy. *Gastroenterology*, 76, 362–4.

Freeman, H.J., Shnitka, T.K., Piercey. J.R.A., Weinstein, W.M. (1977) Cytomegalovirus infection of the gastrointestinal tract in a patient with late onset immunodeficiency syndrome. *Gastroenterology*, 73, 1397–1403.

Galiatsatos, P., Shrier, I., Lamoureux, E., Szilagyi, A. (2005) Meta-analysis of outcome of cytomegalovirus colitis in immunocompetent hosts. *Dig. Dis. Sci.*, 50, 609–16.

Gebbers, J-O., Ferguson, D.J.P., Mason, C., Kelly, P., Jewell, D.P. (1987) Spirochaetosis of the human rectum associated with an intraepithelial mast cell and IgE plasma cell response. *Gut*, 28, 588–93.

George, L.W., Nakata, M.M., Thompson, J., White, M.L. (1985) *Aeromonas*-related diarrhoea in adults. *Arch. Intern. Med.*, 145, 2207–11.

Gleason, T.H., Patterson, S.D. (1982) The pathology of *Yersinia enterocolitica* ileocolitis. *Am. J. Surg. Pathol.*, 6, 347–55.

Goldmeier, D., Sargeaunt, P.G., Price, A. B. *et al.* (1986) Is *Entamoeba histolytica* in homosexual men a pathogen? *Lancet*, i, 641–4.

Goodell, S.E., Quinn, T.C., Mkrtichian, E., Schuffier, M.D., Holmes, K.K., Corey, L. (1983) Herpes simplex virus proctitis in homosexual men: clinical, sigmoidoscopic and histopathological features. *N. Engl. J. Med.*, 287, 868–71.

Goodman, Z.D., Boitnott, J.K., Yardley, J.H. (1979) Perforation of the colon associated with cytomegalovirus infection. *Dig. Dis. Sci.*, 24, 376–80.

Griffiths, J.K., Gorbach, S.L. (1993) Other bacterial diarrhoeas. *Baillieres Clin. Gastroenterol.*, 7(2), 263–305.

Gui, L., Subramony, C., Fratkin, J., Hughson, M.D. (2002) Fatal enteritis necroticans (pigbel) in a diabetic adult. *Mod. Pathol.*, 15, 66–70.

Guthrie, S.O., Gordon, P.V., Thomas, V., Thorp, J.A., Peabody, J., Clark, R.H. (2003) Necrotizing enterocolitis among neonates in the United States. *J. Perinatol.*, 23, 278–85.

Gutierrez, Y., Bhatia, P., Garbadawala, S.T., Dobson, J.R., Wallace, T.M., Carey, T.E. (1996) Strongyloides stercoralis eosinophilic granulomatous enterocolitis. *Am. J. Surg. Pathol.*, 20, 603–12.

Hing, M.C., Goldschmidt, C., Mathijs, J.M., Cunningham, A.L., Cooper, D.A. (1992) Chronic colitis associated with human immunodeficiency virus infection. *Med. J. Aust.*, 156, 683–7.

Hinton, N.A., Taggart, J.G., Orr, J.H. (1960) The significance of the isolation of coagulase positive staphylococci from stool. *Am. J. Clin. Pathol.*, 33, 505–10.

Hommes, D.W., Sterringa, G., van Deventer, S.J., Tytgat, G.N., Weel, J. (2004) The pathogenicity of cytomegalovirus in inflammatory bowel disease: a systematic review and evidence-based recommendation for future research. *Inflamm. Bowel Dis.*, 10, 245–50.

Hovind-Hougen, K., Birch-Andersen. A., Nielsen, R.H., Orholm, M., Pedersen, J.O., Teglbjaerg, P.S,, Thaysen, E.H. (1982) Intestinal spirochaetosis: morphological characterization and cultivation of *Brachyspira aalborgi*, gen. nov. sp. nov. *J. Clin. Microbiol.*, 16, 1127–36.

Isaacs, D., Hunt, G.H., Phillips, A.D., Price, E.H., Raafat, F., Walker-Smith. J.A. (1985) Cryptosporidiosis in immunocompetent children. *J. Clin. Pathol.*, 38, 76–81.

Janoff, E.N., Orenstein, J.M., Manischewitz, J.F., Smith, P.D. (1991) Adenovirus colitis in the acquired immunodeficiency syndrome. *Gastroenterology*, 100, 976–9.

Jenkins, D., Goodall, A., Scott, B.B. (1997) Simple objective criteria for the diagnosis of acute diarrhoea on rectal biopsy. *J. Clin. Pathol.*, 50, 580–5.

Jewkes, J., Larson, H.E., Price, A.B., Sanderson, P.J., Davies, H.A. (1981) Aetiology of acute diarrhoea in adults. *Gut*, 22, 388–92.

Jokipii, L., Polyola, S., Jokipii, A.M.M. (1983) *Cryptosporidium*: a frequent finding in patients with gastrointestinal symptoms. *Lancet*, ii, 358–60.

Juniper, K. (1978) Amoebiasis. *Clin. Gastroenterol.*, 7(1), 3–29.

Kacker, P.P. (1973) A case of *Giardia lamblia* proctitis presenting in a V.D. clinic. *Br. J. Ven. Dis.*, 49, 318–19.

Kafetzis, D.A., Skevaki, C., Costalos, C. (2003) Neonatal necrotizing enterocolitis: an overview. *Curr. Opin. Infect. Dis.*, 16, 349–55.

Kamham, N., Vij, R., Cartwright, C.A., Longacre, T. (2004) Cytomegalovirus infection in steroid-refractory ulcerative colitis: a case control study. *Am. J. Surg. Pathol.*, 28, 365–73.

Kaufman, H.S., Kahn, A.C., Iacobuzio-Donahue C., Talamini, M.A., Lillemoe, K.D., Hamilton, S.R. (1999) Cytomegalovirus enterocolitis: clinical associations and outcomes. *Dis. Colon Rectum*, 42, 24–30.

Kaur, G., Raj, S.M., Naing, N.N. (2002) Trichuriasis: localized inflammatory response in the colon. *Southeast Asian J. Trop. Med. Public Health.*, 33, 224–8.

Khalil, M., Iwatt, A.R., Gugnani, H.C. (1989) African histoplasmosis masquerading as carcinoma of the colon. Report of a case and review of the literature. *Dis. Colon Rectum*, 32, 518–20.

Kirsch, R., Pentecost, M., de M Hall, P., Epstein, D.P., Watermeyer, G., Freiderich, P.W. (2006) Role of colonoscopic biopsy in distinguishing between Crohn's disease and intestinal tuberculosis. *J. Clin. Pathol.*, 59, 840–4.

Klausner, J.D., Kohn, R., Kent, C. (2004) Etiology of clinical proctitis among men who have sex with men. *Clin. Infect. Dis.*, 15, 300–2.

Klein, E.J., Fisher. L.S., Chow, A.W. (1977) Anorectal gonococcal infection. *Ann. Intern. Med.*, 86, 340–6.

Kliegman, R.M. (1979) Neonatal necrotizing enterocolitis. Implications for an infectious disease. *Paediatr. Clin. N. Am.*, 26(2), 327–44.

Klotz, S.A., Drutz, D.J., Tam, M.R., Reed, K.H. (1983) Hemorrhagic proctitis due to lymphogranuloma venereum serogroup LZ. Diagnosis by fluorescent monoclonal antibody. *N. Engl. J. Med.*, 308, 1563–5.

Knight, R. (1978) Giardiasis, isosporiasis and balantidiasis. *Clin. Gastroenterol.*, 71(1), 31–47.

Koplan, J.P., Fineberg, H.V., Ferraro, M.J.B., Rosenberg, M. (1980) Value of stool cultures. *Lancet*, ii, 413–16.

Kostianovsky, M., Orenstein, J.M., Schaff, Z., Grimley, P.M. (1987) Cytomembranous inclusions observed in acquired immunodeficiency syndrome. Clinical and experimental review. *Arch. Path. Lab. Med.*, 111, 218–23.

Kostman, J.R., Patel, M., Catalano, E., Camacho, J., Hoffpauir, J., DiNubile, M.J. (1995) Invasive colitis and hepatitis due to previously uncharacterized spirochaetes in patients with advanced human immunodeficiency virus infection. *Clin. Infect. Dis.*, 21, 1159–65.

Kotler, D.P., Gaetz, H.P., Lange, M., Klein, E.B., Holt, P.R. (1984) Enteropathy associated with the Acquired Immunodeficiency Syndrome. *Ann. Intern. Med.*, 101, 421–8.

Kotler, D.P., Weaver, S.C., Terzakis, J.A. (1986) Ultrastructural features of epithelial cell degeneration in rectal crypts of patients with AIDS. *Am. J. Surg. Pathol.*, 18, 531–8.

Kumar, N.B., Nostrant, T.T., Appelman, H.D. (1982) The histopathologic spectrum of acute self-limited colitis (acute infectious-type colitis). *Am. J. Surg. Pathol.*, 6, 523–9.

Ladas, S.D., Savva, S., Frydas, A., Kalovidiris, A., Hatzioannou, J., Raptis, S. (1989) Invasive balantidiasis presented as chronic colitis and lung involvement. *Dig. Dis. Sci.*, 34, 1621–3.

Lambert, M.E., Schofield, P.F., Ironside, A.G., Mandal, B.K. (1979) *Campylobacter* colitis. *Br. Med. J.*, 1, 857–9.

Larsson, P.A., Olling, S., Darle, N. (1991) Amebic colitis presenting as acute inflammatory bowel disease. Case report. *Eur. J. Surg.*, 157, 553–5.

Laughon, B.E., Druckman, D.A., Vernon, A. *et al.* (1988) Prevalence of enteric pathogens in homosexual men with and without acquired immunodeficiency syndrome. *Gastroenterology*, 94, 984–93.

Lee, F.D., Kraszewski, A., Gordon, J., Howie, J.G.R., McSeveney, D., Harland, N.A. (1971) Intestinal spirochaetosis. *Gut*, 12, 126–33.

Lee, S.C., Hwang, K.P., Tsai, W.S., Lin, C.Y., Lee, N. (2002) Detection of *Enterobius vermicularis* eggs in the submucosa of the transverse colon of a man presenting with colon carcinoma. *Am. J. Trop. Hyg.*, 69, 233.

Lee, S.D., Surawicz, C.M. (2001) Infectious causes of diarrhoea. *Gastroenterol. Clin. N. Am.*, 30(3), 697–707.

Lemos, L.B., Qu, Z., Laucirica, R., Fred, H.L.K. (2003) Hyperinfection syndrome in strongyloidiasis: report of two cases. *Ann. Diagn. Pathol.*, 7, 87–94.

Leprince, E., Durous, E., Francois, Y. *et al.* (1993) Ileocolitis caused by Herpes simplex virus type 2. *Gastroenterol. Clin. Biol.*, 17, 855–8.

Levin, I., Rornano, S., Steinberg, M. (1964) Lymphogranuloma venereum: rectal stricture and carcinoma. *Dis. Col. Rectum*, 7, 129–34.

Lo, T.C., Heading, R.C., Gilmour, H.M. (1994) Intestinal spirochaetosis. *Postgrad. Med. J.*, 70, 134–7.

Loosli, J., Gyr, K., Stalder, H., Vischer, W., Voegtlin, J., Gasser, M., Reichlin, B. (1985) Etiology of acute infectious diarrhoea in a highly industrialized area of Switzerland. *Gastroenterology*, 88, 75–9.

Lysy, J., Zimmerman, J., Sherman, Y., Feigin, R., Ligumsky, M. (1991) Crohn's colitis complicated by superimposed invasive amoebic colitis. *Am. J. Gastroenterol.*, 86, 1063–5.

Maayan-Metzger, A., Itzchak, A., Mazkereth, R., Kuint, J. (2004) Necrotizing enterocolitis in full-term infants: case-control study and review of the literature. *J. Perinatol.*, 24, 494–9.

McGovern, V.J., Slavutin, L.J. (1979) Pathology of *Salmonella* colitis. *Am. Surg. Pathol.*, 3, 483–90.

McMillan, A., Lee, F.D. (1981) Sigmoidoscopic and microscopic appearance of the rectal mucosa in homosexual men. *Gut*, 22, 1035–41.

McMillan, A., Gilmour, H.M., Slatford, K, McNeillage, G.J.C. (1983) Proctitis in homosexual men. *Br. J. Vener. Dis.*, 59, 260–4.

McMillan, A., Gilmour, H.M., McNeillage, G.J.C., Scott, G.R. (1984) Amoebiasis in homosexual men. *Gut*, 25, 356–60.

Maddox, A., Francis, N., Moss, J., Blanshard, C., Gazzard, B. (1992) Adenovirus of the large bowel in HIV positive patients. *J. Clin. Pathol.*, 45, 684–8.

Makinen, M., Niemala, S., Lehtola, J. and Karttunen, J. (1998) Collagenous colitis and Yersinia enterocolitica infection. *Dig. Dis. Sci.*, 43, 1341–6.

Maliha, G.M., Hepps, K.S., Maia D.M., Gentry, K.R., Fraire, A.E., Goodgame, R.W. (1991) Whipple's disease can mimic chronic AIDS enteropathy. *Am. J. Gastroenterol.*, 86, 79–81.

Mandal, B.K, Mani, V. (1976) Colonic involvement in salmonellosis. *Lancet*, i, 887–8.

Marshall, J.B. (1993) Tuberculosis of the gastrointestinal tract and peritoneum. *Am. J. Gastroenterol.*, 88, 989–99.

Mathan, M.M., Mathan, V.L. (1985) Local Shwartzman reaction in the rectal mucosa in acute diarrhoea. *J. Pathol.*, 146, 179–87.

Matsumoto, T., Iida, M., Matsui, T., Sakamoto, K., Fuchigami, T., Haraguchi, Y., Fujishima, M. (1990) Endoscopic findings in *Yersinia enterocolitica* enterocolitis. *Gastrointest. Endosc.*, 36, 583–7.

Matsumoto, T., Iida, M., Kimura, Y., Fujishima, M. (1994) Culture of colonoscopically obtained biopsy specimens in acute colitis. *Gastrointest. Endosc.*, 40, 184–7.

Meiselman, M.S., Cello, J.P., Margaretten, W. (1985) Cytomegalovirus colitis. Report of the clinical, endoscopic and pathologic findings in two patients with the acquired immune deficiency syndrome. *Gastroenterology*, 88, 171–5.

Mikosza, A.S., Hampson, D.J. (2001) Human intestinal spirochaetosis: *Brachyspira aalborgi* and/or *Brachyspira pilosicoli*. *Anim. Health Res. Rev.*, 2, 101–10.

Ming-Chai, C., Pei-Yu, C., Chi-Yuan, C. *et al.* (1981) Colorectal cancer and schistosomiasis. *Lancet*, i, 971–3.

Morandi, E., Grassi, C., Cellerino, P., Massaro, P.P., Corsi, F., Trabucchi, E. (2003) Verocytotoxin-producing *Escherichia coli* EH O157:H7 colitis. *J. Clin. Gastroenterol.*, 36, 44–6.

de la Monte, S.M., Hutchins, G.M. (1985) Follicular proctocolitis and neuromatous hyperplasia with lymphogranuloma venereum. *Hum. Pathol.*, 16,1025–32.

Muldoon, J., O'Riordan, K., Rao, S., Abecassis, M. (1996) Ischemic colitis secondary to venous thrombosis. A rare presentation of cytomegalovirus vasculitis following renal transplantation. *Transplantation*, 61, 1651–3.

Munday, P.E., Dawson, S.G., Johnson, A.P. *et al.* (1981) A microbiological study of non-gonococcal proctitis in passive male homosexuals. *Postgrad. Med. J.*, 57, 705–11.

Murray, K.F., Patterson, K. (2000) *Escherichia coli* O157:H7-induced hemolytic–uremic syndrome: histopathologic changes in the colon over time. *Pediatr. Dev. Pathol.*, 3, 232–9.

Murrell, T.G., Walker, P.D. (1991) The pigbel story of Papua New Guinea. *Trans. R. Soc. Trop. Med. Hyg.*, 85, 119–22.

Murrell, T.G.C., Roth, L., Egerton, I., Samels, J., Walker, P.D. (1966) Pig-bel: enteritis necroticans. A study in diagnosis and management. *Lancet*, i, 215–22.

Neafie, R.C., Connor, D.H. (1976) Trichuriasis. In: Binford, C.H., Connor, D.H. (eds) *Pathology of tropical and extraordinary diseases, vol. II*, Washington, DC: Armed Forces Institute of Pathology, Ch. 4.

Neafie, R.C., Connor, D.H., Meyers, W.M. (1976) Enterobiasis. In: Binford, C.H., Connor, D.H. (eds) *Pathology of tropical and extraordinary diseases, vol. II*, Washington, DC: Armed Forces Institute of Pathology, pp. 455–9.

Nguyen, H.N., Frank, D., Handt, S., Rieband, H.C., Maurin, N., Sieberth, H.G., Matern, S. (1999) Severe gastrointestinal haemorrhage due to *Mycobacterium avium* complex in a patient receiving immunosuppressive therapy. *Am. J. Gastroenterol.*, 94, 232–5.

Nielsen, R.H., Orholm, M., Pedersen, J.O., Hovind-Hougen, K., Teglbjaerg, P.S., Thaysen, E.H. (1983) Colorectal spirochaetosis: clinical significance of the infestation. *Gastroenterology*, 85, 62–7.

Nime, F.A., Burek, J.D., Page, D.L., Holscher, M.A., Yardley, J.H. (1976) Acute enterocolitis in a human being infected with the protozoan *Cryptosporidium. Gastroenterology*, 70, 592–6.

Nostrant, T.T., Kumar, N.B., Appelman, H.D. (1987) Histopathology differentiates acute self-limiting colitis from ulcerative colitis. *Gastroenterology*, 92, 318–28.

Orenstein, J.M, Dieterich, D.T. (2001) The histopathology of 103 consecutive biopsies from 82 symptomatic patients with acquired immunodeficiency syndrome: original and look-back diagnoses. *Arch. Pathol. Lab. Med.*, 125, 1042–6.

Padmanabhan, V., Dahlstrom, J., Maxwell, L., Kaye, G., Clarke, A., Barratt, P.J. (1996) Invasive intestinal spirochaetosis: a report of three cases. *Pathology*, 28, 283–6.

Pai, C.H., Gordon, R., Sims, H.V., Bryan, L.B. (1984) Sporadic cases of haemorrhagic colitis associated with *Escherichia coli*. O157:H7. *Ann. Intern. Med.*, 101, 738–42.

Papagrigoriadis, S., Rennie, J.A. (1998) Lymphogranuloma venereum as a cause of rectal strictures. *Postgrad. Med. J.*, 74, 168–9.

Patel, N., Amarapurkar, D., Agal, S., Baijal, R., Kulshrestha, P., Pramanik, S., Gupte, P. (2004) Gastrointestinal luminal tuberculosis: establishing the diagnosis. *J. Gastroenterol. Hepatol.*, 19, 1240–6.

Pauwels, A., Meyohas, M.C., Eliaszawicz, M., Legendre, C., Mougeot, G., Frottier, J. (1992) Toxoplasma colitis in the acquired immuno-deficiency syndrome. *Am. J. Gastroenterol.*, 87, 518–19.

Powell, S.J., Wilmot, A.J. (1966) Ulcerative post-dysenteric colitis. *Gut*, 7, 438–43.

Prata, A. (1978) *Schistosomiasis mansoni. Clin. Gastroenterol.*, 7(1), 77–85.

Prathap, I.C., Gilman, R. (1970) The histopathology of acute intestinal amoebiasis. *Am. J. Pathol.*, 60, 229–45.

Price, A.B. (1985) Histology of clostridial gut diseases in man. In: Borriello S.P. (ed.) *Clostridia in gastrointestinal disease.* Boca Raton: CRC Press, pp. 177–94.

Price, A.B., Jewkes, J., Sanderson, P.J. (1979) Acute diarrhoea, *Campylobacter* colitis and the role of rectal biopsy. *J. Clin. Pathol.*, 32, 990–7.

Prior, A., Lessells, A.M., Whorwell, P.J. (1987) Is biopsy necessary if colonoscopy is normal? *Dig. Dis. Sci.*, 332, 673–6.

Pulimood, A.B., Ramakrishna, B.S., Kurian, G., Peter, S., Patra, S., Mathan, V.I., Mathan, N.N. (1999) Endoscopic mucosal biopsies are useful in distinguishing granulomatous colitis due to Crohn's disease from tuberculosis. *Gut*, 45, 537–41.

Pulimood, A.B., Peter, S., Ramakrishna, B., Chacko, A., Jeyamani, R., Jeyaseelan, L., Kurian, G. (2005) Segmental colonoscopic biopsies in the differentiation of ileocolic tuberculosis from Crohn's disease: *J. Gastroenterol. Hepatol.*, 20, 688–96.

Quinn, T.C., Goodell, S.E., Mkrtichian, E., Schuffler, M.D., Wang, S-P., Stamm, W.E., Holmes, K.K. (1981) *Chlamydia trachomatis* proctitis. *N. Engl. J. Med.*, 305, 195–200.

Quinn, T.C., Stamm, W.E., Goodell, S.E. *et al.* (1983) The polymicrobial origin of intestinal infection in homosexual men. *N. Engl. J. Med.*, 309, 576–82.

Quinn, T.C., Goodell, S.E., Fennell, C., Wang, S.P., Schuffler, M.D., Holmes, K.K., Stamm, W.E. (1984) Infections with *Campylobacter jejuni* and *Campylobacter*-like organisms in homosexual men. *Ann. Intern. Med.*, 101, 187–92.

Radhakrishnan, S., Al Nakib, B., Shaikh, H., Menon, N.K. (1986) The value of colonoscopy in schistosomal, tuberculous and amebic colitis. Two-year experience. *Dis. Colon Rectum*, 29, 891–5.

Rodgers, F.G., Rodgers, C., Shelton, A.P., Hawkey, C.J. (1986) Proposed pathogenic mechanism for the diarrhoea associated with human intestinal spirochaetosis. *Am. J. Clin. Pathol.*, 86, 679–82.

Rosen, S.A., Wexner, S.D., Woodhouse, S. *et al.* (2005) Not all inflammation in the right lower quadrant is appendicitis: a case report of *Escherichia coli* O157:H7 with a review of the literature. *Am. Surg.*, 71, 532–6.

Roskell, D.E., Hyde, G.M., Campbell, A.P., Jewell, D.P., Gray, W. (1995) HIV associated cytomegalovirus colitis as a mimic of inflammatory bowel disease. *Gut*, 37, 148–50.

Roth, R.I., Owen, R.L., Keren, D.F., Volberding, P.A. (1985) Intestinal infection with *Mycobacterium avium* in acquired immunodeficiency syndrome (AIDS): histological and clinical comparison with Whipple's disease. *Dig. Dis. Sci.*, 30, 497–504.

Sachdev, H.P., Chadha, V., Malhotra, V., Verghese, A, Puri, R.K. (1993) Rectal histopathology in endemic *Shigella* and *Salmonella* diarrhoea. *J. Pediatr. Gastroenterol. Nutr.*, 16, 33–8.

Sargeaunt, P.G., Williams, J.E. (1979) Electrophoretic isoenzyme patterns of the pathogenic and non-pathogenic intestinal amoebae of man. *Trans. R. Soc. Trop. Med. Hyg.*, 73, 225–7.

Scarce, M. (1997) Harbinger of plague: a bad case of gay bowel syndrome. *J. Homosex.* 34, 1–35.

Schumacher, G., Sandstedt, R., Mollby, R., Kollberg, B. (1991) Clinical and histological features differentiating non-relapsing colitis from first attacks of inflammatory bowel disease. *Scand. J. Gastroenterol.*, 26, 151–61.

Schwab, K.S., Shaw, R. (1993) Infectious diarrhoea. Viruses. *Baillieres Clin. Gastroenterol.*, 7(2), 307–31.

Serra, S., Chetty, R. (2005) Bizarre stromal cells in ischemic bowel disease. *Ann. Diagn. Pathol.*, 9, 193–6.

Shah, S., Thomas, V., Mathan, M., Chacko, A., Chandy, G., Ramakrishna, B.S., Rolston, D.D. (1992) Colonoscopic study of 50 patients with colonic tuberculosis. *Gut*, 33, 347–51.

Simmonds, S.D., Noble, M.A., Freeman, H.J. (1987) Gastrointestinal features of culture positive *Yersinia enterocolitica* infection. *Gastroenterology*, 92, 112–17.

Singh, V., Kumar, P., Kamal, J., Prakash, V., Vaiphei, K., Singh, K. (1996) Clinicocolonoscopic profile of colonic tuberculosis. *Am. J. Gastroenterol.*, 91, 565–8.

Smith, H.R., Rowe, B., Gross, R.J., Fry, N.K., Scotland, S.M. (1987) Haemorrhagic colitis and Vero-cytotoxin-producing *Escherichia coli* in England and Wales. *Lancet*, i, 1062–4.

Smith, J. (1969) Mycosis of the alimentary tract. *Gut*, 10, 1035–40.

Soave, R., Danner, R.L., Honig, C.L., Pearl, M.A., Hart, C.C., Nash, T., Roberts, R.B. (1984) Cryptosporidiosis in homosexual men. *Ann. Intern. Med.*, 100, 504–11.

Sobel, J., Mixter, C.G., Kohle, P. *et al.* (2005) Necrotizing enterocolitis associated with *Clostridium perfringens* type A in previously healthy North American adults. *J. Am. Coll. Surg.*, 201, 48–56.

Speelman, P., Kabir, I., Islam, M. (1984) Distribution and spread of colonic lesions in shigellosis. A colonoscopic study. *J. Infect. Dis.*, 150, 899–903.

Surawicz, C.M., (1988) The role of rectal biopsy in infectious colitis. *Am. J. Surg. Pathol.*, 12(Suppl. 1), 82–8.

Surawicz, C.M., Belic, L. (1984) Rectal biopsy helps to distinguish acute self-limited colitis from idiopathic inflammatory bowel disease. *Gastroenterology*, 86, 104–13.

Surawicz, C.M., Goodell, S.E., Quinn, T.C. *et al.* (1986) Spectrum of rectal biopsy abnormalities in homosexual men with intestinal symptoms. *Gastroenterology*, 91, 651–9.

Taylor, D.N., Echeverria, P., Blaser, M.J., Pitarangsi, C., Blacklow, N., Cross, J., Weniger, B.G. (1985) Polymicrobial aetiology of traveller's diarrhoea. *Lancet*, i, 381–3.

Therkilsden, M.H., Jensen, B.N., Teglbjaerg, P.S., Rasmussen, S.N. (1989) The final outcome in patients presenting with their first episode of acute diarrhoea and an inflamed rectal mucosa with preserved crypt architecture. A clinicopathologic study. *Scand. J. Gastroenterol.*, 24, 158–64.

Thomas, M.E., Tillet, H.E. (1975) Diarrhoea in general practice: a sixteen-year report of investigations in a microbiology laboratory with epidemiological assessment. *J. Hyg. (Camb.)*, 74, 183–94.

Thomas, P.D., Pollok, R.C., Gazzard, B.D. (1999) Enteric viral infections as a cause of diarrhoea

in the acquired immunodeficiency syndrome. *HIV Med.* 1, 19–24.

Trivett-Moore, N.L., Gilbert, G.L., Law, C.L., Trott, D.J., Hampson, D.J. (1998) Isolation of *Serpulina pilosicoli* from rectal biopsy specimens showing evidence of intestinal spirochaetosis. *J. Clin. Microbiol.*, 36, 261–5.

Ustun, S., Dagci, H., Aksoy, U., Guruz, Y., Ersoz, G. (2003) Prevalence of amebiasis in inflammatory bowel disease in Turkey. *World J. Gastroenterol.* 9, 1834–5.

van Loon, F.P., van Schaik, S., Banik, A.K., Ahmed, T., Zaman, A., Kay, B.A. (1990) *Clostridium perfringens* type C and watery diarrhoea in Bangladesh. *Trop. Geogr. Med.*, 42, 123–7.

van Mook, W.N.K.A., Koek, G.H., van der Ven, A.J.A.M., Ceelan, T.L., Bos, R.P. (2004) Human intestinal spirochaetosis: any clinical significance? *Eur. J. Gastroenterol. Hepatol.*, 16, 83–7.

van Spreeuwel, J.P., Duursma, G.C., Meijer, C.J., Bax, R., Rosenkrans, P.C., Lindeman, J. (1985) *Campylobacter colitis*: histological immunohistochemical and ultrastructural findings. *Gut*, 26, 945–51.

Vantrappen, G., Agg, H.O., Ponette, E., Geboes, K., Bertrand, P.H. (1977) *Yersinia* enteritis and enterocolitis: gastroenterological aspects. *Gastroenterology*, 72, 220–7.

Warren, K.S. (1978) *Schistomiasis japonica*. *Clin. Gastroenterol.*, 7(1), 77–85.

Weir, W.R.C. (1985) *Campylobacter* infection. *Curr. Opin. Gastroenterol.*, 1, 130–4.

Weller, I.V.D. (1985) The gay bowel. *Gut*, 26, 869–75.

Wilcox, C.M., Chalasani, N., Lazenby, A., Schwartz, D.A. (1998) Cytomegalovirus colitis in acquired immunodeficiency syndrome: a clinical and endoscopic study. *Gastrointest. Endosc.*, 48, 39–43.

Wolke, A., Meyers, S., Adelsberg, B.R., Bottone, E.J., Damsker, B., Schwartz, I.S., Janowitz, H.D. (1984) *Mycobacterium avium-intracellulare*-associated colitis in a patient with the acquired immunodeficiency syndrome. *J. Clin. Gastroenterol.*, 6, 225–9.

CHAPTER 5

ULCERATIVE COLITIS

5.1 Introduction	90	
5.2 The biopsy for diagnosis	91	
5.2.1 Active phase of ulcerative proctocolitis	91	
5.2.2 Resolving phase of ulcerative proctocolitis	96	
5.2.3 The phase of remission	98	
5.2.4 Lectins, adhesion molecules and mucins	100	
5.2.5 Summary	100	
5.3 The equivocal biopsy	101	
5.4 Sequential biopsies	101	
5.5 Colonoscopic biopsy	102	
5.5.1 The colonoscopist's report	102	

5.5.2 Colonoscopic biopsies – variable patterns of involvement 103
5.5.3 Interpretation of colonoscopic biopsies 103
5.5.4 Biopsy interpretation and treatment 104
5.6 Inflammatory polyps ('pseudopolyps') 106
5.7 Fulminant acute colitis (toxic dilatation) 106
5.8 Follicular proctitis 107
5.9 Conclusions 107
References 107

5.1 INTRODUCTION

Ulcerative colitis is characteristically a chronic intermittent disease of the large bowel mucosa. Less commonly, symptoms are low grade and continuous (Moum *et al.*, 1997a). Rarely, patients suffer only a single attack (Edwards and Truelove, 1963). This chapter is based on the assumption that the disease has a characteristic histological appearance which develops during its course. In general this allows a confident biopsy diagnosis to be made in established disease but usually only a suggested diagnosis at the initial presentation (Goldman and Antonioli, 1982; Therkildsen *et al.*, 1989) when a distinction from infectious colitis [acute self-limiting colitis (ASLC)] or Crohn's disease is the commonest diagnostic dilemma confronting

the pathologist (Chapters 4 and 6). Moum *et al.* (1997b) found up to 10 per cent of patients initially thought to have chronic inflammatory bowel disease needed reclassification. The development of a characteristic pattern over a variable period makes sequential biopsy part of the diagnostic work-up (Goldman, 1994; Schumacher *et al.*, 1994a; Geboes, 2001). Because of the inherent prolonged and paroxysmal nature of ulcerative colitis it is best to avoid the labels 'acute' and 'chronic' but to consider the disease in terms of three phases; **active, resolving** and **in remission** (quiescent). We feel the term 'acute colitis' should be restricted to clinical use and has no pathological specificity.

In this book, idiopathic proctitis (haemorrhagic proctitis, granular proctitis and ulcerative proctitis) is assumed to be part of the spectrum of ulcerative colitis (Ritchie *et al.*, 1978a; Day *et al.*, 2003), but with characteristic sigmoidoscopic and histological changes restricted to the rectum. The term is not strictly synonymous with non-specific proctitis (Ritchie *et al.*, 1978b; Farmer, 1987; Day *et al.*, 2003) which, in our opinion, has broader connotations and we feel should be avoided unless qualified by helpful pointers to a likely diagnosis, or comment on unlikely diagnoses (Section 12.3). Of patients presenting with proctitis or proctosigmoiditis more extensive disease will have developed in 10–20 per cent at 5 years and in 30 per cent at 10 years (Ayres *et al.*, 1996).

Biopsy in ulcerative colitis is used to ascertain one of two main issues: to establish the diagnosis or to assess progress both anatomically and in relation to onset of complications. The biopsy also acts as a permanent record of the state of disease at one point in time. Because ulcerative colitis was understood to invariably commence in the rectum, spreading proximally and in continuity in a diffuse manner, a rectal biopsy was accepted as an adequate initial diagnostic step, relatively free of sampling error. This dogma about the first attack still stands (Day *et al.*, 2003; Robert *et al.*, 2004a) but there is now a realization that in chronic disease, especially once treatment has started, that the rectum can return to normal (Odze *et al.*, 1993; Levine *et al.*, 1996) and, moreover, the colonic inflammation can be patchy (Bernstein *et al.*, 1995; Kleer and Appelman, 1998; Kim *et al.*, 1999). The pattern of inflammation in children can also be atypical and, at the onset of disease, the rectum manifests fewer characteristic features (Markovitz *et al.*, 1993; Washington *et al.*, 2002), leading to possible erroneous diagnoses of Crohn's disease. Children are also atypical in that a proportion with ulcerative colitis, though more with Crohn's disease, will also have gastritis and a gastric biopsy has become part of the work-up in the investigation of paediatric inflammatory bowel disease (Domizio, 1994; Sharif *et al.*, 2002; Kundhal *et al.*, 2003). Colonoscopic biopsy offers more scope for comments on severity, extent, etc. (Waye, 1980). The individual microscopic criteria described below for rectal biopsy interpretation apply equally to colonoscopic material and the special considerations applicable to colonoscopic biopsies considered in Sections 5.5.3 and 5.5.4.

5.2 THE BIOPSY FOR DIAGNOSIS

The changes in crypt pattern and the nature of the inflammatory infiltrate are the prime abnormalities to be considered in making the diagnosis. However, the prominence and reliability of these abnormalities depend on the length of the clinical history, the phase of the disease at the time of the biopsy and the influence of any therapy administered (Geboes, 2001; Schumacher *et al.*, 1994a). These points are rarely appreciated by clinicians the history from whom is often little more than '?ulcerative colitis/?Crohn's disease'. Here the biopsy features are considered in three discrete phases.

5.2.1 Active phase of ulcerative proctocolitis

It is helpful to know the sigmoidoscopic changes and these should be documented on the request form. The mucosa loses its vascular pattern and is characteristically granular and friable. Ulceration may be absent. There may be histological evidence of disease even when the sigmoidoscopic appearances are normal (Das *et al.*, 1977; Spiliadis *et al.*, 1987). However, this is uncommon, compared, for example, with microscopic colitis where it is the norm (Chapter 9).

5.2.1a The epithelium and crypts

The major impact of the disease is reflected in the crypts (Surawicz and Belic, 1984). In active disease the goblet cells are depleted of mucin (Hellstrom and Fisher, 1967; Cook and Dixon, 1973; McCormick *et al.*, 1990). The crypts may initially appear elongated and the surface epithelium takes on an undulating or low villiform pattern (Seldenrijk *et al.*, 1991). Subsequently, and gradually, the regular architecture is lost and the crypts become branched and distorted (Price and Morson, 1975; Nostrant *et al.*, 1987; Seldenrijk *et al.*, 1991; Schumacher *et al.*, 1994a). There is accompanying infiltration by acute and chronic inflammatory cells which identify the active phase (Figs 5.1 and 5.2). This is considered

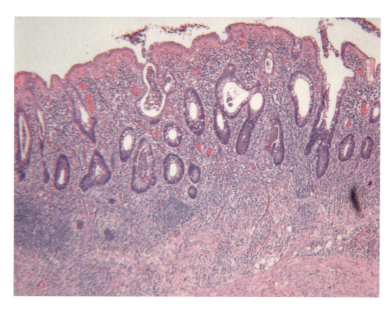

Figure 5.1 Active ulcerative colitis. The lamina propria is expanded by a diffuse heavy infiltrate of chronic inflammatory cells. There are scattered crypt abscesses present, mucin depletion and the crypt architecture is beginning to become distorted. In the deep mucosa some lymphoid collections are present.

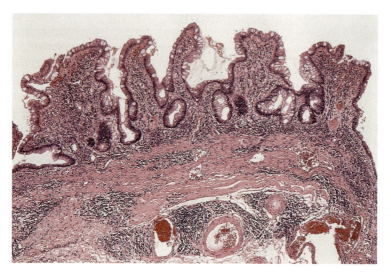

Figure 5.2 Active ulcerative colitis. In this biopsy a characteristic feature, in addition to the diffuse inflammation, is the villiform mucosal configuration and crypt irregularity. There is also some reduplication of the muscularis mucosae that can be a feature of long-standing disease.

in more detail below. The epithelium shows varying degrees of degeneration and regeneration which contribute to the visual abnormality of crypt histology. Mitoses are increased. Shortening of crypts, a feature of atrophy, occurs later (Fig. 5.3).

It must be remembered that glandular irregularity follows re-epithelialization of ulcerated mucosa from any cause and must not automatically be labelled ulcerative colitis.

As mentioned, the dogma that the rectum is invariably in the vanguard of the pathology, while

true for the most part, is no longer an absolute. This adds to the difficulties in the differential diagnosis of inflammatory bowel disease, particular caution in interpretation being required in the paediatric population (Markowitz *et al.*, 1993; Washington *et al.*, 2002; Robert *et al.*, 2004b). However, the damage to the cryptal epithelium and structure is unique to ulcerative colitis and in a biopsy the ensuing crypt distortion is the most specific pointer to the diagnosis. Its degree, at least in part, depends on the time from onset of symptoms to biopsy.

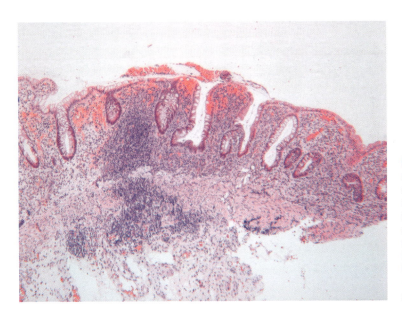

Figure 5.3 Long-standing chronic ulcerative colitis with established architectural distortion and crypt atrophy manifest by fewer and shorter crypts. Some lymphoid aggregates involve the muscularis mucosae and on-going treatment has led to the inflammation becoming patchy with partial resolution seen towards the left side of the figure.

Schumacher *et al.* (1994a) showed that if this was less than 15 days, crypt distortion was not seen. Its incidence increased as this interval lengthened so that it was present in 78 per cent of their biopsies taken 121–300 days after symptoms commenced. Surawicz and Belic (1984) claimed to see distortion in their biopsy series within 1 month. Such data cannot be too precise since, unlike ASLC, which has a predominantly acute onset, the onset of ulcerative colitis is more commonly insidious (Schumacher *et al.*, 1994b) and mucosal damage may therefore be ongoing during any initial subclinical phase. Moreover, there is likely to be variation between individual patients with regard to the speed of onset and the permanence of damage, irrespective of treatment regimens (Dick and Grayson, 1961; Whitehead, 1985). We are increasingly seeing biopsies, usually in the context of the cancer surveillance programme, which have to be passed as normal but are from patients with a confident diagnosis of long-standing ulcerative colitis based on prior biopsy evidence (Fig. 5.4).

5.2.1b The lamina propria and its inflammatory cells

In addition to crypt architectural changes, the assessment of the other accompanying histological features is also necessary for differentiation from certain transient causes of crypt damage that accompany healing ulceration of any cause. In active ulcerative colitis there is typically a heavy mixed diffuse inflammatory cell infiltrate throughout the lamina propria at the commencement of the disease. It may be focal very early on but involvement of the lower one-third of the lamina propria, especially a basal plasmacytosis, is claimed to distinguish the pattern from ASLC (Nostrant *et al.*, 1987; Schumacher *et al.*, 1991; Jenkins *et al.*, 1997) though not of course from Crohn's disease. The infiltrate quickly progresses to an even distribution throughout the biopsy and comprises plasma cells, lymphocytes and neutrophils. Although large numbers of neutrophil polymorphs are present, they are often less striking than in infectious colitis (Price *et al.*, 1979; Kumar *et al.*, 1982) as they are masked by large numbers of other cell types. This, together with capillary congestion and oedema, tends to make the mucosa look thicker than normal and often imparts an undulating villiform pattern to the surface mentioned earlier (Fig. 5.5). This villiform configuration was also found to be one of the key distinguishing attributes when attempting to distinguish ASLC from ulcerative colitis (Surawicz and Belic, 1984; Nostrant *et al.*, 1987; Schumacher *et al.*, 1994a). Lymphoid follicles can be seen and

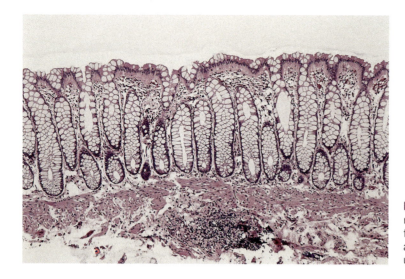

Figure 5.4 A rectal biopsy that might be considered normal yet from a patient with an established and biopsy proven history of ulcerative colitis.

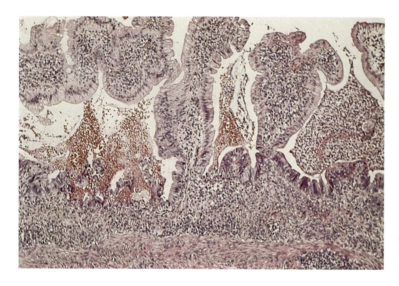

Figure 5.5 Severe active ulcerative colitis with a florid villiform configuration and focal ulceration.

are normally present in rectal mucosa (Dukes and Bussey, 1926) but their number may be increased to give a pattern of follicular proctitis (Section 5.8). The low-power impression of the biopsy in active disease is therefore one of dense cellularity. On closer inspection, neutrophils are seen infiltrating and lying free on the surface epithelium. In addition, many penetrate the cryptal epithelium with the formation of crypt abscesses. The latter are common in active disease and may be found anywhere in the mucosa (Fig. 5.6). In large numbers they are an important

discriminating attribute of ulcerative colitis but are certainly not exclusive to the disease (Schachter *et al.*, 1970; Schumacher *et al.*, 1994a). It is the proportion of crypt abscesses measured against other features that is the useful sign. Some crypts may contain but a few neutrophils whereas others are greatly distended by large numbers.

Other important constituents of the inflammatory response include eosinophils and mast cells (Anthonisen and Rus, 1971). Their presence or absence helps little in making an initial diagnosis

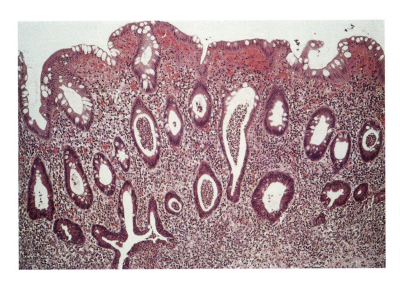

Figure 5.6 In this illustration crypt abscesses are clearly seen in conjunction with goblet cell depletion and diffuse chronic inflammation.

though it has been suggested that a prominent infiltrate of eosinophils is associated with a better-than-average prognosis (Heatley and James, 1978). More recent studies have failed to confirm this (Paoluzi *et al.*, 1984; Sarin *et al.*, 1987) and it seems more likely that an apparent excess of eosinophils could result from their relative persistence in an otherwise resolving inflammatory reaction. When eosinophils predominate parasitic disease or eosinophilic colitis should also be considered (Sections 3.8.5, 4.7 and 12.5.10).

The granularity of the mucosa in the acute attack is accounted for by large numbers of congested capillaries throughout the lamina propria. This also explains the mucosal friability and bleeding tendency commonly experienced during sigmoidoscopy (Fig. 5.7).

5.2.1c Muscularis mucosae and submucosa

A few inflammatory cells are often observed in the submucosa but when they are numerous, there are two explanations to consider. First the diagnosis may be wrong and the pattern is one of 'disproportionate inflammation', characteristic of Crohn's disease (Section 6.3.6). Second, the biopsy may have been taken adjacent to an area of severe ulceration.

The muscularis mucosae can become thickened in ulcerative colitis (Fig. 5.2) but this is usually in a long-standing case (Goulston and McGovern, 1969) and is difficult to appreciate in biopsy material.

5.2.1d Difficulties with diagnosis

The above description applies to the active phase of inflammation in the first attack. Before the onset of architectural distortion a confident opinion is rarely justified (Goldman and Antonioli, 1982; Surawicz and Belic, 1984; Nostrant *et al.*, 1987; Schumacher *et al.*, 1994a), though with a full house of goblet cell depletion, full-thickness diffuse heavy infiltration by plasma cells, lymphocytes and neutrophil polymorphs, together with numerous crypt abscesses and a villiform undulating surface (Figs 5.2 and 5.6), ulcerative colitis must be the pathologist's first choice. The differential diagnosis is considered later, but it is the biopsy taken early on, in the initial attack, which presents the greatest interpretative problems. In practice, the majority of patients are treated by the general practitioner for a few weeks before referral to hospital. In terms of the biopsy this delay is diagnostically useful (Schumacher *et al.*, 1994a). In the interpretation of first biopsies there is a subtle balance to take into account for, with time, although the architectural damage becomes more evident, the inflammation diminishes and becomes more focal. The former sign increases the confidence one can place on the diagnosis but the latter opens up other possibilities, in particular Crohn's disease

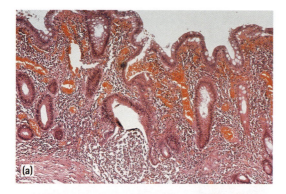

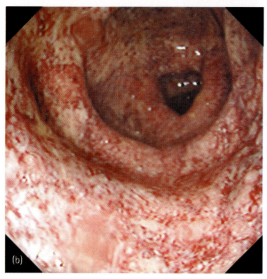

Figure 5.7 (a) This inflamed biopsy also illustrates the capillary engorgement that accompanies active disease and which is the basis of the friable congested mucosa observed at colonoscopy (see b). (b) A colonoscopic view of the friable congested granular mucosa of active ulcerative colitis reflected in the biopsy characteristics seen in (a).

and resolving ASLC. Attention must also be drawn to the occurrence of crypt-associated giant cells and crypt-associated granulomas (Mahadeva *et al.*, 2002) (Fig. 5.8), which can occur at any stage in the natural history of the disease. If the granulomas are free-standing in the lamina propria or submucosa the diagnosis of ulcerative colitis can be excluded but this is not the case if they are seen as part of the inflammatory reaction to a damaged crypt (Fig. 3.40; Section 3.8.10a).

5.2.2 Resolving phase of ulcerative proctocolitis

5.2.2a Sequential changes

The waxing and waning nature of ulcerative colitis means that the biopsy picture varies with time. Although, as mentioned already, this complicates the issue when interpreting a single biopsy taken for diagnostic purposes, the sequential changes seen across a succession of biopsies can add a useful diagnostic dimension.

As resolution commences, the goblet cell population returns towards normal. The surface epithelial cells also regain their normal configuration. Depending on the severity of the attack the crypt architecture will show evidence of damage, some crypts may be lost, some become shortened and some become branched. There may even be an increase in size of both crypts and goblet cells suggesting transformation to transitional mucosa (Franzin *et al.*, 1983) (Figs 5.9 and 5.10).

As resolution proceeds, the numbers of both neutrophils and chronic inflammatory cells in the lamina propria diminish, in particular neutrophils. Only an occasional crypt abscess will remain and as the plasma cells and lymphocyte numbers recede their distribution becomes more focal.

5.2.2b Difficulties with diagnosis

In the resolving phase, therefore, the inflammation is focal, the goblet cell population is restored and the crypt architecture might be only minimally altered. Such a pattern can be seen in many conditions, such as Crohn's disease (Morson, 1971) and infection. It is not safe to make a firm diagnostic commitment to ulcerative colitis with the above picture if this is the patient's first biopsy. The degree of residual crypt damage will determine the confidence of the opinion. Obviously, if there is an earlier series of biopsies, the diagnosis may have already been established and then it is reasonable to comment on the resolving nature of the inflammation. The pathologist should remember that the natural history of the disease and its histology are modified by treatment (Geboes, 2001) (Section 5.5.4).

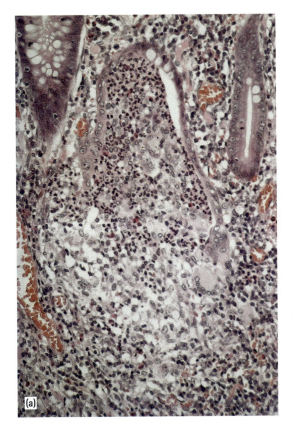

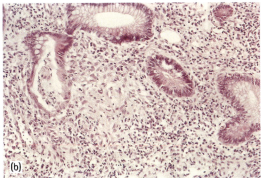

Figure 5.8 (a) An obvious crypt associated granuloma showing a disrupted crypt with histiocytes and giant cells as well as other inflammatory cells. Eosinophils are prominent. (b) A cluster of histiocytes forming a granuloma with a more subtle association with the adjacent crypt than seen in (a). The crypt architectural distortion can be appreciated even in this limited view. (a) and (b) are from cases of established ulcerative colitis.

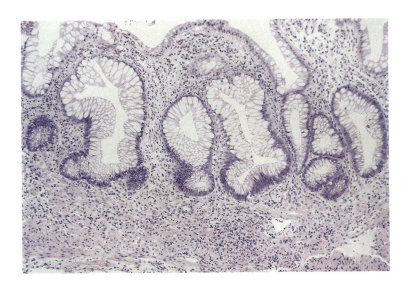

Figure 5.9 Resolving ulcerative colitis. The inflammatory cell infiltrate is minor, no crypt abscesses are evident with the crypts themselves being distorted and lined by enlarged mucin secreting cells.

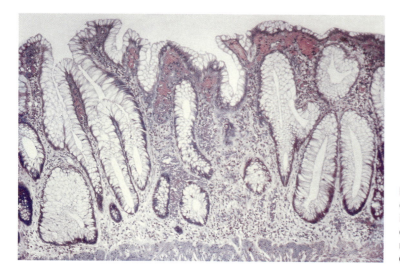

Figure 5.10 Resolving ulcerative colitis. The inflammatory cell infiltrate is now minimal but the crypt architectural deformity remains the hallmark of ulcerative colitis.

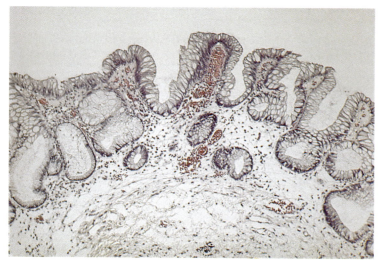

Figure 5.11 Quiescent ulcerative colitis. There is no inflammation and the crypts are distorted and short.

5.2.3 The phase of remission

5.2.3a The epithelium and crypts

Atrophy is the hallmark of this phase of the disease. In the typical case the mucosa appears thinned and the crypts are short and stubby (Fig. 5.11). This is best appreciated from the gap between the muscularis mucosae and the crypt bases. There is also a reduction in numbers of crypts per unit length of mucosa. The goblet cell population is usually normal at this stage and the surface flat. Paneth cell metaplasia is common within crypts and, while not a specific marker for ulcerative colitis, is helpful in indicating chronic damage (Watson and Roy, 1960; Dundas *et al.*, 1997) (Fig. 5.12). The crypts may also contain increased numbers of endocrine cells (Skinner *et al.*, 1971; Gledhill *et al.*, 1986). Care should be taken in distinguishing true atrophy from the artefact of over-zealous stretching of a biopsy and from the normally reduced numbers of crypts in biopsies taken close to the anal margin (Section 3.6.2).

5.2.3b The lamina propria

As expected, there is no active inflammatory cell component, in the form of neutrophils, in the phase of remission. Lymphocytes and plasma cells may

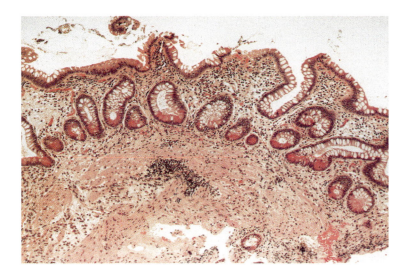

Figure 5.12 Chronic ulcerative colitis showing well-marked Paneth cell metaplasia.

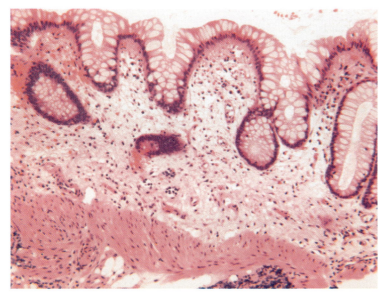

Figure 5.13 Ulcerative colitis in remission. There is hypocellularity of the lamina propria with crypt loss and those remaining are short, failing to extend to the muscularis mucosae.

be present in slightly raised numbers but often the lamina propria appears to have a reduced cellular component (Fig. 5.13). This is not the effect of oedema and no satisfactory explanation has been put forward for this observation. It may result from steroid therapy given to many patients by this time in the natural history of their disease. Multiple small vacuoles of fat or gas (Snover *et al.*, 1985; Gagliardi *et al.*, 1996) can replace much of the lamina propria in quiescent disease but are of no diagnostic value as they may be seen in otherwise normal biopsies (Section 3.8.12). While fibrosis

is not typically a feature of ulcerative colitis in remission we have seen cases in which a band of collagen is present in the mucosa between the base of the crypts and the muscularis mucosae (Fig. 5.14). This suggests scarring as a reaction to previous damage. There can also be reduplication of the muscularis mucosae (Fig. 5.2).

5.2.3c Difficulties with diagnosis

When seen in a biopsy the picture described above points strongly to a diagnosis of long-standing

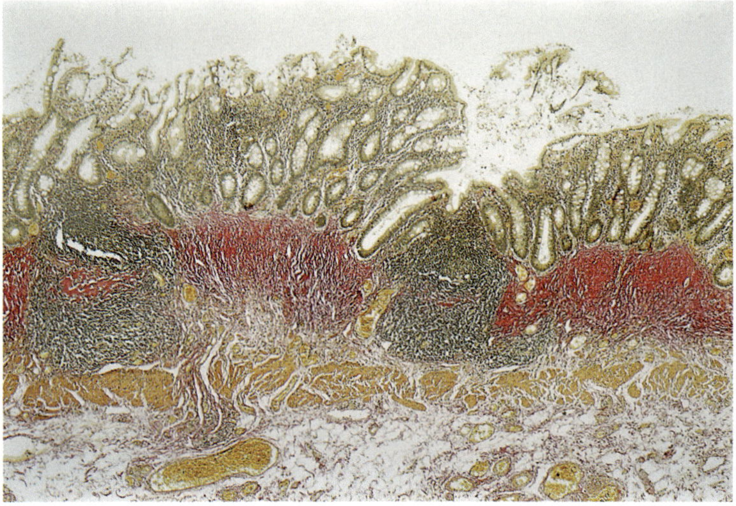

Figure 5.14 Details from a colectomy specimen in a case of chronic ulcerative colitis to demonstrate the unusual finding of fibrosis deep in the lamina propria. This could cause diagnostic confusion if sampled in a routine biopsy (Haematoxylin-van Gieson).

ulcerative colitis as the other common causes of colitis do not produce this atrophic picture. Healed ulceration of whatever cause may produce mucosal simplification but in such instances there is accompanying fibrosis within the lamina propria and the muscularis mucosae may also appear interrupted. It is unusual to see this picture during the initial presentation of the disease. However not all patients with long-standing disease progress to an overtly atrophic pattern; in some, irrespective of therapy, atrophy may be minimal and hard to appreciate. This is a particular diagnostic problem if the patient is presenting for the first time, despite a long history of chronic diarrhoea.

5.2.4 Lectins, adhesion molecules and mucins

Histopathologists yearn for some form of stain technology that will distinguish ulcerative colitis from Crohn's disease, at the least, and preferably from other forms of inflammatory bowel disease also. Much of the work has revolved around aspects of mucin histochemistry (Jass *et al.*, 1986), lectins, adhesion molecules and differences in mucosal immunoglobulins (Scott *et al.*, 1983) (Section 12.4.2). For example, it was shown that patients with chronic inflammatory bowel disease have significantly higher levels of mucosal IgG containing cells than those with ASLC (van Spreeuwel *et al.*, 1985).

While all have stimulated considerable interest and contributed significantly to the understanding of the pathogenesis of chronic inflammatory bowel disease no single distinguishing marker has emerged. There are much interesting data (Podolsky and Isselbacher, 1984; Jacobs and Huber, 1985; van Spreeuwel *et al.*, 1985; Yoshioka *et al.*, 1989; Jones *et al.*, 1995) but of the various methodologies it is still fair to state that none play a significant role in an individual case.

5.2.5 Summary

In the foregoing sections the bias has been towards the pathologist studying the initial rectal biopsy in a patient with typical ulcerative colitis. Of the three basic patterns – active disease, resolving disease and disease in remission – a confident opinion can be ventured on the first and last, always bearing in mind it is the combination of appearances, rather than any one feature, which distinguishes ulcerative colitis from the other conditions considered to be part of the differential diagnosis (Chapter 12). The combinations that the pathologist must seek in active ulcerative colitis are diffuse transmucosal inflammation, an abnormal crypt pattern, an undulating villous mucosal configuration and the dominance of crypt abscesses. In quiescent disease, crypt atrophy and the depleted cellular content of the lamina propria are key features. What is unknown is what determines the expression of each of the criteria. Riley *et al.* (1991) showed that that the presence of acute inflammation in rectal biopsies was associated with a more frequent relapse rate and that this was independent of the presence of chronic inflammation.

5.3 THE EQUIVOCAL BIOPSY

In a study at St Mark's Hospital, London, UK, a correct and confident diagnosis was given in 67 per cent of first biopsies in patients who, at subsequent surgery, had proven ulcerative colitis (Frei and Morson, 1982). This gives some idea of the likelihood of obtaining a typical biopsy at the first attempt using the subsequent surgical specimen as the outcome standard. Several purely biopsy studies focus on the criteria for distinguishing ASLC from ulcerative colitis (Section 4.2.5). If the criteria for selection of the diagnostic parameters are stringent the diagnostic accuracy is reported as over 90 per cent (Nostrant *et al.*, 1987; Dundas *et al.*, 1997). In their paper Nostrant *et al.* (1987) relied on crypt destruction with cryptal inflammation, architectural distortion, mucus depletion and transmural diffuse mixed inflammation, claiming a 100 per cent success rate in separating the two conditions. The variation in diagnostic success rates between authors is in part due to definitions of particular features, in particular crypt distortion versus crypt branching. Thus merely requiring the identification in a biopsy of two as opposed to one vertically branched crypts considerably alters the specificity and sensitivity of the success rate in distinguishing ulcerative colitis from ASLC (Schumacher *et al.*, 1994a; Dundas *et al.*, 1997). Whatever the definitions and selection of criteria, when the combination of these selected signs are insufficient a differential must be considered and this is discussed in Chapter 12. Having considered and rejected the other possibilities, if the overall picture still falls short of a confident opinion of ulcerative colitis, then it is only by sequential biopsies, accompanied by careful clinical and radiological assessment, that a diagnosis may eventually be reached. Use of the terms colitis indeterminate, colitis unspecified, colitis not further classified, etc.,

in such circumstances is discussed later (Section 12.3.3). Given the relative ease of obtaining sequential biopsies it is better to err on the side of diagnostic caution than attach a life-long label of chronic inflammatory bowel disease to a patient with all the accompanying social and economic implications that such a diagnosis carries.

5.4 SEQUENTIAL BIOPSIES

Sequential biopsy is part and parcel of the management of ulcerative colitis (Goldman, 1984). The aim of follow-up biopsies is usually one of the following: (a) to substantiate the diagnosis, (b) to monitor the activity of the disease, (c) to check on the effectiveness of therapy or (d) to detect the onset of precancerous changes. There is proportionately less concern with the diagnostic criteria, although in some cases it may take several biopsies over a period of time to form a confident opinion. Many will have experienced the chagrin of finding a granuloma in a patient previously believed safely classified as suffering from ulcerative colitis but care needs to be taken not to change the diagnosis solely because of identifying a cryptal granuloma (Mahadeva *et al.*, 2002). Follow-up biopsies should always be compared with earlier ones, commenting particularly on the change in inflammatory infiltrate, the degree of architectural damage and, when relevant, the presence or absence of dysplasia.

The typical sequence is of a diagnostic biopsy showing florid acute inflammation, followed several weeks later by a biopsy to assess treatment. The picture will usually have changed from that of the active phase of disease to that of a resolving pattern (Schumacher *et al.*, 1994a) (Fig. 5.15). It is not known why some patients have chronic intermittent disease with a near-normal biopsy between attacks (Fig. 5.4), whereas others experience continuous low-grade disease and correspondingly abnormal biopsies. In general, in ulcerative colitis the colorectal biopsy mirrors the clinical situation with the exception of the fulminant attack (Section 5.7). In the colon as a whole, the depth of ulceration correlates well with the likelihood of toxic dilatation (Buckall *et al.*, 1980).

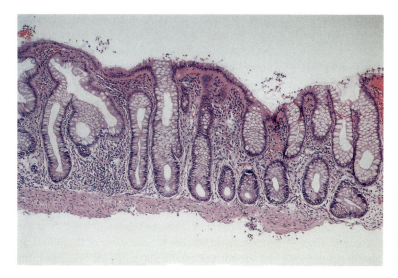

Figure 5.15 Resolving ulcerative colitis showing the start of crypt architectural damage, but with the goblet cell population restored, inflammation is minor and less uniform.

While the inevitability of permanent rectal damage in ulcerative colitis is no longer dogma, if a follow-up rectal biopsy is entirely normal there should still be a careful reassessment of the original findings and of the clinical and radiological data, as the occurrence is still uncommon.

5.5 COLONOSCOPIC BIOPSY

Most of the remarks applicable to the interpretation of rectal biopsy in the diagnosis of ulcerative colitis also apply to colonoscopic biopsy. A colonoscopic examination will have been undertaken to help establish the diagnosis, if rectal biopsy was equivocal, to assess the extent of disease or to monitor treatment and onset of complications (Waye, 1980). To be able to map the distribution and extent of disease individually sited biopsies should either be placed in separate containers or placed in order on a cellulose strip. This technique considerably reduces a laboratory's workload (Chapter 1; Figs 1.1–1.3). It is important that the endoscopic findings are also sent to the pathologist.

5.5.1 The colonoscopist's report

A good colonoscopist will provide a macroscopic account that is equivalent to examining the surgical specimen. In active ulcerative colitis the rectum, with rare exceptions that are mainly in children (Markowitz *et al.*, 1993; Washington *et al.*, 2002; Robert *et al.*, 2004b), will be involved with disease spreading proximally for a varying distance. When the presenting history is short, disease is limited to the rectum and sigmoid in 58 per cent of patients, in 2 per cent the whole left colon is involved and in 14 per cent a total colitis is present (Ritchie *et al.*, 1978a). The mucosa is red, granular and friable (Fig. 5.7b). Ulcers appear as thin layers of slough on this abnormal background. Overall, there is an even pattern of disease in the involved areas.

Spontaneous rectal sparing is rare and has been discussed previously but is mimicked if healing is promoted by steroid enemas. Not all areas of the affected colon need be equally active, especially after treatment and this may give a false impression of segmental disease (Bernstein *et al.*, 1995; Kleer and Appelman, 1998; Kim *et al.*, 1999). It is accepted that radiology underestimates the extent of disease compared with colonoscopy, which, in turn, underestimates involvement compared with histology (Gabrielsson *et al.*, 1979). The endoscopist must not believe that, because he sees no changes, the mucosa is normal (Myren *et al.*, 1976; Rhodes, 2001). Moum *et al.* (1999) found that microscopy showed more extensive disease at diagnosis than direct visualization and this had risen to 28 per cent at follow-up examination. Having gone to the trouble of colonoscopic examination, biopsies should always be taken (Holdstock *et al.*, 1984). It is also important to take a rectal biopsy at the time of colonoscopy. The diagnostic importance, if this is normal, is reconsidered in Section 12.2.

5.5.2 Colonoscopic biopsies – variable patterns of involvement

The belief that ulcerative colitis invariably exhibits an even, continuous pattern of proximal spread that commences in the rectum, like the dogma that rectal damage is inevitable and permanent, has had to be modified in recent years (Bernstein *et al.*, 1995; Kleer and Appelman, 1998; Kim *et al.*, 1999). Nevertheless, this still remains the commonest pattern of involvement for the large majority of cases and should still be considered the working rule.

5.5.2a The 'skip' lesion

This is a term that used to herald a diagnosis of Crohn's disease but is now also used to describe a particular pattern of inflammation in ulcerative colitis. It denotes rectal or left-sided disease in conjunction with a segment of right-sided disease particularly involving the caecum and/or appendix (D'Haens *et al.*, 1997; Hill *et al.*, 2002) (Fig. 5.16). The intervening mucosa is normal. Alone, such a discontinuous pattern of inflammation does not denote Crohn's disease. A critical assessment of the individual histological features, as outlined in this chapter, must still be made to determine the correct diagnosis. It is claimed that this discontinuous pattern of colonic involvement in ulcerative colitis has a similar natural history to left-sided disease (Mutinga *et al.*, 2004).

5.5.2b Patchy disease

Several authors draw attention to the point that patchy disease, be it between biopsy sites or within a single biopsy, can occur in ulcerative colitis (Bernstein *et al.*, 1995; Kleer and Appelman, 1998; Kim *et al.*, 1999). This is most often the case in patients on treatment (Odze *et al.*, 1993) and is not necessarily a marker for Crohn's disease.

5.5.3 Interpretation of colonoscopic biopsies

Exactly the same diagnostic attributes apply to each colonoscopic biopsy as to a rectal biopsy. The biopsy is usually smaller, making evaluation more difficult, but the sampling error is reduced by including tissue from multiple sites. In diagnostic terms, colonoscopic biopsies are most useful when the rectal biopsy has failed to show sufficient criteria for a confident opinion. A series of diffusely inflamed colonoscopic biopsies throughout the left side of the colon and a normal right colon, or at least a lesser degree of inflammatory change, put more weight behind a diagnosis of ulcerative colitis than would be possible if only an equivocal rectal biopsy were available (Bentley *et al.*, 2002). As already discussed, some variation in activity from site to site is allowed, especially in treated patients, but a completely normal biopsy among a series of abnormal ones should lead to a questioning of the diagnosis and review of the other diagnostic data, having taken account of the possibility of the caecal/appendiceal skip lesion discussed in the preceding section (Section 5.5.2). Perhaps the biggest discrepancy in involvement is seen in the fulminant attack (Section 5.7).

A colonoscopic series of biopsies gives the true extent of disease (Farmer *et al.*, 1980; Moum *et al.*, 1999). Coupled with this, the degree of inflammatory activity and mucosal architectural damage provide accurate data of severity. However, as with microscopic colitis, where normal endoscopy does not equal normal histology, mucosal disease can be overlooked at endoscopy in ulcerative colitis (Kleer and Appelman, 1998; Rhodes, 2001). This is particularly the case when defining the proximal extent of disease and was appreciated in the early studies on ulcerative colitis (Truelove and Richards, 1956). As mentioned earlier (Section 5.1) between 10 per cent and 20 per cent of patients presenting with disease limited to the rectum progress to more extensive left-sided colitis at 5 years. The cumulative risk for total colitis eventually rises to 30 per cent (Ritchie *et al.*, 1978a; Ayres *et al.*, 1996). It is well known that patients with total or extensive colitis have an increased risk of developing cancer and precancer (Lennard-Jones *et al.*, 1977; Axon,

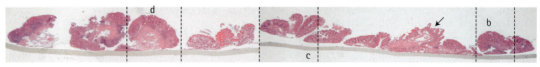

(a)

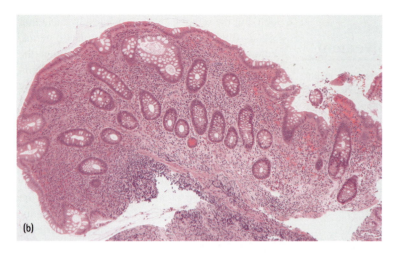

(b)

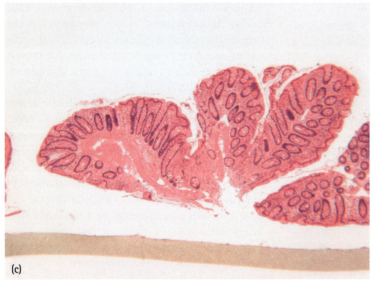

(c)

Figure 5.16 (a–d) This series of illustrations demonstrates the 'skip' lesion or caecal patch seen in some instances of ulcerative colitis. (a) The entire colonoscopic series is seen aligned on a cellulose strip: Even at this low magnification it is clear that the caecal biopsies (b), to the right of the ileal biopsy (arrow) with its villi evident, are inflamed, the mid colonic biopsies are not involved (c) and the recto-sigmoid mucosa is inflamed (d). The caecal biopsy (b) shows inflammation and some crypt distortion. (c) The biopsies from the region of the transverse colon not involved.

1997) but there is also evidence to show a small but significant increased risk in those with only left-sided disease (Nugent *et al.*, 1991; Sugita *et al.*, 1991). This makes accurate assessment of extent by colonoscopic biopsy mandatory in the long-term management of ulcerative colitis. Colonoscopic screening for dysplastic changes is discussed in Chapter 17.

5.5.4 Biopsy interpretation and treatment

Treatment has an influence on biopsy morphology which has been alluded to on several occasions in this chapter. For example, 5-amino salicylic acid can normalize the rectal histology (Odze *et al.*, 1993). When reporting biopsies it is important to be aware

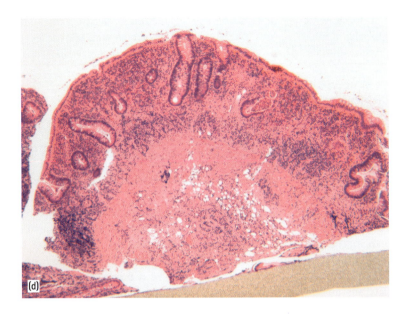

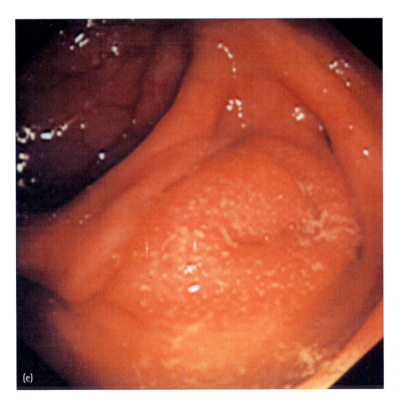

Figure 5.16 (d) The sigmoid biopsy shows severe diffuse inflammation, crypt distortion, crypt abscesses and goblet depletion. (e) The granular appearance of the inflamed caecum and peri-appendicular region is seen on colonoscopy.

of treatment regimens, especially if faced with atypical microscopy in what was thought to be a typical case of ulcerative colitis, and certainly before changing a previous diagnostic opinion. The changes produced depend on the type of treatment, whether topical or systemic, and on the individual as responses vary (Geboes and Dalle, 2002). In ulcerative colitis the aim is to overcome the inflammatory response but the outcome is not necessarily uniform around the colon. This results in patchy disease both on endoscopy and microscopy (Bernstein *et al.*, 1995; Kleer and Appelman, 1998; Kim *et al.*, 1999; Geboes, 2001). The unwary might be misled to diagnose resolving infection or Crohn's disease. Generally, in those that respond to treatment, the neutrophil polymorphs disappear rapidly in days or a short number of weeks. The chronic inflammatory cell infiltrate takes more time to resolve and diminishes over weeks or months and in some cases persists as a permanent low-grade infiltrate. The architectural damage is mostly permanent with some exceptions, as discussed earlier (Bernstein *et al.*, 1995; Levine *et al.*, 1996). In clinical practice the rate of histological resolution of inflammation can be adapted to act as a scoring system to measure drug efficacy (Geboes and Dalle, 2002) and to predict the likelihood of relapse (Riley *et al.*, 1991).

5.6 INFLAMMATORY POLYPS ('PSEUDOPOLYPS')

Polyps are a frequent finding on barium enema or at colonoscopy in patients with ulcerative colitis and are usually of the inflammatory type ('pseudopolyps') (Day *et al.*, 2003). They indicate a prior severe bout of mucosal ulceration, with irregular healing, leaving a tag of mucosa protruding from the surface (Price, 1978a; Kelly and Gabos, 1987). Biopsy is the only acceptable way to make the distinction from true neoplastic polyps (adenomas).

Inflammatory polyps may comprise granulation tissue, a mixture of glands and granulation tissue, or a tag of virtually normal mucosa. There is no dysplasia and these polyps are of no significance; they are simply a reflection of the patient's past

and not an omen for the future. Occasionally large localized masses of such polyps form and can even be a cause of obstruction (Munchar *et al.*, 2001; Yada *et al.*, 2005).

5.7 FULMINANT ACUTE COLITIS (TOXIC DILATATION)

This occurs in from 1.6 per cent to 17 per cent of patients with ulcerative colitis, depending on the population studied (Edwards and Truelove, 1964; Jalan *et al.*, 1969; Gan and Beck, 2003). No histological features have been described which forecast the outcome in any one case. Colonoscopy is contraindicated in toxic dilatation and a rectal biopsy is the only practical procedure available for a tissue diagnosis. Unfortunately, however, the main impact of the fulminant attack is most often on the transverse colon and the rectum is relatively spared (Lumb *et al.*, 1955), failing to provide diagnostic changes. Thus, being confronted with minimal changes in a rectal biopsy in a clinical case of fulminant colitis does not necessarily indicate Crohn's disease or, indeed, rule out ulcerative colitis.

Care must also be exercised in interpreting a colonoscopic series in patients developing dilatation but in whom colonoscopy is not yet contraindicated. The pattern of inflammation in such cases is misleading. Ulcerated areas occur adjacent to 'polypoid' islands of surviving mucosa (Fazio, 1980). The latter show surprisingly little inflammation despite the proximity to severe disease. The crypt architecture may also often be intact (Price, 1978b). Biopsies from areas of ulceration are unhelpful, showing only slough or granulation tissue. Further misleading features in fulminant colitis are the transmural nature of the inflammation and the regular pattern of fissuring common to all causes of toxic dilatation (Lumb *et al.*, 1955; Price, 1978b). They are not diagnostic of Crohn's disease in this clinical situation (Yantiss *et al.*, 2006). These misleading features have led to the use of the term 'indeterminate colitis' (Price, 1978b; Geboes *et al.*, 2003; Guindi and

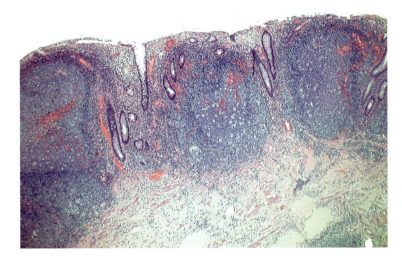

Figure 5.17 Follicular proctitis in ulcerative colitis. The mucosa is thickened and expanded by large lymphoid follicles displacing the crypts.

Riddell, 2004) in surgical cases and the use of this term in biopsy work is discussed in Section 12.3.3.

(Section 18.3) when considering this follicular pattern in biopsy work.

5.8 FOLLICULAR PROCTITIS

Lymphoid follicles are part of the normal histology of the rectal mucosa. In many biopsies from patients with established ulcerative colitis large numbers of follicles lie in the mucosa and there is atrophy of the crypts (Fig. 5.17). The follicles are usually accompanied by a diffuse infiltrate of plasma cells, neutrophil polymorphs and crypt irregularity, characteristic of ulcerative colitis. The reason for the predominant follicles is not known but it has been accepted as a pattern from which to diagnose ulcerative colitis or limited idiopathic proctitis. Lymphoid follicles are also a prominent feature of biopsies from the defunctioned rectum, when they become hyperplastic.

A form of follicular proctitis distinct from the above may exist (Flejou *et al.*, 1988). Here, there is no accompanying inflammation, apart from the follicular hyperplasia, and, clinically, the patient's only complaint is rectal bleeding. Follicles are clearly visible as a nodular mucosa with a sharp proximal rectal margin. Whether or not this is a separate entity remains to be documented. Care must be taken to exclude lymphoid polyps (Section 15.13), lymphomatous polyposis and lymphoma

5.9 CONCLUSIONS

This chapter has been primarily restricted to the diagnostic features of ulcerative colitis and assessment of its extent and progress. Much is written about the various histological attributes in inflammatory bowel disease of all types. In our view only a select few are critical when compiling any individual patient's report. Colonoscopy, by providing information on the distribution of disease, increases diagnostic accuracy, whereas any one biopsy may be equivocal. Since the first edition of this book, an appreciation has developed that a small but significant number of cases of ulcerative colitis may yield normal rectal biopsies at some stage in their course, may exhibit right-sided skip lesions and that the inflammatory infiltrate may show variability both within and between individual biopsies.

REFERENCES

Anthonisen, P., Rus, P. (1971) Eosinophilic granulocytes in the rectal mucosa of patients with ulcerative colitis and Crohn's disease of ileum and colon. *Scand. J. Gastroenterol.*, 6, 731–4.

Axon, A.T. (1997) Screening and surveillance of ulcerative colitis. *Gastrointest. Endosc. Clin. N. Am.*, 7, 129–45.

Ayres, R.C., Gillen, C.D., Walmsley, R.S., Allen, R.N. (1996) Progression of ulcerative proctosigmoiditis: incidence and factors influencing progression. *Eur. J. Gastroenterol. Hepatol.*, 8, 555–8.

Bentley, E., Jenkins, D., Campbell, F., Warren, B. (2002) How could pathologists improve the initial diagnosis of colitis? Evidence from an international workshop. *J. Clin. Pathol.*, 55, 955–60.

Bernstein, C.N.B., Shanahan, F., Anton, P.A., Weinstein, W.M. (1995) Patchiness of mucosal inflammation in treated ulcerative colitis: a prospective study. *Gastrointest. Endosc.*, 42, 232–7.

Buckall, N.A., Williams, C.T., Bartram, C.L., Lennard-Jones, J.E. (1980) Depth of ulceration in acute colitis. *Gastroenterology*, 79, 19–25.

Cook, M.C., Dixon, M.F. (1973) An analysis of the reliability of detection and diagnostic value of various pathological features in Crohn's disease and ulcerative colitis. *Gut*, 14, 255–62.

Das, K.M., Morecki, R., Nair, P., Berkowitz, J.M. (1977) Idiopathic proctitis: the morphology of proximal colonic mucosa and its clinical significance. *Am. Dig. Dis.*, 22, 524–8.

Day, D.W., Jass, J.R., Price, A.B. *et al.* (2003) *Morson and Dawson's gastrointestinal pathology*, 4th edn. Oxford: Blackwell.

D'Haens, G., Genoes, K., Peeters, M., Baert, F., Ectors, N., Rutgeerts, P. (1997) Patchy and caecal inflammation associated with distal ulcerative colitis, a prospective endoscopic study. *Am. J. Gastroenterol.*, 92, 1275–9.

Dick, A.P., Grayson, M.J. (1961) Ulcerative colitis. A follow up investigation with mucosal biopsy studies. *Br. Med. J.*, 1, 160–5.

Domizio, P. (1994) Pathology of chronic inflammatory bowel disease in children. *Baillieres Clin. Gastroenterol.*, 8(1), 35–63.

Dukes, C., Bussey, H.J.R. (1926) The number of lymphoid follicles in the human large intestine. *J. Pathol. Bacteriol.*, 29, 111–16.

Dundas, S.A.C., Dutton, J., Skipworth, P. (1997) Reliability of rectal biopsy in distinguishing between chronic inflammatory bowel disease and acute self-limiting colitis. *Histopathology*, 31, 60–6.

Edwards, F.C., Truelove, S.C. (1963) The course and prognosis of ulcerative colitis, Parts I and II. *Gut*, 4, 299–315.

Edwards, F.C., Truelove, S.C. (1964) The course and prognosis of ulcerative colitis, Parts III and IV. *Gut*, 5, 1–22.

Farmer, R.G., (1987) Non-specific ulcerative proctitis. *Gastroenterol. Clin. N. Am.*, 16, 157–74.

Farmer, R.G., Whelan, G., Swak, M.V. (1980) Colonoscopy in distal ulcerative colitis. *Clin. Gastroenterol.*, 9, 297–306.

Fazio, V.W. (1980) Toxic megacolon in ulcerative colitis and Crohn's colitis. *Clin. Gastroenterol.*, 9(2), 389–408.

Flejou, J-F., Potet, F., Bogomoletz, W.V. *et al.* (1988) Lymphoid follicular proctitis. A condition different from ulcerative proctitis? *Dig. Dis. Sci.*, 33, 314–20.

Franzin, G., Grigioni, W.F., Dina, R., Scarpa, A., Zamboni, G. (1983) Mucin secretion and morphological changes of the mucosa in non-neoplastic diseases of the colon. *Histopathology*, 7, 707–18.

Frei, J.V., Morson, B.C. (1982) Medical audit of rectal biopsy diagnosis of inflammatory bowel disease. *J. Clin. Pathol.*, 35, 341–4.

Gabrielsson, N., Granquist, S., Sundelin, P., Thorgeirsson, T. (1979) Extent of inflammatory lesions in ulcerative colitis assessed by radiology, colonoscopy and endoscopic biopsies. *Gastrointest. Radiol.*, 4, 395–400.

Gagliardi, G., Thompson, I.W., Hershman, M.J., Forbes, A., Hawley, P.R., Talbot, I.C. (1996) Pneumatosis coli: a proposed pathogenesis based on study of 25 cases and review of the literature. *Int. J. Colorectal Dis.*, 11, 111–18.

Gan, S.I., Beck, P.L. (2003) A new look at toxic megacolon: an update and review of incidence, etiology, pathogenesis, and management. *Am. J. Gastroenterol.*, 98, 2363–71.

Geboes, K. (2001) Pathology of inflammatory bowel disease (IBD): variability with time and treatment. *Colorectal Dis.*, 3, 2–12.

Geboes, K., Dalle, I. (2002) Influence of treatment on morphological features of mucosal inflammation. *Gut*, 50(Suppl. 3), III, 37–42.

Geboes, K., Joossens, S., Prantera, C., Rutgeerts, P. (2003) Indeterminate colitis in clinical practice. *Curr. Diagn. Pathol.*, 9, 179–87.

Gledhill, A., Enticott, M.E., Howe, S. (1986) Variation in the argyrophil cell population of the rectum in ulcerative colitis and adenocarcinoma. *J. Pathol.*, 149, 287–91.

Goldman, H. (1984) Acute versus chronic colitis: how and when to distinguish by biopsy. *Gastroenterology*, 86, 199–201.

Goldman, H. (1994) Interpretation of large intestinal mucosal biopsy specimens. *Hum. Pathol.*, 25, 1150–9.

Goldman, H., Antonioli, D.A. (1982) Mucosal biopsy of the rectum, colon and distal ileum. *Hum. Pathol.*, 13, 981–1012.

Goulston, S.J.M., McGovern, V.J. (1969) The nature of benign strictures in ulcerative colitis. *N. Engl. J. Med.*, 281, 290–5.

Guindi, M., Riddell, R.H. (2004) Indeterminate colitis. *J. Clin. Pathol.*, 57, 1233–44.

Heatley, R.V., James, P.D. (1978) Eosinophils in the rectal mucosa. A simple method of predicting the outcome of ulcerative proctitis. *Gut*, 20, 787–91.

Hellstrom, H.R., Fisher, E.R. (1967) Estimation of mucosal mucin as an aid in the differentiation of Crohn's disease of the colon and chronic ulcerative colitis. *Am. J. Clin. Pathol.*, 48, 259–68.

Hill, M.D., Davies, G., McIntyre, A.S., Gerard, D.A. (2002) Proctitis with caecitis: an atypical presentation of ulcerative colitis. *Endoscopy*, 34, 664–6.

Holdstock, G., DuBoulay, C.E., Smith, C.L. (1984) Survey of the use of colonoscopy in inflammatory bowel disease. *Dig. Dis. Sci.*, 29, 731–4.

Jacobs, L.R., Huber, P.W. (1985) Regional distribution and alterations of lectin binding to colorectal mucin in mucosal biopsies from controls and subjects with inflammatory bowel disease. *J. Clin. Invest.*, 75, 112–18.

Jalan, K.N., Sircus, W., Card, W.I. *et al.* (1969) An experience of ulcerative colitis. 1, Toxic dilation in 55 cases. *Gastroenterology*, 57, 68–82.

Jass, J.R., England, J., Miller, K. (1986) Value of mucin histochemistry in follow-up surveillance of patients with long standing ulcerative colitis. *J. Clin. Pathol.*, 39, 393–8.

Jenkins, D., Goodall, A., Scott, B.B. (1997) Simple objective criteria for diagnosis of causes of acute diarrhoea on rectal biopsy. *J. Clin. Pathol.*, 50, 580–5.

Jones, S.C., Banks, R.E., Haidar, A. *et al.* (1995) Adhesion molecules in inflammatory bowel disease. *Gut*, 36, 724–30.

Kelly, J.K., Gabos, S. (1987) The pathogenesis of inflammatory polyps. *Dis. Colon Rectum*, 30, 251–4.

Kim, B., Barnett, J.L., Kleer, C.G., Appelman, H.D. (1999) Endoscopic and histological patchiness in treated ulcerative colitis. *Am. J. Gastroenterol.*, 84, 3258–62.

Kleer, C.G., Appelman, H.D. (1998) Ulcerative colitis: patterns of involvement in colorectal biopsies and changes with time. *Am. J. Surg. Pathol.*, 22, 983–9.

Kumar, N.B., Nostrant, T.T., Appelman, H.D. (1982) The histopathological spectrum of acute self-limited colitis (acute infectious-type colitis). *Am. J. Surg. Pathol.*, 6, 523–9.

Kundhal, P.S., Stormon, M.O., Zachos, M., Critch, J.N., Cutz, E., Griffiths, A.M. (2003) Gastral antral biopsy in the differentiation of pediatric colitides. *Am. J. Gastroenterol.*, 98, 557–61.

Lennard-Jones, J.E., Morson, B.C., Ritchie, J.K., Shove, D.C., Williams, C.B. (1977) Cancer in colitis: assessment of the individual risk by clinical and histological criteria. *Gastroenterology*, 73, 1280–9.

Levine, T.S., Tzardi, M., Mitchell, S., Sowter, C., Price, A.B. (1996) Diagnostic difficulty arising from rectal recovery in ulcerative colitis. *J. Clin. Pathol.*, 50, 319–23.

Lumb, C., Protheroe, R.H.B., Ramsay, C.S. (1955) Ulcerative colitis with dilatation of the colon. *Br. J. Surg.*, 43, 182–8.

McCormick, D.A., Horton, L.W., Mee, A.S. (1990) Mucin depletion in inflammatory bowel disease. *J. Clin. Pathol.*, 43, 143–6.

Mahadeva, U., Martin, J.P., Patel, N.K., Price, A.B. (2002) Granulomatous ulcerative colitis: a re-appraisal of the mucosal granuloma in the distinction of Crohn's disease from ulcerative colitis. *Histopathology*, 41, 50–5.

Markowitz, J., Kahn, E., Grancher, K., Hyams, J., Treem, W., Daum, F. (1993) Atypical rectosigmoid histology in children with newly diagnosed ulcerative colitis. *Am. J. Gastro-enterol.*, 88, 2034–7.

Morson, B.C. (1971) Histopathology of Crohn's disease, *Scand. J. Gastroenterol.*, 6, 573–5.

Moum, B., Ekbom, A., Vatn, M.H. *et al.* (1997a) Clinical course during the 1st year after diagnosis in ulcerative colitis and Crohn's disease. Results of a large, prospective population-based study in south eastern Norway, 1990–93. *Scand. J. Gastroenterol.*, 32, 1005–12.

Moum, B., Ekbom, A., Vatn, M.H. *et al.* (1997b) Inflammatory bowel disease: re-evaluation of the diagnosis in a prospective population based study in south eastern Norway. *Gut*, 40, 328–32.

Moum, B., Ekbom, A., Vatn, M.H., Elgjo, K. (1999) Change in the extent of colonoscopic and histological involvement in ulcerative colitis over time. *Am. J. Gastroenterol.*, 94, 1564–9.

Munchar, J., Rahman, H.A., Zawawi, M.M. (2001) Localised giant pseudopolyposis in ulcerative colitis. *Eur. J. Gastroenterol. Hepatol.*, 13, 1385–7.

Mutinga, M.L., Odze, R.D., Wang, H.H., Hornick, J.L., Farraye, F.A. (2004) The clinical significance of right-sided colonic inflammation in patients with left-sided chronic ulcerative colitis. *Inflamm. Bowel Dis.*,10, 215–19.

Myren, J., Serek-Hanssen, A., Solberg, L. (1976) Routine and blind histological diagnoses on colonoscopic biopsies compared to clinical colonoscopic observations in patients without and with colitis. *Scand. J. Gastroenterol.*, 11, 135–40.

Nostrant, T.T., Kumar, N.B., Appelman, H.D. (1987) Histopathology differentiates acute self-limiting colitis from ulcerative colitis. *Gastroenterology*, 92, 318–28.

Nugent, F.W., Haggitt, R.C., Gilpin, P.A. (1991) Cancer surveillance in ulcerative colitis. *Gastroenterology*, 100, 1241–8.

Odze, R., Antonioli, D., Peppercorn, M., Goldman, H. (1993) Effect of topical 5-aminosalycylic acid (5-ASA) therapy on rectal mucosal biopsy morphology in chronic ulcerative colitis. *Am. J. Surg. Pathol.*, 17, 869–75.

Paoluzi, P., Iannoni, C., Marcheggiano, A. *et al.* (1984) Tissue eosinophils count in ulcerative colitis. *Ital. J. Gastroenterol.*, 16, 99–101.

Podolsky, D.K., Isselbacher, K.J. (1984) Glycoprotein composition of colonic mucosa. Specific alterations in ulcerative colitis. *Gastroenterology*, 87, 991–8.

Price, A.B. (1978a) Benign lymphoid polyps and inflammatory polyps, In: Morson, B.C. (ed.) *Pathogenesis of colorectal cancer (major problems in pathology)*. Philadelphia and London: Saunders, pp. 33–42.

Price, A.B. (1978b) Overlap in the spectrum of non–specific inflammatory bowel disease – 'colitis indeterminate'. *J. Clin. Pathol.*, 31, 567–77.

Price, A.B., Morson, B.C. (1975) Inflammatory bowel disease: the surgical pathology of Crohn's disease and ulcerative colitis. *Hum. Pathol.*, 6, 7–29.

Price, A.B., Jewkes, J., Sanderson, P.J. (1979) Acute diarrhoea: *Campylobacter* colitis and the role of rectal biopsy. *J. Clin. Pathol.*, 32, 990–7.

Rhodes, J.M. (2001) Ulcerative colitis extent varies with time but endoscopic appearances may be deceptive. *Gut*, 49, 322–3.

Riley, S.A., Mani, V., Goodman, M.J., Dutt, S., Herd, M.E. (1991) Microscopic activity in ulcerative colitis. *Gut*, 32, 174–8.

Ritchie, J.K., Powell-Tuck, J., Lennard-Jones, J.E. (1978a) Clinical outcome of the first ten years of ulcerative colitis and proctitis. *Lancet*, i, 1140–4.

Ritchie, J.K., Powell-Tuck, J., Lennard-Jones, J.E. (1978b) The prognosis of idiopathic proctitis. *Scand. J. Gastroenterol.*, 12, 727–32.

Robert, M.E., Skacel, M., Ullman, T., Bernstein, C.N. Easley, K., Goldblum, J.R. (2004a) Patterns of colonic involvement at initial presentation in ulcerative colitis: a retrospective study of 46 newly diagnosed cases. *Am. J. Clin. Pathol.*, 122, 94–9.

Robert, M.E., Tang, L., Hao, L.M., Reyes-Mugica, M. (2004b) Patterns of mucosal inflammation in mucosal biopsies of ulcerative colitis: perceived differences in pediatric populations are limited to children younger than 10 years. *Am. J. Surg. Pathol.*, 28, 183–9.

Sarin, S.K., Malhotra, Y., Sen Gupta, S., Karol, A., Gaur, S.K., Anand, B.S. (1987) Significance of eosinophils and mast cell counts in rectal mucosa in ulcerative colitis. A prospective controlled trial. *Dig. Dis. Sci.*, 32, 363–7.

Schachter, H., Goldstein, M.J., Rappaport, H., Fennessy, M.B., Kirsner, J.B. (1970) Ulcerative and 'granulomatous' colitis – validity of differential diagnostic criteria: a study of 100 patients treated by total colectomy. *Ann. Intern. Med.*, 72, 841–51.

Schumacher, G., Sandstedt, B., Mollby, R., Kollberg, B. (1991) Clinical and histological features differentiating non-relapsing colitis from first attacks of inflammatory bowel disease. *Scand. J. Gastroenterol.*, 26, 151–61.

Schumacher, G., Kollberg, B., Sandstedt, B. (1994a) A prospective study of first attacks of inflammatory bowel disease and infectious colitis: Histologic course during the first year after presentation. *Scand. J. Gastroenterol.*, 29, 318–32.

Schumacher, G., Sandstedt, B., Kollberg, B. (1994b) A prospective study of first attacks of inflammatory bowel disease and infectious colitis: clinical findings and early disease. *Scand. J. Gastroenterol.*, 29, 265–74.

Scott, B.B., Goodall, A., Stephenson, P., Jenkins, D. (1983) Rectal mucosal plasma cells in inflammatory bowel disease. *Gut*, 24, 519–24.

Seldenrijk, C.A., Morson, B.C., Meuwissen, S.G., Schipper, N.W., Lindeman, J., Meijer, C.J. (1991) Histopathological evaluation of colonic mucosal biopsy specimens in chronic inflammatory bowel disease: diagnostic implications. *Gut*, 32, 1514–20.

Sharif, F., McDermott, M., Dillon, M. *et al.* (2002) Focally enhanced gastritis in children with Crohn's disease and ulcerative colitis. *Am. J. Gastroenterol.*, 97, 1415–20.

Skinner, J.M., Whitehead, R., Piris, J. (1971) Argentaffin cells in ulcerative colitis. *Gut*, 12, 636–8.

Spiliadis, C.A., Spiliadis, C.A., Lennard-Jones, J.E. (1987) Ulcerative colitis with relative sparing of the rectum. Clinical features, histology, and prognosis. *Dis. Colon Rectum*, 30, 334–6.

Snover, D.C., Sandstad, J., Hutton, S. (1985) Mucosal pseudolipomatosis of the colon. *Am. J. Clin. Pathol.*, 84, 575–80.

Sugita, A., Sachar, D.B., Bodian, C., Ribeiro, M.B., Aufses, A.H. Jr., Greenstein, A.J. (1991) Colorectal cancer in ulcerative colitis. Influence of anatomical extent and age of onset on colitis–cancer interval. *Gut*, 32, 167–9.

Surawicz, M.C., Belic, L. (1984) Rectal biopsy helps to distinguish acute self-limited colitis from idiopathic inflammatory bowel disease. *Gastroenterology*, 86, 104–13.

Truelove, S.C., Richards, W.C.D. (1956) Biopsy studies in ulcerative colitis. *Br. Med. J.*, i, 1315–8.

Therkildsen, M.H., Jensen, B.N., Teglbjaerg, P.S., Rasmussen, S.N. (1989) The final outcome of patients presenting with their first episode of acute diarrhoea and an inflamed rectal mucosa with preserved crypt architecture. A clinicopathologic study. *Scand. J. Gastroenterol.*, 24, 158–64.

van Spreeuwel, J.P., Lindeman, J., Meijer, C.J. (1985) A quantitative study of immuno-globulin containing cells in the differential diagnosis of acute colitis. *J. Clin. Pathol.*, 38, 774–7.

Washington, K., Greenson, J.K., Montgomery, E. *et al.* (2002) Histopathology of ulcerative colitis in initial rectal biopsy in children. *Am. J. Surg. Pathol.*, 26, 1441–9.

Watson, A.J., Roy, A.D. (1960) Paneth cells in the large intestine in ulcerative colitis. *J. Pathol. Bacteriol.*, 80, 309–16.

Waye, J.D. (1980) Endoscopy in inflammatory bowel disease. *Clin. Gastroenterol.*, 9(2), 279–96.

Whitehead, R. (1985) Mucosal biopsy of the gastrointestinal tract. In: Bennington, J.L. (ed.) *Major problems in pathology*, Vol. 3. Philadelphia and London: Saunders, p. 215.

Yada, S., Matsumoto, T., Kudo, T., Hirahashi, M., Yaop, T., Mibu, R., Iida, M. (2005) Colonic obstruction due to giant inflammatory polyposis in a patient with ulcerative colitis. *J. Gastroenterol.*, 40, 536–9.

Yantiss, R.K., Farraye, F.A., O'Brien, M.J. *et al.* (2006) Prognostic significance of superficial fissuring ulceration in patients with severe 'indeterminate' colitis. *Am. J. Surg. Pathol.*, 30, 165–70.

Yoshioka, H., Inada, M., Ogawa, K., Ohshio, G., Yamabe, H., Hamashima, Y., Miyake, T. (1989) Lectin histochemistry in ulcerative colitis and Crohn's disease. *J. Exp. Pathol.*, 4, 69–78.

CHAPTER 6

CROHN'S DISEASE

6.1 Introduction	113	
6.2 Making the diagnosis	113	
6.3 Histopathology	114	
6.3.1 Epithelial and crypt changes	114	
6.3.2 Lamina propria and inflammation	115	
6.3.3 The granuloma	115	
6.3.4 The aphthoid ulcer	117	
6.3.5 Fissures	118	
6.3.6 Submucosa: disproportionate inflammation and neural hyperplasia	118	
6.4 Differential diagnosis	118	
6.4.1 Pre-pouch ileitis	119	

6.5 Disease activity	119
6.6 Indicators of prognosis	120
6.7 Colonoscopic biopsy in Crohn's disease	120
6.7.1 The colonoscopist's report	120
6.7.2 The colonoscopic biopsy	120
6.8 Complications	121
6.8.1 Inflammatory polyps ('pseudopolyps')	121
6.8.2 Toxic megacolon	121
6.9 Conclusions	121
References	121

6.1 INTRODUCTION

Crohn's disease may affect any part of the gastro-intestinal tract (Basu et al., 1975; Dunne et al., 1977), though it most commonly presents as regional ileitis (Higgens and Allan, 1980), ileocolitis, colitis or perianal disease. The disease is frequently focal in distribution and, unlike ulcerative colitis, involves the full thickness of the bowel wall. In contrast to ulcerative colitis, the rectum is frequently spared. For these reasons, there is an inherent sampling error in biopsy work and biopsy is comparatively less useful than in the diagnosis of ulcerative colitis (Morson, 1972a; Hill et al., 1979). However, the uneven distribution is itself an important sign which can be appreciated both in a series of biopsies and macroscopically by the examining endoscopist.

6.2 MAKING THE DIAGNOSIS

The diagnostic process should begin with details of the sigmoidoscopic (or colonoscopic) examination. The description by the endoscopist of the sigmoidoscopic appearance provides a macroscopic picture as important to the pathologist as the resected surgical specimen (Axon and Dickinson, 1983). In contradistinction to ulcerative colitis the rectum may appear normal in about half of all cases. Tiny aphthoid ulcers are believed to be the first lesions to develop in newly involved areas (Morson, 1972b). In time, the ulceration becomes serpiginous, longitudinal and eccentric within the bowel. Oedema and linear ulceration combine to produce the classical picture of 'cobblestoning' (Geboes and Vantrappen, 1975; Waye, 1980). Inflammatory polyps may occur as in ulcerative

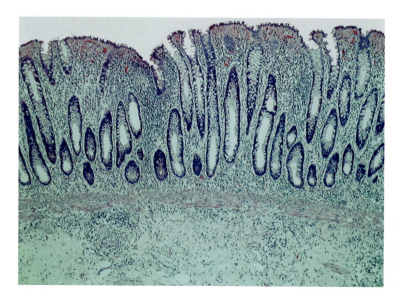

Figure 6.1 Crohn's disease. The crypts are straight and somewhat elongated. The goblet cells are well preserved, both in crypts and on the surface. There is patchy mucosal inflammation and a submucosal granuloma is present.

colitis and, between abnormal areas ('skip' lesions), the mucosa usually appears normal. Anal lesions are painless fissures, ulcerated pile-like complexes or ulcers in the anal canal. Fistulae, skin tags and perianal abscesses may develop as complications of these primary events.

6.3 HISTOPATHOLOGY

There are two principal questions. First, assuming the patient has idiopathic inflammatory bowel disease, do the features favour Crohn's disease, rather than ulcerative colitis? Second, is it specifically Crohn's disease to the exclusion of all other forms of inflammation? For example, a granuloma within a biopsy, unrelated to crypt rupture, is strongly suggestive of Crohn's disease when the only possible alternative is ulcerative colitis (Mahedeva *et al.*, 2002). It is not diagnostic, however, in the wider context of inflammatory conditions (Section 3.8.11). Obviously, the differential diagnosis from ulcerative colitis only relates to cases limited to the large bowel. Significant small intestinal disease rules out ulcerative colitis as a diagnosis, with the caveat of a limited back-wash ileitis.

6.3.1 Epithelial and crypt changes

The key epithelial feature, predominant but not invariable in Crohn's disease, is the preservation of crypt architecture and the goblet cell population despite considerable inflammation (Cook and Dixon, 1973; Yardley and Donowitz, 1977). The crypts maintain their length and the surface epithelial cells show only minor degenerative changes (Fig. 6.1), a feature accounting for the high surface cell/crypt cell ratio noted by Thompson *et al.* (1985) which was found to be of value in differentiating Crohn's disease from ulcerative colitis. Crypt branching may occur but it is not a dominant feature (Morson, 1972a; Whitehead, 1985). For any degree of inflammation in the lamina propria there is relatively little goblet cell depletion (Morson, 1971), though not all agree with the value of goblet cell changes (Surawicz *et al.*, 1981). There is one exception, namely, that close to ulceration or in the subsequent early healing phase the crypt architecture can be distorted to the degree seen in ulcerative colitis (Fig. 6.2). It is important to have clinical information about any adjacent ulceration and so avoid misinterpretation. This stresses again the need for accurate anatomical localization of the biopsy by the

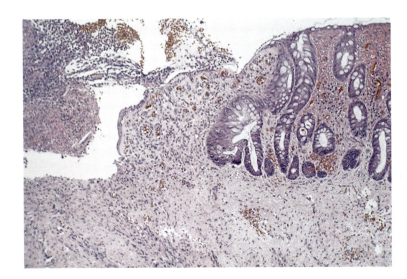

Figure 6.2 Crypt distortion in Crohn's disease. This biopsy, from the edge of a rectal ulcer, shows bifurcation of crypts.

clinician and transmission of this information to the pathologist.

6.3.2 Lamina propria and inflammation

Macroscopically, the distribution of Crohn's disease is patchy and this is also reflected histologically in the mucosal inflammatory infiltrate. Rather than the constituents of this inflammatory infiltrate it is therefore its distribution that is characteristic (Yardley and Donowitz, 1977; Goldman and Antonioli, 1982). Lymphocytes, plasma cells and polymorphs are the main components and a variation in their density across the biopsy is an important sign (Fig. 6.1). Between groups of crypts or between one crypt and the next, the density of inflammation may vary. This is the histological counterpart of the gross 'skip lesion'. Such focality can be best appreciated using *en face* orientation (Hamilton *et al.*, 1980).

Looking at the inflammatory infiltrate in more detail, the neutrophil polymorphs in a biopsy of Crohn's disease are usually less conspicuous (Fig. 6.3) than in the acute stages of the other main forms of inflammatory bowel disease, namely ulcerative colitis and also infection. Crypt abscesses do occur but never dominate the biopsy picture (Morson, 1972a). When present, a particular pattern of basal invasion by polymorphs is believed by some (McGovern and Goulston, 1968) to typify Crohn's disease but this is not our experience. Seldenrijk *et al.* (1991) suggested that histiocytes were prominent within the crypt abscesses in Crohn's disease but we have not found this to be sufficiently consistent to be diagnostically useful.

Coupled with patchy inflammation the diagnosis of Crohn's disease becomes more likely if small collections (basal aggregates) of lymphocytes can be found alongside the bases of crypts (Fig. 6.4) (McGovern and Goulston, 1968). It is difficult, but necessary, to distinguish such collections from more structured lymphoid follicles. Examination of additional levels often helps to make this distinction by revealing the larger size or germinal centre of a definite follicle. A follicular pattern of colitis is not a feature of Crohn's disease. Alteration of the other inflammatory cell components, i.e. mast cells, eosinophils, histiocytes, etc., in the lamina propria, does occur in Crohn's disease but the changes have not been shown to be of value in the differential diagnosis.

6.3.3 The granuloma

When present, the granuloma is the key sign and perhaps the only diagnostic one, with the provisos just mentioned about patchy distribution and

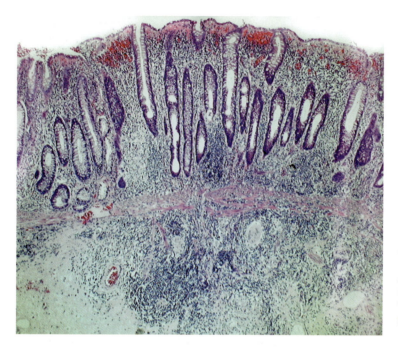

Figure 6.3 Crohn's disease. In this biopsy there is patchy inflammation of mucosa and submucosa, the predominant cells being lymphocytes. A small crypt abscess is present but neutrophils are inconspicuous. Note the submucosal granuloma and giant cells.

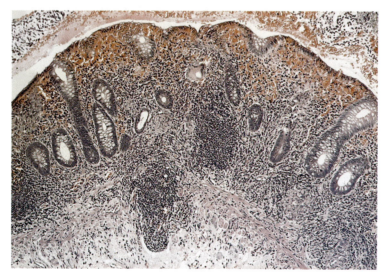

Figure 6.4 Crohn's disease. Prominent basally situated mucosal lymphoid aggregates. There are also mucosal granulomas and giant cells are associated with damaged crypts.

lymphoid aggregates being suggestive of Crohn's disease. Typical granulomas in Crohn's disease comprise collections of epithelioid cells and a cuff of lymphocytes, with or without Langhans giant cells (Figs 3.43 and 6.4). Granulomas may be seen in inflamed mucosa and in sigmoidoscopically normal mucosa (Rotterdam *et al.*, 1977). For example, patients with disease restricted to the ileum may exhibit a granuloma in an otherwise normal rectal biopsy (Surawicz *et al.*, 1981). The granulomas occur throughout the bowel wall in Crohn's disease and, in a biopsy, must also be looked for in any superficial submucosa present (Fig. 6.5). In the submucosa, granulomas are clearly unrelated to crypt rupture so this interpretative problem is avoided. Caseation does not occur but, rarely, a focus of central necrosis may be seen. The granulomas are normally single, but two or three may lie in close proximity.

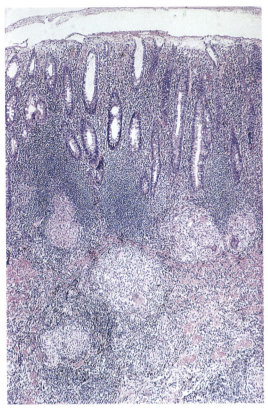

Figure 6.5 Crohn's disease. This section from a resected colon shows how even florid submucosal and basal mucosal granulomas could be missed by a superficial mucosal biopsy.

Confluent granulomas are not found and should suggest tuberculosis as, of course, should florid central caseation. In addition to the typical granuloma with giant cells described, microgranulomas occur (Rotterdam *et al.*, 1977). These consist of clusters of histiocytes and small numbers of inflammatory cells (Fig. 3.42). They are easily overlooked but can also be overdiagnosed, as similar appearances are produced by sections passing tangentially through pericryptal areas (Fig. 3.45) or the walls of small blood vessels (Fig. 3.44). Furthermore, giant cells, sometimes accompanying ill-formed granulomas, can also be seen in relation to ruptured crypts and associated mucin (Fig. 3.40). These 'granulomatous crypt abscesses' are most frequently associated with infective colitis and must not be misinterpreted as

indicating Crohn's disease (Surawicz *et al.*, 1981; Goldman and Antonioli, 1982). Moreover, Mahadeva *et al.* (2002) describe such lesions in cases confidently indexed as ulcerative colitis. Sections from deeper levels often help to clarify this situation. However, it should be remembered that collections of epithelioid cells can be found in relation to crypt abscesses (Seldenrijk *et al.*, 1991) and damaged crypts (Lee *et al.*, 1997) in patients with Crohn's disease and require careful evaluation in the context of all the other signs present in the biopsy series.

The incidence of granulomas in Crohn's disease varies according to whether biopsies or surgically resected specimens are being considered. In a series of 188 consecutive patients, Heresbach *et al.* (2005) found granulomas in 37 per cent of a combined biopsy and surgical series. In biopsy work, the quoted incidence of granulomas is variable, dependent on the site of major disease (Rotterdam *et al.*, 1977; Surawicz *et al.*, 1981). As mentioned earlier, they can be found in the rectum even when disease seems restricted to the ileum. The figures for overall incidence range from 0 to nearly 30 per cent (Anderson and Bogoch, 1968; Petri *et al.*, 1982). When multiple levels through biopsies are cut, the incidence is maintained above 20 per cent (Surawicz *et al.*, 1981, Seldenrijk *et al.*, 1991). However, such a routine markedly increases a departmental workload. We compromise by examining multiple levels through the biopsy only in cases in which there is a strong clinical suspicion or when other features seen in the first three routine levels point towards Crohn's disease. Such a regimen yielded granulomas in 15 per cent of biopsies in the series of Iliffe and Owen (1981).

6.3.4 The aphthoid ulcer

These are believed by some to be the initial lesions of Crohn's disease (Brooke, 1959). In a biopsy they are seen as small areas of ulceration situated immediately over a lymphoid follicle (Fig. 6.6) (McGovern and Goulston, 1968). The adjacent mucosa shows only minimal abnormality. On sigmoidoscopy they appear as tiny punched-out lesions with a white base, resembling oral aphthae. They have been described in *Campylobacter* colitis and yersiniosis

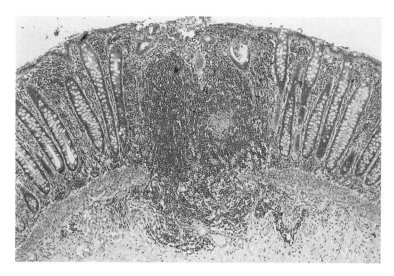

Figure 6.6 Aphthoid ulcer in Crohn's disease. The epithelium overlying a lymphoid follicle is eroded. A small mucosal granuloma lies in the follicle. There is a crypt abscess but the goblet cells and crypt architecture are preserved.

(Vantrappen *et al.*, 1977) and as a result of bowel preparation for colonoscopy (Rejchrt *et al.*, 2004) but, in the context of ulcerative colitis versus Crohn's disease, are important markers of the latter. Even smaller microerosions have been described by Poulsen *et al.* (1984). These are closely associated with granulomas and should be the target of biopsy procedures.

6.3.5 Fissures

Penetration by a narrow ulcer, or the base of a wider ulcer, down through the submucosa and into the muscle represents fissuring ulceration, a feature characteristic of Crohn's disease but, owing to the superficial nature of biopsy material, one which is rarely seen. It is necessary to exclude two possible sources of confusion. First, that a lymphoma is not present, as fissuring may be a feature of this condition (Lee *et al.*, 1986), and, second, the clinical situation is not that of acute fulminant colitis from any cause (Price and Morson, 1975).

6.3.6 Submucosa: disproportionate inflammation and neural hyperplasia

The clinician should make every effort to provide a biopsy that includes the superficial half of the submucosa, essential for the assessment of 'disproportionate inflammation'. This refers to a mixed infiltrate within the submucosa (Fig. 3.57). The sign is only of value when the biopsy is from intact mucosa for, when ulceration is present from whatever cause, the adjacent superficial submucosa may become involved. Disproportionate inflammation reflects the transmural nature of the inflammatory process and/or the propensity for the ulceration of Crohn's disease to track deeply and undermine adjacent mucosa. Again, the usefulness of this sign is devalued when reporting on a case of fulminant colitis. Granulomas in the submucosa are important because, as already mentioned, they are free of the interpretative difficulties associated with the inflammatory crypt damage considered earlier (Section 6.3.3). There is often neural hyperplasia and, in deep biopsies, large nerve bundles can be seen.

6.4 DIFFERENTIAL DIAGNOSIS

When granulomatous inflammation is found in colorectal biopsies, the possibility of tuberculosis has to be borne in mind, especially in patients of Asian origin (Pulimood *et al.*, 2005; Kirsch *et al.*, 2006). The endoscopist may suspect tuberculosis because of certain endoscopic features (Sato *et al.*, 2004), such as circumferential ulceration with nodules, small discrete circumferentially arranged, round or irregular ulcers, multiple erosions restricted to the large bowel or small ulcers or erosions restricted to the ileum. Healed tuberculous lesions may produce a patulous ileocaecal valve, pseudodiverticula and mucosal atrophy and scarring. Tuberculosis is considered in more detail in Section 4.2.7b.

In practice, there is little diagnostic problem when a granuloma is present, taking account of the above caveat and remembering that crypt damage can evoke granuloma formation (Section 6.3.3). However, in the absence of a granuloma, what can be the degree of diagnostic confidence? It is reasonable to make Crohn's the diagnosis of choice from a rectal biopsy when there is patchy inflammation along the mucosa, the crypts and their goblet cell components show little derangement and basal lymphoid aggregates are present (Morson, 1974). Shallow ulcers, often multiple, can be produced at the ileocaecal valve and in the terminal ileum by non-steroidal anti-inflammatory drugs (Lengeling *et al.*, 2003). The histology of these ulcers is described in Chapter 11. If other features of colitis are present, clues to the diagnosis are likely to be found. Submucosal involvement, aphthoid ulceration and fissures strengthen the diagnostic conviction for Crohn's disease considerably but, as mentioned, fissures are rarely taken in biopsies. When curetted tissue from a fistula is available, the presence of granulomas composed of epithelioid cells, as opposed to foreign body giant cells, raises the level of suspicion of Crohn's disease. Bataille and colleagues (2004) have interestingly shown that CD68-positive macrophages are scanty in the granulation tissue lining fistulas in Crohn's disease, whereas these cells are numerous in the lining of fistulas from non-Crohn's patients.

Because of the patchy distribution of Crohn's disease, examination of a colonoscopic biopsy series yields more diagnostic accuracy than a rectal biopsy. Bentley *et al.* (2002) showed that expert gastrointestinal pathologists correctly diagnosed Crohn's disease from a colonoscopic series in 64 per cent of cases, compared with only 24 per cent of cases from rectal biopsies alone; interestingly, the corresponding figures for non-gastrointestinal specialist pathologists were 60 per cent and 12 per cent. Different diagnostic rates in the older literature may reflect the larger size of rectal biopsies taken at rigid sigmoidoscopy than are now taken using flexible endoscopy. Thus, Dyer *et al.* (1970) claimed a confident opinion of Crohn's disease in 23 per cent from a rectal biopsy study, relying on the above features, with granulomas in 19 per cent. Equivalent figures for Korelitz and Sommers (1977) were 30 per cent and 18 per cent and, for Illife and Owen (1981) 28 per cent and 14 per cent. Morson (1974) found that as many as 41 per cent of initial rectal biopsies were diagnostic from patients subsequently shown to have Crohn's disease at surgery. When all the biopsies available from each patient are examined, abnormalities have been documented in 40–70 per cent of biopsies overall, regardless of site (Dyer *et al.*, 1970; Korelitz and Sommers, 1977; Iliffe and Owen, 1981). Consideration of the clinical situation, the endoscopic findings and the radiology add a final vital dimension which compensates for the absence of any diagnostic granuloma. Paradoxically, with the correct distribution of proximal disease a normal rectal biopsy can be the key to establishing the diagnosis.

6.4.1 Pre-pouch ileitis

A small proportion of patients with ileoanal pouches after colectomy for ulcerative colitis develop severe inflammation of the neoterminal ileum, with ulceration (Goldstein *et al.*, 1997). This can resemble Crohn's disease but should not trigger a change in diagnosis if the preoperative biopsies and the colectomy specimen show typical features of ulcerative colitis (Chapter 5 and Section 11.5).

6.5 DISEASE ACTIVITY

In the equivalent discussion in the chapter dealing with ulcerative colitis (Section 5.2) it was possible to recognize active disease, a phase of remission and quiescent disease. This does not apply to

Crohn's disease. To date, no study has been able to successfully correlate specific features with clinical activity (Gomes *et al.*, 1986). As mentioned, granulomas may occur in otherwise normal mucosa and, presumably, signify involvement but do not relate to any symptomatology. Fibrosis in the submucosa and splaying of the muscularis mucosae, appreciated in a well-taken biopsy, indicate long-standing disease. Ulceration, with a predominantly acute inflammatory cell infiltrate, in the presence of other pointers to Crohn's disease, can be taken to mean tissue activity, but there is poor correlation with clinical activity. However localized the disease may seem, Crohn's disease may affect the whole of the gastrointestinal tract (Goodman *et al.*, 1976; Dunne *et al.*, 1977). Abnormal jejunal mucosa has been demonstrated in patients with disease which is apparently localized to the terminal ileum and colon. Mention has already been made of rectal granulomas in patients with disease restricted to the terminal ileum.

6.6 INDICATORS OF PROGNOSIS

Several studies have attempted to identify prognostic histological features, mostly using surgical material. Granulomas are claimed to exert a favourable prognosis (Glass and Baker, 1976; Chambers and Morson, 1979), but this has not been corroborated by others (Wilson *et al.*, 1980; Wolfson *et al.*, 1982). In a biopsy study Ward and Webb (1977) suggested that ulceration and fissuring indicated a poor prognosis. Overall, however, there is no universally accepted prognostic microscopic feature worth documenting, as such, in a biopsy report.

The view that the likelihood of recurrence of Crohn's disease is reduced if surgical resection of the affected bowel is complete has been superseded by a realization that, provided severely ulcerated or strictured bowel is not left in place, anastomotic recurrence bears no relation to microscopic features of disease (Kotanagi *et al.*, 1991) and there is little value in taking biopsies for frozen section during surgery for Crohn's (Hamilton *et al.*, 1985).

6.7 COLONOSCOPIC BIOPSY IN CROHN'S DISEASE

6.7.1 The colonoscopist's report

Although a distinction can often be made from ulcerative colitis, firm separation of Crohn's disease from other forms of inflammation cannot be justified from a single biopsy in the absence of a granuloma unless there is good supporting macroscopic evidence from the endoscopic report (Waye, 1980; Axon and Dickinson, 1983). In a classical case the endoscopist will see segmental disease and asymmetrical involvement of the mucosa in the affected area. The disease may predominate on the right and rectal sparing is characteristic. The latter must be interpreted with care for, occasionally, in ulcerative colitis there may be only minimal rectal involvement, particularly following treatment with steroid enemas. Conversely, patterns of Crohn's disease that diffusely affect the rectum are well recognized (Goldman and Antonioli, 1982). Strictures, cobblestone mucosa and linear ulceration are all macroscopic features of Crohn's disease, as are skip areas of normal-looking bowel. Indeed, the colonoscopic picture of the gross features, previously available only from the surgical resection, may provide a better diagnostic tool than biopsies in a significant number of cases.

6.7.2 The colonoscopic biopsy

A series of biopsies is usually taken. Colonoscopic biopsies are small and superficial and not ideal to see the transmural features of Crohn's disease. Indeed, granulomas are also rare in colonoscopic series (Geboes *et al.*, 1978; Waye, 1980). It is the variation in intensity of inflammation and the occasional normal biopsy in the series that form the most useful aids. To have colitis, other than Crohn's disease, with such a combination is unusual. For this reason, biopsies should be taken at intervals along the length of the colon and rectum, as well as from the terminal ileum, from endoscopically normal as well as from abnormal areas. It is more difficult for a pathologist to interpret what may in themselves be non-specific inflammatory changes in biopsies solely from the parts of the bowel which are focally grossly affected by Crohn's disease. Provided that these caveats are recognized by the clinician, and they inform his practice, we feel the pathologist should be prepared to make a confident diagnosis of Crohn's disease. Ischaemia is the most likely alternative and is dealt with in Chapter 10.

6.8 COMPLICATIONS

6.8.1 Inflammatory polyps ('pseudopolyps')

Although inflammatory polyps (Section 15.9) may be more common in ulcerative colitis it should be remembered that they are also found in Crohn's disease. They are of no diagnostic importance in a particular case.

6.8.2 Toxic megacolon

This is reported to occur in between 6 per cent and 12 per cent of patients with Crohn's disease (Buzzard *et al.*, 1974; Farmer *et al.*, 1975). It is a more common complication of colonic than ileal disease and it is possible that the presence of granulomas has a 'protective' role.

Biopsy has little value in the diagnosis and management of toxic megacolon and, as in ulcerative colitis, may even be misleading (Sections 5.7 and 12.3.3b).

6.9 CONCLUSIONS

In the absence of a granuloma a confident diagnosis from a single colorectal biopsy is rarely made. The combination of focal inflammation, acute and chronic, with regular crypt architecture, normal goblet cells and basal lymphoid aggregates is highly suggestive (Jones *et al.*, 1973) and this strong bias should be reflected in the report (Morson, 1974). The level of confidence in the diagnosis is increased if a colonoscopic series confirms the typical distribution of inflammatory changes. Regardless of the anatomical site of involvement, colorectal and ileal biopsy is a valuable diagnostic procedure in Crohn's disease.

REFERENCES

Anderson, F.H., Bogoch, A. (1968) Biopsies of large bowel in regional enteritis. *Can. Med. Assoc. J.*, 98, 150–3.

Axon, A.J.R., Dickinson, R.J. (1983) Endoscopy in Crohn's disease. In: Allan, R.N., Keighley, M.R.B., Alexander-Williams, J., Hawkins, C. (eds) *Inflammatory bowel disease*. Edinburgh: Churchill Livingstone, pp. 412–17.

Basu, M.K., Asquith, P., Thompson, R.A., Cooke, W.T. (1975) Oral manifestations of Crohn's disease. *Gut*, 16, 249–54.

Bataille, F., Klebl, F., Rummele, P. *et al.* (2004) Morphological characterization of Crohn's disease fistulae. *Gut*, 53, 1314–21.

Bentley, E., Jenkins, D., Campbell, F., Warren, B. (2002) How could pathologists improve the initial diagnosis of colitis? Evidence from an international workshop. *J. Clin. Pathol.*, 55, 955–60.

Brooke, B.M. (1959) Granulomatous diseases of the intestine. *Lancet*, ii, 745–9.

Buzzard, A.J., Baker, W.N.W., Neeham, P.R.C., Warren, R.C. (1974) Acute toxic dilation of the colon in Crohn's disease. *Gut*, 15, 416–19.

Chambers, T.J., Morson, B.C. (1979) The granuloma in Crohn's disease. *Gut*, 20, 269–74.

Cook, M.C., Dixon, M.F. (1973) An analysis of the reliability of detection and diagnostic value of various pathological features in Crohn's disease and ulcerative colitis. *Gut*, 14, 255–62.

Dunne, W.T., Cooke, W.T., Allan, R.N. (1977) Enzymatic and morphometric evidence for Crohn's disease as a diffuse lesion of the gastrointestinal tract. *Gut*, 18, 290–4.

Dyer, N.H., Stansfeld, A.C., Dawson, A.M. (1970) The value of rectal biopsy in the diagnosis of Crohn's disease. *Scand. J. Gastroenterol.*, 5, 491–6.

Farmer, R.C., Hawk, W.A., Turnbull, R.B. (1975) Clinical patterns in Crohn's disease: a statistical study of 615 cases. *Gastroenterology*, 68, 627–35.

Geboes, K., Desmet, V.J., De Wolf-Peeters, C., Vantrappen, C. (1978) The value of endoscopic biopsies in the diagnosis of Crohn's disease. *Am. J. Proctol.*, 29, 21–8.

Geboes, M., Vantrappen, G. (1975) The value of colonoscopy in the diagnosis of Crohn's disease. *Gastrointest. Endoscopy*, 22, 18–23.

Glass, R.G., Baker, W.N.W. (1976) Role of the granuloma in recurrent Crohn's disease. *Gut*, 17, 75–7.

Goldman, H., Antonioli, D.A. (1982) Mucosal biopsy of the rectum, colon and distal ileum. *Human Pathol.*, 13, 981–1012.

Goldstein, N.S., Sanford, W.W., Bodzin, J.H. (1997) Crohn's-like complications in patients with ulcerative colitis after total proctocolectomy and ileal pouch–anal anastomosis. *Am. J. Surg. Pathol.*, 21, 1343–53.

Gomes, P., Du Boulay, C., Smith, C.L., Holdstock, G. (1986) Relationship between disease activity indices and colonoscopic findings in patients with colonic inflammatory bowel disease. *Gut*, 27, 92–5.

Goodman, M.J., Skinner, J.M., Truelove, S.C. (1976) Abnormalities in the apparently normal bowel mucosa in Crohn's disease. *Lancet*, i, 275–8.

Hamilton, S.R., Bussey, H.J.R., Morson, B.C. (1980) *En face* histologic technique to demonstrate mucosal inflammatory lesions in macroscopically uninvolved colon of Crohn's disease resection specimens. *Lab. Invest.*, 42, 121.

Hamilton, S.R., Reese, J., Pennington, L., Boitnott, J.K., Bayless, T.M., Cameron, J.L. (1985) The role of resection margin frozen section in the surgical management of Crohn's disease. *Surg. Gynecol. Obstet.*, 160, 57–62.

Heresbach, D., Alexandre, J.L., Branger, B. *et al.* (2005) Frequency and significance of granulomas in a cohort of incident cases of Crohn's disease. *Gut*, 54, 215–22.

Higgens, S.C., Allan, R.N. (1980) Crohn's disease of the distal ileum. *Gut*, 21, 933–40.

Hill, R.B., Kent, T.H., Hansen, R.N. (1979) Clinical usefulness of rectal biopsy in Crohn's disease. *Gastroenterology*, 77, 938–44.

Iliffe, G.D., Owen, D.A. (1981) Rectal biopsy in Crohn's disease. *Dig. Dis. Sci.*, 26, 321–4.

Jones, J.H., Lennard-Jones, J.E., Morson, B.C. *et al.* (1973) Numerical taxonomy and discriminant analysis applied to non-specific colitis. *Q. J. Med.*, 42, 715–32.

Kirsch, R., Pentecost, M., de M Hall, P., Epstein, D.P., Watermeyer, G., Freiderich, P.W. (2006) Role of colonoscopic biopsy in distinguishing between Crohn's disease and intestinal tuberculosis. *J. Clin. Pathol.*, 59, 840–4.

Korelitz, B.I., Sommers, S.C. (1977) Rectal biopsy in patients with Crohn's disease. *J. Am. Med. Assoc.*, 237, 2742–4.

Kotanagi, H., Kramer, K., Fazio, V.W., Petras, R.E. (1991) Do microscopic abnormalities at resection margins correlate with increased anastomotic recurrence in Crohn's disease? Retrospective analysis of 100 cases. *Dis. Colon Rectum*, 34, 909–16.

Lee, F.D., Maguire, C., Obeidat, W., Russell, R.I. (1997) Importance of cryptolytic lesions and pericryptal granulomas in inflammatory bowel disease. *J. Clin. Pathol.*, 50, 148–52.

Lee, M.H., Waxman, M., Gillooley, J.F. (1986) Primary malignant lymphoma of the anorectum in homosexual men. *Dis. Colon Rectum*, 29, 413–16.

Lengeling, R.W., Mitros, F.A., Brennan, J.A., Schulze, K.S. (2003) Ulcerative ileitis encountered at ileo-colonoscopy: likely role of nonsteroidal agents. *Clin. Gastroenterol. Hepatol.*, 1, 160–9.

Mahadeva, U., Martin, J.P., Patel, N.K., Price, A. B. (2002) Granulomatous ulcerative colitis: a re-appraisal of the mucosal granuloma in the distinction of Crohn's disease from ulcerative colitis. *Histopathology*, 41, 50–5.

McGovern, V.J., Goulston, S.J.M. (1968) Crohn's disease of the colon. *Gut*, 9, 164–76.

Morson, B.C. (1971) Histopathology of Crohn's disease. *Scand. J. Gastroenterol.*, 6, 57–5.

Morson, B.C. (1972a) Rectal biopsy in inflammatory bowel disease. *N. Engl. J. Med.*, 287, 1337–9.

Morson, B.C. (1972b) The early histological lesion of Crohn's disease. *Proc. R. Soc. Med.*, 65, 71–2.

Morson, B.C. (1974) Rectal biopsy in inflammatory bowel disease. *Pathol. Ann.*, 9, 209–30.

Petri, M., Poulsen, S.S., Christensen, K., Jarnum, S. (1982) The incidence of granulomas in serial sections of rectal biopsies from patients with Crohn's disease. *Acta Pathol. Micro. Immunol. Scand. A*, 90, 145–7.

Poulsen, S.S., Tinggaard-Pedersen, N., Jarnum, S. (1984) Microerosions in rectal biopsies in Crohn's disease. *Scand. J. Gastroenterol.*, 19, 607–12.

Price, A., Morson, B.C. (1975) Inflammatory bowel disease: the surgical pathology of Crohn's disease and ulcerative colitis. *Hum. Pathol.*, 6, 7–29.

Pulimood, A.B., Peter, S., Ramakrishna, B., Chacko, A., Jeyamani, R., Jeyaseelan, L. (2005) Segmental colonoscopic biopsies in the differentiation of ileocolic tuberculosis from Crohn's disease. *J. Gastroenterol. Hepatol.*, 20, 688–96.

Rejchrt, S., Bures, J., Siroky, M., Kopacova, M., Slezak, L., Langr, F. (2004) A prospective, observational study of colonic mucosal abnormalities associated with orally administered sodium phosphate for colon cleansing before colonoscopy. *Gastrointest. Endosc.*, 59, 651–4.

Rotterdam, H., Korelitz, B.L., Sommers, S.C. (1977) Microgranulomas in grossly normal rectal mucosa in Crohn's disease. *Am. J. Clin. Pathol.*, 67, 550–4.

Sato, S., Yao, K., Yao, T., Schlemper, R.J., Matsui, T., Sakurai, T., Iwashita, A. (2004) Colonoscopy in the diagnosis of intestinal tuberculosis in asymptomatic patients. *Gastrointest. Endosc.*, 59, 362–8.

Seldenrijk, C.A., Morson, B.C., Meuwissen, S.G., Schipper, N.W., Lindeman, J., Meijer, C.J.

(1991) Histopathological evaluation of colonic mucosal biopsy specimens in chronic inflammatory bowel disease: diagnostic implications. *Gut*, 32, 1514–20.

Surawicz, C.M., Meisel, J.L., Ylvisaker, T., Saunders, D.R., Rubin, C.E. (1981) Rectal biopsy in the diagnosis of Crohn's disease: Value of multiple biopsies and serial sectioning. *Gastroenterology*, 81, 66–71.

Thompson, M., Sowter, C., Altman, D., Slavin, G., Price, A.B. (1985) Rectal biopsy in inflammatory bowel disease: a study using computerised interactive image analysis. *J. Clin. Pathol.*, 38, 631–8.

Vantrappen, G., Agg, H.O., Ponette, E., Ceboes, K., Bertrand, P.H. (1977) *Yersinia* enteritis and enterocolitis: Gastroenterological aspects. *Gastroenterology*, 72, 220–7.

Ward, M., Webb, J.N. (1977) Rectal biopsy as a prognostic guide in Crohn's colitis. *J. Clin. Pathol.*, 30, 126–31.

Waye, J.D. (1980) Endoscopy in inflammatory bowel disease. *Clin. Gastroenterol.*, 9, 297–306.

Whitehead, R. (1985) Mucosal biopsy of the gastrointestinal tract. In: Bennington, J.L. (ed.) *Major problems in pathology vol. 3.* Philadelphia: Saunders.

Wilson, J.A.P., Burkhardt, R.T., Kumar, N., Appelman, H.D. (1980) Relationship of granulomas to clinical parameters in Crohn's disease. *Gastroenterology*, 78, A 1292.

Wolfson, D.M., Sachar, D.B., Cohen, A. *et al.* (1982) Granulomas do not affect postoperative recurrence rates in Crohn's disease. *Gastroenterology*, 83, 405–9.

Yardley, J.H., Donowitz, M. (1977) Colorectal biopsy in inflammatory bowel disease. In: Yardley, J.H., Morson, B.C., Abell, M.R. (eds) *The gastrointestinal tract. International Academy of Pathology monograph.* Baltimore: Williams and Wilkins, pp. 50–94.

CHAPTER 7

ILEOANAL POUCH PATHOLOGY

7.1 Introduction: clinical indications for pouch surgery	124	7.5 Pre-pouch ileitis — 128
7.2 Normal adaptive changes: ileal mucosa vs. residual rectal cuff mucosa	124	7.6 Differential diagnosis of pouchitis — 128
7.3 Inflammation and pouchitis	125	7.7 Neoplasia — 130
7.4 Risk factors for pouchitis	126	7.7.1 Adenoma — 130
		7.7.2 Dysplasia — 131
		References — 131

7.1 INTRODUCTION: CLINICAL INDICATIONS FOR POUCH SURGERY

Ileoanal pouches were first introduced to restore anal continence in patients who had undergone proctocolectomy for ulcerative colitis (Parks and Nicholls, 1978). Pouch surgery is now offered to patients as an alternative to permanent ileostomy following proctocolectomy for a variety of conditions, including, in particular, familial adenomatous polyposis (Nicholls *et al.*, 1985); ileoanal pouches have also been fabricated following proctocolectomy for intractable constipation (Nicholls and Kamm, 1988), juvenile polyposis, necrotizing enterocolitis, extensive Hirschsprung's disease and indeterminate colitis (Pishori *et al.*, 2004). Rarely, a patient with Crohn's disease will have a pouch (Panis *et al.*, 1996), although Crohn's disease is usually regarded as a contraindication to pouch surgery. Another contraindication is the presence of a low rectal carcinoma.

7.2 NORMAL ADAPTIVE CHANGES: ILEAL MUCOSA VS. RESIDUAL RECTAL CUFF MUCOSA

In the majority of pouches the mucosa rapidly undergoes morphological changes towards a colon-like morphology. Biopsies show varying degrees of villous atrophy, often total, accompanied by crypt hyperplasia and diffuse infiltration of the lamina propria by chronic inflammatory cells (Fig. 7.1). The morphology closely resembles colorectal mucosa, although it has been shown that this is not a complete metaplasia, as small bowel specific disaccharidase–sucrase isomaltase expression is retained (de-Silva *et al.*, 1991). These changes can be regarded as a physiological adaptation to mucosal stress, analogous to the changes that occur in the small bowel mucosa in coeliac patients in response to the toxic influence of gluten. The adverse influence in the case of ileal pouch mucosa is the replacement of the normal

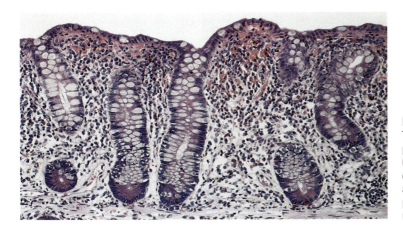

Figure 7.1 Adaptive colonization. This is a mucosal biopsy of an ileal pouch showing a flat surface ('sub-total villous atrophy') with a diffuse infiltrate of lymphocytes and plasma cells within the lamina propria. Note that Paneth cells are retained.

semisterile small intestinal chyme by bacteria-laden faecal material.

There is a tendency for inflammatory changes to be most prominent in the more distal and posterior part of a pouch. Multiple biopsies should therefore be taken to adequately assess ileal pouch histology. In addition to inflammation of the pouch itself, there can sometimes be quite severe inflammation in the neoterminal ileum, proximal to the pouch (Goldstein *et al.*, 1997). Biopsies from here and from different parts of the pouch should be clearly identified, preferably keeping them in separate, labelled pots, to avoid confusion.

When examining pouch mucosal biopsies, it is important to avoid mistaking a biopsy from a distal cuff of residual rectum for ileal pouch mucosa (Thompson-Fawcett *et al.*, 1999). Surgical practice varies and some surgeons intentionally leave a short rectal cuff, to which the ileal pouch is anastomosed, rather than directly to the anus. Residual rectal mucosa, however small in amount, can be severely inflamed in a patient with ulcerative colitis. This will continue to pose a risk of neoplasia. The pathologist can suspect that a biopsy may be of rectal cuff mucosa if one of a series of biopsies, particularly a distal biopsy, shows markedly more severe inflammation than the others. In these circumstances, markers of small bowel origin, such as Paneth cells or villi, may be unreliable. It is therefore important that the pouch biopsies are

sufficiently labelled by the endoscopist to enable the pathologist to identify the most distal, which may be contenders for tissue from a rectal cuff.

7.3 INFLAMMATION AND POUCHITIS

Superimposed on the above 'physiological' changes there can be acute inflammatory changes, with neutrophil polymorphs infiltrating the surface and crypt epithelium and focal superficial ulceration (Fig. 7.2). Interpretation of this can be difficult. The presence of chronic inflammatory cells and even acute inflammation, with neutrophils within surface or crypt epithelium, does not necessarily indicate that there is significant pouchitis (Evgenikos *et al.*, 2001). It should be noted that the term pouchitis is a clinicopathological label given to a chronic relapsing condition in which diarrhoea, bleeding, abdominal bloating and pain, urgency, discharge and systemic symptoms occur, as well as endoscopic evidence of pouch mucosal inflammation and histological evidence of acute inflammation. It is useful to grade the inflammation in biopsies of pouch mucosa, according to the severity of the acute inflammatory cell infiltration and ulceration. A pathological scoring system was devised by Moskowitz and colleagues (Moskowitz *et al.*, 1986; Shepherd *et al.*, 1987)

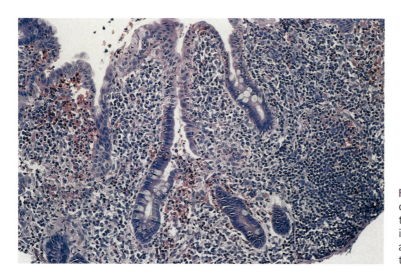

Figure 7.2 Acute inflammatory cells (score 2). Superimposed on the diffuse infiltrate of chronic inflammatory cells there is cryptitis and a few polymorphs have found their way into a crypt lumen.

Table 7.1 Pathological scoring system (after Moskowitz *et al.*, 1986)

Histological feature	Score
Acute	
Infiltration of epithelium by neutrophils	
None	0
Mild and patchy infiltrate in the surface epithelium	1
Moderate with crypt abscesses	2
Severe with crypt abscesses	3
Ulceration (per low power field)	
None	0
Mild superficial (>25%)	1
Moderate (25–50%)	2
Extensive (>50%)	3
Chronic	
Chronic inflammatory cells infiltration	
None	0
Mild and patchy	1
Moderate	2
Severe	3
Villous atrophy	
None	0
Minor abnormality of villous architecture	1
Partial villous atrophy	2
Subtotal villous atrophy	3

(Table 7.1). For clinical purposes the histological acute inflammatory markers (epithelial infiltration by neutrophils and ulceration) from this system are incorporated into a 'Pouchitis Disease Activity Index' (PDAI), based on a collection of symptoms, presence of fever, endoscopic findings and histology (Sandborn *et al.*, 1994). A PDAI of 7 or greater is taken as the definition of pouchitis. In pouchitis, the histological acute inflammatory cell (neutrophil) score is usually at least 2 (Fig. 7.3). Ulceration (Fig. 7.4) is not invariably seen in biopsies, although so-called ulcer-associated cell lineage may be present (Fig. 7.5).

7.4 RISK FACTORS FOR POUCHITIS

Pouchitis occurs almost exclusively in patients with ulcerative colitis but only half of all ulcerative colitis patients are likely ever to develop pouchitis (Cheifetz and Itzkowitz, 2004) and one-third of these will have only one episode (Meagher *et al.*, 1998). Chronic refractory pouchitis develops in only 5 per cent of ulcerative colitis patients and pouch excision is required in only a small minority of these (Cheifetz and Itzkowitz, 2004). Pouchitis can be regarded as the homologue of ulcerative colitis affecting ileal mucosa which has already been primed by colorectal adaptation to the pouch environment. Patients with extra-intestinal manifestations (EIM) of inflammatory bowel disease have a greater risk of developing pouchitis than those without EIM (Lohmuller *et al.*, 1990). This is especially true when primary sclerosing cholangiitis (PSC) is present, when the risk of

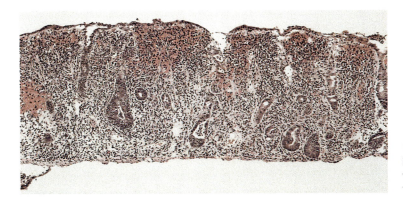

Figure 7.3 Severe acute inflammation (score 3). In addition to chronic inflammatory changes there are numerous crypt abscesses.

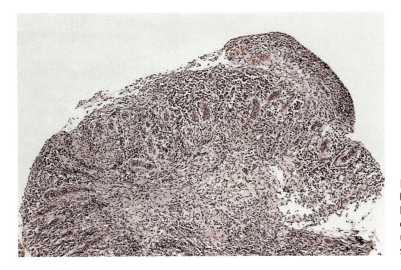

Figure 7.4 Ulceration seen in a biopsy of ileoanal pouch mucosa. From a patient who had had colectomy and pouch surgery for ulcerative colitis, with relapsing symptoms of pouchitis.

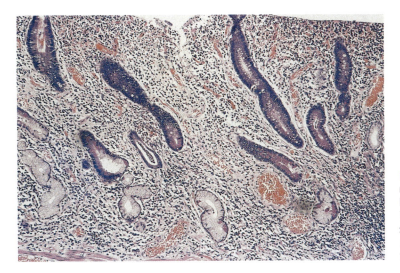

Figure 7.5 Pseudo-pyloric metaplasia (ulcer-associated cell lineage – UACL) in a biopsy of an ileoanal pouch with a high acute score (crypt abscesses and ulceration). The original diagnosis was ulcerative colitis.

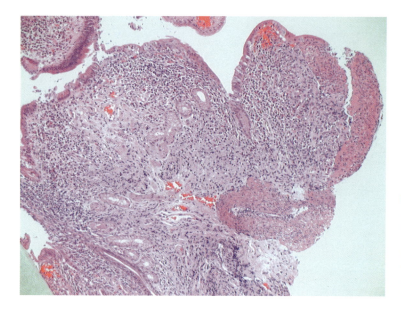

Figure 7.6 Severe pre-pouch ileitis, with ulceration. Biopsy of mucosa from neo-terminal ileum, showing active chronic inflammation with ulcer slough and ulcer-associated cell lineage (UACL). This condition, which is not uncommon, should be distinguished from Crohn's disease.

pouchitis is doubled (Penna *et al.*, 1996). Other risk factors are smoking (Merrett *et al.*, 1996) and constitutional IL-1ra (interleukin 1 receptor antagonist) gene allele 2 (Carter *et al.*, 2001).

It might be expected that patients with indeterminate colitis, based on the appearances in the resected colon, would be a source of diagnostic difficulty. However, several studies have shown that such cases tend to behave as ulcerative colitis and there is no contraindication to pouch surgery (Pishori *et al.*, 2004).

In our experience, pouchitis is rare in FAP. The published incidence in FAP is 3 to 14 per cent, depending on the series (Cheifetz and Itzkowitz, 2004). The severity of chronic inflammation is unrelated to clinical pouchitis and, whatever the original diagnosis, the normal adaptive, chronic inflammatory changes may be equally pronounced.

7.5 PRE-POUCH ILEITIS

Some patients with a history of typical ulcerative colitis can have particularly troublesome pouchitis and neoterminal ileitis of the pre-pouch bowel which mimics Crohn's disease, including stricturing and even fistulation. Sometimes this appears to be caused

by ischaemia. There may be severe ulceration (Fig. 7.6) but specific histological features are rarely found (Goldstein *et al.*, 1997). This is not a rare condition, having been seen in 15 of 661 patients who had undergone surgery for inflammatory bowel disease (Bell *et al.*, 2006). In only four of these patients was pouch excision necessary and the remainder either resolved spontaneously or responded to antibiotic or anti-inflammatory therapy. A diagnosis of Crohn's disease should not be made merely from examination of pouch and neoterminal ileal biopsies in such patients. Only after review of the surgical pathology of the colectomy specimen and any preoperative biopsies can any change in the diagnosis to Crohn's disease be contemplated.

7.6 DIFFERENTIAL DIAGNOSIS OF POUCHITIS

As mentioned previously, biopsies of distal mucosa from pouch patients can be actively inflamed even in the absence of inflammation of the more proximal mucosa, owing to persisting ulcerative colitis in a residual rectal cuff (Thompson-Fawcett *et al.*, 1999). Provided that cuffitis is excluded, symptoms of pouchitis can be mimicked by other conditions,

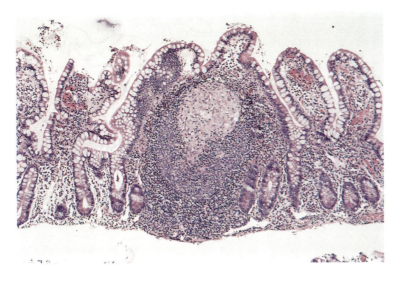

Figure 7.7 Granuloma in ileal pouch mucosa. Sporadic granulomas, often in lymphoid follicles, can sometimes be found in pouch mucosal biopsies, unrelated to other pathological or clinical features of inflammation.

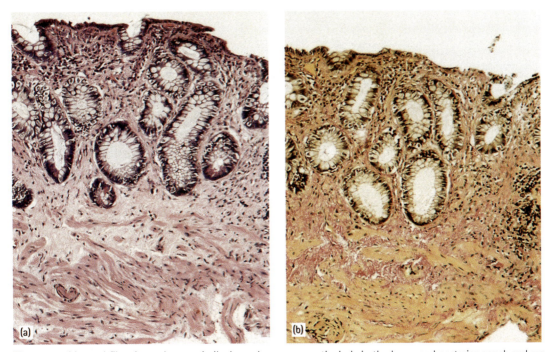

Figure 7.8 Mucosal fibrosis can be seen in ileal pouch mucosa, particularly in the lower and posterior pouch and may be due to chronic trauma, possibly from instrumentation. (a) Haematoxylin and eosin; (b) van Gieson.

including pouch–anal fistulas, abscesses, outlet obstruction or anastomotic leak.

Other inflammatory features that can be seen in pouch mucosa are granulomas (Fig. 7.7) and fibrosis. An occasional small or sometimes quite large and well-formed granuloma can be found,

whatever the original diagnosis and, taken in isolation, is not diagnostic of Crohn's disease (Shepherd *et al.*, 1989). Fibrosis may be present, particularly in the posterior or inferior pouch mucosa (Fig. 7.8) and, again is not a specific diagnostic feature. It can be the result of repetitive trauma, caused

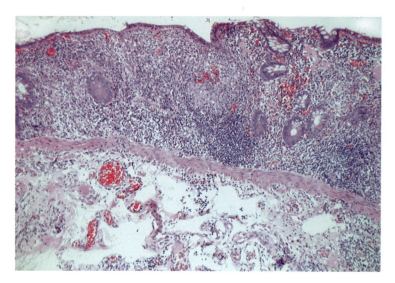

Figure 7.9 Ileal pouch biopsy from a patient with Crohn's disease, showing patchy chronic inflammation, granuloma formation and mucosal and submucosal lymphangiectasis.

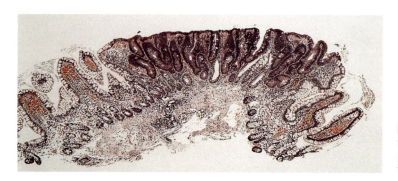

Figure 7.10 A flat mildly dysplastic tubular adenoma in a biopsy of ileal pouch mucosa from a patient with familial adenomatous polyposis.

either by mucosal prolapse or by repeated catheterization. This is sometimes practised in patients that have postoperative difficulty with pouch evacuation.

Despite all efforts, an occasional patient with Crohn's disease will have undergone pouch surgery. The outcome for these patients is unpredictable; severe pouch inflammation, with stricturing and fistulation are not inevitable (Panis *et al.*, 1996). When the pouch does become affected by Crohn's disease, patchy inflammation and oedema, fissuring ulceration and granulomas may be seen in biopsies (Fig. 7.9), rather than the more diffuse pouchitis described above.

7.7 NEOPLASIA

7.7.1 Adenoma

Adenomas frequently develop in the pouch mucosa of patients with familial adenomatous polyposis (FAP) and are usually tubular in type, small and mildly dysplastic (Fig. 7.10) but may occasionally be large and villous (Beveridge *et al.*, 2004). Thus, patients with FAP who have had prophylactic proctocolectomy and ileoanal pouch surgery remain at risk for the development of tumours in the pouch and still require careful follow-up.

7.7.2 Dysplasia

Very few instances of epithelial dysplasia have been described in pouch mucosa in patients with ulcerative colitis (Veress *et al.*, 1995) and molecular genetic changes have been found with low prevalence (Gullberg *et al.*, 2002). However, we have not seen an example of dysplasia in these circumstances in our own practice (Setti-Carraro *et al.*, 1994) and it is probably a rare event (Thompson-Fawcett *et al.*, 2001), suggesting that surveillance need not be instituted in these patients (Herline *et al.*, 2003). It should, however, be remembered that any residual rectal mucosa, for example in an anorectal cuff, remains at risk of neoplasia following colectomy. The anal transitional zone mucosa is particularly prone to undergo dysplasia (O'Riordain *et al.*, 2000).

REFERENCES

Bell, A.J., Price, A.B., Forbes, A., Ciclitera, P.J., Groves, C., Nicholls, R.J. (2006) Pre-pouch ileitis: a disease of the ileum in ulcerative colitis after restorative proctocolectomy. *Colorectal Dis.*, 8(5), 401–10.

Beveridge, I.G., Swain, D.J., Groves, C.J. *et al.* (2004) Large villous adenomas arising in ileal pouches in familial adenomatous polyposis: report of two cases. *Dis. Colon Rectum*, 47, 123–6.

Carter, M.J., Di Giovine, F.S., Cox, A. *et al.* (2001) The interleukin 1 receptor antagonist gene allele 2 as a predictor of pouchitis following colectomy and IPAA in ulcerative colitis. *Gastroenterology*, 121, 805–11.

Cheifetz, A., Itzkowitz, S. (2004) The diagnosis and treatment of pouchitis in inflammatory bowel disease. *J. Clin. Gastroenterol.*, 38, S44–50.

de-Silva, H.J., Millard, P.R., Kettlewell, M., Mortensen, N.J., Prince, C., Jewell, D.P. (1991) Mucosal characteristics of pelvic ileal pouches. *Gut*, 32, 61–5.

Evgenikos, N., Bartolo, D.C., Hamer-Hodges, D.W., Ghosh, S. (2001) Comparison of the Moskowitz criteria and the pouchitis disease activity index (PDAI) for diagnosis of ileoanal pouch inflammation. *Colorectal Dis.*, 3, 161–4.

Goldstein, N.S., Sanford, W.W., Bodzin, J.H. (1997) Crohn's-like complications in patients with ulcerative colitis after total proctocolectomy and ileal pouch–anal anastomosis. *Am. J. Surg. Pathol.*, 21, 1343–53.

Gullberg, K., Lindforss, U., Zetterquist, H. *et al.* (2002) Cancer risk assessment in long-standing pouchitis. DNA aberrations are rare in transformed neoplastic pelvic pouch mucosa. *Int. J. Colorectal Dis.*, 17, 92–7.

Herline, A.J., Meisinger, L.L., Rusin, L.C. *et al.* (2003) Is routine pouch surveillance for dysplasia indicated for ileoanal pouches? *Dis. Colon Rectum*, 46, 156–9.

Lohmuller, J.L., Pemberton, J.H., Dozois, R.R., Ilstrup, D., van Heerden, J. (1990) Pouchitis and extraintestinal manifestations of inflammatory bowel disease after ileal pouch–anal anastomosis. *Ann. Surg.*, 211, 622–7.

Meagher, A.P., Farouk, R., Dozois, R.R., Kelly, K.A., Pemberton, J.H. (1998) J ileal pouch–anal anastomosis for chronic ulcerative colitis: complications and long-term outcome in 1310 patients. *Br. J. Surg.*, 85, 800–3.

Merrett, M.N., Soper, N., Mortensen, N., Jewell, D.P. (1996) Intestinal permeability in the ileal pouch. *Gut*, 39, 226–30.

Moskowitz, R.L., Shepherd, N.A., Nicholls, R.J. (1986) An assessment of inflammation in the reservoir after restorative proctocolectomy with ileoanal ileal reservoir. *Int. J. Colorectal Dis.*, 1, 167–74.

Nicholls, R.J., Kamm, M.A. (1988) Proctocolectomy with restorative ileoanal reservoir for severe idiopathic constipation. Report of two cases. *Dis. Colon Rectum*, 31, 968–9.

Nicholls, R.J., Moskowitz, R.L., Shepherd, N.A. (1985) Restorative proctocolectomy with ileal reservoir. *Br. J. Surg.*, 72(Suppl.), S76–9.

O'Riordain, M.G., Fazio, V.W., Lavery, I.C. *et al.* (2000) Incidence and natural history of dysplasia of the anal transitional zone after ileal pouch–anal anastomosis: results of a five-year to ten-year follow-up. *Dis. Colon Rectum*, 43, 1660–5.

Panis, Y., Poupard, B., Nemeth, J., Lavergne, A., Hautefeuille, P., Valleur, P. (1996) Ileal pouch/anal anastomosis for Crohn's disease. *Lancet*, 347, 854–7.

Parks, A.G., Nicholls, R.J. (1978) Proctocolectomy without ileostomy for ulcerative colitis. *Br. Med. J.*, 2, 85–8.

Penna, C., Dozois, R., Tremaine, W., Sandborn, W., LaRusso, N., Schleck, C., Ilstrup, D. (1996) Pouchitis after ileal pouch-anal anastomosis for ulcerative colitis occurs with increased frequency in patients with associated primary sclerosing cholangitis. *Gut*, 38, 234–9.

Pishori, T., Dinnewitzer, A., Zmora, O. *et al.* (2004) Outcome of patients with indeterminate colitis undergoing a double-stapled ileal pouch–anal anastomosis. *Dis. Colon Rectum*, 47, 717–21.

Sandborn, W.J., Tremaine, W.J., Batts, K.P., Pemberton, J.H., Phillips, S.F. (1994) Pouchitis after ileal pouch–anal anastomosis: a Pouchitis Disease Activity Index. *Mayo Clin. Proc.*, 69, 409–15.

Setti-Carraro, P., Ritchie, J.K., Wilkinson, K.H., Nicholls, R.J., Hawley, P.R. (1994) The first 10 years' experience of restorative proctocolectomy for ulcerative colitis. *Gut*, 35, 1070–5.

Shepherd, N.A., Jass, J.R., Duval, I., Moskowitz, R.L., Nicholls, R.J., Morson, B.C. (1987). Restorative proctocolectomy with ileal reservoir: pathological and histochemical study of biopsy specimens. *J. Clin. Pathol.*, 40, 601–7.

Shepherd, N.A., Hulten, L., Tytgat, G.N. *et al.* (1989) Pouchitis. *Int. J. Colorectal Dis.*, 4, 205–29.

Thompson-Fawcett, M.W., Mortensen, N.J., Warren, B.F. (1999) 'Cuffitis' and inflammatory changes in the columnar cuff, anal transitional zone, and ileal reservoir after stapled pouch–anal anastomosis. *Dis. Colon Rectum*, 42, 348–55.

Thompson-Fawcett, M.W., Marcus, V., Redston, M., Cohen, Z., McLeod, R.S. (2001) Risk of dysplasia in long-term ileal pouches and pouches with chronic pouchitis. *Gastroenterology*, 121, 275–81.

Veress, B., Reinholt, F.P., Lindquist, K., Lofberg, R., Liljeqvist, L. (1995) Long-term histomorphological surveillance of the pelvic ileal pouch: dysplasia develops in a subgroup of patients. *Gastroenterology*, 109, 1090–7.

CHAPTER 8

PSEUDOMEMBRANOUS COLITIS

8.1 Introduction: pseudomembranous colitis, antibiotic–associated colitis and diarrhoea — 133
   8.1.1 Terminology — 134
8.2 The biopsy diagnosis — 134
   8.2.1 Pseudomembranous colitis — 134
   8.2.2 Antibiotic-associated colitis — 138
   8.2.3 Antibiotic-associated diarrhoea — 139

8.3 Problems in the differential diagnosis — 140
8.4 *Clostridium difficile* and its toxin — 140
8.5 The pathologist's role in the diagnosis of pseudomembranous colitis — 142
8.6 Conclusions — 142
References — 142

8.1 INTRODUCTION: PSEUDOMEMBRANOUS COLITIS, ANTIBIOTIC-ASSOCIATED COLITIS AND DIARRHOEA

The appearances of typical pseudomembranous colitis (PMC) present no diagnostic problems to the pathologist (Goulston and McGovern, 1965; Price and Davies, 1977). Problems arise because PMC can be a patchy lesion producing sampling errors and because of the complex relationship between diarrhoea, antibiotics and the spectrum of pathological changes. While for many in the community antibiotic-associated diarrhoea (AAD) is little more than nuisance value, in the elderly hospitalized patient established PMC is a cause of significant mortality. Especially if there is comorbid disease, the patient is immunocompromised or there is a delay in diagnosis (Morris *et al.*, 2002; Andrews *et al.*, 2003).

When *Clostridium difficile* was identified as one of the major causes of PMC, if not the only cause, its presence or that of its toxin seemed to provide a simple diagnostic test (Rifkin *et al.*, 1977; Bartlett *et al.*, 1978a; George *et al.*, 1978; Larson and Price, 1977). It is now evident that the relationships between the organism and its toxins, antibiotics and mucosal pathology are complex, resulting in a wide spectrum of disease patterns from combinations of pathogenic factors (Lishman *et al.*, 1981; Kyne *et al.*, 2001; Wilcox and Minton, 2001). Isolated case reports also exist which suggest that other organisms may occasionally produce the picture of PMC (Schwartz *et al.*, 1980; Phillips *et al.*, 1981; Dickinson *et al.*, 1985; Battaglino and Rockey, 1999; Olofinlade and Chiang, 2001).

A characteristic morphological feature is the inflammatory pseudomembrane but, in general terms, this could result from many causes of inflammatory mucosal damage. It is perhaps not surprising therefore that the term 'pseudomembranous' may be used more broadly being incorporated into the descriptive terminology that includes other patterns of inflammatory bowel disease, for example pseudomembranous collagenous colitis (Section 9.3.1) (Byrne *et al.*, 2003; Yuan *et al.*, 2003).

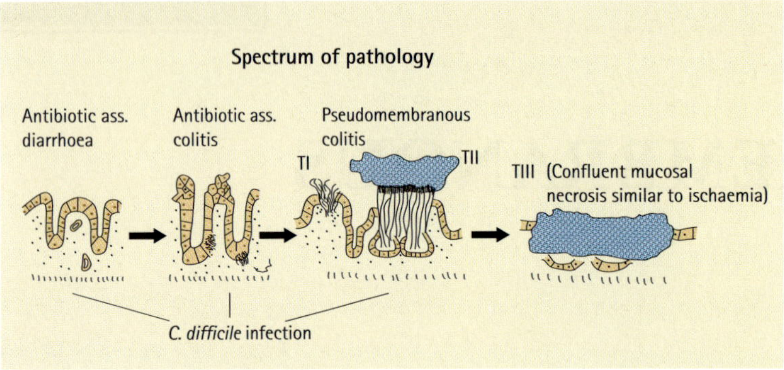

Figure 8.1 Diagrammatic representation of the spectrum of changes associated with antibiotics and *Clostridium difficile* infection (Figs 8.3a,b, 8.6a,b, 8.8, 8.10).

8.1.1 Terminology

Pseudomembranous colitis, antibiotic-associated colitis (AAC) and AAD are closely linked terms. They are not, however, synonymous and each encompasses a different part of the overall spectrum.

8.1.1a Pseudomembranous colitis

We feel that this is solely a morphological diagnosis based on histological appearances in the biopsy. It is not an absolute requirement to have a history of antibiotics (Bartlett *et al.*, 1980; Perkin *et al.*, 1980; Wald *et al.*, 1980) or to isolate *C. difficile* with or without its toxin (Dickinson *et al.*, 1985; Olafinlade and Chiang 2001). In the large majority of cases, however, there will be a history of antibiotics and *C. difficile* and/or its toxin will be present (Bartlett, 1979). Virtually any antibiotic, with the possible exceptions of vancomycin and the aminoglycosides should be considered potential offenders.

8.1.1b Antibiotic-associated colitis

This term implies a clear history of recent antibiotics and biopsy evidence of colitis, sometimes with features in common with infectious colitis (see below), but without pseudomembrane formation.

8.1.1c Antibiotic-associated diarrhoea

This is best reserved for patients recently prescribed antibiotics who develop diarrhoea but have normal rectal biopsies. It is less closely linked to the presence of *C. difficile* than PMC and AAC (Bartlett, 2000) (Section 8.2.3).

8.1.1d *Clostridium difficile*-associated diarrhoea

Clostridium difficile-associated diarrhoea (CDAD) is defined by the presence of the organism and its toxins and can occur in all three of the conditions described above, the association being strongest with PMC and weakest with AAD.

8.1.1e Summary

The above terms should be qualified by a statement on the presence of *C. difficile* and its toxins (Fig. 8.1).

The value of these definitions is limited by the extent of the clinical examination. For strict accuracy a diagnosis of PMC can only be excluded after a full colonoscopic examination. It is a patchy disease which, when severe, involves the rectum, but rectal sparing often occurs. Thus Tedesco *et al.* (1982) found that only 77 per cent of cases were identified if investigation was limited to rigid sigmoidoscopy and this was as low as 31 per cent in the series of Seppala *et al.* (1981). With the greater range of the flexible sigmoidoscope 85 per cent of cases could be detected.

8.2 THE BIOPSY DIAGNOSIS

8.2.1 Pseudomembranous colitis

A helpful clinician will document that there are discrete yellow plaques to be seen on sigmoidoscopy (Fig. 8.2). Often, however, the view is obscured by a torrent of faeces. Furthermore, the developing

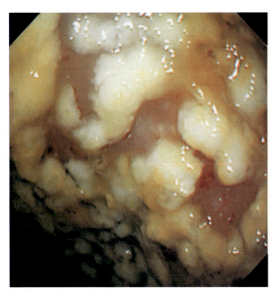

Figure 8.2 Endoscopic view of the yellow plaques separated by normal mucosa typical of the type II lesions of pseudomembranous colitis.

lesion, although recognizable on microscopy may not be apparent macroscopically.

The biopsy patterns have been divided into three (Price and Davies, 1977), reflecting pathological, but not necessarily clinical, severity. There is some evidence that the changes can be progressive, with the typical lesions not seen until the third or fourth biopsy (Keighley *et al.*, 1978). It is also known that patients with established PMC have higher faecal toxin titres and white cell counts and more profuse diarrhoea (Burdon *et al.*, 1981).

8.2.1a Type I lesion

This comprises a small surface erosion between the crypts. There is commonly a luminal spray of nuclear debris, polymorphs and mucus (Figs 3.5 and 8.3). The immediately adjacent lamina propria is usually oedematous with clusters of polymorphs and capillary ectasia. Local crypts can show some infiltration by polymorphs and there may be an eosinophilic subepithelial exudate. Intact surface epithelial cells often appear grouped into tufts, giving the mucosa a crenated appearance (Fig. 3.4). Several discrete lesions may be apparent in the same biopsy. It is important that other adjacent

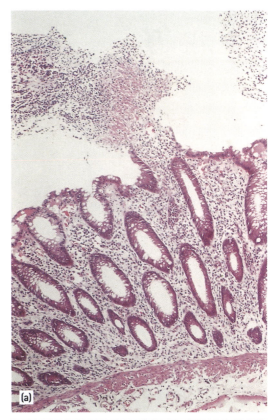

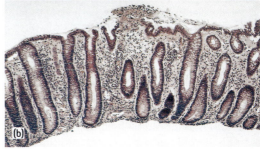

Figure 8.3 (a, b) The type I lesion. A luminal spray of mucus and polymorphs, the latter often with a linear configuration, on a background mucosa with minimal inflammatory changes.

abnormalities are limited to those of a minor nature as described here; surface erosions are a common response to any mucosal trauma or mucosal prolapse (du Boulay *et al.*, 1983) and the distinction of the *Type I* focus from an early developing ulcer of whatever cause may be difficult (Fig. 8.4). The adjacent mucosa should provide the clues that allow the correct evaluation of the erosive lesions (Fig. 8.5).

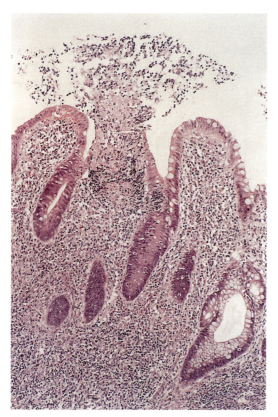

Figure 8.4 A superficial erosion in a biopsy from a patient with ulcerative colitis mimicking a type I lesion. The intense accompanying acute and chronic inflammation is not seen in pseudomembranous colitis and is the clue to considering an alternative diagnosis. In this particular biopsy there was some adjacent crypt architectural distortion.

This Type I change, or 'summit' lesion (Price and Davies, 1977), is the earliest from which a confident diagnosis of PMC can be given. It is essential to cut levels through a biopsy to try and identify such a lesion in all suspected cases. Misinterpretation of the non-specific nature of miscellaneous tiny erosions, whatever the site, has resulted in PMC being described in unusual locations, such as in adenomas or even in the bladder (Goulston and McGovern, 1980).

8.2.1b Type II lesion

This is the classical picture of PMC and corresponds to the yellow plaque seen on the colonic and rectal mucosa (Fig. 8.2). It is important for the clinician to

biopsy the plaque as the intervening mucosa is virtually normal. Focal groups of disrupted crypts are present. Any biopsy may contain two or three such groups, each comprising two to six crypts. These are dilated and have usually shed the superficial half of the crypt epithelium (Fig. 8.6). Mucin, fibrin and polymorphs stream out of the dilated crypts and sit as a cap over the surface. The adjacent mucosa shows only minimal inflammation and the crypt architecture is intact. When submucosa is present in the biopsy it is often oedematous. In some cases capillary microthrombi may be observed in the mucosa. Margination of polymorphs is also a common observation within dilated capillaries.

Interestingly, the classical type II appearance of PMC with the disruption of crypts and loss of cellular adhesion may result in the appearance of signet ring cells (Fig. 8.7) (Schiffman, 1996). These should not be mistaken for malignant cells and are always contained within the crypt boundaries. In difficult cases immunostaining may help. In benign signet ring cell change the cells are all negative for p53 and Ki6, and all positive with E cadherin (Wang *et al.*, 2003). By contrast, signet ring carcinoma cells are only weakly positive for E-cadherin and positive for p53 and Ki67 in over 50 per cent of the cases.

8.2.1c Type III lesion

Biopsies from this stage show the most destruction (Fig. 8.8). Endoscopically, a pseudomembrane is clearly visible and individual plaques are beginning to coalesce to give a confluent membrane.

A biopsy may be unhelpful when there is complete mucosal ulceration with a covering of inflammatory slough, the histology being identical to that at any site of mucosal necrosis from whatever cause. The presence of relatively normal mucosa at one edge is a helpful clue to the diagnosis of PMC. However, caution is required in toxic megacolon, as the surviving mucosal islands appear relatively normal in the face of severe adjacent ulceration (Fig. 12.6 on page 208) (Price, 1978).

At a stage prior to complete necrosis the ghost outlines of the disrupted crypts may be discernible in a background of inflammatory cells and degenerate lamina propria. Again, cautious interpretation is

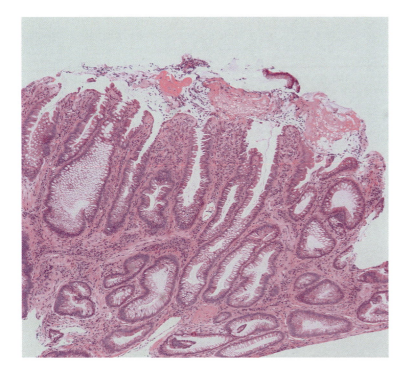

Figure 8.5 A biopsy in a case of the mucosal prolapse syndrome with surface features that mimic a type I lesion. In this case the background features were of fibrosis and arborization of the muscularis mucosae into the overlying lamina propria.

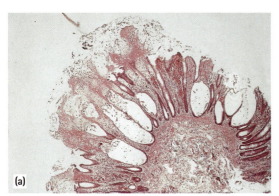

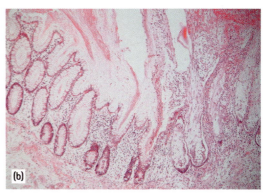

Figure 8.6 (a,b) These two micrographs illustrate typical type II lesions of pseudomembranous colitis. There is cystic dilatation of groups of crypts which have shed the superficial half of their epithelial linings into the overlying exudates. The latter forms the yellow membranes seen in Fig. 8.2.

necessary as ischaemic necrosis produces a similar picture (Figs 8.9 and 10.4; Section 10.9) and autolysis in a poorly fixed biopsy can be misinterpreted by the unwary. Capillary thrombi, perhaps a guide to primary ischaemic disease, are frequently seen at this stage (Whitehead, 1971). But these too are difficult to evaluate for they may well be secondary to the ulcerative events (Section 10.6.2). This can be resolved if they are found beneath intact mucosa. Signet ring cell change (Fig. 8.7), referred to above, within the type III pattern is also a source of misinterpretation since the margins of the crypts, within which the signet ring cells are contained and which provide a useful delineation from the pattern in malignancy, are no longer as easily discernible.

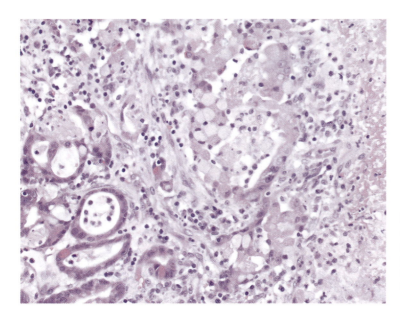

Figure 8.7 Distended mucin-containing cells with loss of cell cohesion in a case of pseudomembranous colitis – an appearance not to be misinterpreted as a signet ring cell carcinoma.

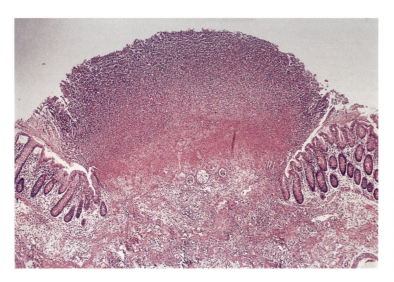

Figure 8.8 Pseudomembranous colitis, type III lesion. The mucosa is almost entirely necrotic. Distinction from ischaemic colitis can be difficult at this stage, though the finding of normal mucosa on either side is often a useful clue.

8.2.2 Antibiotic-associated colitis

By definition, there is no membrane and the three patterns of PMC are absent. However, the mucosa often shows changes akin to those described in infective proctocolitis (Section 4.2.1), though of a more muted nature (Price and Day, 1981; Rocca *et al.*, 1984). Mild focal inflammation of the mucosa is present with clusters of polymorphs and only a minimal increase in plasma cells. The polymorphs are usually superficial and infiltrate the upper halves of the crypts and surface epithelium. The latter can appear crenated, as described earlier, owing to heaping up of 'nests' of epithelium (Fig. 8.10). Nuclear debris is seen, with capillary dilatation and focal subepithelial oedema. The impression is that, close by, there is a Type I summit lesion and examination of levels through the block is mandatory

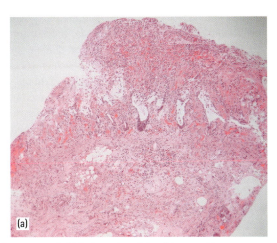
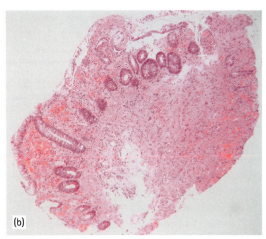

Figure 8.9 (a,b) Ischaemic colitis with resemblance to pseudomembranous colitis. (a) There is partial necrosis of the crypts and a surface membrane resembling a late type II lesion. The background mucosa shows the homogeneous eosinophilia characteristic of ischaemia and this is most evident to the left side where there is also typical crypt drop out and crypt withering. (b) The distinction from pseudomembranous colitis is helped by the features in an adjacent biopsy. Here there is crypt drop-out, eosinophilia of the lamina propria and haemorrhage, all characteristic of ischaemic damage.

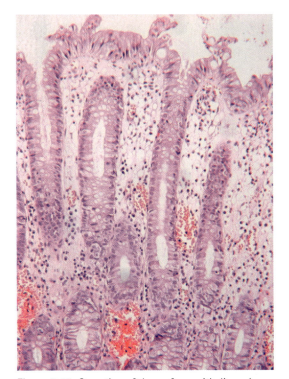

Figure 8.10 Crenation of the surface epithelium along with oedema and mild inflammatory changes. This picture is far from diagnostic but if this is the only abnormality seen then infection, in particular *Clostridium difficile*, should be included in the differential diagnosis.

when these features are present. The clinician should be reminded to double-check the antibiotic history.

However, the above pattern is by no means diagnostic. It may be seen in any one of the infective diarrhoeas and, it must be said, in many patients with diarrhoea for whom no explanation is found. However, it forms the basis for what is usually a helpful clinical suggestion. In the majority of patients with AAC the picture is simply one of acute non-specific inflammation, as described in Section 12.3, where even the subtle clues of tufting, nuclear debris and subepithelial oedema are absent.

A transient right-sided haemorrhagic AAC has been described in relation to ampicillin and penicillin (Sakurai *et al.*, 1979; Toffler *et al.*, 1978) but, to date, no pathological details have been documented. This could be related to the verotoxin producing *Escherichia coli* (Section 4.2.4a).

8.2.3 Antibiotic-associated diarrhoea

Within the scope of this book this term is restricted to patients with a relevant history and diarrhoea, but with a normal biopsy. It is frustrating to realize that the majority of patients with diarrhoea related to recent antibiotics will fall into this category, indeed *C. difficile* is responsible for only a small percentage of the cases of AAD in the community (Beaugerie *et al.*, 2003). There is an association with *C. difficile* toxin in 10–20 per cent of cases (Bartlett, 1984, 2002). Obviously, the group is difficult to evaluate and only colonoscopic biopsies can confidently exclude a colitis, an investigation seldom justified in such cases.

The enigmatic cases of AAD are more likely to be dose related, less likely to experience accompanying systemic symptoms and usually resolve on stopping the drug or reducing the dose. In contrast, *C. difficile*-associated cases may persist following cessation of the drug and are more likely to be recategorized as AAC if a biopsy is undertaken (Demaio and Bartlett 1995; Bartlett 2002).

8.3 PROBLEMS IN THE DIFFERENTIAL DIAGNOSIS

The Type II lesion of PMC should present no difficulty. When AAC and PMC are clinically suspected multiple levels need to be examined. With the summit lesions (Type 1) care is needed to exclude non-specific erosions due to local mucosal damage (Section 3.4) or early ulceration, as seen in other inflammatory disease processes. Inspection of the whole biopsy is usually sufficient to do this. In ulcerative colitis (Section 5.2.1) glandular irregularity and goblet cell depletion can be appreciated. Crohn's disease (in the absence of a granuloma) may be harder to eliminate but usually carries a heavier infiltrate of chronic inflammatory cells (Section 6.3.2). In ischaemic colitis the pathology is determined by the rate of onset and it is the distinction between the type III lesion of PMC and the pathology seen with an acute onset of ischaemic damage (Sections 10.6.1 and 10.6.2), rather than the chronic patterns (Sections 10.6.3 and 10.6.4), that is the most difficult to make (Fig. 8.9). In both an inflammatory membrane can be present reflecting the extensive mucosal damage. In the comparative study by Dignan and Greenson (1997) the significant findings favouring ischaemia in such circumstances were a hyalinized lamina propria, signs of atrophic

crypts, lamina propria haemorrhage and a greater likelihood of full thickness necrosis. Indeed, until the discovery of *C. difficile*, PMC was simply considered a variant of ischaemic colitis and the occasional presence of microthrombi may explain at least some of the ischaemic-like features sometimes encountered in PMC. Furthermore it is likely that the pathogenesis of clostridial toxins occurs in part through an ischaemic mechanism.

The typical changes of AAC, as stated, resemble to some degree those in other forms of infectious proctocolitis and stool culture is necessary. This will also detect *C. difficile* and a faecal toxin test must be done.

In the perspective of all such specimens encountered in the histopathology department, it must be repeated that from the majority of patients with diarrhoea following a recent course of antibiotics, a biopsy will be normal or show only minor abnormalities (AAC) and *C. difficile* and its toxins will be undetectable (Beaugerie *et al.*, 2003). However, because diarrhoea can commence many weeks after such a course has been completed, the clinician may not even be aware of the drug history (Tedesco *et al.*, 1974).

In general, the clinician can have some indication whether the antibiotic-associated diarrhoea is *C. difficile* related or due to other causes (Bartlett, 1996) apart from the microbiology result. Thus, as mentioned earlier (Section 8.2.3), in enigmatic AAC, in contrast to *C. difficile*-associated AAC, systemic symptoms are uncommon, there is evidence of dose dependency and usually the diarrhoea will stop if the antibiotic is discontinued (Bartlett, 2002).

8.4 *CLOSTRIDIUM DIFFICILE* AND ITS TOXIN

Following the initial discovery of the association of toxigenic *C. difficile* with PMC (Larson and Price, 1977; Larson *et al.*, 1977; Bartlett *et al.*, 1978b) it has been realized that the association of the organism and antibiotic-associated intestinal disease is complex (Starr, 2005). Toxigenic *C. difficile* is found in over 90 per cent of cases of PMC, 30–40 per cent of cases of AAC and only 6–10 per cent of cases of

AAD (Bartlett, 1979; Burdon *et al.*, 1981; Borriello *et al.*, 1987; Wilcox and Spencer, 1992; Demaio and Bartlett, 1995). This emphasizes that the cause of the majority of cases of AAD is unknown (George *et al.*, 1982; Bartlett, 1996; Beaugerie *et al.*, 2003). In most patients the diarrhoea begins within days of commencing antibiotics, but with the caveat that on a few occasions AAD can develop many weeks after they have finished (Tedesco *et al.*, 1974). In such instances the association might go undetected. Neither the dose nor the route of administration of the antibiotic seems to have any predictive role (Tedesco, 1984). The complex relationship between organism and disease is best appreciated from the observation that toxigenic organisms are carried by up to 64 per cent of healthy neonates (Holst *et al.*, 1981; Lyerly and Wilkins, 1984) and by a small percentage of the normal adult population (Lishman *et al.*, 1981; Demaio and Bartlett, 1995; Dodson and Borriello, 1996; Ozaki *et al.*, 2004). It is clear that, following antibiotic treatment, some individuals harbour the organism and its toxin without developing diarrhoea and that in some patients with diarrhoea, the organism can be isolated, yet there is no detectable toxin (George *et al.*, 1982; Nash *et al.*, 1982; Kyne *et al.*, 2000; Wilcox and Minton, 2001). Moreover the first stool test may be negative (Johal *et al.*, 2004). Asymptomatic carriage is highest in the hospitalized population (Demaio and Bartlett, 1995) and in one study on AAD it was found that, even if the symptoms began in the community, the majority had been hospitalized in the preceding 12 months (Johal *et al.*, 2004). In general, the higher the faecal toxin, the more likely a membrane is to be found (Burdon *et al.*, 1981). It is not understood why some patients after exposure to antibiotics and colonization by *C. difficile*, will develop PMC, whereas others suffer only mild diarrhoea. However, evidence is emerging to show that IgA and IgA antibodies play a role in moderating disease and relapse (Barclay and Borriello, 1984; Kelly, 1996; Kyne *et al.*, 2001; Wilcox and Minton, 2001). This is supported by Johal *et al.* (2004) who have shown that in biopsies from patients with *C. difficile*-associated diarrhoea there were reduced numbers of IgA-producing plasma cells and macrophages in the lamina propria compared with controls. Moreover, this was most marked in

the cases in which a pseudomembranous morphology was present and in those with recurrent disease.

The organism produces two principal toxins classically referred to as A and B (Mitchell *et al.*, 1986; Wren *et al.*, 1987). Some species may produce a binary toxin but its role in human disease is uncertain (Geric *et al.*, 2003). Toxin A is an enterotoxin, responsible for fluid accumulation in the gut, damage to enterocolonic mucosa in animal models and damage to tight junctions in epithelial monolayers. Toxin B is a labile, motility-altering cytotoxin toxin, causing fluid accumulation in rabbit ileal loops (Banno *et al.*, 1984). Toxin B was originally thought only to cause a cytopathic effect (Taylor *et al.*, 1981; Sullivan *et al.*, 1982) but more recent data shows that A negative–B positive strains can cause disease (Borriello *et al.*, 1992; Limaye *et al.*, 2000) and toxin B does have enteropathic effects (Savidge *et al.*, 2003). Both are lethal in the experimental animal (Libby *et al.*, 1982). In addition to variations in antibody responses in individuals and other risk factors (Starr, 2005), variations in the balance between toxin A and B may account for some of the vagaries in the pattern of *C. difficile*-associated colonic disease (Wren *et al.*, 1987). At a cellular level the disruption of tight junctions by toxin A helps toxin B enter epithelial cells. After internalization by the mucosal epithelial cells, their effects on the actin microfilament system are broadly similar (Pothoulakis, 1996).

Because of the spectrum of findings in antibiotic-associated disease, the biopsy and the microbiological findings should be evaluated separately (Samra *et al.*, 2002*)*. Only in established PMC is there a correlation of over 90 per cent. Negative microbiology in such cases is therefore likely to be a false result. As already mentioned, the first stool sample in the clinical situation may be negative and worth repeating (Johal *et al.*, 2004).

Clostridium difficile has been associated with exacerbations of ulcerative colitis and Crohn's disease (Meyers *et al.*, 1981; Trnka and Lamont, 1981; Dorman *et al.*, 1982; Keighley *et al.*, 1982). Though never specifically tested, our experience is that the biopsies in such situations reflect these two conditions (Nash *et al.*, 1997). The organism also has a minor role as a pathogen in cases of sporadic diarrhoea as seen in community studies (Falsen et al., 1980; Brettle et al., 1982; Nash et al., 1982; Beaugerie et al., 2003), but is now recognized as one of the major infective causes of hospital acquired diarrhoea (Starr, 2005). As already noted above, many patients with AAD presenting from the community have been hospitalized within the previous 12 months (Johal et al., 2004).

8.5 THE PATHOLOGIST'S ROLE IN THE DIAGNOSIS OF PSEUDOMEMBRANOUS COLITIS

The gold standard for the diagnosis of *C. difficile* is a positive toxin test (Bartlett 2002), which is positive in 97 per cent of patients with classical histological PMC, 27 per cent of patients with antibiotic-associated diarrhoea and 2 per cent of asymptomatic patients that have received antibiotics (Counihan and Roberts, 1993). Thus, this is a more sensitive test than endoscopic biopsy and allows treatment of a wider range of patients. However, there is still a role for the histopathologist in the clinically unsuspected case in which membranes have not been appreciated, are obscured by poor bowel preparation or where tests are inconclusive. Furthermore, it is the histopathologist's role to flag up a toxin test as the next appropriate investigation in biopsies in which the picture conforms to that of AAC. Finally, remember that a biopsy with no characteristic features of PMC does not necessarily exclude the diagnosis as the colonoscopist may have misdirected the biopsy and sampled between lesions or failed to appreciate that the left colon can be spared (Tedesco et al., 1982; Johal et al., 2004).

8.6 CONCLUSIONS

No one test alone, be it biopsy or culture, can establish the diagnosis of antibiotic-associated disease. Usually, a rectal biopsy, a faecal toxin test and the clinical story are adequate for patient management. While the majority of investigations in clinical antibiotic-associated diarrhoea are negative, ultimately, only total colonoscopic examination and biopsy can exclude either plaque formation or lesser degrees of inflammation.

REFERENCES

Andrews, C.N., Raboud, J., Kassen, B.O., Enns, R. (2003) *Clostridium difficile*-associated diarrhoea: predictors of severity in patients presenting to the emergency department. *Can. J. Gastroenterol.*, 17, 379–73.

Banno, Y., Kobyashi, T., Kono, H., Watanabe, K., Uena, K., Nozawa, Y. (1984) Biochemical characterization and biologic actions of two toxins (D-1 and D-2) from *Clostridium difficile*. *Rev. Infect. Dis.*, 6, S11–S20.

Barclay, F.E., Borriello, S.P. (1984) *Clostridium difficile* and colonization resistance. In: Borriello, S.P. (ed.) *Antibiotic associated diarrhoea and colitis*. Boston: Martinus Nijhoff, pp. 79–87.

Bartlett, J.G. (1979) Antibiotic associated colitis. *Clin. Gastroenterol.*, 8, 783–801.

Bartlett, J.G. (1984) Pseudomembranous colitis and antibiotic-associated colitis. In: Bouchier, I.A.D., Allan, R.N., Hodgson, H.J.F., Keighley M.R.B. (eds) *Textbook of gastroenterology*. London: Balliere Tindall, pp. 1091–7.

Bartlett, J.G. (1996) Management of *Clostridium difficile* infection and other antibiotic-associated diarrhoeas. *Eur. J. Gastroenterol. Hepatol.*, 8, 1054–61.

Bartlett, J.G. (2000) Antibiotic-associated diarrhoea. *N. Engl. J. Med.*, 346, 334–9.

Bartlett, J.G. (2002) *Clostridium difficile*-associated enteric disease. *Curr. Infect. Dis. Rep.*, 4; 477–83.

Bartlett, J.G., Moon, N., Chang, T.W., Taylor, N., Onderdonk, A.B. (1978a) Role of *Clostridium difficile* in antibiotic-associated pseudo-membranous colitis. *Gastroenterology*, 75, 778–82.

Bartlett, J.G., Chang, T.W., Gurwith, M., Gorbach, S.L., Onderdonk, A.B. (1978b) Antibiotic-associated pseudomembranous colitis due to toxin–producing clostridia. *N. Engl. J. Med.*, 298, 531–4.

Bartlett, J.G., Taylor, N.S., Chang, T.W., Dyink, J. (1980) Clinical and laboratory observations in *Clostridium difficile* colitis. *Am. J. Clin. Nutr.*, 33, 2521–6.

Battaglino M.P., Rockey D.C. (1999) Cytomegalovirus colitis presenting with the endoscopic appearance of pseudomembranous colitis. *Gastrointest. Endosc.*, 50, 697–700.

Beaugerie, L., Flahault, A., Barbut, F. *et al.* (2003) Antibiotic-associated diarrhoea and *Clostridium difficile* in the community. *Aliment. Pharmacol. Therap.*, 17, 905–12.

Borriello, S.P., Ketley J.M., Mitchell T.J., Barclay F.E., Welch A.R., Price A.B., Stephen J. (1987) *Clostridium difficile* – a spectrum of virulence and analysis of putative virulence determinants in the hamster model of antibiotic-associated colitis. *J Med. Microbiol.*, 24, 53–64.

Borriello, S.P., Wren, B.W., Hyde, S. *et al.* (1992) Molecular, immunological, and biological characterization of a Toxin A-negative, Toxin-B positive strain of *Clostridium difficile*. *Inf. Immun.*, 60, 4191–9.

du Boulay, C.E.H., Fairbrother, J., Isaacson, P. (1983) Mucosal prolapse syndrome – a unifying concept for solitary ulcer syndrome and related disorders. *J. Clin. Pathol.*, 36, 1264–8.

Brettle, R.P., Poxton, I.R., Murdoch, J.McC., Brown, R., Bryne, M.D., Collee, J.G. (1982) *Clostridium difficile* in association with sporadic diarrhoea. *Br. Med. J.*, 284, 230–3.

Burdon, D.W., George, R.H., Mogg, G.A.G. *et al.* (1981) Faecal toxin and severity of antibiotic–associated pseudomembranous colitis. *J. Clin. Pathol.*, 34, 548–51.

Byrne, M.F., Royston, D., Patchett, S.E. (2003) Association of common variable immuno-deficiency with atypical collagenous colitis. *Eur. J. Gastroenterol. Hepatol.*, 15, 1051–3.

Counihan, T.C., Roberts P.L. (1993) Pseudomem-branous colitis. *Surg. Clin. N. Am.* 73, 1063–74.

Demaio, J., Bartlett, J.G. (1995) Update on diagnosis of *Clostridium difficile*-associated diarrhoea. *Curr. Clin. Top. Infect. Dis.*, 15, 97–114.

Dickinson, R.J., Rampling, A., Wight, D.G.D. (1985) Spontaneous pseudomembranous colitis not associated with *Clostridium difficile*. *J. Infect.*, 10, 252–5.

Dignan, C.R., Greenson, J.K. (1997) Can ischaemic colitis be differentiated from *C. difficile* colitis in biopsy specimens. *Am. J. Surg. Pathol.*, 21, 706–10.

Dodson, A.P., Borriello, S.P. (1996) *Clostridium difficile* infection of the gut. *J. Clin. Pathol.*, 49, 529–32.

Dorman, S.A., Liggoria, E., Winn, W.C., Beeken, W.L. (1982) Isolation of *Clostridium difficile* from patients with inactive Crohn's disease. *Gastroenterology*, 82, 1348–51.

Falsen, E., Kayser, B., Rehls, L., Nygren, B., Svedhem, A. (1980) *Clostridium difficile* in relation to enteric bacterial pathogens. *J. Clin. Microbiol.*, 12, 297–300.

George, R.H., Symonds, J.M., Dimock, F. *et al.* (1978) Identification of *Clostridium difficile* as a cause of pseudomembranous colitis. *Br. Med. J.*, i, 695.

George, W.L., Rolfe, R.D., Finegold, S.M. (1982) *Clostridium difficile* and its cytotoxin in faeces of patients with antimicrobiol agent associated diarrhoea and miscellaneous conditions. *J. Clin. Microbiol.*, 15, 1049–53.

Geric, B., Johnson, S., Gerding, G.N., Grabnar, N., Rupnik, M. (2003) Frequency of binary toxin genes among *Clostridium difficile* strains that do not produce large clostridial toxins. *J. Clin. Microbiol.*, 41, 5227–32.

Goulston, S.J.M., McGovern, V.J. (1965) Pseudo-membranous colitis. *Gut*, 6, 207–12.

Goulston, S.J.M., McCovern, V.J. (1980) Clinical settings in pseudomembranous colitis. *Aust. N.Z. J. Med.*, 10, 139–45.

Holst, E., Helin, I., Mardh, P.A. (1981) Recovery of *Clostridium difficile* from children. *Scand. J. Infect. Dis.*, 13, 41–5.

Johal, S.S., Hammond, J., Solomon, K., James, P.D., Mahida, Y.R. (2004) *Clostridium difficile*-associated diarrhoea in hospitalised patients: onset in the community and hospital and role of flexible sigmoidoscopy. *Gut*, 53, 673–7.

Keighley, M.R.B., Burdon, D.W., Alexander-Williams, J. *et al.* (1978) Diarrhoea and pseudomembranous colitis after gastro-intestinal operations. A prospective study. *Lancet*, ii, 1165–7.

Keighley, M.R.B., Youngs, D., Johnson, M., Allan, R.N., Burdon, D.W. (1982) *Clostridium difficile* toxin in acute diarrhoea complicating inflammatory bowel disease. *Gut*, 23, 410–14.

Kelly, C.P. (1996) Immune response to *Clostridium difficile* infection. *Eur. J. Gastroenterol. Hepatol.*, 8, 1048–53.

Kyne, L., Warny, M., Qamar, A., Kelly, C.P. (2000) Asymptomatic carriage of *Clostridium difficile* and serum levels of IgG antibody against toxin A. *N. Engl. J. Med.*, 342, 390–7.

Kyne, L., Farrell, R.J., Kelly, C.P. (2001) *Clostridium difficile*. *Gastroenterol. Clin. N. Am.*, 30(3), 753–77.

Larson, H.E., Price, A.B. (1977) Pseudomembranous colitis: presence of clostridial toxin. *Lancet*, ii, 1312–14.

Larson, H.E., Parry, J.V., Price, A.B., Davies, D.R., Dolby, J., Tyrell, D.A.J. (1977) Undescribed toxin in pseudomembranous colitis. *Lancet*, i, 1063–6.

Libby, J.M., Jortner, B., Wilkins, T.D. (1982) Effects of the two toxins of *Clostridium difficile* in antibiotic associated cecitis in hamsters. *Infect. Immun.*, 36, 822–9.

Limaye, A.P., Turgeon, D.K., Cookson, B.T., Fritsche, T.R. (2000) Pseudomembranous colitis caused by a toxin A(−) B(+) strain of *Clostridium difficile*. *J. Clin. Microbiol.*, 38, 1696–7.

Lishman, A.H., Al-Jumaili, I.J., Record, C.O. (1981) Spectrum of antibiotic-associated diarrhoea. *Gut*, 22, 34–7.

Lyerly, D.M., Wilkins, T.D. (1984) Characteristics of the toxins of *Clostridium difficile*. In: Borriello, S.P. (ed.), *Antibiotic associated diarrhoea and colitis*. Boston: Martinus Nijhoff, pp. 90–102.

Meyers, S., Mayer, L., Boltone, E., Desmond, E., Janowitz, H.D. (1981) Occurrence of *Clostridium difficile* toxin during the course of inflammatory bowel disease. *Gastroenterology*, 80, 697–700.

Mitchell, T.J., Ketley, J.M., Haslam, S.C., Stephen, J., Burdon, D.W., Candy, D.C.A.,

Daniel, R. (1986) Effect of toxin A and B of *Clostridium difficile* on rabbit ileum and colon. *Gut*, 27, 78–85.

Morris, A.M., Jobe, B.A., Stoney, M., Sheppard, B.C., Deveney, C.W., Deveney, K.E. (2002) *Clostridium difficile* colitis: an increasingly aggressive iatrogenic disease? *Arch. Surg.* 137, 1096–100.

Nash, J.Q., Chattopadhyay, B., Honeycombe, J., Tabaqchali, S. (1982) *Clostridium difficile* and cytotoxin in routine faecal specimens. *J. Clin. Pathol.*, 35, 561–5.

Nash, S.V., Bourgeault, R., Sands, M. (1997) Colonic disease associated with a positive assay for Clostridium difficile toxin: a retrospective study. *J. Clin. Gastroenterol.*, 25, 476–9.

Olofinlade, O., Chiang, C. (2001) Cytomegalovirus infection as a cause of pseudomembranous colitis; a report of four cases. *J. Clin. Gastroenterol.*, 32, 82–4.

Ozaki, E., Kato, H., Kito, H. *et al.* (2004) *Clostridium difficile* colonization in healthy adults: transient colonization and correlation with enterococcal colonization. *J. Med. Microbiol.*, 53, 167–72.

Perkin, S.R., Galdibini, J., Bartlett, J.C. (1980) Role of *Clostridium difficile* in a case of non-antibiotic-associated pseudomembranous colitis. *Gastroenterology*, 79, 948–51.

Phillips, R.K.S., Glazer, C., Borriello, S.P. (1981) Non-*Clostridium difficile* pseudomembranous colitis responding to both vancomycin and metronidazole. *Br. Med. J.*, 283, 823.

Pothoulakis, C. (1996) Pathogenesis of *Clostridium difficile*-associated diarrhoea. *Eur. J. Gastroenterol. Hepatol.*, 8, 1041–7.

Price, A.B. (1978) Overlap in the spectrum of non-specific inflammatory bowel disease – 'colitis indeterminate'. *J. Clin. Pathol.*, 31, 567–77.

Price, A.B., Davies, D.R.D. (1977) Pseudo-membranous colitis. *J. Clin. Pathol.*, 30, 1–12.

Price, A.B., Day, D.W. (1981) Pseudomembranous and infective colitis. In: Anthony P.P., MacSween R.N.M. (eds) *Recent advances in histopathology* 11. Edinburgh: Churchill Livingstone, pp. 99–117.

Rifkin, G.D., Fekety, F.R., Silva, J. Jr (1977) Antibiotic induced colitis, implication of a toxin neutralized by *Clostridium sordellii* antitoxin. *Lancet*, ii, 1103–6.

Rocca, J.M., Heckor, R., Pieterse, A.S., Rich, G.E., Rowland, R. (1984) *Clostridium difficile* colitis. *Aust. N.Z. J. Med.*, 14, 606–10.

Sakurai, Y., Tsuchiya, H., Ikegami, F., Funatomi, T., Takesu, S., Uchikoshi, T. (1979) Acute right-sided haemorrhagic colitis associated with oral administration of ampicillin. *Dig. Dis. Sci.*, 24, 910–15.

Samra, Z., Talmor, S., Bahar, J. (2002) High prevalence of Toxin A-negative toxin B-positive Clostridium difficile in hospitalized patients with gastrointestinal disease. *Diagn. Microbiol. Infect. Dis.*, 43, 189–92.

Savidge, T.C., Pan, W.H., Newman, P., O'Brien, M., Anton, P.M., Pothoulakis, C. (2003) *Clostridium difficile* toxin B is an inflammatory in the human intestine. *Gastroenterology*, 125, 423–20.

Schiffman R. (1996) Signet-ring cells associated with pseudomembranous colitis. *Am. J. Surg. Pathol.* 20, 599–602.

Schwartz, J.M., Hamilton, J.P., Fekety, R. (1980) Clindamycin associated enterocolitis: implications of toxigenic *Clostridium perfringens* type C. *J. Paediatr.*, 97, 661–3.

Seppala, K., Hjelt, L., Sipponon, P. (1981) Colonoscopy in the diagnosis of antibiotic-associated colitis. A prospective study. *Scand. J. Gastroenterol.*, 16, 465–8.

Starr, J. (2005) *Clostridium difficile*-associated diarrhoea: diagnosis and treatment. *Br. Med. J.*, 331, 499–501.

Sullivan, N.M., Pellett, S., Wilkins, T.D. (1982) Purification and characterization of Toxin A and B of *Clostridium difficile*. *Infect. Immun.*, 35, 1032–40.

Taylor, N.S., Thorne, G.M., Bartlett, J.G. (1981) Comparison of two toxins produced by *Clostridium difficile*. *Infect. Immun.*, 34, 1036–43.

Tedesco, F.J. (1984) Antibiotics associated with *Clostridium difficile*-mediated diarrhoea and/or colitis. In: Borriello, S.P. (ed.) *Antibiotic associated diarrhoea and colitis*. Boston: Martinus Nijhoff, pp. 4–8.

Tedesco, F.J., Barton, R.W., Alpers, D.H. (1974) Clindamycin-associated colitis. *Ann. Intern. Med.*, 81, 429–33.

Tedesco, F.J., Corless, J.K., Brownstein, R.E. (1982) Rectal sparing in antibiotic-associated pseudomembranous colitis: a prospective study. *Gastroenterology*, 83, 1259–60.

Toffler, R.B., Pingoud, E.G., Burrell, M.I. (1978) Acute colitis related to penicillin and penicillin derivatives. *Lancet*, ii, 707–9.

Trnka, Y.M., Lamont, J.T. (1981) Association of *Clostridium difficile toxin* with symptomatic relapse of chronic inflammatory bowel disease. *Gastroenterology*, 80, 693–6.

Wald, A., Mendelow, H., Bartlett, J.G. (1980) Non-antibiotic associated pseudomembranous colitis due to toxin producing clostridia. *Ann. Intern. Med.*, 92, 798–9.

Wang, K., Weinrach, D., Lal, A. *et al.* (2003) Signet-ring cell change versus signet-ring cell carcinoma: a comparative analysis. *Am. J. Surg. Pathol.*, 27, 1429–33.

Whitehead, R. (1971) Ischaemic enterocolitis: an expression of the intravascular coagulation syndrome. *Gut*, 12, 912–17.

Wilcox, M., Minton, J. (2001) Role of antibody response in outcome of antibiotic-associated diarrhoea. *Lancet*, 357, 158–9.

Wilcox, M., Spencer, R.C. (1992) *Clostridium difficile* infection; responses, relapses and re-infections. *J. Hosp. Infect.*, 22, 85–92.

Wren, B. Heard, S.R., Tabaqchali, S. (1987) Association between production of toxin A and B and types of *Clostridium difficile*. *J. Clin. Pathol.*, 40, 1397–401.

Yuan, S., Reyes, V., Bronner, M.P. (2003) Pseudomembranous collagenous colitis. *Am. J. Surg. Pathol.*, 27, 1375–9.

CHAPTER 9

MICROSCOPIC COLITIS – COLLAGENOUS COLITIS, LYMPHOCYTIC COLITIS AND THEIR VARIANTS

9.1 Introduction	**146**	
9.2 Terminology	**147**	
9.2.1 Microscopic colitis	147	
9.2.2 Collagenous colitis	147	
9.2.3 Lymphocytic colitis	147	
9.2.4 Overlap forms	147	
9.2.5 Non-collagenous, non-lymphocytic microscopic colitis	147	
9.3 The biopsy diagnosis	**148**	
9.3.1 Collagenous colitis	148	
9.3.2 Lymphocytic colitis	153	
9.3.3 Overlap forms – one disease or two?	155	
9.3.4 The small bowel and microscopic colitis	155	

9.3.5 Differential diagnosis	156
9.3.6 Microscopic colitis; non-lymphocytic, non-collagenous	159
9.3.7 Pitfalls in the diagnosis of microscopic colitis	160
9.4 Aetiology and pathogenesis	**161**
9.4.1 Autoimmunity	161
9.4.2 Pericryptal fibroblasts	161
9.4.3 Lumenal toxins	161
9.4.4 Drugs	162
9.4.5 Pathophysiology	162
9.4.6 Epidemiology	162
9.5 Course and therapy	**162**
9.6 Conclusions	**163**
References	**163**

9.1 INTRODUCTION

Colorectal biopsy finds a unique role in the diagnosis of lymphocytic and collagenous colitis, the two main conditions within the spectrum of disease commonly referred to as microscopic colitis. This latter term, as used in this book, will by definition incorporate both conditions. The majority of patients within this spectrum have chronic watery diarrhoea, a string of normal laboratory tests and,

significantly, a normal or near-normal colonoscopic examination. The diagnosis depends entirely on the taking of a biopsy, which itself depends on a clinician appreciating that a normal-appearing colonic mucosal surface does not necessarily indicate normal microscopy. Variability in clinical awareness on this issue may account for the large range in reporting incidence between centres (Kitchen *et al.*, 2002).

The emergence of this group of diseases began with the descriptive case report of collagenous colitis by Lindstrom in 1976. This highlighted the subepithelial collagenous band in a rectal biopsy from a patient with chronic watery diarrhoea. The microscopy was akin to that of collagenous sprue in the small intestine (Weinstein *et al.*, 1970). Indeed there are several links between microscopic colitis and small bowel pathology (Section 9.3.4). The first use of the term microscopic colitis was by Read *et al.* in 1980 and applied to 'a mild increase in the number of inflammatory cells on colonic or rectal biopsy' in a group of eight patients with chronic diarrhoea probably caused by laxative abuse and in whom the authors judged the inflammation too mild to be ulcerative colitis. The clinical implications of the term became better established from the paper of Kingham *et al.* (1982) reporting six patients with chronic watery diarrhoea all of whom had normal investigations, including radiology and endoscopy. Coincidentally, in two there was also small bowel pathology. However, from subsequent review of the pathology of those patients (Levison *et al.*, 1993) and the studies of other groups microscopic colitis has become the umbrella term predominantly referring to collagenous colitis and lymphocytic colitis (Bogomoletz, 1994). It has the scope to incorporate any inflammatory mucosal changes in colonic biopsy work within the clinical triad of chronic watery diarrhoea, normal radiology and a normal or close to normal, endoscopic picture.

9.2 TERMINOLOGY

9.2.1 Microscopic colitis

In this book this term is used to cover the entities of collagenous and lymphocytic colitis plus a small group of cases that fulfil certain other clinical criteria but histologically lack the lymphocytic and collagenous elements. These criteria, as mentioned above, are chronic watery diarrhoea alongside the existence of biopsy-proven colitis with normal colonic radiology, normal laboratory investigations and a normal endoscopic examination or one with only minimal abnormality. It is further assumed the colitis present does not conform to any other of the recognized patterns of inflammatory bowel disease. The term requires to be qualified by the variety of microscopic colitis present, e.g. lymphocytic type, collagenous type or non-lymphocytic non-collagenous.

9.2.2 Collagenous colitis

The presence of the above criteria in which the colitis includes a thickened subepithelial collagen band in some or all of the biopsies (Fig. 9.1). Between $4\,\mu m$ and $7\,\mu m$ is generally taken as the normal range; this is discussed below.

9.2.3 Lymphocytic colitis

Again the clinical criteria for microscopic colitis must be present plus a raised intraepithelial lymphocyte count and no increase in the collagen plate (Fig. 9.2). The normal intraepithelial lymphocyte count is in the range of 5–10 per 100 epithelial cells. An issue, discussed later, is whether the finding of raised intraepithelial lymphocytes, or for that matter a thickened collagen plate, in one biopsy of a series is sufficient for a confident diagnostic opinion (Section 9.3.5).

9.2.4 Overlap forms

Because patterns of overlap between these definitions are common and will be discussed, it is a practical policy to categorize certain cases of microscopic colitis as of mixed collagenous and lymphocytic type (Section 9.3.3).

9.2.5 Non-collagenous, non-lymphocytic microscopic colitis

The clinical criteria given in Section 9.2.1 must be present plus a colitis lacking the lymphocytic and collagenous components and with insufficient criteria for a diagnosis of other forms of inflammatory bowel disease. These criteria separate this group

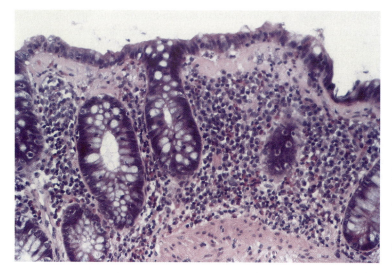

Figure 9.1 Collagenous colitis. The subepithelial collagen band is greater than 10 μm thick. A helpful scale is to compare it with any included or nearby red blood cells (diameter 7 μm). The colitis manifests as a diffuse infiltrate of lymphocytes and plasma cells in the lamina propria.

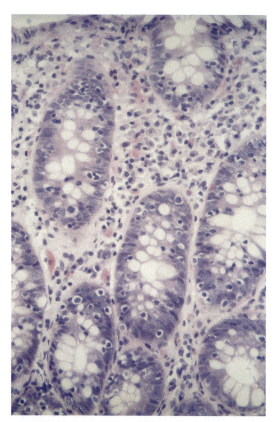

Figure 9.2 Lymphocytic colitis. Against a background of mildly increased inflammatory cells in the lamina propria the crypts show large numbers of intraepithelial lymphocytes. There is no cryptal destruction and no increase in the subepithelial collagen plate.

from what would otherwise be part of the diagnostic discussion of unclassifiable/indeterminate colitis, minimal change colitis (Elliot *et al.*, 1982) and biopsies referred to by some as non-specific colitis (Section 12.3).

9.3 THE BIOPSY DIAGNOSIS

9.3.1 Collagenous colitis

Fundamental to the diagnosis of collagenous colitis is the identification of a thickened and abnormal subepithelial collagen plate along with the presence of a colitis (Figs 3.6b, 9.1 and 9.3). The latter is necessary (Lazenby *et al.*, 1990) because a thickened collagen plate can be found in hyperplastic polyps, occasional carcinomas and some other conditions (Gledhill and Cole, 1984), as well as the result of artefacts of section preparation (Figs 3.6a and 9.4). The colitis and the collagen band abnormality are subject to considerable topographical and quantitative variations. Most series (Lee *et al.*, 1992), with a few exceptions, accept a thickness of $>10\,\mu m$ as abnormal but Wang *et al.* (1988), like Gledhill and Cole (1984), point out it is the quantity of collagen present rather than its mere presence that is a determinant in whether chronic watery diarrhoea

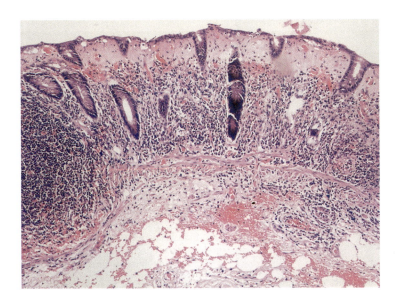

Figure 9.3 Collagenous colitis. There is a grossly thickened subepithelial collagen plate and background colitis. The abnormal band occupies approximately one-third of the mucosal thickness.

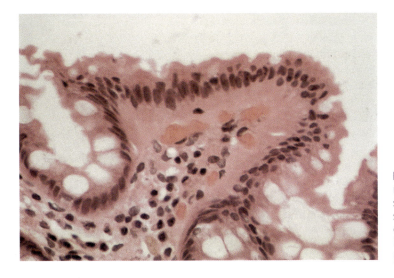

Figure 9.4 An artefact not to be misinterpreted as a collagen band is shown here. There is an eosinophilic subnuclear cytoplasmic band, the consequence of the nuclei becoming located away from their normal basal position.

is present. Moreover, the lower border of the plate should be irregular (Lazenby *et al.*, 1990) with capillaries, red cells, occasional inflammatory cells and apoptotic debris embedded within it. The normal subepithelial collagen band is mostly collagen type IV but in collagenous colitis it is predominantly type VI, some type III and reduced amounts of type I (Flejou *et al.*, 1984; Aigner *et al.*, 1997; Gunther *et al.*, 1999). An interesting paper suggests that the abnormal collagen results in a loss of flexibility of the mucosa such that in some cases it may

'fracture' during colonoscopic air insufflation with characteristic linear tears being observed (Sherman *et al.*, 2004) (Fig. 9.5).

Different studies yield conflicting results on the optimal sites to biopsy to detect the abnormal band. Armes *et al.* (1992) claim a 90 per cent diagnostic rate from recto-sigmoid biopsies whilst Carpenter *et al.* (1992) state procto-sigmoid examination alone would have missed the diagnosis in 40 per cent of their series. On occasions, only a caecal biopsy may be diagnostic (Tanaka *et al.*, 1992).

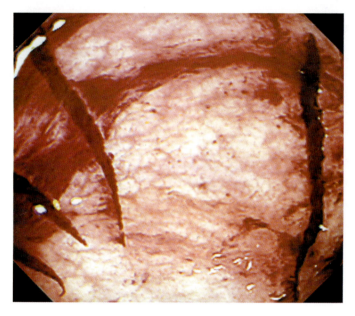

Figure 9.5 Linear tears in the mucosa. On rare occasions in collagenous colitis the unavoidable trauma of a colonoscopy can result in striking mucosal tears. It is presumably related to the collagen band and changes in mucosal elasticity, easily appreciated from the florid abnormality seen in Fig. 9.3. (Photograph courtesy Dr B. Saunders.)

In such cases inflammatory changes were present on flexible sigmoidoscopic biopsy, a useful initial clue that some form of inflammatory bowel disease might be present as a prompt to request more extensive biopsies. The transverse colon is claimed to be the optimal site for demonstrating the collagen band (Offner *et al.*, 1999). Occasionally, it may involve the terminal ileum (Lewis *et al.*, 1991). Overall, what emerges from the literature is the need for clinicians and pathologists to be aware of the possible variations and that, in the correct clinical setting, the identification of the thickened collagen band, though not usually the accompanying background colitis, may require a total colonoscopy. There is a general consensus that for both the identification of the collagen band and the inflammation the rectum is unreliable and that the abnormal collagen is more prominent proximally than distally (Lazenby *et al.*, 1989; Jawhari and Talbot, 1996; Offner *et al.*, 1999). However while not to the same degree at all sites, and with the exceptions mentioned, the abnormalities tend to be diffuse in the majority of cases.

9.3.1a Diagnostic aids

Help with the diagnosis and appreciation of the abnormality of the collagen plate (Section 9.3.7a) can be obtained by use of a simple trichrome stain

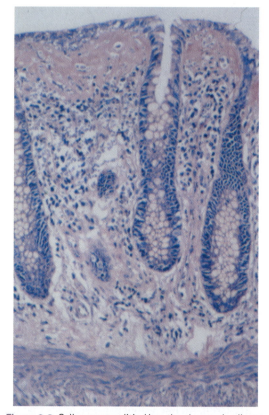

Figure 9.6 Collagenous colitis. Here the abnormal collagen band is accentuated by staining with phosphotungstic acid haematoxylin. Trapped inflammatory cells and a tiny capillary are present within the abnormal layer.

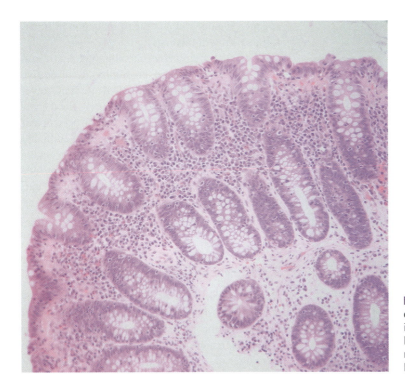

Figure 9.7 In this example of collagenous colitis there is an increase in intraepithelial lymphocytes in the crypts but it is not usually to the extent as in pure lymphocytic colitis (see Fig. 9.2).

or phosphotungstic acid haematoxylin (Fig. 9.6). Tenascin is a more specific immunostain (Aigner *et al.*, 1997). The latter is a glycoprotein involved in the morphogenesis of the extracellular matrix and its increase in a specifically subepithelial position has been shown to be a sensitive marker in collagenous colitis, especially when light microscopy is equivocal. It is therefore of particular use when only a single, low left-sided biopsy has been provided (Anagnostopoulos *et al.*, 1999; Muller *et al.*, 2001; Salas *et al.*, 2003).

9.3.1b The accompanying colitis

The background colitis, which can be very mild (Fig. 9.7), usually mirrors the distribution of the collagen band and has also been shown to have a maximum density in the transverse colon (Offner *et al.*, 1999). The inflammation is mainly one of mononuclear cells, lymphocytes and plasma cells, with the plasma cells often clustered around the base of crypts (Lazenby *et al.*, 1990; Jawhari and Talbot, 1996) just above the muscularis mucosae. This latter distribution helps recognition of mild cases since

it accentuates the loss of the cellular gradient from superficial to deep, a feature of normal mucosa. Lymphocytes, in addition to being found in the lamina propria, are also found in increased numbers in intraepithelial positions, though the former are CD4 type and the latter CD8 (Armes *et al.*, 1992; Mosnier *et al.*, 1996). The intraepithelial counts are not usually as high (Fig. 9.7) as in lymphocytic colitis but there is a considerable overlap in the range (Lazenby *et al.*, 1989) (Section 9.3.3) necessitating reference to mixed types (Armes *et al.*, 1992; Veress *et al.*, 1995) (Fig. 9.8). It is this, plus the overlap in other pathological and clinical parameters, that fuels the debate as to whether collagenous colitis and lymphocytic colitis are merely different profiles within a spectrum of a single disease (Lamps and Lazenby, 2000). It is the abnormal collagen band that is the only reliable defining histological difference, if one is to consider the two as separate diseases (Section 9.3.3).

There is a variable increase in both neutrophils and eosinophils with the latter more prominent in collagenous colitis (Lazenby *et al.*, 1990) than lymphocytic colitis. Stahle-Backdahl *et al.* (2000) suggest that the eosinophils may have a role in

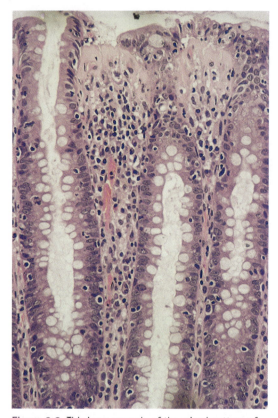

Figure 9.8 This is an example of the mixed pattern of microscopic colitis with a marked increase in both the subepithelial collagen plate and the cryptal intraepithelial lymphocyte count.

collagen remodelling via their production of transforming growth factor-β1.

The cryptal architecture remains intact, a useful sign if considering the possibility of ulcerative colitis, but there can be variable degrees of goblet cell depletion. A characteristic feature is the degeneration of the surface epithelium in the presence of the abnormal collagen band. The surface epithelial cells are often shed or clumped and show degenerative cytological features (Fig. 9.9). This surface loss exposes the underlying collagen plate but, unlike an eroded surface, it is rare to see overlying acute inflammation.

9.3.1c Variations in pattern

As the number of documented case series of microscopic colitis of either main type increases so variants of the typical pathological picture have emerged (Treanor and Sheahan, 2002). Within the spectrum of collagenous colitis, inflammatory changes that overlap with the microscopy of chronic inflammatory bowel disease (ulcerative colitis and Crohn's disease) are accepted, a pseudomembranous pattern, although rare, may also be seen.

Cryptitis, crypt abscesses and Paneth cell metaplasia – common features in chronic inflammatory bowel disease – can be seen in up to one-third

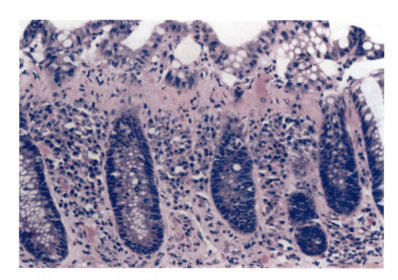

Figure 9.9 Collagenous colitis. The subepithelial collagen band is thickened and contains inflammatory cells. There are degenerative changes in the surface epithelium which is becoming detached and may often appear lost from the biopsy surface.

of cases of both major patterns of microscopic colitis but crypt atrophy and irregularity are found in less the 10 per cent (Ayata *et al.*, 2002). Given the presence, on occasions, of acute inflammation coupled with the more common finding of surface epithelial degeneration or loss, it is perhaps no surprise to come across biopsies in which inflammatory pseudomembranes are present and have been deemed pseudomembranous collagenous colitis (Byrne *et al.*, 2003; Yuan *et al.*, 2003). If such a pattern is found it is worth prompting a search for *Clostridium difficile*, as this combination is documented (Khan *et al.*, 2000; Vesoulis *et al.*, 2000), though most cases will be negative (Giardiello *et al.*, 1990; Yuan *et al.*, 2003).

Several accounts of microscopic colitis document the presence of giant cells or granulomas in the superficial aspect of the lamina propria (Fig. 9.10), the latter associated with crypt damage (Libbrecht *et al.*, 2002; Sandmeier and Bouzourene, 2004; Saurine *et al.*, 2004). The association is more common with collagenous colitis than the lymphocytic variant. The obvious question is whether this is Crohn's disease and this question is even harder to answer when seen in the context of lymphocytic colitis (Section 9.3.2a).

9.3.2 Lymphocytic colitis

The sole reliable biopsy feature distinguishing lymphocytic colitis from collagenous colitis is the presence of an abnormally thick collagen band

in the latter and its absence in the former. While increased intraepithelial lymphocytes are the key feature of lymphocytic colitis they are not specific to that condition. The diagnosis has to be made in the context of the following: the appropriate clinical scenario (Section 9.2.1), a background colitis that is generally but not always diffuse, no abnormal collagen band and intact mucosal crypt architecture (Figs 9.2 and 9.11). These criteria must be carefully appraised since colonic epithelial lymphocytosis can be a feature of not only the overlap with collagenous colitis but also coeliac disease, a specific form of epidemic infective diarrhoea (Brainerd diarrhoea) (Bryant *et al.*, 1996), seen in stages of both acute (infective) and chronic inflammatory bowel disease (Crohn's disease and ulcerative colitis; Chapters 5 and 6) and, remarkably, even in occasional patients with constipation (Wang *et al.*, 1999). They are also increased over lymphoid follicles in the mucosa and such areas should be avoided in the biopsy assessment of this parameter. For this reason Lazenby *et al.* (1989) recommend diagnostic assessment be on material distal to the ascending colon where lymphoid follicles become less common and this might account for some workers finding right-sided colonic counts in lymphocytic colitis to be higher than in the left colon (Ayata *et al.*, 2002).

The normal intraepithelial lymphocyte count is in the region of 5/100 epithelial cells (Dobbins, 1986). Lazenby *et al.* (1989) in one of the major early descriptions of the condition quote a mean count of

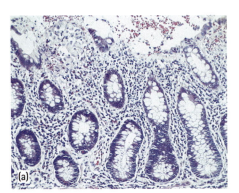
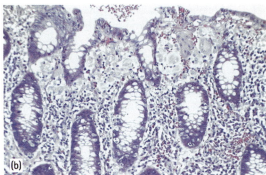

Figure 9.10 Collagenous colitis with giant cells and a granulomatous reaction. (a) The thickened collagen band is evident towards the right. To the left the surface epithelium is disrupted and giant cells and macrophages are present. (b) From the same case, subepithelial giant cells are clearly seen.

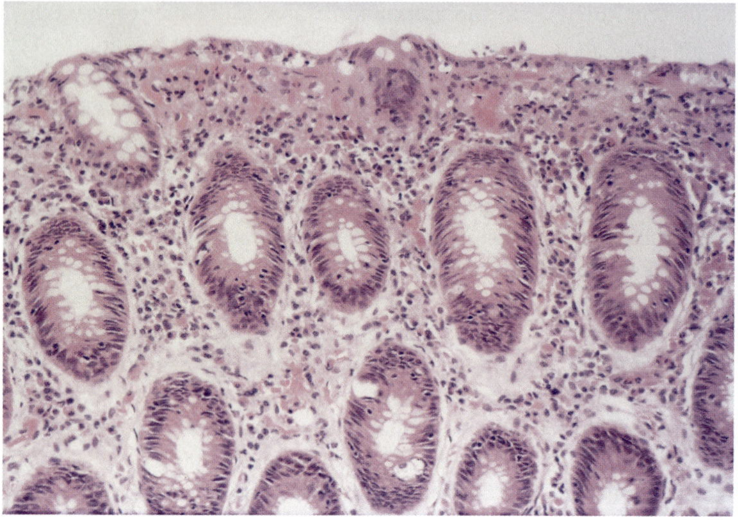

Figure 9.11 Lymphocytic colitis. Increased numbers of lymphocytes are present within the cryptal epithelium. Typically, there is no associated crypt destruction and, in this case, the background inflammation in the lamina propria is relatively minor.

24 per cent but the range is large. At the lower end of this range the distinction between the normal and the pathological is not clear cut and a borderline area exists. Moreover, a raised count, as just mentioned above, can accompany many conditions unrelated to microscopic colitis. In collagenous colitis the counts tend to be lower but in a useful study by Veress et al. (1995) three patient groups were identified within the spectrum of what these authors termed the microscopic colitis syndrome. They describe a pure group with epithelial lymphocytosis and counts in the region of 50 per cent, a mixed group or overlap group that had a thickened collagenous band and mean counts of around 34 per cent and third, a solely collagenous group with no epithelial lymphocytosis. The increase in numbers was evenly distributed around the colonic biopsy sites and in their follow up of six of their patient cohort there was no change in pattern over a 4- to 7-year period. The intraepithelial lymphocytes, whatever the pattern, are cytotoxic/suppressor CD8 in type with the α–β form of T-cell receptor (Armes et al., 1992; Mosnier et al., 1996).

9.3.2a The accompanying colitis

This is very similar to that seen in the collagenous variant of microscopic colitis but generally more uniform in distribution (Jawhari and Talbot, 1996).

There is usually a mild to moderate increase in the cellularity of the lamina propria with mononuclear cells and the loss of the normal lamina propria gradient. Eosinophils are less apparent than in collagenous colitis but acute inflammation and crypt abscesses do occur with a similar frequency (in around one-third of cases; Ayata et al., 2002). The degeneration of the surface epithelial cells is again similar to that seen in collagenous colitis. With the loss of the columnar configuration the cells become flattened and syncytial arrangements can be seen. There is no distortion of the crypt architecture. Macrophages can be a feature of the superficial lamina propria and the same variants of giant cell and granulomatous patterns occur as in collagenous colitis (Fig. 9.10) (Libbrecht et al., 2002; Sandmeier and Bouzourene, 2004; Saurine et al., 2004). However, the reporting of this variant of lymphocytic colitis requires careful correlation with the clinical data to ensure that the criteria for microscopic colitis are met if Crohn's disease is to be excluded. It is especially problematic if the intraepithelial lymphocyte count is only mildly raised. Indeed, definite exclusion of Crohn's disease may then have to depend on follow-up patterns of disease. Nevertheless, the current literature suggests that giant cells and granulomas do comprise a distinct variant within the patterns of microscopic colitis with a clinical course and colonoscopic scenario very different from Crohn's disease. To complicate the issue further both diseases can coexist (Chandratre *et al.*, 1987; Goldstein and Gyorfi, 1999; Pokorny *et al.*, 2001) and the pathology report may need careful wording to convey such possibilities.

9.3.3 Overlap forms – one disease or two?

It is clear from the account so far that the histological and clinical features of the two conditions are similar and that the abnormal and thickened collagen band is the only hard criterion distinguishing the two. Much of the debate on whether collagenous and lymphocytic colitis are a spectrum of one disease or are separate diseases, and on the use of the term microscopic colitis, is clouded by earlier semantic discussions and limited appreciation of the problems posed by restricted sampling.

Within the clinical scenario of chronic watery diarrhoea, the presence of normal colonic radiology, normal laboratory investigations, normal or near normal colonoscopic examination and a colitis, not characteristic of any other major cause of inflammatory bowel disease, plus an increase in subepithelial collagen thickness defines collagenous colitis, whether or not accompanied by an epithelial lymphocytosis. However, a full colonoscopy may be required to identify what could be a solitary biopsy focus of such thickening or its presence in just a minority number (Tanaka *et al.*, 1992).

If the majority also show a florid intraepithelial lymphocytosis should one restrict the diagnosis to collagenous colitis or use both terms? In an opposite scenario if only one or two biopsies in a total series have mildly raised intraepithelial lymphocyte counts, does that warrant a diagnosis of lymphocytic colitis (Section 9.3.5b)? These questions are confounded by the natural history of the two characteristics, the collagen band and epithelial lymphocytosis, which wax and wane irrespective of treatment (Carpenter *et al.*, 1992). Until more is known about all aspects of these entities it is not possible to place each in a watertight diagnostic compartment

or be in a position to know if such a separation is aetiologically justified.

Our own basic definitions are stated in Section 9.2 and our custom when biopsies show both patterns is to report it as such, namely 'microscopic colitis with both collagenous and lymphocytic features' (Fig. 9.8). This has some practical use as there are cases in which, contrary to the findings of Veress *et al.* (1995), one pattern has apparently evolved into the other (Perri *et al.*, 1996). Such examples are used to argue that lymphocytic colitis and collagenous colitis are merely part of the spectrum of one disease. However, they could equally be the result of a simple sampling bias. Armes *et al.* (1992) adopt the term mixed collagenous and lymphocytic colitis and Baert *et al.* (1999) classified their 96 patients according to the predominant histological finding but state overlap occurred in 26–28 per cent of cases.

Overall, there are trends towards seeing collagenous colitis as an entity that occurs in an older age group than lymphocytic colitis, as having a higher female to male sex ratio and a greater association with autoimmune manifestations. On microscopy the trend is to consider it to have a more patchy distribution than lymphocytic colitis, to incorporate more eosinophils and, when intraepithelial lymphocytes are raised, it is not to the same degree. Such generalizations are, however, of limited value in the individual case. Provided that one is confident that the biopsy diagnosis falls under the umbrella of microscopic colitis, and the other colitides have been given careful consideration, the exact phraseology is unimportant as long as it is understood by the clinician managing the case. In the larger studies where sampling may have been more thorough, the impression is that, where the diagnostic criteria are typical of either entity, progression from one to the other does not occur (Veress *et al.*, 1995; Mullhaupt *et al.*, 1998).

9.3.4 The small bowel and microscopic colitis

9.3.4a The terminal ileum

There are case reports of biopsies from the terminal ileum in which an abnormal collagen band has been identified in collagenous colitis (Lewis *et al.*, 1991; Meier *et al.*, 1991) also reports linking both major patterns of microsopic colitis with primary ileal villous atrophy (Veress *et al.*, 1995; Marteau *et al.*, 1997) and with other small bowel abnormalities (Moayyedi *et al.*, 1997). Indeed, villous abnormalities were documented in the original account of microscopic colitis by Kingham *et al.* (1982). Gastric abnormalities have also been documented with both varieties of microscopic colitis (Groisman *et al.*, 1996; Pulimood *et al.*, 1999).

Careful studies of the terminal ileum in lymphocytic colitis are few (Marteau *et al.*, 1997; Sapp *et al.*, 2002; Padmanabhan *et al.*, 2003). The normal count of intraepithelial lymphocytes is quoted as in the region of 3 per 100 enterocytes by Sapp *et al.* (2002) and around 8 per 100 enterocytes by Padmanabhan *et al.* (2003). Sapp *et al.* (2002) claim that counts of over 5/100 had specificities of over 90 per cent for microscopic colitis of either pattern, sensitivities of 73 per cent and 56 per cent for lymphocytic colitis and collagenous colitis, respectively, and corresponding negative predictive values of 71 per cent and 84 per cent. In that study the intraepithelial lymphocyte counts in the villi in disease were in the region of 10 per 100 enterocytes while counts in 'control' cases of Crohn's disease and ulcerative colitis remained down in the region of 2–3 per cent. Padmanabhan *et al.* (2003) found 78 per cent of patients with lymphocytic colitis and 50 per cent of those with collagenous colitis had raised counts with means of 22.3 per 100 enterocytes and 16.7 per 100 enterocytes respectively. Accompanying enterocyte damage occurred but was uncommon.

These abnormalities in terminal ileal biopsies, while mild and far from diagnostic if considered alone, nevertheless provide useful additional evidence if judging a colonic series in what might be an equivocal case. It is worth appreciating in this respect (Sciarretta *et al.*, 1994) that uncomplicated bile acid malabsorption is not associated with raised counts or other pathology in the terminal ileum or colon, though others do document villous atrophy in some instances (Popovic *et al.* 1987).

9.3.4b The duodenum and coeliac disease

Increased duodenal intraepithelial lymphocytes are one of the diagnostic signs of coeliac disease and they can also be increased in the colon. Indeed a rectal gluten challenge (Austin and Dobbin, 1988) has been shown to raise the count. There may be aetiological links between coeliac disease and lymphocytic colitis with quotes of between 24 per cent and 41 per cent of patients having both pathologies (Wolber *et al.*, 1990; Saul, 1993). Fine *et al.* (1998) dispute whether there is a true colitis in coeliac disease rather than merely a qualitative colonic lymphocytosis with no true increase in cellularity in the lamina propria and barely raised intraepithelial lymphocyte counts. However, in refractory sprue they did find a true colitis present in a small percentage of their cases. In certain clinical situations it would seem appropriate for the pathologist, on diagnosing lymphocytic colitis, to suggest the need for a duodenal or jejunal biopsy to exclude accompanying coeliac disease. This probably also applies to collagenous colitis for Armes *et al.* (1992), in an Australian series, found 4 of 10 of their cases with collagenous colitis had coeliac disease. This is a high rate when considered against the national prevalence of coeliac disease in that country of 1 in 3000.

9.3.5 Differential diagnosis

Both clinically and pathologically the differential is broad. First, and outside the scope of this book, are all the causes of chronic secretory watery diarrhoea (Schiller, 1999), such as bile salt malabsorption (Sciarretta *et al.*, 1994), pancreatic insufficiency, the endocrine diarrhoeas and the irritable bowel syndrome. Overall, the colonic biopsy is usually normal, though one study did show almost one-quarter of cases of irritable bowel syndrome may have microscopic colitis (Tuncer *et al.*, 2003). Certainly until the above diagnoses are established it is probably prudent to take a colonoscopic biopsy series to exclude one of the patterns of microscopic colitis. Second are the accepted patterns of inflammatory bowel disease plus the unsatisfactory group with inflammatory appearances that cannot be confidently classified, being deemed indeterminate or referred to by some as non-specific. As with all aspects of diagnostic pathology clinico-pathological liaison is essential for an accurate diagnosis. The pathologist can narrow the field dramatically if pre-armed with the information that the patient has chronic watery diarrhoea, normal intestinal radiology and had a normal or near-normal colonoscopy. Without this information, and in the absence of an abnormal collagen band, the differential enlarges to encompass the pathology of the whole gambit of inflammatory bowel disease.

9.3.5a A collagen band is present

The identification of a thickened collagen band helps focus the diagnostic choice. It is important to ensure that it is not an artefact (see below) and that there is an accompanying colitis. The absence of a colitis, irrespective of the collagen band, is felt to exclude the diagnosis of microscopic colitis of either main type (Lazenby *et al.*, 1990). A thickened collagen layer can occasionally accompany carcinoma, be present in metaplastic polyps or even diverticular disease (Gledhill and Cole, 1984). The accompanying pathology in these conditions means that there is seldom a diagnostic dilemma. Staining for amyloid will prevent an error as it can appear to be a localized collagen-like eosinophilia and mimic the collagen band (Fig. 9.12) (Garcia-Gonzalez *et al.*, 1998). In ischaemic colitis the lamina propria may take on a homogeneous slightly hyaline-like eosinophilia (Figs 8.9b, 9.13 and 12.8) similar to that seen with radiation damage. Both of these may need to be considered but the accompanying pathology is very different (Sections 10.6.2 and 11.1). Fibrosis of the lamina propria can also be a source of diagnostic confusion, being a component of scarring in regions of healed ulceration, a part of the pathology of Crohn's disease, seen in the ischaemic damage of the solitary ulcer syndrome, in systemic sclerosis (Hoare, 1976) and even a rare feature in ulcerative colitis (Balazs *et al.*, 1988). A trichrome stain will accentuate the fibrous pattern and help emphasize the band-like nature of the collagen in collagenous colitis (Fig. 9.6), in contrast to a more

diffuse distribution in these other conditions. However, it will be the other accompanying characteristics in the biopsy that will lead one to the correct diagnosis.

9.3.5b The collagen band is absent

In the absence of a collagen band and even within the correct clinical setting, the differential is harder to resolve and encompasses a wide spectrum. At one end are the inflammatory patterns associated with an intact crypt architecture and a clearly raised intraepithelial lymphocyte count. At the other is the dilemma of distinguishing normal lamina propria cellularity from that with a minimal but significant increase in inflammatory cells. A case such as the latter, if the criteria are fulfilled, might be categorized as microscopic colitis non-collagenous, non-lymphocytic (Section 9.3.6). Furthermore a raised intraepithelial lymphocyte count is not an absolute criteria comparable to the diagnostic implication of an abnormal collagen band. The clinical context remains a critical factor. Thus Wang *et al.* (1999) describe atypical lymphocytic colitis in which, of a series of 40 patients with the microscopic criteria for the diagnosis, the symptomatology and the endoscopic appearances were outside the accepted pro-file of the disease. They concluded that the typical pathology also incorporates a heterogeneous group that includes some patients that may have chronic inflammatory bowel disease, some with infectious diarrhoea and even quote one patient with idiopathic constipation. This last symptomatology mirrors a report of a similar clinical situation in a patient with collagenous colitis (Leigh *et al.*, 1993).

Obviously, lymphoma is included in the differential diagnosis but here the intraepithelial lymphocyte count is usually well above the range ever seen in lymphocytic colitis, there is often infiltrative destruction of the crypts and a monomorphic population in the lamina propria. A more common differential is with Crohn's disease. This is because in lymphocytic colitis, as in Crohn's disease, the inflammation and the lymphoepitheliosis may not be uniform and the architecture remains intact. Moreover Crohn's disease has been associated with

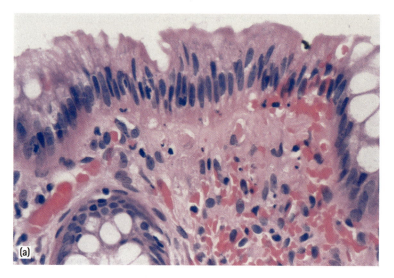

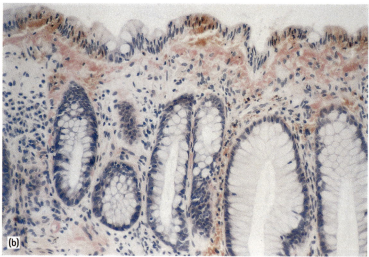

Figure 9.12 Amyloid disease. (a,b) It is important to be certain that any apparent increase in the subepithelial collagen band is not caused by amyloid as in this example. The positive Congo red stain is seen in (b).

a prior diagnosis of lymphocytic colitis (Goldstein and Gyorfi, 1999) and we have seen classical Crohn's pathology in the company of a raised intraepithelial lymphocyte count, a circumstance also mentioned by Lazenby *et al.* (1989). Ulcerative colitis too has been documented in the course of microscopic colitis, mainly the collagenous variant (Giardiello *et al.*, 1991; Pokorny *et al.*, 2001; Robert, 2004). As noted above (Section 9.3.1c) (Ayata *et al.*, 2002) up to one-third of cases of either main variety of microscopic colitis can share some of the features of chronic inflammatory bowel disease, such as crypt abscesses, cryptitis and Paneth cell metaplasia.

Usually, however, the symptomatology and endoscopic features make the distinction from Crohn's disease and ulcerative colitis clear and any overlap in intraepithelial lymphocyte counts is a rarity (Lazenby *et al.*, 1989). The problem of the granulomatous variants of microscopic colitis has been discussed earlier (Section 9.3.2a). The distinction from acute infective colitis is made from the dominant neutrophil infiltration of the crypts and surface, alongside the pattern of crypt withering (Section 4.2.1), characteristic of that condition. The distinction from a resolving case of infection, however, can be more difficult.

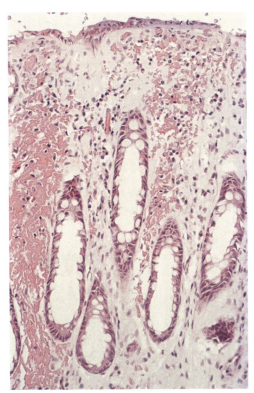

Figure 9.13 Ischaemic damage. In this biopsy there is acute ischaemic damage resulting in an appearance that might be mistaken for an abnormal collagen layer. The lamina propria, in the superficial one-third, has taken on a hyaline slightly glassy eosinophilic character but there is no accompanying inflammatory infiltrate. There is also oedema, haemorrhage and the crypts show degenerative features and slight dilatation. None of the latter are features of collagenous colitis.

There is a rare form of infectious diarrhoea (Bryant et al., 1996) characterized by intraepithelial lymphocytosis. It is known as Brainerd diarrhoea after the town in the USA in which the first recorded outbreak occurred. The counts and any colitis are less pronounced than in non-epidemic lymphocytic colitis. However, it is probably only an epidemiologist armed with the public health data who is in a position to make the distinction, not a pathologist handling an individual biopsy series.

It is our experience that the most problematic area in the differential diagnosis surrounds that end of the spectrum with only mild changes present

when the pathologist is struggling to decide whether the biopsies are normal or genuinely but minimally inflamed. In these cases it is important to appreciate that the cellularity of the lamina propria in the right colon is greater than that on the left (Lazenby et al., 1989; Saul, 1993; Proctor, 2004) and avoid overdiagnosing colitis (Fig. 12.1). However, there is a borderline area (Lazenby et al., 1989). In such cases it is crucial to know the clinical details. Such a picture in the presence of the classical triad (normal endoscopy, chronic watery diarrhoea and normal radiology) warrants different emphasis in the report than if the patient has merely a slight change in bowel habit. There will be occasions when it is best to issue an equivocal report and await follow-up biopsies, if and when the clinician feels the symptoms warrant it. Relevant at all times, but especially in these circumstances, is knowledge of the patient's drug intake in particular of the widely prescribed non-steroidal anti-inflammatory agents (Proctor, 2004).

9.3.6 Microscopic colitis; non-lymphocytic, non-collagenous

This is a contentious category (Warren et al., 2002) and one that many feel could be more misleading than helpful. We, however, find it a useful one provided that the criteria are met (Section 9.2.5). The picture is one of a definite extensive histological colitis, without an accompanying collagen band or intraepithelial lymphocytosis, accompanied by intact mucosal architecture and the clinical picture required for a diagnosis of microscopic colitis (Goldstein and Bhanot, 2004) (Fig. 9.14). It is important to ensure the clinical criteria as well as the histological ones are fulfilled for the category to have meaning. The differential must necessarily be broad to encompass that of inflammatory bowel disease in which there is intact mucosal architecture. This is covered more fully in Chapter 12.

Twelve such cases were documented by Jawhari et al. (1995) and Kitchen et al. (2002) found seven examples in a series of 62 biopsy diagnoses designated microscopic colitis. Interestingly, the majority of this group had a recent history of receiving non-steroidal anti-inflammatory drugs. Saurine *et al.* (2004) also concluded their four cases of microscopic colitis (non-collagenous, non-lymphocytic) were most likely drug related, with non-steroidal anti-inflammatory drugs being involved in two.

Symptoms and inconclusive biopsies can certainly precede the one that establishes the diagnosis and such time-courses have been documented (Teglbjaerg *et al.*, 1984; Shaz *et al.*, 2004). It may also be that chronic inflammatory bowel disease of Crohn's or ulcerative colitis type evolves (Chandratre *et al.*, 1987; Giardiello *et al.*, 1991; Goldstein and Gyorfi, 1999; Pokorny *et al.*, 2001). Either way, when appropriately used we believe this category a helpful one for clinicians. It transmits to them a perspective of where in the spectrum of the pathology of inflammatory bowel disease, at that moment in time, an individual's set of biopsies can be placed. Goldstein and Bhanot (2004) describe atypical forms of lymphocytic colitis in which not all the criteria are met and patients may even be symptomless. These would seem part of this category and non-steroidal anti-inflammatory drugs were again implicated.

9.3.7 Pitfalls in the diagnosis of microscopic colitis

9.3.7a The collagen band

First, pathologists need to be sure that the apparent thickened collagen band is not merely the result of tangential sectioning and to make any measurements in a well-orientated area. It is recommended to avoid the edge of crypts, polyps and peridiverticular regions (Treanor and Sheahan, 2002). Second, pathologists need to be certain that the band is collagen and not, for example, amyloid (Section 20.8) (Fig. 9.12). Third, pathologists need be sure that one is not misinterpreting the band-like eosinophilia seen in certain biopsies produced by prominent subnuclear cytoplasm in the surface colonocytes (Figs 3.6a and 9.4). Lazenby *et al.* (1990) stress that when the collagen increase is borderline particular attention should be given to the lower margin of the band. It ought to be irregular and have entrapped capillaries plus nuclear debris and an occasional inflammatory cell (Figs 3.6b and 9.15). The presence of colitis is also necessary and the difficulties of assessing mild changes have been discussed. A final problem is to appreciate that the distribution of the changes can be patchy. If the clinical story sounded appropriate the pathologist may need to remind the clinician that there has to be adequate sampling from around the whole colon to avoid missing the diagnosis.

9.3.7b The epithelial lymphocytosis

An increase in intraepithelial lymphocytes is seen in the surface epithelium overlying lymphoid follicles and counting in such areas should be

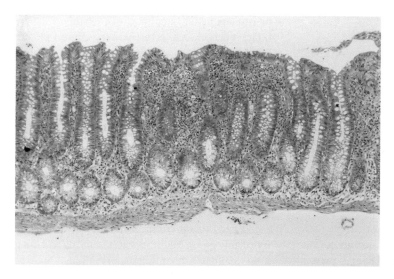

Figure 9.14 Microscopic colitis, non-collagenous, non-lymphocytic. This biopsy is from a patient with the appropriate clinical story of watery diarrhoea and a normal colonoscopy. It shows a colitis manifest as moderate inflammation throughout the lamina propria with some focal cryptal inflammation but insufficient features of either collagenous colitis, lymphocytic colitis or other pattern of chronic inflammatory bowel disease to warrant a confident diagnosis. The remaining biopsies in the colonoscopic series were similar.

avoided. If this is not possible because of the nature of the biopsy, signs of epithelial degeneration would be in favour of genuine pathology.

Overdiagnosis of lymphocytic colitis in circumstances where the abnormalities in the intraepithelial count and changes in lamina propria cellularity are only just outside the normal range have been discussed previously. Again, extensive sampling from around the colon is good clinical practice to overcome any variability in distribution of the changes, coupled with an acceptance that there will be patients with borderline counts on whom a confident diagnosis cannot be made.

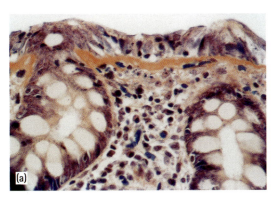

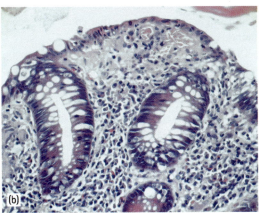

Figure 9.15 The figures illustrate in (a) the apoptotic debris often associated with the abnormal collagen band [phosphotungstic acid–haematoxylin (PTAH) stain] and in (b) the association with inflammatory cells and sometimes capillaries within the band.

9.4 AETIOLOGY AND PATHOGENESIS

9.4.1 Autoimmunity

While neither the precise aetiology nor pathogenesis of the main patterns of microscopic colitis are known some clues exist. Both conditions are strongly associated with diseases believed to be of autoimmune origin, the two commonest being rheumatoid arthritis and thyroid disease. In Swedish studies (Bohr *et al.*, 1996a; Olesen *et al.*, 2004) up to 40 per cent had associated disease regarded as autoimmune. However, apart from some cases of collagenous colitis being antinuclear antibody (ANA)-positive and having raised IgM levels (Bohr *et al.*, 1996b) no specific antibodies have been implicated.

9.4.2 Pericryptal fibroblasts

The role of the pericryptal fibroblast in the dynamics of collagen production has been an area of interest with a decreased rate of collagen degeneration proposed by Aigner *et al.* (1997). A role for tenascin has already been alluded to (Section 9.3.1a) and is involved in collagen remodelling (Treanor and Sheahon, 2002).

9.4.3 Lumenal toxins

Jarnerot *et al.* (1995) suggested that luminal agents may hold the key to the aetiology and pathogenesis when they demonstrated that the collagen band in patients with uncontrollable diarrhoea disappeared if a temporary ileostomy was performed. Moreover, it recurred when the ileostomy was reversed. Dietary factors, bacterial components (Andersen *et al.*, 1993) and drugs might be among many luminal provoking agents. These factors are all incorporated into an attractive hypothesis of specific immunity that links those gastrointestinal diseases characterized by epithelial lymphocytosis (e.g. lymphocytic gastritis, coeliac disease, lymphocytic colitis) (Yardley *et al.*, 1990).

9.4.4 Drugs

There are reports in the literature (Fernandez-Benares *et al.*, 2003) presenting convincing evidence that some cases of microscopic colitis are drug induced, such that symptoms and pathology resolve when the drug is withdrawn and re-appear on a subsequent challenge with the specific drug (Beaugerie *et al.*, 1994). The pathology is also accompanied by appropriate immunological changes. The commonest drugs cited are non-steroidal anti-inflammatory agents (Giardiello *et al.*, 1990; Riddell *et al.*, 1992), proton pump inhibitors (Thompson *et al.*, 2002; Mukherjee, 2003), H₂ receptor antagonists (Beaugerie *et al.*, 1995; Duncan *et al.*, 1997), cyclo3 fort and ticlopidine (Berrebi *et al.*, 1998). Saurine *et al.* (2004) suggest that the granulomatous variety of non-lymphocytic, non-collagenous microscopic colitis they describe may also be drug related citing non-steroidal anti-inflammatory drugs, antibiotics and allopurinol as candidates in their cases. A useful pointer to drug involvement is often the presence of prominent apoptosis (Lee, 1993). Drug-induced colitis is covered more generally in Section 11.4.

9.4.5 Pathophysiology

It seems likely that products generated by the inflammatory cell infiltrate play the major role in causing the diarrhoea of microscopic colitis (Lee *et al.*, 1992), a view supported by the observation that a collagen band or raised intraepithelial lymphocytes can be present in the absence of diarrhoea (Beaugerie *et al.*, 1995; Leigh *et al.*, 1993). At a molecular level there is impairment of NaCl and H₂0 with a leak flux diarrhoea (Rask-Madden *et al.*, 1983; Bo-Linn *et al.*, 1985; Burgel *et al.*, 2002).

Bile acids, although thought to have a role at one time are probably not primarily involved as many diarrhoeal illnesses have increased bile acid malabsorption, yet no evidence of any of the forms of microscopic colitis (Sciarretta *et al.*, 1994; Fernandez-Banares *et al.*, 2001).

9.4.6 Epidemiology

Both collagenous colitis and lymphocytic colitis disease are common in the elderly and in women, with the female to male ratio being higher in collagenous colitis than lymphocytic colitis (Fernandez-Banares *et al.*, 1999). Swedish studies (Olesen *et al.*, 2003) report an increasing incidence in the last decade and a Spanish study (Fernandez-Banares *et al.*, 1999) found a pick-up rate of microscopic colitis of 9.5 per cent in patients complaining of watery diarrhoea. This rose to 20 per cent in those over 70 years old referred for non-bloody diarrhoea. These studies showed that the incidence of microscopic colitis approaches that of Crohn's disease in Sweden and that in those over 70 years of age collagenous colitis has an incidence equal to that of ulcerative colitis.

The rising incidence may be partly explained by increasing biopsy rates on normal mucosa as clinicians have come to appreciate that normal endoscopic mucosa does not equal normal microscopy.

9.5 COURSE AND THERAPY

Unlike chronic inflammatory bowel disease (Crohn's disease and ulcerative colitis) patients with microscopic colitis, despite severe watery diarrhoea, will seldom pursue an unremitting course resistant to therapy and come to surgery (Bowling *et al.*, 1996). Up to 85 per cent in the cohort studied by Bohr *et al.* (1996a) had a chronic intermittent course while Olesen *et al.* (2004) found that 63 per cent had a single attack, but one that could last several months.

Therapy is basically symptomatic commencing with simple anti-diarrhoeal agents before moving on to anti-inflammatory drugs such as 5-aminosalicylic acid or sulfasalazine (Saul, 1993; Bohr *et al.*, 1996a; Mullhaupt *et al.*, 1998; Schiller, 1999; Fernandez-Banares *et al.*, 2003). Bismuth salicylate is claimed to have a 75 per cent success rate (Fine and Lee, 1998) and from Cochrane reviews (Chande *et al.*, 2004) budesonide emerged as the most successful steroid. The beneficial effect of bile acid-binding resins is likely to reflect concomitant bile acid malabsorption and microscopic colitis (Schiller, 2000; Fernandez-Banares *et al.*, 2001).

Relapse rates from a series of studies are in the region of 30 per cent (Goff *et al.*, 1997).

9.6 CONCLUSIONS

The biopsy diagnoses of the main patterns of microscopic colitis, namely collagenous colitis and lymphocytic colitis, when typical, are relatively straightforward. Both have similar well-defined clinical profiles and, the collagen band apart, similar microscopic profiles. Either will be seen regularly in hospital practice where clinicians appreciate both the importance of biopsying normal mucosa and the need for a complete colonoscopic biopsy series if the diagnoses are to be entirely excluded. Diagnostic difficulty arises when the intraepithelial lymphocyte count is only mildly raised and/or when one of the variant patterns described in this chapter is evident.

Several theories of pathogenesis and aetiology exist, that implicating a role for autoimmunity being among the strongest. There is also a clear association, in selected cases, with certain drugs. However, much remains to be unravelled and particularly intriguing is the relationship with conditions characterized by an intraepithelial lymphocytosis in the small intestine and in the stomach.

REFERENCES

Aigner, T., Neureiter, D., Muller, S., Kuspert, G., Belke, J., Kirchner, T. (1997) Extracellular matrix composition and gene expression in collagenous colitis. *Gastroenterology*, 113, 136–43.

Anagnostopoulos, I., Schuppan, D., Riecken, E.O., Gross, U.M., Stein, M. (1999) Tenascin labelling in colorectal biopsies: a useful marker in the diagnosis of collagenous colitis. *Histopathology*, 34, 425–31.

Andersen, T., Andersen, J.R., Tvede, M., Franzmann, M-B. (1993) Collagenous colitis: are bacterial cytotoxins responsible? *Am. J. Gastoenterol.*, 88, 375–77.

Armes, J., Gee, D.C., Macrae, F.A., Schroeder, W., Bhathal P.S. (1992) Collagenous colitis: Jejunal and colorectal pathology. *J. Clin. Pathol.*, 45, 784–87.

Austin, L., Dobbin, W.O. (1988) Studies of the rectal mucosa in coeliac sprue: the intraepithelial lymphocyte. *Gut*, 29, 200–5.

Ayata, G., Ithamukkala, S., Sapp, H. *et al.* (2002) Prevalance and significance of inflammatory bowel disease-like morphologic features in collagenous and lymphocytic colitis. *Am. J. Surg. Pathol.*, 26, 1414–23.

Baert, J., Wouters, K., D'Haens, G. *et al.* (1999) Lymphocytic colitis: a distinct clinical entity? A clinicopathological confrontation of lymphocytic and collagenous colitis. *Gut*, 45, 375–81.

Balazs, M., Egerszegi, P., Vadaz, G., Kovacs, A. (1988) Collagenous colitis: an electron microscopic study including comparison with the chronic fibrotic stage of ulcerative colitis. *Histopathology*, 13, 319–28.

Beaugerie, L., Luboinski, J., Brousse, N., Cosnes, J., Chatelet, F-P., Gendre, J-P., Le Quintrec, Y. (1994) Drug induced lymphocytic colitis. *Gut*, 35, 426–28.

Beaugerie, L., Patey, N., Brousse, N. (1995) Ranitidine, diarrhoea and lymphocytic colitis. *Gut*, 37, 708–11.

Berrebi, D., Sautet, A., Flejou, J-F., Dauge, M-C., Peuchmaur, M., Potet, F. (1998) Ticlopidine induced colitis: a histopathological study including apoptosis. *J. Clin. Pathol.*, 51, 280–83.

Bogomoletz, V. (1994) Collagenous, microscopic and lymphocytic colitis. An evolving concept. *Virchows Arch.*, 424, 573–9.

Bohr, J., Tysk, C., Eriksson, S., Abrahamsson, H., Jarnerot, G. (1996a) Collagenous colitis: a retrospective study of clinical presentation and treatment in 163 patients. *Gut*, 39, 846–51.

Bohr, J., Tysk, C., Yang, P., Danielsson, D., Jarnerot, G. (1996b) Autoantibodies and immunoglobulins in collagenous colitis. *Gut*, 39, 73–76.

Bo-Linn, G.W., Vendrell, D.D., Lee, E., Fordtran, J.S. (1985) An evaluation of the significance of microscopic colitis in patients with chronic diarrhoea. *J. Clin. Invest.*, 75, 1559–69.

Bowling, T.E., Price, A.B., Al Adnani, M., Fairclough, P.D., Menzies-Gow, N., Silk, D.B.

(1996) Interchange between collagenous colitis and lymphocytic colitis in severe disease with autoimmune associations requiring colectomy: a case report. *Gut*, 38, 788–91.

Bryant, D.A., Mintz, E.D., Puhr, N.D., Griffin, P.M., Petras, R.E. (1996) Colonic epithelial lymphocytosis associated with an epidemic chronic diarrhoea. *Am. J. Surg. Pathol.*, 20, 1102–9.

Burgel, N., Bojarski, C., Mankertz, J., Zeitz, M., Fromm, M., Schulzke, J.D. (2002) Mechanisms of diarrhoea in collagenous colitis. *Gastroenterology*, 123, 433–43.

Byrne, M.F., Royston, D., Patchett, S.E. (2003) Association of common variable immuno-deficiency with atypical collagenous colitis. *Eur. J. Hastroenterol. Hepatol.*, 15, 1051–3.

Carpenter, H.A., Tremaine, W.J., Batts, K.P., Czaja, A.J. (1992) Sequential histologic evaluations in collagenous colitis: correlations with disease behaviour and sampling strategy. *Dig. Dis. Sci.*, 37, 1903–09.

Chande, N., McDonald, J.W., MacDonald, J.K. (2004) Interventions for treating collagenous colitis. *Cochrane Database Syst. Rev.*, 1, CD003575.

Chandratre, S., Bramble, M.G., Cooke, W.M., Jones, R.A. (1987) Simultaneous occurrence of collagenous colitis and Crohn's disease. *Digestion*, 36, 55–60.

Dobbins, W.O. (1986) Progress report. Human intraepithelial lymphocytes. *Gut*, 27, 972–85.

Duncan, H.D., Talbot, I.C., Silk, D.B. (1997) Collagenous colitis and cimetidine. *Eur. J. Gastroenterol. Hepatol.*, 9, 819–20.

Elliot, P.R., Williams, C.B., Lennard-Jones, J.E., Dawson, A.M., Bartram, C.I., Thomas, B.M., Morson, B.M. (1982) Colonoscopic diagnosis of minimal change colitis in patients with normal sigmoidoscopy and normal air–contrast enema. *Lancet*, i, 650–1.

Fernandez-Banares, F., Salas, A., Esteve, M., Espinos, J., Forne, M., Viver, J.M. (1999) Incidence of collagenous and lymphocytic colitis: a 5-year population–based study. *Am. J. Gastroenterol.*, 94, 418–23.

Fernandez-Banares, F., Esteve, M., Salas, A., Forne, M., Espinos, J.C., Martin-Comin, J., Viver, J.M. (2001) Bile acid malabsorption in microscopic colitis and in unexplained functional chronic diarrhoea. *Dig. Dis. Sci.*, 46, 2231–38.

Fernandez-Banares, F., Salas, A., Esteve, M., Espinos, J., Forne, M., Viver, J.M. (2003) Collagenous and lymphocytic colitis. Evaluation of clinical and histological features, response to treatment, and long-term follow-up. *Am. J. Gastroenterol.*, 98, 340–7.

Fine, K.D., Lee, E.L. (1998) Efficacy of open-label bismuth salicylate for the treatment of microscopic colitis. *Gastroenterology*, 114, 29–36.

Fine, K.D., Meyer, R., Lee, E.L. (1998) Colonic histopathology in untreated coeliac sprue and refractory sprue: is it lymphocytic colitis or colonic lymphocytosis. *Hum. Pathol.*, 29, 1433–40.

Flejou, J., Grimaud, J., Molas, G., Baviera, E., Potet, F. (1984) Collagenous colitis: ultrastructural study and collagen immunotyping of four cases. *Arch. Pathol. Lab. Med.*, 108, 977–82.

Garcia-Gonzalez, R., Fernandez, F.A., Garijo, M.F., Fernando Val-Bernal, J. (1998) Amyloidosis of the rectum mimicking collagenous colitis. *Pathol. Res. Pract.*, 194, 731–5.

Giardiello, F.M., Hansen, F.C., Lazenby, A.Z., Hellman, D.B., Milligan, F.D., Bayless, T.H., Yardley, J.H., (1990) Collagenous colitis in the setting of non-steroidal anti-inflammatory drugs and antibiotics. *Dig. Dis. Sci.*, 35, 257–60.

Giardiello, F.M., Jackson, F.W., Lazenby, A.J. (1991) Metachronous occurrence of collagenous colitis and ulcerative colitis. *Gut*, 32, 447–9.

Gledhill, A., Cole, F.M. (1984) Significance of basement membrane thickening in the human colon. *Gut*, 25, 1085–8.

Goff, J.S., Barnett, J.L., Pelke, T., Appelman, H.D. (1997) Collagenous colitis: histopathology and clinical course. *Am. J. Gastroenterol.*, 92, 57–60.

Goldstein, N.S., Bhanot, P. (2004) Paucicellular and asymptomatic lymphocytic colitis: expanding the clinicopathologic spectrum of lymphocytic colitis. *Am. J. Clin. Pathol.*, 122, 405–11.

Goldstein, N.S., Gyorfi, T. (1999) Focal lymphocytic colitis and collagenous colitis: patterns of Crohn's colitis? *Am. J. Surg. Pathol.* 23, 1075–81.

Groisman, G.M., Meyers, S., Harpaz, N. (1996) Collagenous gastritis associated with lymphocytic colitis. *J. Clin. Gastroenterol.*, 22, 134–7.

Gunther, U., Schuppan, D., Bauer, M. *et al.* (1999) Fibrogenesis and fibrolysis in collagenous colitis. Patterns of procollagen types 1 and IV, matrix-metalloproteinase-1 and -13, and TMP-1 gene expression. *Am. J. Pathol.*, 155, 493–503.

Hoare, A. (1976) Connective tissue disorders affecting the gastrointestinal tract. *Recent Adv. Gastroenterol.*, 3, 96–123.

Jarnerot, J., Fysk, C., Bohr, J., Eriksson, S. (1995) Collagenous colitis and faecal stream diversion. *Gastroenterology*, 109, 449–55.

Jawhari, A., Talbot, I.C. (1996) Microscopic, lymphocytic and collagenous colitis. *Histopathology*, 29, 101–10.

Jawhari, A., Sheaf, M., Forbes, A., Kamm, M.A., Talbot, I.C. (1995) Microscopic colitis widening the definition. *Gut*, 36 (Suppl.), A26.

Khan, M.A., Brunt, E.M., Longo, W.E., Presti, M.E. (2000) Persistent clostridium difficile colitis: a possible aetiology for the development of collagenous colitis. *Dig. Dis. Sci.*, 45, 998–1001.

Kingham, J., Levison, D., Ball, J., Dawson, A. (1982) Microscopic colitis – a cause of chronic watery diarrhoea. *Br. Med. J.*, 105, 1601–4.

Kitchen, P.A., Levi A.J., Domizio, P., Talbot, I.C., Forbes, A., Price, A.B., London Inflammatory Bowel Disease Forum (2002) Microscopic colitis: the tip of the iceberg. *Eur. J. Gastroenterol. Hepatol.*, 14, 1199–204.

Lamps, L.W., Lazenby, A.J. (2000) Colonic epithelial lymphocytosis and lymphocytic colitis: descriptive histopathology versus distinct clinicopathological entities. *Adv. Anat. Pathol.*, 7, 210–13.

Lazenby, A.J., Yardley, J.H., Giardiello, F.M., Jessurun, J., Bayless, T.M. (1989) Lymphocytic ('microscopic') colitis: a comparative histopathologic study with particular reference to collagenous colitis. *Hum. Pathol.*, 20, 18–28.

Lazenby, A.J., Yardley, J.H., Giardiello, F.M., Bayless, T.M. (1990) Pitfalls in the diagnosis of collagenous colitis: experience with 75 cases from a registry of collagenous colitis at the John Hopkins Hospital. *Hum. Pathol.*, 21, 905–10.

Lee, E., Schiller, L.R., Vendrell, D., Carol, A., Santa, A., Fordtran, J.S. (1992) Subepithelial collagen table thickness in colon specimens from patients with microscopic colitis and collagenous colitis. *Gastroenterology*, 103, 1790–6.

Lee, F.D. (1993) Importance of apoptosis in the histopathology of drug related lesions in the large intestine. *J. Clin. Pathol.*, 46, 118–22.

Leigh, C., Elahmady, A., Mitros, F.A., Metcalf, A., Al-Jurf, A. (1993) Collagenous colitis associated with chronic constipation. *Am. J. Surg. Pathol.*, 17, 81–4.

Levison, D., Lazenby, A., Yardley, J.H. (1993) Microscopic colitis cases revisited. *Gastroenterology*, 105, 1594–6.

Lewis, F.W., Warren, G.H., Goff, J.S. (1991) Collagenous colitis with involvement of the terminal ileum. *Dig. Dis. Sci.*, 36, 1161–3.

Libbrecht, L., Croes, R., Ectors, N., Staels, F., Geboes, K. (2002) Microscopic colitis with giant cells. *Histopathology*, 40, 335–8.

Lindstrom, J. (1976) Collagenous colitis with watery diarrhoea – a new entity. *Pathol. Eur.*, 11, 87–9.

Marteau, P., Lavergne-Slove, A., Lemann, M., Bouhnik, Y., Bertheau, P., Becheur, H., Galian, A., Rambaud, J.C. (1997) Primary villous atrophy is often associated with microscopic colitis. *Gut*, 41, 561–4.

Meier, P.N., Otto, P., Ritter, M., Stolte, M. (1991) Collagenous duodenitis and ileitis in a patient with collagenous colitis. *Leber Magen. Darm.*, 21, 231–2.

Moayyedi, P., O'Mahoney, S., Jackson, P., Lynch, D.A., Dixon, M.F., Axon, A.T. (1997) Small intestine in lymphocytic and collagenous colitis: mucosal morphology, permeability and secretory immunity to gliadin. *J. Clin. Pathol.*, 50, 527–29.

Mosnier, J-F., Larvol, L., Barge, J., Dubois, S., De La Bigne, S., Henin, D., Cerf, M. (1996) Lymphocytic and collagenous colitis: An immunohistochemical study. *Am. J. Gastroenterol.*, 91, 709–13.

Mukherjee, S. (2003) Diarrhoea associated with lansoprazole. *J. Gastroenterol. Hepatol.*, 18, 602–3.

Muller, S., Neureiter, D., Stolte, M., Verbeke, C., Heuschmann, P., Kirchner, T., Aigner, T. (2001) Tenascin: a sensitive and specific diagnostic marker of minimal collagenous colitis. *Virchows Arch.*, 438, 435–41.

Mullhaupt, B., Guller, U., Anabitarte, M., Guller, R., Fried, M. (1998) Lymphocyitc colitis: clinical presentation and long term course. *Gut*, 43, 629–33.

Offner, F.A., Jao, R.V., Lewin, K.J., Havelec, L., Weinstein, W.M. (1999) Collagenous colitis: a study of the distribution of morphological abnormalities and their histological detection. *Hum. Pathol.*, 30, 451–7.

Olesen, M., Eriksson, S., Bohr, J., Jarnerot, G., Tysk, C. (2003) Microscopic colitis: a common diarrhoeal disease. An epidemiological study in Orebro, Sweden, 1993–1998. *Gut*, 53, 346–50.

Olesen, M., Eriksson, S., Bohr, J., Jarnerot, G., Tysk, C. (2004) Lymphocytic colitis: a retrospective study of 199 Swedish patients. *Gut*, 54, 536–41.

Padmanabhan, V., Callas, P.W., Li, S.C., Trainer, T.D. (2003) Histopathological features of the terminal ileum in lymphocytic and collagenous colitis: A study of 32 cases and review of the literature. *Mod. Pathol.*, 16, 115–19.

Perri, F., Annese, V., Pastore, M., Andriulli, A. (1996) Microscopic colitis progressed to collagenous colitis: a morphometric study. *Ital. J. Gastroenterol.*, 28, 147–51.

Pokorny, C.S., Kneale, K.I., Henderson, C.J. (2001) Progression of collagenous colitis to ulcerative colitis. *J. Clin. Gastroenterol.*, 32, 435–8.

Popovic, O.S., Kostic, K.M., Milovic, B.V. *et al.* (1987) Primary bile acid malabsorption, histologic and immunologic study in three patients. *Gastroenterology*, 92, 1851–8.

Proctor, D.D. (2004) The clinical and pathological significance of microscopic colitis. *Int. J. Surg. Pathol.*, 38, S31.

Pulimood, A.B., Ramakrishna, B.S., Mathan, M.M. (1999) Collagenous gastritis and collagenous colitis: a report with sequential histological and ultrastructural findings. *Gut*, 44, 881–5.

Rask-Madden, J., Grove, O., Hansen, M.G., Bukhave, K., Scient, C., Henrik-Nielson, R. (1983) Colonic transport of water and electrolytes in a patient with secretory diarrhoea due to collagenous colitis. *Dig. Dis. Sci.*, 28, 1141–6.

Read, N.W., Krejs, G.J., Read, M.G., Santa Ana, C.A., Morawski, S.G., Fordtran, J.S. (1980) Chronic diarrhoea of unknown origin. *Gastroenterology*, 78, 264–71.

Riddell, R., Tanaka, M., Mazzoleni, G. (1992) Non-steroidal anti-inflammatory drugs as a possible cause of collagenous colitis – a case control study. *Gut*, 33, 683–6.

Robert, M.E. (2004) Microscopic colitis, pathologic considerations and changing dogma. *J. Clin. Gastroenterol.*, 38., S18–S26.

Salas, A., Fernandez-Benares, F., Casalots, J., Gonzalez, C., Tarroch, X., Forcada, P., Gonzalez, G. (2003) Subepithelial myofibroblasts and tenascin expression in microscopic colitis. *Histopathology*, 43, 48–54.

Sandmeier, D., Bouzourene, H. (2004) Microscopic colitis with giant cells: a rare new histopathologic subtype? *Int. J. Surg. Pathol.*, 12, 45–8.

Sapp, H., Ithamukkala, S., Brien, T.P., *et al.* (2002) The terminal ileum is affected in patients with lymphocytic or collagenous colitis. *Am. J. Surg. Pathol.*, 26, 1484–92.

Saul, S.H. (1993) The watery diarrhoea–colitis syndrome. *Int. J. Surg. Pathol.*, 1, 65–82.

Saurine, T.J., Brewer, J.M., Eckstein, R.P. (2004) Microscopic colitis with granulomatous inflammation. *Histopathology*, 45, 82–6.

Schiller, L.C. (1999) Microscopic colitis syndrome: lymphocytic colitis and collagenous colitis. *Semin. Gastrointest. Dis.*, 10, 145–55.

Schiller, L.C. (2000) Pathophysiology and treatment of microscopic-colitis syndrome. *Lancet*, 355, 243–8.

Sciarretta, G., Furno, A., Morrone, B., Malaguti, P. (1994) Absence of histopathological changes of ileum and colon in functional diarrhoea associated with bile acid malabsorption by SeHCAT test: a prospective study. *Am. J. Gatroenterol.*, 89, 1058–61.

Shaz, B.H., Reddy, S.I., Ayata, G. *et al.* (2004) Sequential clinical and histopathological changes in collagenous and lymphocytic colitis over time. *Mod. Pathol.*, 17, 395–401.

Sherman, A., Ackert, J.J., Rajapaksa, R., West, A.B., Oweity, T. (2004) Fractured colon: an endoscopically distinctive lesion associated with colonic perforation following colonoscopy in patients with collagenous colitis. *J. Clin. Gastroenterol.*, 38, 341–5.

Stahle-Backdahl, M., Maim, J., Veress, B., Benoni, C., Bruce, K., Egesten, A. (2000) Increased presence of eosinophilic granulocytes expressing transforming growth factor beta-1 in collagenous colitis. *Scand. J. Gastroenterol.*, 35, 742–6.

Tanaka, M., Mazzoleni, G., Riddell, R.H. (1992) Distribution of collagenous colitis: utility of flexible sigmoidoscopy. *Gut*, 33, 65–70.

Teglbjaerg, P.S., Thaysen, E.H., Jensen, H.H. (1984) Development of collagenous colitis in sequential biopsy specimens. *Gastroenterology*, 87, 703–9.

Thomson, R.D., Lestina, L.S., Bensen, S.P., Toor, A., Maheshwari, Y., Ratcliffe, N.R. (2002) Lansoprazole-associated microscopic colitis: a case series. *Am. J. Gastroenterol.*, 97, 2908–13.

Treanor, D., Sheahan, K. (2002) Microscopic colitis: lymphocytic and collagenous colitis. *Curr. Diagn. Pathol.*, 8, 33–41.

Tuncer, C., Cindoruk, M., Dursun, A., Karakan, T. (2003) Prevalence of microscopic colitis in patients with symptoms suggesting irritable bowel syndrome. *Acta Gastroenterol. Belg.*, 66, 133–6.

Veress, B., Lofberg, R., Bergman, L. (1995) Microscopic colitis syndrome. *Gut*, 36, 880–6.

Vesoulis, Z., Lozanski, Z., Loiudice, T. (2000) Synchronous occurrence of collagenous colitis and pseudomembranous colitis. *Can. J. Gastroenterol.*, 14, 353–.

Wang, H.H., Owings, D.V., Antonioli, D.A., Goldman, H. (1988) Increased subepithelial deposition is not specific for collagenous colitis. *Mod. Pathol.*, 1, 329–35.

Wang, N., Dumont, J.A., Achkar, E., Easley, K.A., Petras, R.E., Goldblum, J.R. (1999) Colonic epithelial lymphocytosis without a thickened subepithelial collagen table: a clinicopathological study of 40 cases supporting a heterogeneous entity. *Am. J. Surg. Pathol.*, 23, 1068–74.

Warren, B.F., Edwards, C.M., Travis, S.P.L. (2002) 'Microscopic colitis' classification and terminology. *Histopathology*, 40, 374–6.

Weinstein, G.D., Saunders, D.R., Tytgat, G.M., Rubin, C.E. (1970) Collagenous sprue – an unrecognized cause of malabsorption. *N. Engl. J. Med.*, 283, 1297–301.

Wolber, R., Owen, D., Freeman, H. (1990) Colonic lymphocytosis in patients with celiac sprue. *Hum. Pathol.*, 21, 1092–6.

Yardley, J.H., Lazenby, A.J., Giardiello, F.M., Bayless, T.M. (1990) Collagenous, 'microscopic', lymphocytic, and other gentler and more subtle forms of colitis. *Hum. Pathol.*, 21, 1089–91.

Yuan, S., Reyes, V., Bronner, M.P. (2003) Pseudomembranous collagenous colitis. *Am. J. Surg. Pathol.*, 27, 1375–9.

CHAPTER 10

ISCHAEMIC COLITIS

10.1 Introduction	168	
10.2 Anatomical considerations	168	
10.3 Precipitating causes	169	
10.4 Natural history of ischaemic bowel disease	171	
10.4.1 Occlusive disease	171	
10.4.2 Non-occlusive disease	171	
10.5 Endoscopic features	171	
10.6 Biopsy appearances	172	
10.6.1 Gangrenous ischaemia	172	

10.6.2 Non-gangrenous ischaemic colitis	172
10.6.3 The reparative phase	174
10.6.4 The phase of stricture	175
10.7 Difficulties with diagnosis	175
10.8 Vasculitis	176
10.9 Necrotizing colitis syndromes	177
References	177

10.1 INTRODUCTION

Ischaemic colitis is a major cause of large intestinal problems requiring medical attention and it is our impression that its frequency is increasing in hospital biopsy practice. The overall incidence of ischaemic colitis in general populations is small, ranging from 4.5 to 44 cases per 100 000 person-years (Higgins *et al.*, 2004). However, it is the second or third commonest cause of acute lower gastrointestinal haemorrhage (Longstreth, 1997; Vernava *et al.*, 1997), and results from approximately half of all cases of mesenteric vasculopathy (Cappell, 1998). In the elderly, ulcerative colitis and Crohn's disease are probably overdiagnosed at the expense of ischaemic colitis. Brandt *et al.* (1981) felt this to be the case in up to 35 per cent of their series of elderly colitics after critical review.

The aetiology of an ischaemic insult and its rate of onset determine the pathology of ischaemic colitis (Price, 1990). The spectrum ranges from infarction and gangrene of the bowel (McGovern and Coulston, 1965) to transient fleeting episodes (Boley *et al.*, 1963; Dawson and Schaefer, 1971). Between the two

extremes is a slow onset pattern, usually chronic and progressing to a stricture (Marston *et al.*, 1966; Brown, 1968). The role of biopsy depends on the clinical pattern. Clearly, in gangrene of the bowel, a surgical emergency, biopsy is clinically inappropriate. Although ischaemic colitis is typically a disease of the elderly (Shoji and Becker, 1994), it can also present in young patients, in both gangrenous and self-limiting forms (the latter, so-called transient ischaemic colitis, is commoner in women on oestrogen or oral contraceptive therapy) (Newell and Deckert, 1997).

A knowledge of the vascular anatomy, the likely precipitating events and the endoscopic and radiological data are required if the diagnosis of ischaemia is to be made with confidence from a biopsy.

10.2 ANATOMICAL CONSIDERATIONS

The superior mesenteric artery supplies the proximal half of the large bowel, the inferior mesenteric and iliac arteries the distal half. A marginal artery forms an anastomosis between the two and, following occlusion of one of the major vessels of supply, viability depends on its patency. The supply is believed by some to be most susceptible at the splenic flexure (Griffith's point), a 'watershed' zone between the superior and the inferior mesenteric arteries and, in the rectum, at the junctional zone between the inferior mesenteric and iliac arteries (Marston, 1972). However, injection studies have failed to substantiate the concept of a watershed area at the splenic flexure (Binns and Isaacson, 1978) and Alschibaja and Morson (1977) point out that ischaemia is commoner in the lower left colon (Sudeck's point) than at the splenic flexure. The ileocaecal region is also at risk (Yamazaki et al., 1997a) and the right colon can be affected (Bower, 1993). The rectum is involved in only 4–16 per cent of cases (Reeders et al., 1984) and rectosigmoid ischaemia has clear precipitating factors (Sharma et al. 1995).

10.3 PRECIPITATING CAUSES

It is not appropriate to discuss in detail here the aetiology of large intestinal ischaemia. The subject was well reviewed by Reeders et al. (1984). It is customary to classify the causes into arterial occlusions, small vessel disease, venous occlusions and non-occlusive factors. However, it is probable that more than one factor frequently operates and that non-occlusive factors play a dominant role in over 30 per cent of patients (Renton, 1972). While Table 10.1 indicates the more important physiopathological precipitating factors of ischaemic colitis, a more detailed list of causes is presented in Table 10.2. On a molecular level, it appears that both platelet-activating factor (Hsueh et al., 1986; Nagahata et al., 1999) and antioxidants (Thomson et al., 1998) play their part in the development of ischaemic colitis.

Ischaemic colitis is a spectrum of disease (Arnott et al., 1999). Occlusive disease of the inferior mesenteric artery is often iatrogenic, occurring in the course of reconstructive aortic surgery but, in atherosclerotic subjects, the inferior mesenteric artery is less of a trap for emboli than the superior vessel. The incidence of bowel ischaemia after surgery of the

Table 10.1 Precipitating factors in large intestinal ischaemia

Arterial occlusion
Superior mesenteric artery (commonly thrombo-atheromatous disease)
Inferior mesenteric artery (commonly surgical intervention)

Small vessel disease
Diabetes mellitus
Amyloidosis
Irradiation vasculopathy
Arteritis (e.g. rheumatoid arthritis)
Renal transplantation/immunosuppression

Venous occlusion
Thrombosis: idiopathic
  in portal hypertension
  acute pancreatitis
  hypercoagulability states
Mechanical compression

Non-occlusive factors (low flow states)
Shock
Dehydration
Drugs (see Table 10.2)
Increased luminal pressure (large bowel obstruction): tumours
Hirschsprung's disease volvulus/strangulation diverticular disease

abdominal aorta is 2.8 per cent or, in the context of shock associated with ruptured aortic aneurysm, 7.3 per cent (Bjorck et al., 1996). In 95 per cent of patients the lesion affects the left colon within the reach of a sigmoidoscope (Bjorck et al., 1996). The occurrence of gradual stenoses and occlusions to a critical level is surprisingly rare (Croft et al., 1981). The most common clinical predisposing factors are atherosclerosis, shock and congestive heart failure but in elderly patients ischaemic colitis can appear with no predisposing factors (Alapati and Mihas, 1999). Most patients respond favourably to conservative measurements within 48 hours, although massive bleeding and perforation are not infrequent (Chou et al., 1989), and surgery may be necessary in approximately 20 per cent of cases (Cappell, 1998). Non-occlusive ischaemia occurs because haemoperfusion of the large bowel is susceptible to hypotension; mesenteric arterial tone rises and blood flow falls during the homeostatic response in states of shock, dehydration or in the 'fight or flight' reaction (Bergstein et al., 1995). Drugs such as vasopressin, digoxin, anti-hypertensive agents and ergot have a

Table 10.2 Causes of large intestinal ischaemia

Cause	References
Aortoiliac–femoral surgery	
By itself	Bjorck *et al.* (1996), Mackay *et al.* (1994), Piotrowski *et al.* (1996)
With previous irradiation	Israeli *et al.* (1996)
Other surgery	Greenwald and Brandt (1998), Sakorafas and Tsiotos (1999), Yamazaki *et al.* (1997b)
Colonoscopy	Cremers *et al.* (1998), Wheeldon and Grundman (1990)
Phlebosclerosis	Maruyama *et al.* (1997)
Atheroemboli/cholesterol crystals	Gramlich and Hunter (1994), Moolenaar and Lamers (1996), O'Briain *et al.* (1991)
Renal impairment	
Nephrotic syndrome	Yasumori *et al.* (1995)
Chronic renal failure and dialysis	Flobert et al. (2000), Wellington and Rody (1993)
Acute pancreatitis	Yamagiwa *et al.* (1993)
Infective	
Schistosomiasis	Neves *et al.* (1993)
Vasculitis	
Wegener's	Storesund *et al.* (1998)
Systemic lupus erythematosus	Ho *et al.* (1987)
Polyarteritis nodosa	Okada *et al.* (1999)
Others	Greenwald and Brandt (1998)
Toxic megacolon	Markoglou *et al.* (1993)
Amyloidosis	Kaiserling and Krober (1995), Trinh *et al.* (1991)
Drugs	
In general	Neitlich and Burrell (1999)
Interferon-α	Tada *et al.* (1996)
NSAIDs	Carratu *et al.* (1993)
Oral contraceptive	Deana and Dean (1995)
Premarin	Gurbuz *et al.* (1994)
Amphetamines	Beyer *et al.* (1991), Johnson and Berenson (1991)
Psychotropic drugs in general	Patel *et al.* (1992)
Laxatives	Oh *et al.* (1997)
Crack and cocaine abuse	Yang *et al.* (1991), Boutros *et al.* (1997), Brown *et al.* (1994)
Others	Greenwald and Brandt (1998)
Haematological disorders	Bower (1993), Scholz (1993)
Enema	Berenguer *et al.* (1981)
Hypotension/shock	Bower (1993), Ludwig *et al.* (1995)
Colorectal cancer	Seow-Choen *et al.* (1993)
Phaeochromocytoma	Sharma *et al.* (1995)
Mechanical	Bower (1993), Greenwald and Brandt (1998)
Long-distance running	Heer *et al.* (1987)

similar effect and alcohol has also been implicated, in combination with other drugs (Reeders *et al.*, 1984). Ischaemic colitis is a recognized consequence of abuse of drugs such as amphetamines (Beyer *et al.*, 1991; Johnson and Berenson, 1991) and cocaine (Brown *et al.*, 1994; Boutros *et al.*, 1997) (Section 11.4.8).

In large intestinal obstruction there is overdistension of the bowel owing to increased luminal contents under pressure and mucosal perfusion is reduced by the tension acting on the bowel wall. This can have important local or diffuse ischaemic effects (i.e. obstructive colitis, also discussed in Section 13.6.2). The mechanism has been confirmed by animal experiments (Gatch and Gulbertson, 1935). It should be remembered that obstructive colitis may develop not only in relation to a carcinoma (Schwartz and Boley, 1972), megacolon or adhesions, but also proximal to diverticular disease (probably an underestimated cause of this problem). Chlorpromazine, given in large doses for long periods, as it often is in psychiatric patients, has a similar effect through inhibition of peristalsis (Clarke *et al.*, 1972).

Since a combination of two or more of these factors is very commonly present in the elderly, it is not surprising that 80 per cent of cases of ischaemic colitis occur in patients over the age of 50 years (Reeders *et al.*, 1984).

10.4 NATURAL HISTORY OF ISCHAEMIC BOWEL DISEASE

To interpret the biopsy in ischaemic disease of the colon it is necessary to appreciate the natural history of the changes (Whitehead, 1976; Alschibaja and Morson, 1977). In general, acute ischaemic colitis usually runs a benign course; however, when the right colon is involved it tends to be more severe (Medina *et al.*, 2004). The sequelae are also more severe if there is an underlying peripheral vasculopathy (Medina *et al.*, 2004).

10.4.1 Occlusive disease

The consequences of vascular occlusion depend on the size of vessel affected and the effectiveness of a collateral circulation. If the latter is insufficient the immediate result is cell death. The superficial half of the mucosa is the most vulnerable (Whitehead, 1972). The extent of the vascular deprivation determines the length and depth involved and, indeed, the clinical presentation (Swerdlow *et al.*, 1981).

Following acute mucosal damage a phase of repair occurs. Granulation tissue is produced, followed by fibrosis and re-epithelialization (Whitehead, 1976). This can then lead to the final phase of stricture formation if damage was severe, or complete recovery if damage was limited. The above patterns apply to occlusive events of large and small vessels. The rate of onset of the occlusion will affect the outcome so that, with a gradual diminution in blood supply, many patients may not present until late on, at the stage when they already have a stricture (Alschibaja and Morson, 1977).

10.4.2 Non-occlusive disease

The pattern in non-occlusive, low flow states is different. Damage to the bowel is more extensive, taking the form of acute haemorrhagic infarction or one of the various forms of 'necrotizing colitis' (Marston, 1962, 1986). Surgical intervention is the rule. In the rare cases where conservative management is possible strictures subsequently develop, demonstrating the same natural evolution of ischaemic damage.

Transient disease ('evanescent' colitis; Miller *et al.*, 1971) has been referred to and is related to limited vascular events from which swift uncomplicated recovery is possible (Barcewicz and Welch, 1980; Heron *et al.*, 1981).

The ascending or transverse colon are particularly affected (Clarke *et al.*, 1972). The nature of the vascular lesion in these cases is uncertain. Venous thrombosis and an association with oral contraceptives have been suggested (Kilpatrick *et al.*, 1968; Cotton and Thomas, 1971), but men are equally afflicted.

10.5 ENDOSCOPIC FEATURES

Clinically, the differential diagnosis of colonic ischaemia is broad, including infectious colitis, inflammatory bowel disease, pseudomembranous colitis, diverticulitis and colonic carcinoma (Greenwald and Brandt, 1998). The histological appearance can therefore be of paramount importance in establishing the diagnosis. This is also important in cases in which the radiological imaging is rather featureless and non-specific (Robson *et al.*, 1992; Toursarkissian and Thompson, 1997).

Like the pathology, the endoscopic appearances depend on the rate of onset of ischaemia. In acute episodes the clinician will normally see focally swollen, bluish-purple mucosa with oedema and contact bleeding (Dawson and Schaefer, 1971; Scowcroft *et al.*, 1981). Scattered isolated ulceration occurs, predominantly in the left half of the colon. The appearances are unlike those of either ulcerative colitis or Crohn's disease and this knowledge is helpful if the biopsy features are inconclusive. It may be difficult to distinguish an ischaemic stricture from Crohn's disease if no adjacent mucosal abnormalities are present. In chronic ischaemic proctitis white mucosal scars can be detected at sigmoidoscopy (Devroede *et al.*, 1982). Atheroemboli leading to localized ischaemia can produce a polypoidal appearance (Gramlich and Hunter, 1994).

Early colonoscopy and biopsy can diagnose ischaemic colitis, particularly if performed by day three from onset of symptoms (Habu *et al.*, 1996). Evaluation of the extent of the disease is necessary, with cases of total ischaemic colitis having a worse prognosis than those with segmental colonic ischaemia (Longo *et al.*, 1997). A computed tomography (CT) scan evaluation can be useful in confirming the diagnosis, to suggest it when clinically unsuspected or to assess complications, but cannot predict the development of infarction (Balthazar *et al.*, 1999). Computed tomography scanning can also be of help in identifying areas of ischaemic colitis proximal to colonic cancer (Ko *et al.*, 1997).

10.6 BIOPSY APPEARANCES

In their review on biopsy diagnosis of colitis, Tsang and Rotterdam (1999) indicate that although pathologists are good at describing the features of ischaemic colitis, in half of the cases they do not translate them into the right diagnosis, and more awareness is therefore necessary. In general, the importance of tight clinicopathological correlation to establish this diagnosis cannot be overemphasized (Carpenter and Talley, 2000).

10.6.1 Gangrenous ischaemia

As this is a surgical emergency, biopsy is seldom performed or, indeed, warranted. On the rare occasions when a biopsy is taken, the mucosa and muscularis mucosae appear completely necrotic and suffused with blood (Fig. 10.1). The crypts are lost and only their positional outlines remain (Whitehead, 1976). The submucosa frequently contains free blood.

10.6.2 Non-gangrenous ischaemic colitis

Biopsy is most frequently undertaken in the non-resolving form of the disease, but similar features are described in evanescent colitis (Dawson and Schaefer, 1971).

The characteristic feature of the milder episode is damage restricted to the superficial half of the mucosa (Whitehead, 1976). The upper halves of the crypts show varying degrees of degeneration and may even be sloughed off, along with the surface epithelium (Fig. 10.2). Small erosions may be seen. If

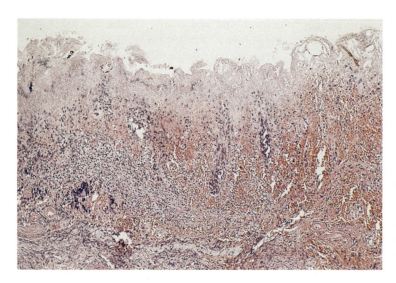

Figure 10.1 Gangrenous ischaemia. Biopsy of left colon from an elderly patient who presented with bloody diarrhoea. The mucosa is almost completely necrotic and there is haemorrhage into both mucosa and submucosa.

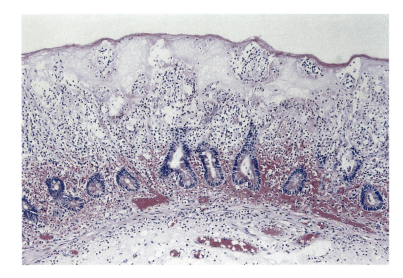

Figure 10.2 Acute ischaemic colitis. In this relatively mild case there is necrosis and sloughing of the surface and upper crypt epithelium only. A fibrinous exudate covers the surface. The residual crypt epithelium shows goblet cell loss and regenerative hyperchromatism. The lamina propria is oedematous and oedema masks the presence of neutrophils.

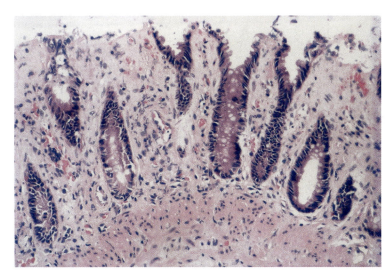

Figure 10.3 Acute ischaemic colitis. The surface and crypt epithelium is degenerate and flattened rather than sloughed away. There is mucosal oedema with a hyaline eosinophilic appearance, not to be confused with collagenous colitis.

intact, the crypt cells will have lost their mucin, are flattened and basophilic and have hyperchromatic nuclei (Fig. 10.3). Depending on severity, the basal halves of the crypts survive. Accompanying this cryptal and epithelial damage is a varying, though moderate, inflammatory cell infiltrate. Polymorphs are usually present, infiltrating between the upper crypt cells. Occasionally, focal active colitis with no accompanying architectural change, may be the only abnormality in biopsies from ischaemic colitic patients (Greenson *et al.*, 1997; Volk *et al.*, 1998).

The lamina propria is oedematous but often has a deeply eosinophilic quality (Fig. 10.3). Indeed, the superficial lamina propria frequently takes on a hyalinized appearance, which can be mistaken for a collagen band. Fibrin plugs may be noted in mucosal capillaries. In the lower half of the mucosa the cryptal epithelium may be hyperchromatic and show increased numbers of mitoses.

In more severe cases, the crypt base epithelium is degenerate and damaged, and if no intact muscularis mucosae is noted, distinction from gangrene may be impossible (Fig. 10.1). Mild to moderate

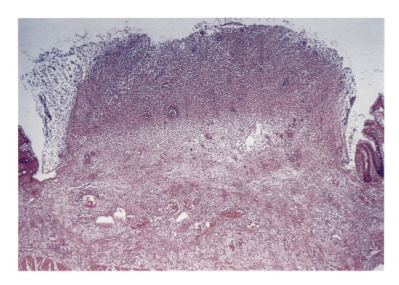

Figure 10.4 Ischaemic ulcer. The fibrino-purulent exudate and granulation tissue forming the floor of this ulcer show no specific features.

collections of acute inflammatory cells, plasma cells and lymphocytes, are present. Ulceration and infection supervene on this damaged mucosa (Fig. 10.4). At this stage, unless some intact mucosa has been biopsied the ulceration shows no distinguishing qualities from ulceration of any other cause, e.g. pseudomembranous colitis (Fig. 8.8 on page 138).

If submucosa is included in the biopsy it is usually oedematous. A careful inspection of the larger submucosal vessels may reveal evidence of vasculitis or an embolus (Fig. 10.5). When ischaemia is suspected it is always worth cutting levels through the biopsy in search of vascular lesions. However, evidence that thrombi in small vessels are the primary cause of ischaemia must be interpreted with caution in ulcerated lesions. To establish that they are not secondary events they must be observed in non-ulcerated areas. Disseminated intravascular coagulation is an important cause of ischaemic disease (Margaretten and McKay, 1971; Whitehead, 1971).

10.6.3 The reparative phase

Although it is convenient to subdivide the changes in the manner laid out here, in the majority of cases both the acute and the reparative changes occur alongside each other.

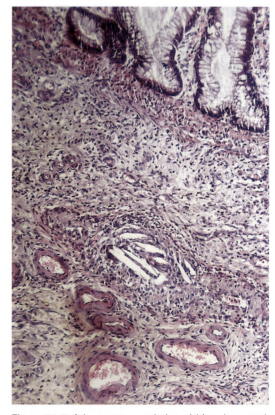

Figure 10.5 Atheromatous embolus within submucosal arteriole.

If the basal epithelium survives, the crypts will regenerate and the mucosa return to normal (Dawson and Schaefer, 1971; Whitehead, 1976). If damage is more severe the end result will be distorted crypts, reduced in number. The surface epithelium will grow over an area of full-thickness mucosal ulceration which may then be completely devoid of crypts. Accompanying the change the lamina propria undergoes fibrosis. There is capillary proliferation and a mild to moderate mixed inflammatory infiltrate which can include iron-laden histiocytes (Marston *et al.*, 1966). The latter are always cited as a common and useful sign for ischaemia but, in our experience, are rarely seen.

Following ischaemic damage to a greater depth – 'mural infarction' (Swerdlow *et al.*, 1981) – the muscularis mucosae is replaced by proliferating fibroblasts which spread down into the superficial submucosa (Day *et al.*, 2003).

10.6.4 The phase of stricture

With only mild disease, as in transient forms of ischaemic colitis, recovery is complete within a few days (Whitehead, 1976). A biopsy would then fail to detect any abnormality. However, after bouts of severe acute disease or in chronic vascular insufficiency, residual abnormality remains. Fibrosis, being the hallmark of healing, leads to stricture formation (Day *et al.*, 2003). The changes predominate in the submucosa, which may be densely fibrotic and thinned. The superficial fibres of the circular muscular coat are often also involved. Biopsy shows

permanent mucosal damage, consisting of thinning with crypt atrophy (Fig. 10.6). A flat epithelium may even rest directly on the fibrotic muscularis propria, the submucosa having been obliterated. This will not be evident in a biopsy. Surviving crypts are irregular and the lamina propria is usually densely fibrotic at this stage; in fact, presence of mucosal elastin and so-called 'diamond-shaped' crypts, a feature of solitary rectal ulcer, can be identified in half of ischaemic colitis cases (Warren *et al.*, 1990). Inflammation is not a striking feature but, again, iron-laden macrophages should be sought. Van Gieson's and Perls' stains highlight these features. Although ischaemia is commoner higher up in the bowel, sacral artery disease affects the rectum and may produce a recognizable syndrome of faecal incontinence and rectal angina (Devroede *et al.*, 1982).

10.7 DIFFICULTIES WITH DIAGNOSIS

The situation is relatively clear-cut when there is an arteritis or vascular occlusion, or if the mucosa is infarcted. When destruction is limited to the superficial half of the mucosa, difficulty arises in making the distinction from pseudomembranous colitis (Chapter 8). Briefly, pseudomembranes can be present in ischaemic colitis; however, specific histological features such as hyalinization

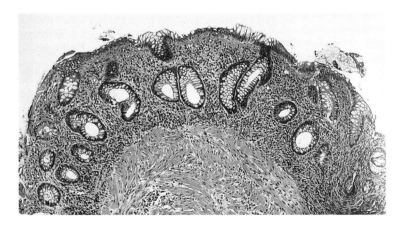

Figure 10.6 Healed ischaemic colitis (phase of stricture). This biopsy, from a high rectal stricture shows atrophy and deformity of crypts. There is no evidence of active ischaemic damage and the picture resembles quiescent ulcerative colitis, apart from fibrosis of the lamina propria, particularly close to the surface.

of the lamina propria, lamina propria haemorrhage, atrophic microcrypts, full-thickness mucosal necrosis and diffuse distribution of pseudomembranes can help in distinguishing them from those of *Clostridium difficile* pseudomembranous colitis (Dignan and Greenson, 1997). There may also be problems with biopsies taken during the reparative phase. Any healing ulcer can re-epithelialize and will then show crypt distortion, granulation tissue and some fibrosis. To be confident of distinguishing crypt distortion, as seen in ulcerative colitis, from the pattern in ischaemia, these other mucosal abnormalities must be carefully assessed. Much depends on having biopsies from other sites and knowing the distribution of the lesion. Ischaemic colitis is usually patchy, predominates on the left side and, as previously mentioned, endoscopy may show focal submucosal haemorrhages (Section 10.5). This combination is unlike anything seen in ulcerative colitis or Crohn's disease. When a stricture is established, the biopsy will reveal dense fibrosis of the lamina propria (Parish *et al.*, 1991), some cryptal simplification and, possibly, haemosiderin-laden macrophages.

Chronic radiation colitis may resemble this picture and, indeed, has a basis in ischaemia, but localization in the rectum, the presence of irradiation fibroblasts, ectatic mucosal capillaries and endarteritis obliterans in the submucosa should suggest the aetiology of irradiation (Section 11.1).

10.8 VASCULITIS

Vasculitis of the small vessels of the colon can occur during the course of the following diseases:

- Polyarteritis nodosa
- Allergic granulomatosis
- Rheumatoid arthritis
- Systemic lupus erythematosus
- Scleroderma
- Behçet's disease.

Vasculitis rarely presents as ischaemic colitis in the first instance and, although there is a report of a patient with previously unsuspected vasculitis who developed an ulcerative colitis-like picture (Burt *et al.*, 1983) gastrointestinal involvement in these conditions is usually just a part of the systemic illness. In rheumatoid arthritis, rectal biopsy demonstrated a vasculitis in 40 per cent of one series of patients in whom there was clinical evidence of vasculitic disease (Tribe *et al.*, 1981). Although rectal and/or colonic biopsies may help establish that a vasculitis is present, the accompanying ulcerative and inflammatory changes in the colon are rarely specific. The diagnosis is made from the overall clinical picture. In severe cases there may be infarction of the colon (Rosenblum *et al.*, 1963) but, more commonly, there is segmental ulceration, causing confusion with Crohn's disease. In Crohn's disease itself, granulomas are often located close to blood vessels, particularly veins, simulating a granulomatous vasculitis. However, this seems to be because granulomas tend to arise in lymphatics, which travel with vascular bundles, rather than primarily a vasculitic process (Talbot *et al.*, 1992; Matson *et al.*, 1995).

As the vasculitis is best appreciated in the submucosal vessels, clinicians should be encouraged to try and take deep biopsies. Tribe *et al.* (1981) recommend biopsy of the posterior rectal wall to avoid problems from perforation. It is important to remember that vessels close to the floor of any ulcer are commonly inflamed and thrombosed and can lead the unwary to overdiagnose vasculitis (Fig. 10.7). Damaged vessels may only be identified with difficulty and, whenever a vasculitis is suspected, multiple levels should be examined through the block; as in temporal arteritis, the lesions can be focal. Indeed, one should not be misled by a normal surface mucosa: an arteritis might not be accompanied by ischaemic damage if the collateral circulation is adequate. Healed ulceration, with its inherent diagnostic problems, is discussed previously.

Either arteries or, less frequently, veins can be involved. The vessels may show one of several patterns: an obvious acute necrotizing vasculitis with fibrinoid necrosis and infiltration by inflammatory cells, with nuclear dust formation; a subacute pattern with cuffing of vessels by lymphocytes; or a chronic or burnt-out vasculitis. The last pattern may be missed, as inflammation is absent, but an elastic-van Gieson stain will demonstrate damage

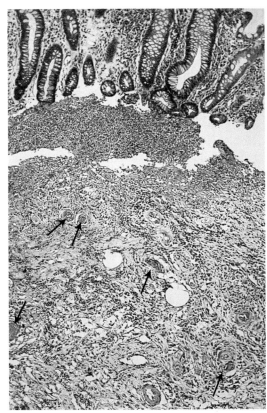

Figure 10.7 Thrombosis of small blood vessels (arrowed) in floor of ulcer. Rectal biopsy from a patient with Crohn's disease.

and interruption of the internal elastic lamina (Tribe *et al.*, 1981).

For further comments on vasculitis see Section 20.1.2.

10.9 NECROTIZING COLITIS SYNDROMES

There is a bewildering array of terms in the literature to describe necrotic and haemorrhagic lesions of the colon, such as enteritis necroticans, haemorrhagic enterocolitis, phlegmonous enterocolitis and neonatal necrotizing enterocolitis (Marston, 1986). Some are clearly ischaemic, with gangrene of the bowel, and caused by low flow. In others the pathogenesis is less clear, with bacteria, particularly

clostridial species, playing a part. All are characterized by extensive mucosal necrosis and have been termed 'acute intestinal failure' by Marston. They are predominantly surgical emergencies and are rarely biopsied. Gradually, this melange of entities may be unravelled; it is only comparatively recently that pseudomembranous colitis has been removed from this category following the discovery of the role of C. *difficile*.

REFERENCES

Alapati, S.V., Mihas, A.A. (1999) When to suspect ischemic colitis. Why is this condition so often missed or misdiagnosed? *Postgrad. Med.*, 105, 177–80.

Alschibaja, T., Morson, B.C. (1977) Ischaemic bowel disease. *J. Clin. Pathol. (R. Coll. Pathol. Symp.)*, 30 (Suppl.), 11, 68–77.

Arnott, I.D., Ghosh, S., Ferguson, A. (1999) The spectrum of ischaemic colitis. *Eur. J. Gastroenterol. Hepatol.*, 11, 295–303.

Balthazar, E.J., Yen, B.C., Gordon, R.B. (1999) Ischemic colitis: CT evaluation of 54 cases. Radiology, 211, 381–8.

Barcewicz, P.A., Welch, J.P. (1980) Ischaemic colitis in young patients. *Dis. Col. Rectum*, 123, 109–14.

Berenguer, J., Cabades, F., Gras, M.D., Pertejo, V., Rayon, M., Sala, T. (1981) Ischemic colitis attributable to a cleansing enema. *Hepatogastroenterology*, 28, 173–5.

Bergstein, J.M., Wallace, J.R., Wittmann, D.H., Aprahamian, C. (1995) Shock-associated right colon ischemia and necrosis. *J. Trauma*, 39, 1171–4.

Beyer, K.L., Bickel, J.T., Butt, J.H. (1991) Ischemic colitis associated with dextroamphetamine use. *J. Clin. Gastroenterol.*, 13, 198–201.

Bjorck, M., Bergqvist, D., Troeng, T. (1996) Incidence and clinical presentation of bowel ischaemia after aortoiliac surgery – 2930 operations from a population-based registry in Sweden. *Eur. J. Vasc. Endovasc. Surg.*, 12, 139–44.

Binns, J.C., Isaacson, P. (1978) Age-related changes in colonic blood supply. Their relevance to ischaemic colitis. *Gut*, 19, 384–90.

Boley, S.J., Schwartz, S., Lash, J., Sternhill, V. (1963) Reversible vascular occlusion of the colon. *Surg. Gynecol. Obstet.*, 116, 53–60.

Boutros, H.H., Pautler, S., Chakrabarti, S. (1997) Cocaine-induced ischemic colitis with small-vessel thrombosis of colon and gallbladder. *J. Clin. Gastroenterol.*, 24, 49–53.

Bower, T.C. (1993) Ischemic colitis. *Surg. Clin. N. Am.*, 73, 1037–53.

Brandt, L., Boley, S., Coldberg, L., Mitsudo, S., Berman, A. (1981) Colitis in the elderly. *Am. J. Gastroenterol.*, 76, 239–45.

Brown, A.R. (1968) Diagnosis and management of non-gangrenous ischaemic colitis. *Gut*, 9, 737.

Brown, D.N., Rosenholtz, M.J., Marshall, J.B. (1994) Ischemic colitis related to cocaine abuse. *Am. J. Gastroenterol.*, 89, 1558–61.

Burt, R.W., Berenson, M.M., Samuelson, C.O., Cathey, W.J. (1983) Rheumatoid vasculitis of the colon presenting as pancolitis. *Dig. Dis. Sci.*, 28, 183–8.

Cappell, M.S. (1998) Intestinal (mesenteric) vasculopathy. II. Ischemic colitis and chronic mesenteric ischemia. *Gastroenterol. Clin. N. Am.*, 27, 827–60, vi.

Carpenter, H.A., Talley, N.J. (2000) The importance of clinicopathological correlation in the diagnosis of inflammatory conditions of the colon: histological patterns with clinical implications. *Am. J. Gastroenterol.*, 95, 878–96.

Carratu, R., Parisi, P., Agozzino, A. (1993) Segmental ischemic colitis associated with nonsteroidal antiinflammatory drugs. *J. Clin. Gastroenterol.*, 16, 31–4.

Chou, Y.H., Hsu, S.C., Wang, C.Y., Chen, C.L., How, S.W. (1989) Ischemic colitis as a cause of massive lower gastrointestinal bleeding and peritonitis. Report of five cases. *Dis. Colon Rectum*, 32, 1065–70.

Clarke, A.W., Lloyd-Mostyn, R.H., de Sadler, M.R. (1972) Ischaemic colitis in young adults. *Br. Med. J.*, 4, 70–2.

Cotton, P.B., Thomas, M.L. (1971) Ischaemic colitis and the contraceptive pill. *Br. Med. J.*, 3, 27–8.

Cremers, M.I., Oliveira, A.P., Freitas, J. (1998) Ischemic colitis as a complication of colonoscopy. *Endoscopy*, 30(4), S54.

Croft, R.J., Menon, G.P., Marston, A. (1981) Does intestinal angina exist? A critical study of obstructed visceral arteries. *Br. J. Surg.*, 68, 316–18.

Dawson, M.A., Schaefer, J.W. (1971) The clinical course of reversible ischaemic colitis – observations on the progression of sigmoidoscopic and histological changes. *Gastroenterology*, 60, 577–80.

Day, D.W., Jass, J.R., Price, A.B. *et al.* (2003) Ischaemic strictures. In: *Morson and Dawson's gastrointestinal pathology*, 4th edn. Oxford, London: Blackwell, pp. 543–4.

Deana, D.G., Dean, P.J. (1995) Reversible ischemic colitis in young women. Association with oral contraceptive use. *Am. J. Surg. Pathol.*, 19, 454–62.

Devroede, G., Vobecky, S., Massé, S., Arhan, P., Léger, C., Duguay, C., Hémond, M. (1982) Ischaemic fecal incontinence and rectal angina. *Gastroenterology*, 83, 970–80.

Dignan, C.R., Greenson, J.K. (1997) Can ischemic colitis be differentiated from *C. difficile* colitis in biopsy specimens? *Am. J. Surg. Pathol.*, 21, 706–10.

Flobert, C., Cellier, C., Berger, A. *et al.* (2000) Right colonic involvement is associated with severe forms of ischemic colitis and occurs frequently in patients with chronic renal failure requiring hemodialysis. *Am. J. Gastroenterol.*, 95, 195–8.

Gatch, W.D., Gulbertson, C.G. (1935) Circulatory disturbances caused by intestinal obstruction. *Ann. Surg.*, 102, 619.

Gramlich, T.L., Hunter, S.B. (1994) Focal polypoid ischemia of the colon: atheroemboli presenting as a colonic polyp. *Arch. Pathol. Lab. Med.*, 118, 308–9.

Greenson, J.K., Stern, R.A., Carpenter, S.L., Barnett, J.L. (1997) The clinical significance of focal active colitis. *Hum. Pathol.*, 28, 729–33.

Greenwald, D.A., Brandt, L.J. (1998) Colonic ischemia. *J. Clin. Gastroenterol.*, 27, 122–8.

Gurbuz, A.K., Gurbuz, B., Salas, L., Rosenshein, N.B., Donowitz, M., Giardiello, F.M. (1994)

Premarin-induced ischemic colitis. *J. Clin. Gastroenterol.*, 19, 108–11.

Habu, Y., Tahashi, Y., Kiyota, K., Matsumura, K., Hirota, M,. Inokuchi, H., Kawai, K. (1996) Reevaluation of clinical features of ischemic colitis. Analysis of 68 consecutive cases diagnosed by early colonoscopy. *Scand. J. Gastroenterol.*, 31, 881–6.

Heer, M., Repond, F., Hany, A., Sulser, H., Kehl, O., Jager, K. (1987) Acute ischaemic colitis in a female long distance runner. *Gut*, 28, 896–9.

Heron, H.C., Khubchandani, I.T., Trimpi, H.D., Sheets, J.A., Starik, J.J. (1981) Evanescent colitis. *Dis. Col. Rectum*, 24, 555–61.

Higgins, P.D., Davis, K.J., Laine, L. (2004) Systematic review: the epidemiology of ischaemic colitis. *Aliment. Pharmacol. Ther.*, 19, 729–38.

Ho, M.S., Teh, L.B., Goh, H.S. (1987) Ischaemic colitis in systemic lupus erythematosus – report of a case and review of the literature. *Ann. Acad. Med. Singapore*, 16, 501–3.

Hsueh, W., Gonzalez–Crussi, F., Arroyave, J.L. (1986) Platelet-activating factor-induced ischemic bowel necrosis. An investigation of secondary mediators in its pathogenesis. *Am. J. Pathol.*, 122, 231–9.

Israeli, D., Dardik, H., Wolodiger, F., Silvestri, F., Scherl, B., Chessler, R. (1996) Pelvic radiation therapy as a risk factor for ischemic colitis complicating abdominal aortic reconstruction. *J. Vasc. Surg.*, 23, 706–9.

Johnson, T.D., Berenson, M.M. (1991) Methamphetamine-induced ischemic colitis. *J. Clin. Gastroenterol.*, 13, 687–9.

Kaiserling, E., Krober, S. (1995) Massive intestinal hemorrhage associated with intestinal amyloidosis. An investigation of underlying pathologic processes. *Gen. Diagn. Pathol.*, 141, 147–54.

Kilpatrick, Z.M., Silverman, J.F., Betancourt, E., Farman, J., Lawson, J.P. (1968) Vascular occlusion of the colon and oral contraceptives. Possible relation. *N. Engl. J. Med.*, 278, 438–40.

Ko, G.Y., Ha, H.K., Lee, H.J. *et al.* (1997) Usefulness of CT in patients with ischemic colitis proximal to colonic cancer. *Am. J. Roentgenol.*, 168, 951–6.

Longo, W.E., Ward, D., Vernava, A.M. 3rd, Kaminski, D.L. (1997) Outcome of patients with total colonic ischemia. *Dis. Colon Rectum*, 40, 1448–54.

Longstreth, G.F. (1997) Epidemiology and outcome of patients hospitalized with acute lower gastrointestinal hemorrhage: a population-based study. *Am. J. Gastroenterol.*, 92, 419–24.

Ludwig, K.A., Quebbeman, E.J., Bergstein, J.M., Wallace, J.R., Wittmann, D.H., Aprahamian, C. (1995) Shock-associated right colon ischemia and necrosis. *J. Trauma*, 39, 1171–4.

McGovern, V.J., Goulston, S.J.M. (1965) Ischaemic enterocolitis. *Gut*, 6, 213–20.

Mackay, C., Murphy, P., Rosenberg, I.L., Tait, N.P. (1994) Case report: rectal infarction after abdominal aortic surgery. *Br. J. Radiol.*, 67, 497–8.

Margaretten, W., McKay, D.G. (1971) Thrombotic ulcerations of the gastrointestinal tract. *Arch. Intern. Med.*, 127, 250–3.

Markoglou, C., Avgerinos, A., Mitrakou, M., Sava, S., Prigouris, S., Hatziyoannou, J., Raptis, S. (1993) Toxic megacolon secondary to acute ischemic colitis. *Hepatogastroenterology*, 40, 188–90.

Marston, A. (1962) The bowel in shock. The role of mesenteric arterial disease as a cause of death in the elderly. *Lancet*, ii, 365–70.

Marston, A. (1972) Basic structure and function of the intestinal circulation. *Clin. Gastroenterol.*, 1, 539–46.

Marston, A. (1986) *Vascular disease of the gut.* London and Melbourne: Edward Arnold, pp. 1–15.

Marston, A., Pheils, M.T., Lea Thomas, M., Morson, B.C. (1966) Ischaemic colitis. *Gut*, 7, 1–15.

Maruyama, Y., Watanabe, F., Kanaoka, S. *et al.* (1997) A case of phlebosclerotic ischemic colitis: a distinct entity. *Endoscopy*, 29, 334.

Matson, A.P., van Kruiningen, H.J., West, A.B., Cartun, R.W., Colombel, J.F., Cortot, A. (1995) The relationship of granulomas to blood vessels in intestinal Crohn's disease. *Modern Pathol.*, 8, 680–5.

Medina, C., Vilaseca, J., Videla, S., Fabra, R., Armengol-Miro, J.R., Malagelada, J.R. (2004) Outcome of patients with ischemic colitis: review of fifty-three cases. *Dis. Colon Rectum*, 47, 180–4.

Miller, W.T., De Poto, D.W., Scholl, H.W., Rattensperger, E.C. (1971) Evanescent colitis in the young adult: a new entity? *Radiology*, 100, 71–8.

Moolenaar, W., Lamers, C.B. (1996) Cholesterol crystal embolisation to the alimentary tract. *Gut*, 38, 196–200.

Nagahata, Y., Azumi, Y., Akimoto, T., Nomura, H., Ichihara, T., Idei, H., Kuroda, Y. (1999) Role of platelet activating factor on severity of ischemic colitis. *Dis. Colon Rectum*, 42, 218–24.

Neitlich, J.D., Burrell, M.I. (1999) Drug-induced disorders of the colon. *Abdom. Imaging*, 24, 23–8.

Neves, J., Raso, P., Pinto, D.deM., da Silva, S.P., Alvarenga, R.J. (1993) Ischaemic colitis (necrotizing colitis, pseudomembranous colitis) in acute *Schistosomiasis mansoni*: report of two cases. *Trans. R. Soc. Trop. Med. Hyg.*, 87, 449–52.

Newell, A.M., Deckert, J.J. (1997) Transient ischemic colitis in young adults. *Am. Fam. Physician*, 56, 1103–8 .

O'Briain, D.S., Jeffers, M., Kay, E.W., Hourihane, D.O. (1991) Bleeding due to colorectal atheroembolism. Diagnosis by biopsy of adenomatous polyps or of ischemic ulcer. *Am. J. Surg. Pathol.*, 15, 1078–82.

Oh, J.K., Meiselman, M., Lataif, L.E. Jr. (1997) Ischemic colitis caused by oral hyperosmotic saline laxatives. *Gastrointest. Endosc.*, 45, 319–22 .

Okada, M., Konishi, F., Sakuma, K., Kanazawa, K., Koiwai, H., Kaizaki, Y. (1999) Perforation of the sigmoid colon with ischemic change due to polyarteritis nodosa. *J. Gastroenterol.*, 34, 400–4.

Parish, K.L., Chapman, W.C., Williams, L.F. Jr. (1991) Ischemic colitis. An ever-changing spectrum? *Am. Surg.*, 57, 118–21.

Patel, Y.J., Scherl, N.D., Elias, S., Chessler, R.K., Zingler, B.M. (1992) Ischemic colitis associated with psychotropic drugs. *Dig. Dis. Sci.*, 37, 1148–9.

Piotrowski, J.J., Ripepi, A.J., Yuhas, J.P., Alexander, J.J., Brandt, C.P. (1996) Colonic ischemia: the Achilles heel of ruptured aortic aneurysm repair. *Am. Surg.*, 62, 557–60.

Price, A.B. (1990) Ischaemic colitis. *Curr. Top. Pathol.*, 81, 229–46.

Reeders, J.W.A.J., Tytgat, G.N.J., Rosenbusch, G., Gratama, S. (1984) *Ischaemic colitis.* Dordrecht: Martinus Nijhoff.

Renton, C.J.C. (1972) Non-occlusive intestinal infarction. *Clin. Gastroenterol.*, 1(3), 655–74.

Robson, N.K., Khan, S.M., Rawlinson, J., Dewbury, K.C. (1992) Ischaemic colitis: clinical, radiological and pathological correlation in three cases. *Clin. Radiol.*, 46, 337–9.

Rosenblum, W.I., Budzilovick, G.N., Solomon, C. (1963) Peri-arteritis nodosa with perforation of the colon. *Am. J. Dig. Dis.*, 8, 463–71.

Sakorafas, G.H., Tsiotos, G.G. (1999) Intra-abdominal complications after cardiac surgery. *Eur. J. Surg.*, 165, 820–7.

Scholz, F.J. (1993) Ischemic bowel disease. *Radiol. Clin. N. Am.*, 31, 1197–218.

Schwartz, S.S., Boley, S.J. (1972) Ischaemic origin of ulcerative colitis associated with potentially obstructing lesions of the colon. *Radiology*, 102, 249–52.

Scowcroft, C.W., Sanowski, R.A., Kozarek, R.A. (1981) Colonoscopy in ischaemic colitis. *Gastrointest. Endosc.*, 27, 156–61.

Seow-Choen, F., Chua, T.L., Goh, H.S. (1993) Ischaemic colitis and colorectal cancer: some problems and pitfalls. *Int. J. Colorectal Dis.*, 8, 210–12.

Sharma, S., Longo, W.E., Baniadam, B., Vernava, A.M. 3rd (1995) Colorectal manifestations of endocrine disease. *Dis. Colon Rectum*, 38, 318–23.

Shoji, B.T., Becker, J.M. (1994) Colorectal disease in the elderly patient. *Surg. Clin. N. Am.*, 74, 293–316.

Storesund, B., Gran, J.T., Koldingsnes, W. (1998) Severe intestinal involvement in Wegener's granulomatosis: report of two cases and review of the literature. *Br. J. Rheumatol.*, 37, 387–90.

Swerdlow, S.H., Antonioli, D.A., Goldman, H. (1981) Intestinal infarction: a new classification. *Arch. Pathol. Lab. Med.*, 105, 218 (Letter).

Tada, H., Saitoh, S., Nakagawa, Y. *et al.* (1996) Ischemic colitis during interferon-alpha treatment for chronic active hepatitis C. *J. Gastroenterol.*, 31, 582–4.

Talbot, I.C., Kamm, M.A., Leaker, B.R. (1992) Pathogenesis of Crohn's disease. *Lancet*, 340, 315–16.

Thomson, A., Hemphill, D., Jeejeebhoy, K.N. (1998) Oxidative stress and antioxidants in intestinal disease. *Dig. Dis.*, 16, 152–8.

Toursarkissian, B., Thompson, R.W. (1997) Ischemic colitis. *Surg. Clin. N. Am.*, 77, 461–70.

Tribe, C.R., Scott, D.G.L., Bacon, P.A. (1981) Rectal biopsy in the diagnosis of systemic vasculitis. *J. Clin. Pathol.*, 34, 843–50.

Trinh, T.D., Jones, B., Fishman, E.K. (1991) Amyloidosis of the colon presenting as ischemic colitis: a case report and review of the literature. *Gastrointest. Radiol.*, 16, 133–6.

Tsang, P., Rotterdam, H. (1999) Biopsy diagnosis of colitis: possibilities and pitfalls. *Am. J. Surg. Pathol.*, 23, 423–30.

Vernava, A.M. 3rd, Moore, B.A., Longo, W.E., Johnson, F.E. (1997) Lower gastrointestinal bleeding. *Dis. Colon Rectum*, 40, 846–58.

Volk, E.E., Shapiro, B.D., Easley, K.A., Goldblum, J.R. (1998) The clinical significance of a biopsy-based diagnosis of focal active colitis: a clinicopathologic study of 31 cases. *Mod. Pathol.*, 11, 789–94.

Warren, B.F., Dankwa, E.K., Davies, J.D. (1990) 'Diamond-shaped' crypts and mucosal elastin: helpful diagnostic features in biopsies of rectal prolapse. *Histopathology*, 17, 129–34.

Wellington, J.L., Rody, K. (1993) Acute abdominal emergencies in patients on long-term ambulatory peritoneal dialysis. *Can. J. Surg.*, 36, 522–4.

Wheeldon, N.M., Grundman, M.J. (1990) Ischaemic colitis as a complication of colonoscopy. *Br. Med. J.*, 301, 1080–1.

Whitehead, R. (1971) Ischaemic enterocolitis; an expression of the intravascular coagulation syndrome. *Gut*, 12, 912–17.

Whitehead, R. (1972) The pathology of intestinal ischaemia. *Clin. Gastroenterol.*, 1. 613–37.

Whitehead, R. (1976) The pathology of ischemia of the intestines. *Pathol. Ann.*, ll, 1–52.

Yamagiwa, I., Obata, K., Hatanaka, Y., Saito, H., Washio, M. (1993) Ischemic colitis complicating severe acute pancreatitis in a child. *J. Pediatr. Gastroenterol. Nutr.*, 16, 208–11.

Yamazaki, T., Shirai, Y., Tada, T., Sasaki, M., Sakai, Y., Hatakeyama, K. (1997a) Ischemic colitis arising in watershed areas of the colonic blood supply: a report of two cases. *Surg. Today*, 27, 460–2.

Yamazaki, T., Shirai, Y., Sakai, Y., Hatakeyama, K. (1997b) Ischemic stricture of the rectosigmoid colon caused by division of the superior rectal artery below Sudeck's point during sigmoidectomy: report of a case. *Surg. Today*, 27, 254–6.

Yang, R.D., Han, M.W., McCarthy, J.H. (1991) Ischemic colitis in a crack abuser. *Dig. Dis. Sci.*, 36, 238–40.

Yasumori, R., Shibata, T., Nasu, M., Ohzono, Y., Harada, T., Hara, K. (1995) A case of nephrotic syndrome associated with ischemic colitis exhibiting thickening of the colon wall. *Nippon Jinzo Gakkai Shi*, 37, 348–52.

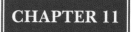

CHAPTER 11

IATROGENIC DISEASE

11.1 Radiation colitis   182
11.2 Barium granuloma   184
11.3 Oleogranuloma   184
11.4 Drug–associated colitis   185
    11.4.1 Introduction   185
    11.4.2 General features   186
    11.4.3 Biopsy clues   186
    11.4.4 Non-steroidal anti-inflammatory drugs   187
    11.4.5 Antibiotics   189
    11.4.6 Gold   190
    11.4.7 Cocaine   190
    11.4.8 Pancreatic enzyme supplements   190
11.5 Diversion proctocolitis   191
11.6 Graft-versus-host disease   192
11.7 Neutropenic colitis   194
11.8 Colitis caused by bowel preparations and instrumentation   194
11.9 Anastomotic ulceration   195
11.10 Melanosis coli and laxative abuse   195
References   196

11.1 RADIATION COLITIS

In biopsy practice the recognition of radiation damage is mainly seen as the chronic effect of the long-term complication of radiotherapy given for bladder and gynaecological cancers. The accuracy of modern equipment has meant that acute radiation injury is rarely encountered (Gelfand *et al.*, 1968), indeed the chronic picture is also becoming less common. Acute damage can still be seen in resections for rectal carcinoma in the context of short term preoperative adjuvant therapy regimens (Leupin *et al.*, 2002). This is seldom a biopsy issue but, because the epithelial damage produced can be mistaken for dysplasia, it is a potential diagnostic pitfall and receives brief coverage below.

The recognition of chronic damage is the main biopsy challenge and the changes can manifest over a wide time-scale from a few weeks to many years after therapy. This delay reflects the ischaemic basis of the damage, which remains subclinical until the sum of the radiation-induced changes and those caused by any progressive background vascular disease, such as diabetes or hypertension (DeCosse *et al.*, 1969), exceed this subclinical threshold. The damage to the large bowel usually presents with bleeding or symptoms from a developing stricture. The rectum and transverse colon are the sites most frequently affected, from exposure to irradiation of the pelvis and para-aortic lymph nodes, respectively.

The diagnostic biopsy features are related to changes in fibroblasts, vessel walls and connective tissue ground substance. Bizarre radiation fibroblasts can be recognized in the submucosa and an obliterative endarteritis in submucosal vessels is a less frequent occurrence. The background connective tissue of both mucosa and submucosa appears eosinophilic and hyaline. Telangiectatic mucosal blood vessels may be a prominent feature and often the only one seen in a small biopsy. These vessels may have thick hyaline walls, which will distinguish

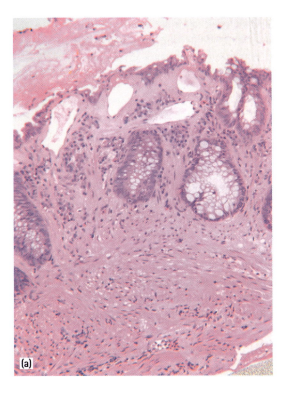

them from the thin-walled angioma-like dilated vessels of angiodysplasia (Fig. 11.1). We have seen severe haemorrhage in such a case (Taverner *et al.*, 1982).

The ischaemic pathogenesis means that some typically ischaemic characteristics (Sections 10.6.2 and 10.6.3) (Hasleton *et al.*, 1985) may also be apparent in a biopsy, features such as degeneration of the upper halves of crypts, ulceration and attempts at healing. This can lead to crypt atrophy which could be mistaken for ulcerative colitis (Fig. 11.2) were it not for the associated changes. Indeed, cases can present as ischaemia-induced emergencies (Tomori *et al.*, 1999). Other documented long-term consequences of chronic radiation are rectal carcinoma (Tamai *et al.*, 1999) and colitis cystica profunda (Gardiner *et al.*, 1984). The latter is presumably the result of abnormal healing following mucosal ischaemic breakdown. The review by Berthrong and Fajardo (1981) of the spectrum of changes to be found in radiation colitis is still useful.

The mucosal pathology of preoperative adjuvant radiotherapy given either days or a few weeks prior to surgery for rectal carcinoma is not usually a biopsy problem but, as mentioned above, epithelial features resembling dysplasia can occur with the potential to be a source of diagnostic error (Fig. 11.3). In the study by Leupin *et al.* (2002), short term preoperative irradiation resulted in severe diffuse mucosal inflammation in which eosinophils

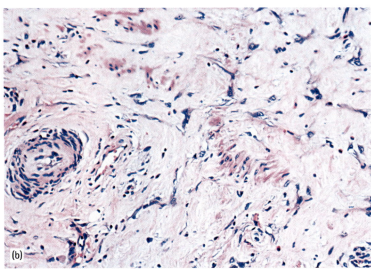

Figure 11.1 In this biopsy (a) from a case of radiation proctitis the telangiectatic blood vessels and hyalinization of the lamina propria are clearly seen beneath the surface epithelium. (b) Detail from the superficial submucosa of a similar case but showing the typical bizarre radiation fibroblasts. The small vessel included shows the characteristic hyaline thickening of the intima and wall.

were prominent. There was also crypt withering, crypt loss, dysplasia-like nuclear atypicality in cryptal epithelium and increased apoptosis. Despite these marked abnormalities the patients remained symptom free. However, should there be an indication for biopsy in such a patient cohort an awareness of this potentially misleading picture becomes important. Chronic inflammatory bowel disease, dysplasia in colitis, infection and even graft-versus-host disease might be mistakenly diagnosed if confronted with the picture but unaware of the clinical context.

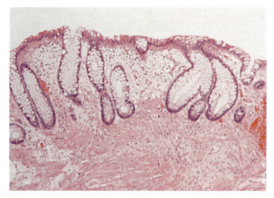

Figure 11.2 In this biopsy, taken many years after pelvic irradiation, the damage has led to crypt atrophy and distortion resulting in a picture that, without the appropriate clinical history, might be mistaken for quiescent chronic ulcerative colitis.

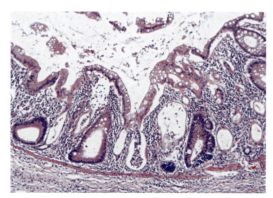

Figure 11.3 Although a biopsy is rarely indicated when preoperative radiotherapy is given, epithelial damage is a common finding and can be mistaken for dysplasia, as in this illustration.

11.2 BARIUM GRANULOMA

This can present as a hard mass at any point along the wall of the large bowel, sometimes with ulceration. It is caused by the accumulation of barium-laden histiocytes – the consequence of barium having been extruded through a defect in the mucosa (Fielding and Lumsden, 1973). This event may precede symptomatic presentation of the lesion by many years (Subramanyam *et al.*, 1988). More frequently, however, small clusters of barium-containing histiocytes are simply an incidental finding in a biopsy performed for other reasons.

However, if the biopsy has been taken because of suspicion of a tumour then sheets of large barium-containing histiocytes will be seen with unstained but highly refractile granular cytoplasm, predominantly in the submucosa (Fig. 11.4). The coarser barium particles are noticeably birefringent, but finely granular barium is less so. There will be some fibrosis. Barium can be stained by the rhodizonate method while the barium gelatine preparations, used to inject colectomy specimens in order to demonstrate vascular abnormalities, stain with an elastic–van Gieson stain (personal observation).

11.3 OLEOGRANULOMA

Biopsies are taken of oleogranulomas because, as with barium granulomas, these lesions sometimes cause a firm indurated mass with an ulcerated surface and can be clinically mistaken for carcinoma (Hernandez *et al.*, 1967). However, oleogranulomas are, unlike barium granulomas, rarely found proximal to the lower rectum.

Histologically, oleogranulomas involve the mucosa but more prominently the submucosa. They show characteristic features of irregularly arranged large, pale macrophages and multinucleate giant cells in relation to round lipid vacuoles (Fig. 11.5). Some of the lipid appears to lie in lymphatic capillaries. The lipid material is usually removed from the tissues during processing and its demonstration requires frozen section preparation. There is also an accompanying variable infiltrate of neutrophil and

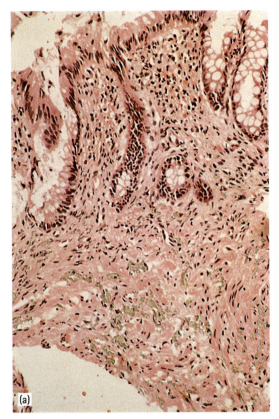

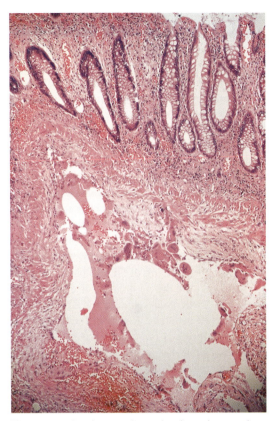

Figure 11.5 An oleogranuloma showing submucosal irregular lipid-containing vacuoles and associated giant cells.

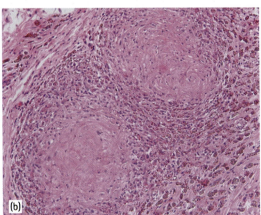

Figure 11.4 (a) The refractile barium-containing macrophages are seen in the lower mucosa and muscularis mucosae. (b) Similar macrophages in the submucosa surround burnt-out fibrotic granulomas. In this case the barium investigation responsible for the damage had been carried out many years previously.

eosinophil polymorphs, mainly in the early lesions. Lesions of long standing contain few polymorphs but are more fibrous with dense collagen fibres.

The lesions are almost always caused by a tissue reaction to injected oil used as a vehicle in the treatment of piles by sclerotherapy. Vegetable oils are the most frequently used (e.g. almond oil; Mazier *et al.*, 1978).

11.4 DRUG-ASSOCIATED COLITIS

11.4.1 Introduction

A wide range of drugs produce clinical gastro-intestinal side-effects (mainly diarrhoea, constipation, nausea and vomiting). Moreover, drugs are associated with a wide range of pathological changes from minor non-specific inflammation to typical colitides such as ischaemic colitis (Deana and Dean, 1995), microscopic colitis (Beaugerie *et al.*, 1994, 1995) and in many cases a focal colitis difficult to distinguish in biopsies from Crohn's disease or infection (Goldstein and Cinenza, 1998). Indirectly they can also be responsible for genuine infections. Can the pathologist recognize specific changes in the colorectal or terminal ileal mucosa that allows the diagnosis of such drug-induced aetiologies? This question is an important aspect of diagnostic biopsy work to prevent an erroneous diagnosis of, for example, chronic inflammatory bowel disease, for what might be a simple condition reversible following withdrawal of the offending drug. Withdrawal of a drug and resolution of the pathology, followed by recurrence of the pathology on a subsequent challenge, is the gold standard for establishing a drug-induced aetiology. However, the latter of the two requirements is rarely undertaken. Moreover, because a drug history is seldom provided the pathologist needs to be alert to the possibility of iatrogenic disease, especially if the picture is unusual and without an obvious explanation. Even the clinician may not have elicited such possibilities as so many 'over the counter' drug sales occur and patients, unaware of the concept of drug-induced disease, often do not consider such purchases as of any relevance to their illness. Two further general points are important. First is the temporal relationship between a drug and the resulting pathology: this may not be immediate but may occur after a period of days or weeks. Second, the resulting pathology may be an indirect consequence of the drug rather than one of direct toxicity. Antibiotics and immunosuppressive agents are such examples. Both these classes of drug can promote a colitis due to opportunistic infection rather than by direct toxicity.

11.4.2 General features

The endoscopist can be confronted by a wide range of appearances none of which are diagnostic, apart from the unique concentric diaphragm-like stricturing due to non-steroidal anti-inflammatory drugs (NSAIDs) (Lang *et al.*, 1988). Drugs can be responsible for ulceration, an ischaemic picture, strictures and a range of inflammatory patterns that, as a generalization, bear more resemblance to infection or Crohn's disease than ulcerative colitis. Drug therapy will modify the typical diagnostic patterns of the inflammatory colitides not only for the endoscopist but also the pathologist. The pathologist reviewing a biopsy that is accompanied by an endoscopy account of puzzling mucosal appearance, describing isolated or apparently randomly distributed ulcers should at least pause to consider iatrogenic drug-induced disease in the differential.

11.4.3 Biopsy clues

Even though it is seldom possible to conclude a biopsy report with dogmatic identification of a specific drug or drug class there are important histological markers (Lee, 1993, 1994; Price, 2003) (Fig. 11.6a–d). These, alongside any endoscopic clues, or pointers in the history, will prompt the clinician to consider such a likelihood and perhaps undertake a trial of drug withdrawal if clinically feasible.

Increased apoptosis (Lee, 1993) (Fig. 11.6a,b) epithelial vacuolation (mainly a small intestinal occurrence), focal intra-epithelial lymphocytosis (Fig. 11.6d) (Beaugerie *et al.*, 1994), eosinophils (Fig. 11.6b) (Lee, 1994; Martin *et al.*, 1981) and of course melanosis (Ghadially and Walley, 1994) are the most useful indicators. None are specific markers of drug-induced pathology. However, when present, either in the situation where the overall microscopic picture is not typical of one of the major patterns of chronic inflammatory bowel disease, or where they are striking in what otherwise seems to be a recognizable pattern of colitis, the report should mention the possibility of a drug-induced aetiology. For example, both collagenous and lymphocytic colitis have been shown to be drug-induced (Section 9.4.4) in some instances (Riddell *et al.*, 1992; Beaugerie *et al.*, 1994).

The well-documented examples of drug-associated colitis are listed in Table 11.1 and the typical picture described in the relevant chapter. This chapter is restricted to comments on certain drugs and some of the more common problems that are faced in biopsy practice.

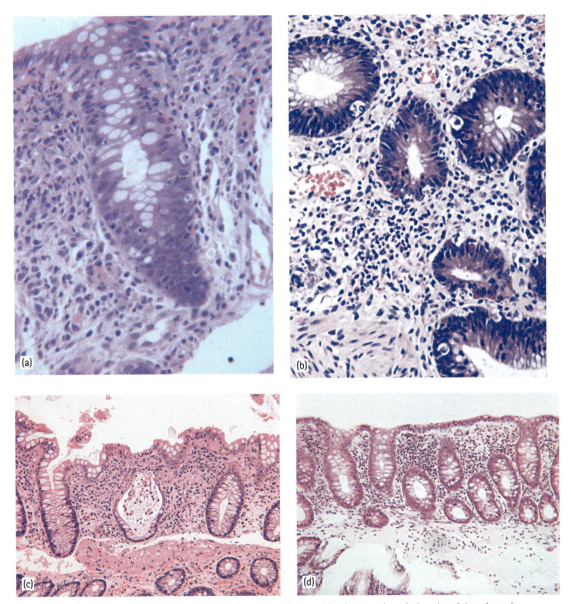

Figure 11.6 (a–d) These figures illustrate some of the clues that could point to a drug-induced aetiology in a given case of colitis. (a) From a patient on diclofenac, there is apoptosis and minor inflammation within the crypt plus a slight increase in surrounding eosinophils. (b) The apoptosis is more evident as is the inflammation. The patient had been receiving gold therapy. (c) Focal inflammation, a dilated crypt and an increase in eosinophils can be seen in this biopsy from a patient receiving non-steroidal anti-inflammatory drugs for rheumatoid arthritis. (d) The biopsy is again from a patient on diclofenac and shows mild focal inflammation in the lamina propria and a slight increase in intraepithelial lymphocytes in the crypts to the right of the picture.

11.4.4 Non-steroidal anti-inflammatory drugs

Concentric diaphragm-like stricturing is believed to be the diagnostic picture of NSAID-induced disease (Lang *et al.*, 1988). It was originally described in the small intestine and beyond the reach of a biopsy but is now well documented in the colon, especially on the right side (Bjarnason and Price, 1994; Byrne *et al.*, 2002). It is essentially

Table 11.1 Drugs or drug groups established as associated with colitis (modified from Cappell, 2004)

Ischaemic colitis (including vasculitis)	NSAIDs,* cocaine, ergotamine-containing preparations, oestrogens (with progesterone)
Microscopic colitis (collagenous and/or lymphocytic)	NSAIDs, ticlopidine, some protein pump inhibitors, some H_2 antagonists
Infectious or necrotizing enterocolitis	
Neutropenic colitis	Chemotherapeutic agents (e.g. adriamycin, 5-fluorouracil)
Pseudomembranous colitis	Antibiotics
Haemorrhagic colitis	Ampicillin, amoxicillin, erythromycin
Opportunistic infections (e.g. cytomegalovirus, adenovirus, cryptosporidiosis, *Mycobacterium avium intracellulare*)	Drugs that cause immunosuppression (e.g. steroids chemotherapy)
Yersiniosis	Deferoxamine (promotes *Yersinia* replication via its role in iron metabolism)
Mimics of chronic inflammatory bowel disease, cytotoxic or allergic colitis	NSAIDs, gold salts, α-methyldopa, sodium phosphate solution
Graft-versus-host disease	Mycophenalate mofetil
Colonic pseudo-obstruction	Narcotics, loperamide, phenothiazines, vincristine
Cathartic colon and colonic obstruction	Anthraquinones (senna, cascara)
Variable patterns and 'focal active colitis'	Glutaraldehyde, detergent enemas, herbal remedies

*NSAIDs, non-steroidal anti-inflammatory drugs.

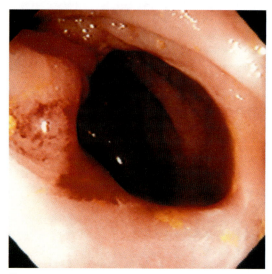

Figure 11.7 This endoscopic view of the right colon shows a diaphragm with ulceration along the rim in a patient who was receiving non-steroidal anti-inflammatory drugs.

a macroscopic endoscopic diagnosis (Fig. 11.7) as the biopsy features will reflect little more than the ulceration that is commonly seen on the crest of the haustra or the local non-specific inflammation in the immediate vicinity. There may be some submucosal fibrosis seen if the biopsy is deep enough.

Diaphragm-like strictures are rare but NSAIDs are associated with several other commoner patterns of colitis and small intestinal ulceration (Madhok *et al.*, 1986). Among these are microscopic colitis (Chapter 9), both the typical patterns of lymphocytic and collagenous (Riddell *et al.*, 1992) plus variants (Sections 9.3.6 and 12.3.2) such as a paucicellular form of lymphocytic colitis (Kitchen *et al.*, 2002; Goldstein and Bhanot, 2004) and collagenous colitis in which ulceration is observed (Kakar *et al.*, 2003). Ischaemic colitis is documented (Carratu *et al.*, 1993) and the drugs can precipitate attacks of diverticulitis (Morris *et al.*, 2003). Even when confronted with the typical features of ulcerative colitis NSAIDs need consideration for they are documented to activate quiescent disease (Kaufman and Taubin, 1987) and may even play a more general role in the pathogenesis of colitis. Thus, Tanner and Raghunath (1988) suggest NSAIDs may account for up to 10 per cent of new cases of colitis while Gleeson and Davis (2003) found a history of recent NSAID ingestion in 74 per cent of new cases of colitis compared with control group values of 30 per cent for hospital inpatients and 20 per cent for community controls attending Accident and Emergency Departments. Perhaps the commonest and most challenging picture is the one of focal inflammation and ulceration (Figs 11.6c and 11.8) that poses problems in making

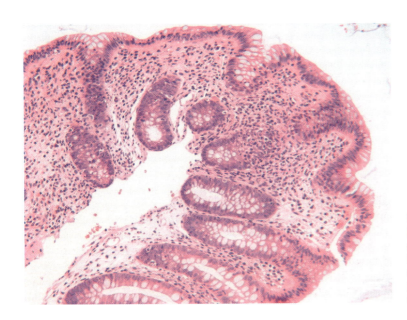

Figure 11.8 Focal inflammation in a biopsy from a patient with colitis on non-steroidal anti-inflammatory drugs which, in the absence of other pathology, is a prompt to consider a drug-induced aetiology for the colitis.

a distinction from Crohn's disease or possible infection (Goldstein and Cinenza, 1998). These authors point out that crypt branching, atrophy and crypt shortening, as in typical ulcerative colitis, are not seen, though they use the subtle term of crypt disarray as a feature. The latter is defined as some variation in crypt size and distribution. By contrast in the series of patients prescribed NSAIDs looked at by Puspok *et al.* (2000) the biopsies were thought to resemble ischaemia. Thus, the literature accounts vary and the clue will be to recognize, in the background of one of the above patterns, those pointers to drug involvement mentioned earlier (Section 11.4.3). These are combinations that involve increased eosinophils and apoptotic bodies perhaps along with focal intraepithelial lymphocytosis. If such a picture is present then the issue of NSAIDs might be raised in the report to the clinician.

As mentioned in Section 12.6.2c, aphthoid ulceration in the terminal ileum is a regular finding during colonoscopic surveillance and screening, with the majority proving to be incidental. However, NSAIDs will cause a significant number of such cases and care must be taken not to overdiagnose Crohn's disease in such situations, especially in asymptomatic patients. It is not merely oral NSAIDs that are problematic but colitis and proctitis, including anal stenosis, can occur as a complication of NSAID suppositories (D'Haens *et al.*, 1993).

11.4.5 Antibiotics

The major pathology associated with antibiotics in colorectal biopsy diagnosis is comprehensively covered in Chapter 8. The pathologist's role centres around the recognition of pseudomembranous colitis and antibiotic-associated colitis, this spectrum of morphology being a consequence of *Clostridium difficile* infection. The role of antibiotics is that of altering the bowel flora such that it becomes susceptible to colonization by *C. difficile*. In the much commoner mere 'nuisance' antibiotic-associated diarrhoea the colonic mucosa is normal, with other mechanisms being responsible for the intestinal disturbance, for example the small intestinal damage caused by neomycin toxicity (Jacobsen *et al.*, 1960).

The literature contains accounts of a haemorrhagic colitis that can occur with penicillin and its derivatives. It is unrelated to *C. difficile* (Kato *et al.*, 1995; Miller *et al.*, 1998) presenting with the sudden onset on bloody diarrhoea and abdominal pain. It is closely related to the course of therapy and self-limiting once the drug is stopped. We have not seen a case but it would seem to be rarely a biopsy problem, being predominantly right-sided with diffuse of focal mucosal haemorrhage seen at colonoscopy. The limited data on biopsies have reported corresponding haemorrhage in the lamina propria and a variable accompanying acute inflammatory cell infiltrate (Moulis and Vender, 1994; Miller *et al.*, 1998).

11.4.6 Gold

Gold salts may be used as therapy to treat intractable rheumatoid arthritis and are a rare cause of severe colitis (White and Major, 1983). Macroscopically, this can resemble ulcerative colitis, even pseudomembranous colitis (Reinhart *et al.*, 1983). On microscopy, however, the crypt architecture and goblet cell population remain intact with eosinophils being prominent (Martin *et al.*, 1981) and apoptosis (Fig. 11.6b) (Jackson *et al.*, 1986: Wong *et al.*, 1993). Accompanying opportunistic infection has been documented (Wong *et al.*, 1993) and a misleading feature can be the onset of colitis after cessation of therapy (Teodorescu *et al.*, 1993). The picture, like that for most drugs, is not specific, as exemplified by some cases being misdiagnosed as Crohn's disease (Lavy *et al.*, 1992).

11.4.7 Cocaine

Appreciation that cocaine may precipitate ischaemic colitis (Linder *et al.*, 2000) is important when confronted by ischaemic features in a biopsy from a young person in whom there is no story of cardiovascular disease and, in the case of females, no history of contraceptive pill use (Deana and Dean, 1995). The ischaemia is caused by activation of α-adrenergic receptors in the mesentery (Gourgoutis and Das, 1994) and the documentation in the literature is mainly case reports in which extensive infarction and often perforation have occurred (Brown *et al.*, 1994; Boutros *et al.*, 1997). The onset of the ischaemic damage following the drug varies from as short as 1 hour to as long as 2 days (Linder *et al.*, 2000).

11.4.8 Pancreatic enzyme supplements

High-dose enteric coated pancreatic enzyme supplements given to patients with cystic fibrosis have been found to produce a fibrosing colopathy

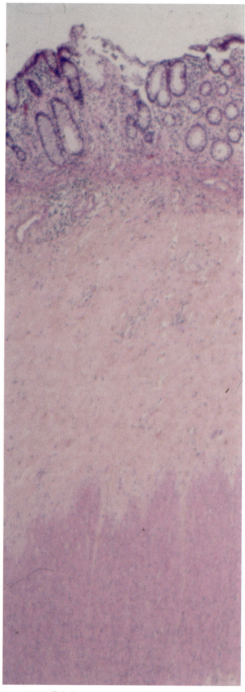

Figure 11.9 This is an example of the submucosal fibrosis that can be a complication of high-dose enteric-coated pancreatic enzyme supplements. It is from a right hemicolectomy but highlights the need for any potential diagnostic biopsy to include submucosa if such a cause was thought to be likely.

(Pawel *et al.*, 1997). The predominant pathology is one of stricturing due to fibrosis of the submucosa. As it is mainly right-sided it may be mistaken for Crohn's disease and potentially be a diagnostic problem in a colonoscopic series. The mucosa shows non-specific inflammation and eosinophils are prominent (Bansi *et al.*, 2000). A deep biopsy must be provided if the submucosal fibrosis is to be appreciated (Fig. 11.9) but the diagnosis should be self evident from the clinical history. The therapeutic change to low-dose regimens has made this an extremely rare complication.

11.5 DIVERSION PROCTOCOLITIS

Because of the misleading histological features biopsy has only a limited diagnostic role in the pathology that follows diversion of the faecal stream. The latter will usually have been undertaken for two main groups of patients. First for those with chronic inflammatory bowel disease (Crohn's disease and ulcerative colitis) in which medical treatment has failed and second, those in which there is no background inflammatory disease but diversion has become a necessary part of the management of that condition. This may apply on occasions to diverticular disease, Hirschsprung's disease or an obstructing carcinoma. The prediversion condition has a major effect on the outcome in the diverted segment and therefore on how a biopsy needs to be interpreted (Warren and Shepherd, 1992; Edwards *et al.*, 1999). The aetiology of diversion changes is considered a consequence of an alteration in the luminal flora with a resulting lack of butyrate production (Harig *et al.*, 1989), this being a fatty acid trophic to the colorectal mucosa. The abnormalities can become apparent within 3 months of diversion surgery (Roe *et al.*, 1993).

There are two basic patterns of pathology. The first is invariable and deemed the chronic diversion reaction by Haque *et al.* (1993). The second is an additional acute inflammatory component the severity of which, by contrast, is highly variable. The diversion reaction, easily appreciated in a biopsy, comprises lymphoid hyperplasia (Yeong *et al.*,

1991), which accounts for the nodular appearance of the rectal mucosa, together with focal overlying erosions (Lusk *et al.*, 1984). There is also an increase in the lamina propria of chronic inflammatory cells, mainly lymphocytes and plasma cells with some macrophages (Roe *et al.*, 1993). Acute inflammation is minimal. The crypt architecture tends to remain intact other than minor misalignment caused by the lymphoid hyperplasia in the mucosa. This is the characteristic picture seen in biopsy material from diverted bowel in which there has been no preexisting chronic inflammatory bowel disease.

The term diversion proctocolitis, as used by Haque *et al.* (1993), in contrast to the chronic diversion reaction, refers to the above picture on which the presence of acute inflammation is superimposed (Fig. 11.10). This can be of variable severity from focal infiltration by neutrophil polymorphs in the lamina propria and in scattered crypts to florid ulceration, extensive cryptitis and crypt abscess formation. Significant crypt architectural distortion with crypt branching and atrophy usually only accompanies cases in which there has been preexisting ulcerative colitis. Its degree will reflect the pre-existing damage to the rectum (Warren and Shepherd, 1992; Roe *et al.*, 1993). In such cases it is not possible to state with certainty how much of the acute inflammation is purely a complication of the diversion and how much an exacerbation of the background inflammatory bowel disease (Geraghty and Talbot, 1991). As already mentioned, the prediversion disease has significant bearing on the picture. In a diverted segment undertaken for Crohn's disease the acute inflammation subsides with only the chronic diversion reaction remaining (Harper *et al.*, 1985), plus a degree of fibrosis. In ulcerative colitis, however, the diversion often exacerbates the inflammatory process. There is one interesting study suggesting that diversion proctocolitis may even predispose to the onset of ulcerative colitis in previously normal on-stream bowel (Lim *et al.*, 1999).

An important principle in the interpretation of diversion pathology, be it of a biopsy or an excised diverted rectum, is not to change the disease classification on the basis of the diversion histological appearances. Always review the original operative specimen on which the diagnosis was made. This is because studies on the diverted rectum have

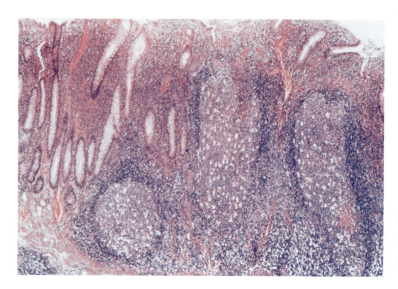

Figure 11.10 This biopsy shows the diversion reaction manifest by the follicular hyperplasia to the right and a superimposed colitis evident to the left of the illustration.

shown features that mimic Crohn's disease even when the original excision was for typical ulcerative colitis (Warren *et al.*, 1993). Thus, there can be transmural inflammation, fissuring ulceration and granuloma formation. Granuloma formation is usually related to damaged crypts or suture material and previous surgical manipulation.

Overall, the diagnostic value of biopsy in a diverted segment is largely restricted to comments on the severity or otherwise of the acute inflammation present. This is generally for immediate management purposes rather than for any primary diagnostic role.

11.6 GRAFT-VERSUS-HOST DISEASE

For organ or bone marrow transplantation, recipients are usually immunosuppressed with a combination of total body irradiation and chemotherapeutic agents, such as cyclophosphamide. In this situation immunocompetent T-cells of the graft can recognize major histocompatibility complex antigens on the surface of the suppressed host cells with resulting graft-versus-host disease. The three main organs involved are the skin, liver and gastrointestinal tract. The disease has an acute phase generally commencing within 50 days (McDonald

et al., 1986a) and a chronic phase, appearing after 100 days. In the latter there has usually been a history of acute graft-versus-host disease but in about 20–30 per cent of cases the chronic phase may occur *de novo* (McDonald *et al.*, 1986b). Biopsy is most useful in the acute stage and rectal biopsy has a high diagnostic yield (Sale *et al.*, 1979; McDonald *et al.*, 1986a), although some studies have found gastric biopsies to be the single most useful site (Cox *et al.*, 1994). Roy *et al.* (1991) found 18 per cent of their cases had upper gastrointestinal disease only.

In colorectal biopsies the cardinal histological feature of graft-versus-host disease is the finding of either single crypt cell necrosis (apoptosis) (Fig. 11.11a) or as small groups and termed the 'exploding crypt lesion' (Sale *et al.*, 1979; Snover, 1990; Shidham *et al.*, 2003). While apoptotic foci are not pathognomonic of graft-versus-host disease and are seen, for example, in radiation damage, cytomegalovirus infection, acquired immunedeficiency syndrome (AIDS), drug-induced colitis and even chronic inflammatory bowel disease, their presence as a prominent feature in the context of otherwise very muted inflammatory parameters is highly suggestive of the condition. There is an accompanying mild increase in chronic inflammatory cells, especially as focal periglandular infiltrates (Bombi *et al.*, 1995) and small numbers

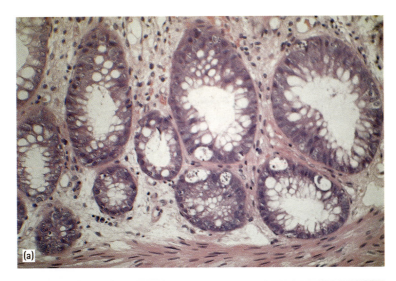

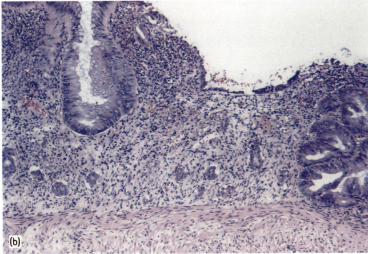

Figure 11.11 (a) There is florid single-cell cryptal apoptosis characteristic of the graft-versus-host reaction, but this is not in itself diagnostic (cf. Fig. 11.6b). Another characteristic of the graft-versus-host reaction is seen in (b) where there is crypt loss but the neuroendocrine cells in the base of the crypts survive.

of eosinophils are present. Some crypt disarray, an increase in muciphages, focal fibrosis and an increase in the microvessel network were also shown to be features of acute graft-versus-host disease. However, in the study of Shidham *et al.* (2003) cryptitis and crypt abscess formation were not significantly increased over their control groups. Especially striking, as mentioned above, is that the cryptal damage and apoptosis are out of proportion to any other accompanying changes. This is a useful distinguishing feature in the differential diagnosis with chronic inflammatory bowel disease (Crohn's disease and ulcerative colitis). When cryptal damage is severe their only remaining

remnants may be clusters of neuroendocrine cells deep in the mucosa (Lampert *et al.*, 1985) (Fig. 11.11b). On occasions severe ulceration and denudation of the mucosa occurs but the diagnosis can only be made from intact mucosa and any biopsy should be directed at the least affected areas. Because the crypt lesions can be focal it is good policy to examine levels if the diagnosis is suspected. Changes caused by cytomegalovirus, a common opportunistic infection in immunosuppressed patients, can mimic graft-versus-host disease (Snover, 1985) and needs careful exclusion (Sale *et al.*, 1979).

Before making the diagnosis it is most important to know the precise date of the transplant in relation to when the biopsy was taken. This is because the pretransplant conditioning regimens cause mucosal damage almost indistinguishable from graft-versus-host disease. However, most studies show this has resolved by about 20 days (Epstein *et al.*, 1980; Iqbal *et al.*, 2000). Thus, a diagnosis of graft-versus-host disease should be confidently made only after this 20-day period has elapsed. Prior to this the value of biopsy is limited to determining if infection is present or not (Snover, 1990).

Chronic graft-versus-host disease is seldom a colorectal biopsy problem and, contrary to acute graft-versus-host disease, the oesophagus is characteristically involved, with submucosal fibrosis being a prominent feature (Shulman *et al.*, 1980). In the large bowel the picture seen is one dominated by gland distortion and atrophy which mimics chronic quiescent atrophic ulcerative colitis (Asplund and Gramlich, 1998). There is also focal fibrosis of the lamina propria which would be an unusual feature in ulcerative colitis.

11.7 NEUTROPENIC COLITIS

This is a fulminant necrotizing and ulcerating inflammatory condition predominantly of the caecum, ascending colon and terminal ileum, which initially clinically resembles appendicitis with abdominal pain and fever. There may be more extensive colonic involvement (Kulaylat *et al.*, 1997; Tokar *et al.*, 2003). It occurs in patients with a low granulocyte count in the peripheral blood (Kies *et al.*, 1979), whether caused by treated leukaemia (King *et al.*, 1984), idiopathic neutropenia (Hopkins and Kushner, 1983), aplastic anaemia (Mulholland and Delany, 1983) or drug-induced agranulocytosis (Braye *et al.*, 1982). King *et al.* (1984) demonstrated, by immunofluorescence, *Clostridium septicum* bacilli invading the mucosa and submucosa and suggested that the condition is a specific opportunistic infection by this organism but other Clostridia may be involved (Newbold *et al.*, 1987).

Most of the documented cases have been diagnosed either at autopsy or at laparotomy and, since the left side of the colon is not usually affected, biopsy plays little part in the diagnosis. Moreover, the state of the colon renders colonoscopy and biopsy a hazardous procedure (Tokar *et al.*, 2003). The histological features are those of mucosal and submucosal oedema with focal or confluent necrosis. There is only a scanty mononuclear cell inflammatory cell infiltrate and a paucity of neutrophils. Vascular thrombi and Gram-positive organisms are common findings (Tokar *et al.*, 2003). The features can closely resemble ischaemia and pseudomembranous colitis.

The disease carries a high mortality but some authors are now advocating early surgery to improve the outcome (Bavaro, 2002; Tokar *et al.*, 2003; Cunningham *et al.*, 2005).

11.8 COLITIS CAUSED BY BOWEL PREPARATIONS AND INSTRUMENTATION

Certain preparatory enemas and colonoscopy cleansing agents can cause limited mucosal histological abnormalities that might be misinterpreted in a biopsy resulting in an overdiagnosis of early chronic inflammatory bowel disease (Meisel *et al.*, 1977).

Hypertonic enemas, such as sodium phosphate, are documented as associated with aphthoid ulceration and minor inflammatory changes that include focal cryptitis (Zwas *et al.*, 1996; Driman and Preiksaitis, 1998; Wong *et al.*, 2000; Watts *et al.*, 2002). From our own experience we suspect that the various preparatory regimens, or vigorous instrumentation, are likely to be responsible for the finding of occasional intraepithelial inflammatory cells, both acute and chronic, in otherwise normal colonoscopic series and for which there is no other explanation. Leriche *et al.* (1978), in a prospective study of rectal biopsies from volunteers given hypertonic enemas, found, as part of the enema reaction, mucus depletion in 90 per cent, mucosal oedema in 88 per cent, extruded mucus in 70 per cent and free red blood cells in the lamina propria in 39 per cent of their volunteer cohort.

A more florid colitis is produced by contamination from instrument cleansing agents such as glutaraldehyde and hydrogen peroxide. This is believed to be the consequence of inadequate washing of the colonoscope following cleaning but prior to any subsequent use. The colitis caused by glutaraldehyde usually presents with tenesmus, frequency and bloody diarrhoea within 12–24 hours of the colonoscopic procedure and the biopsy features have been shown to resemble ischaemic damage (West *et al.*, 1995; Caprilli *et al.*, 1998; Stein *et al.*, 2001). The presence of residual hydrogen peroxide can produce blanching of the mucosal surface (Jonas *et al.*, 1988; Bilotta and Waye, 1989) and even mimic pseudomembranous colitis macroscopically, while gas and air leaking into the lamina propria has been put forward as a possible explanation for the picture of mucosal pseudolipomatosis (Ryan and Potter, 1995; Gagliardi *et al.*, 1996).

11.9 ANASTOMOTIC ULCERATION

A small, regular and frustrating number of biopsies are received from patients during the course of long-term surveillance of anastomotic sites at which ulceration has been identified by the colonoscopist and in whom there may be an associated iron-deficiency anaemia. The preceding resections can have been for a variety of conditions but predominantly tumours, the management of inflammatory

bowel disease or necrotizing enterocolitis in children. The findings are mostly of ulcer slough and accompanying inflamed granulation tissue, leaving the slight anxiety that, depending on the original diagnosis, tumour or recurrent inflammatory bowel disease is being missed. Clearly, these possibilities must be carefully excluded but there is a group in whom no explanation can be found. The aetiology remains speculative but ischaemic damage on a mechanical basis from previous surgical disruption of the local blood supply would seem the most likely cause (Sondheimer *et al.*, 1995; Chari and Keate, 2000).

11.10 MELANOSIS COLI AND LAXATIVE ABUSE

When florid, the granular brown pigment in clusters of macrophages, typical of melanosis coli, is easily seen (Figs 11.12 and 3.38) but, where only single scattered macrophages contain the pigment, it is easily overlooked. The pigmented cells towards the luminal aspect of the mucosa are generally of pale golden brown colour, whereas in the base of the lamina propria the pigment is sometimes a dirty greyish colour. There is frequently increased cellularity of the lamina propria, with a mild excess

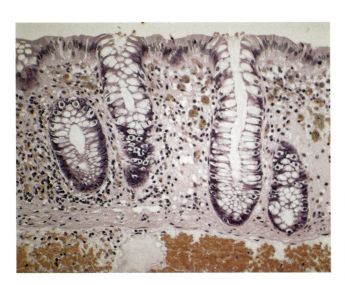

Figure 11.12 A rectal biopsy in which melanosis coli is present. The pigment containing macrophages are clearly seen though, in this example, there is no increase in other inflammatory components in the lamina propria. (Haematoxylin and eosin.)

of lymphocytes, plasma cells and prominent eosinophils. It is likely that this is caused by mild concurrent obstructive colitis (Section 13.6.2). Melanosis coli is commonly associated with the use of anthranoid laxatives, though they are not a prerequisite since it has been observed in ulcerative colitis and Crohn's disease patients with no history of a laxative intake (Pardi et al., 1998). When present there is increased epithelial apoptosis (Benavides et al., 1997) and Byers et al. (1997) suggest that the pigment is an end product of this or a related and degenerative process. It has been documented to appear within 10 months of starting the appropriate laxatives and, following their withdrawal, has resolved within a year (Willems et al., 2003). A striking effect seen by the endoscopist and pathologist, manifest as speckled pale areas down the colonoscope, is because the lamina propria of polyps remains free of pigment containing macrophages despite obvious melanosis of the surrounding mucosa. The explanation for this is unclear.

The pigment is autofluorescent, sudanophilic, acid-fast and stains with the periodic acid–Schiff (PAS) and Schmorl's reaction. Argentaffin positivity is abolished by bleaching, hence the resemblance to melanin. It is, however, lipofuscin and the residual material derived from organelles sequestrated and digested in autolysosomes (Ghadially and Walley, 1994). It should not be mistaken for iron pigment that can be seen as a manifestation of ischaemic colitis; a Perl's stain will make this distinction.

There is a recognized cohort of patients who are laxative abusers with the potential to cause considerable diagnostic problems before the correct diagnosis is made. Biopsy may show melanosis coli, be normal or show minor degrees of inflammation best considered under the umbrella term of focal active colitis (Greenson et al., 1997; Volk et al., 1998). Indeed the term 'microscopic colitis' was originally coined to refer to such minor abnormalities found in a series of patients complaining of diarrhoea but with a normal colonoscopy in whom laxative abuse was eventually uncovered (Read et al., 1980).

Cathartic colon, a condition believed to be caused by neuronal damage of the colonic autonomic nerves and ganglia from laxative abuse seems no longer to be a clinical problem, presumably owing to changing and less damaging laxative preparations (Muller-Lissner, 1996). Podophyllin-containing compounds may have been responsible.

The brown bowel syndrome (Horn et al., 1990) in which lipofuscin pigment is found in the muscularis propria, is believed related to vitamin E deficiency and is not a biopsy problem.

REFERENCES

Asplund, S., Gramlich, T.L. (1998) Chronic mucosal changes in the colon in graft-versus-host disease. *Mod. Pathol.*, 11, 513–15.

Bansi, D.S., Price, A., Russell, C., Sarner, M. (2000) Fibrosing colopathy in an adult owing to over use of pancreatic enzyme supplements. *Gut*, 46, 283–5.

Bavaro, M.F. (2002) Neutropenic enterocolitis. *Curr. Gastroenterol. Rep.*, 4, 297–301.

Beaugerie, L., Luboinski, J., Brousse, N., Cosnes, J., Chatelet, J-P., Gendre, J.P., Le Quintrec, Y. (1994) Drug induced lymphocytic colitis. *Gut*, 35, 426–42.

Beaugerie, L., Patey, N., Brousse, N. (1995) Ranitidine, diarrhoea and lymphocytic colitis. *Gut*, 37, 708–11.

Benavides, S.H., Morgante, P.E., Monserrat, A.J., Zarate, J., Porta, E.A. (1997) The pigment of melanosis coli: a lectin histochemical study. *Gastrointest. Endosc.*, 46, 131–8.

Berthrong, M., Fajardo, L.F. (1981) Radiation injury in surgical pathology. Part II, Alimentary tract. *Am. J. Surg. Pathol.*, 5, 153–78.

Bilotta, J.J., Waye, J.D. (1989) Hydrogen peroxide enteritis: the 'snow white' sign. *Gastrointest. Endosc.*, 35, 428–30.

Bjarnason, I., Price, A.B. (1994) The small and large intestinal pathologies of non-steroidal anti-inflammatory drugs. *Ann. Pathol.*, 14, 326–32.

Bombi, J.A., Nadal, A., Carreras, E., Ramirez, J., Munoz, J., Rozman, C., Cardesa, A. (1995) Assessment of histopathologic changes in the colon biopsies in acute graft-versus-host disease. *Am. J. Clin. Pathol.*, 103, 690–5.

Boutros, H.H., Pautler, S., Chakrabarti, S. (1997) Cocaine-induced ischaemic colitis with small-vessel thrombosis of colon and gallbladder. *J. Clin. Gastroenterol.*, 24, 49–53.

Braye, S.G., Coppplestone, J.A., Gartell, P.C. (1982) Neutropenic enterocolitis during mianserin-induced agranulocytosis. *Br. Med. J.*, 285, 1117.

Brown, D.N., Rosenholtz, M.J., Marshall, J.B. (1994) Ischaemic colitis related to cocaine abuse. *Am. J. Gastroenterol.*, 89, 1558–61.

Byers, R.J., Marsh, P., Parkinson, D., Haboubi, N.Y. (1997) Melanosis coli in association with an increase in colonic epithelial apoptosis and not with laxative abuse. *Histopathology*, 30, 160–4.

Byrne, M.F., McGuiness, J., Smyth, C.M. *et al.* (2002) Nonsteroidal anti-inflammatory drug-induced diaphragms and ulceration in the colon. *Eur. J. Gastroenterol. Hepatol.*, 14, 1265–9.

Cappell, M.S. (2004) Colonic toxicity of administered drugs and chemicals. *Am. J. Gastroenterol.*, 99, 1175–90.

Caprilli, R., Viscido, A., Frieri, G., Latella, G. (1998) Acute colitis following colonoscopy. *Endoscopy*, 30, 428–31.

Carratu, R., Parisi, P., Agozzino, A. (1993) Segmental ischaemia associated with nonsteroidal antiinflammatory drugs. *J. Clin. Gastroenterol.*, 16, 31–4.

Chari, S.T., Keate, R.F. (2000) Ileocolonic anastomotic ulcers: a case series and review of the literature. *Am. J. Gastroenterol.*, 95, 1239–43.

Cox, G.J., Matsui, S.M., Lo, R.S. *et al.* (1994) Etiology and outcome of diarrhoea after marrow transplantation: a prospective study. *Gastroenterology*, 107, 1398–407.

Cunningham, S.C., Fakhry, K., Bass, B.L., Napolitano, L.M. (2005) Neutropenic enterocolitis in adults: case series and review of the literature. *Dig. Dis. Sci.*, 50, 215–20.

Deana, D.G., Dean, P.J. (1995) Reversible ischaemic colitis in young women. Association with oral contraceptive use. *Am. J. Surg. Pathol.*, 19, 454–62.

DeCosse, J.J., Rhodes, R.S., Wentz, W.B., Reagan, J.W., Dwfrken, H.J., Holden, W.D. (1969) The natural history and management of radiation induced injury of the gastrointestinal tract. *Ann. Surg.*, 170, 369–84.

D'Haens, G., Breysem, Y., Rutgeerts, P., van Besien, B., Geboes, K., Ponette, E., Vantrappen, G. (1993) Proctitis and rectal stenosis induced by nonsteroidal antiinflammatory suppositories. *J. Clin. Gastroenterol.*, 17, 207–12.

Driman, D.K., Preiksaitis, H.G. (1998) Colorectal inflammation and increased cell proliferation associated with sodium phosphate bowel preparation solution. *Hum. Pathol.*, 29, 972–8.

Edwards, C.M., George, B., Warren, B.F. (1999) Diversion colitis – new light through old windows. *Histopathology*, 34, 1–5.

Epstein, R.J., McDonald, G.B., Sale, G.E., Shulman, H.M., Thomas, E.D. (1980) The diagnostic accuracy of the rectal biopsy in acute graft-versus-host disease: a prospective study of thirteen patients. *Gastroenterology*, 78, 764–71.

Fielding, J.F., Lumsden, K. (1973) Large bowel perforations in patients undergoing sigmoidoscopy and barium enema. *Br. Med. J.*, 1, 471–3.

Gagliardi, G., Thompson, I.W., Hershman, M.J., Forbes, A., Hawley, P.R., Talbot, I.C. (1996) Pneumatosis coli: a proposed pathogenesis based on study of 25 cases and review of the literature. *Int. J. Colorectal Dis.*, 11, 111–18.

Gardiner, G.W., McAuliffe, W., Murray, D. (1984) Colitis cystica profunda occurring in radiation induced colonic stricture. *Hum. Pathol.*, 15, 295–7.

Gelfand, M.D., Tepper, M., Katz, L.A., Binder, H.J., Yesner, R., Floch, M.H. (1968) Acute irradiation proctitis in man. Development of eosinophilic abscesses. *Gastroenterology*, 54, 401–11.

Geraghty, J.M., Talbot, I.C. (1991) Diversion colitis: histological features in the colon and rectum after defunctioning colostomy. *Gut*, 32, 1020–3.

Ghadially, F.N., Walley, V.M. (1994) Melanosis of the gastrointestinal tract. *Histopathology*, 25, 197–207.

Gleeson, M.H., Davis, A.J. (2003) Non-steroidal anti-inflammatory drugs, aspirin and newly diagnosed colitis: a case control study. *Aliment. Pharmacol. Ther.*, 17, 817–25.

Goldstein, N.S., Bhanot, P. (2004) Paucicellular and asymptomatic lymphocytic colitis: expanding the clinicopathologic spectrum of lymphocytic colitis. *Am. J. Clin. Pathol.*, 122, 405–11.

Goldstein, N.S., Cinenza, A.N. (1998) The histopathology of nonsteroidal anti-inflammatory drug–associatred colitis. *Am. J. Clin. Pathol.*, 110, 622–9.

Gourgoutis, G., Das, G. (1994) Gastrointestinal manifestations of cocaine addiction. *Int. J. Clin. Pharmacol. Ther.*, 32, 136–41.

Greenson, J.K., Stern, R.A., Carpenter, S.L., Barnett, J.L. (1997) The clinical significance of focal active colitis. *Hum. Pathol.*, 28, 729–33.

Haque, S., Eisen, R.N., West, A.B. (1993) The morphologic features of diversion colitis: studies of a pediatric population with no other disease of the intestinal mucosa. *Hum. Pathol.*, 24, 211–19.

Harig, J.M., Soergel, K.H., Komorowski, R.A., Wood, C.M. (1989) Treatment of diversion colitis with short chain fatty acid irrigation. *N. Engl. J. Med.*, 320, 23–8.

Harper, P.H., Lee, E.C., Kettlewell, M.G., Bennett, M.K., Jewell, D.P. (1985) Role of the faecal stream in the maintenance of Crohn's colitis. *Gut*, 26, 279–84.

Hasleton, P.S., Carr, N., Schofield, P.F. (1985) Vascular changes in radiation bowel disease. *Histopathology*, 9, 517–34.

Hernandez, V., Hernandez, I.A., Berthrong, M. (1967) Oleogranuloma simulating carcinoma of the rectum. *Dis. Col. Rectum*, 10, 205.

Hopkins, D.G., Kushner, J.P. (1983) Clostridial species in the pathogenesis of necrotizing enterocolitis in patients with neutropenia. *Am. J. Hematol.*, 14, 289–94.

Horn, T., Svendsen, L.B., Nielsen, R. (1990) Brown bowel syndrome. Review of the literature and presentation of cases. *Scand. J. Gastroenterol.*, 25, 66–72.

Iqbal, N., Salzman, D., Lazenby, A.J., Wilcox, C.M. (2000) Diagnosis of gastrointestinal graft-versus-host disease. *Am. J. Gastroenterol.*, 95, 3034–8.

Jackson, C.W., Haboubi, N.Y., Whorwell, P.J., Schofield, P.F. (1986) Gold induced enterocolitis. *Gut*, 27, 452–6.

Jacobsen, E.D., Priot, J.T., Faloo, W.W. (1960) Malabsorptive syndrome induced by neomycin toxicity. *J. Clin. Lab. Med.*, 56, 245–50.

Jonas, G., Mahoney, A., Murray, J., Gertler, S. (1988) Chemical colitis due to endoscope cleaning solutions: a mimic of pseudomembranous colitis. *Gastroenterology*, 95, 1403–8.

Kakar, S., Pardi, D.S., Burgart, L.J. (2003) Colonic ulcers accompanying collagenous colitis: implications of non-steroidal anti-inflammatory drugs. *Am. J. Gastroenterol.*, 98, 1834–7.

Kaufman, H.J., Taubin, H.L. (1987) Nonsteroidal anti-inflammatory drugs activate quiescent inflammatory bowel disease. *Ann. Intern. Med.*, 107, 513–16.

Kato, S., Ebina, K., Ozawa, A., Naganuma, H., Nakagawa, H. (1995) Antibiotic-associated haemorrhagic colitis without *Clostridium difficile* toxin in children. *J. Pediatr.*, 126, 1008–10.

Kies, M.S., Luedke, D.W., Boyd, J.F., McCue, M.J. (1979) Neutropenic enterocolitis. *Cancer*, 43, 730–4.

King, A., Rampling, A., Wight, D.G.D., Warren, R.E. (1984) Neutropenic enterocolitis due to *Clostridium septicum* infection. *J. Clin. Pathol.*, 37, 335–43.

Kitchen, P.A., Levi, A.J., Domizio, P., Talbot, I.C., Forbes, A., Price, A.B. (2002) Microscopic colitis; the tip of the iceberg? *Eur. J. Gastroenterol. Hepatol.*, 14, 1199–204.

Kulaylat, M., Doerr, R., Ambrus, J. (1997) A case presentation and review of neutropenic enterocolitis. *J. Med.*, 28, 1–19.

Lampert, I.A., Thorpe, P., van Noorden, S., Marsh, J., Goldman, J.M., Gordon-Smith, E.C., Evans, D.J. (1985) Selective sparing of enterochromaffin cells in graft versus host disease affecting the colonic mucosa. *Histopathology*, 9, 875–86.

Lang, J., Price, A.B., Levi, A.J., Burke, M., Gumpel, J.M., Bjarnason, I. (1988) Diaphragm disease: pathology of disease of the small intestine induced by non-steroidal anti-inflammatory drugs. *J. Clin. Pathol.*, 41, 516–26.

Lavy, A., Militianu, D., Eidelman, S. (1992) Diseases of the intestine mimicking Crohn's disease. *J. Clin. Gastroenterol.*, 15, 17–23.

Lee, F.D. (1993) Importance of apoptosis in the histopathology of drug related lesions of the large intestine. *J. Clin. Pathol.*, 46, 118–22.

Lee, F.D. (1994) Drug related lesions of the intestinal tract. *Histopathology*, 24, 303–8.

Leriche, M., Devroede, G., Sanchez, G., Rossano, J. (1978) Changes in the rectal mucosa induced by hypertonic enemas. *Dis. Colon Rectum*, 21, 227–36.

Leupin, N., Curschmann, J., Kranzbuhler, H., Maurer, C.A., Laissue, J.A., Mazzucchelli, I. (2002) Acute radiation colitis in patients treated with short-term preoperative radiotherapy for rectal cancer. *Am. J. Surg. Pathol.*, 26, 498–504.

Lim, A.G., Langmead, F.I., Feakins, R.M., Rampton, D.S. (1999) Diversion colitis: a trigger for ulcerative colitis in the in-stream colon. *Gut*, 44, 279–82.

Linder, J.D., Monkemuller, K.E., Raijman, I., Johnson, L., Wilcox, C.M. (2000) Cocaine-associated ischaemic colitis. *South. Med. J.*, 93, 909–13.

Lusk, L.B., Reichen, J., Levine, J.S. (1984) Aphthous ulceration in diversion colitis. Clinical implications. *Gastroenterology*, 1171–3.

Madhok, R., Mackenzie, J.A., Lee, F.D., Bruckner, F.E., Terry, T.R., Sturrock, R.D. (1986) Small bowel ulceration in patients receiving non-steroidal anti-inflammatory drugs for rheumatoid arthritis. *Q. J. Med.*, 58, 53–8.

Martin, D.M., Goldman, J.A., Gilliam, J., Nasrallah, S.M. (1981) Gold-induced eosinophilic enterocolitis: response to oral cromolyn sodium. *Gastroenterology*, 80, 1567–70.

Mazier, W.P., Sun, K.M., Robertson, W.G. (1978) Oil-induced granuloma (eleoma) of the rectum: report of four cases. *Dis. Col. Rectum*, 21, 292–4.

McDonald, G.B., Shulman, H.M., Sullivan, K.M., Spencer, G.D. (1986a) Intestinal and hepatic complications of human bone marrow transplantation. Part 1. *Gastroenterology*, 90, 460–77.

McDonald, G.B., Shulman, H.M., Sullivan, K.M., Spencer, G.D. (1986b) Intestinal and hepatic complications of human bone marrow transplantation. Part II. *Gastroenterology*, 90, 770–84.

Meisel, J.L., Bergman, D., Graney, D., Saunders, D.R., Rubin, C.E. (1977) Human rectal mucosa: proctoscopic and morphological changes caused by laxatives. *Gastroenterology*, 72, 1274–9.

Miller, A.M., Bassett, M.L., Dahlstrom, J.E., Doe, W.F. (1998) Antibiotic-associated haemorrhagic colitis. *J. Gastroenterol. Hepatol.*, 13, 115–18.

Morris, C.R., Harvey, I.M., Stebbings, W.S., Speakman, C.T., Kennedy, H.J., Hart, A.R. (2003) Anti-inflammatory drugs, analgesics and the risk of perforated diverticular disease. *Br. J. Surg.*, 90, 1267–72.

Moulis, H., Vender, R.J. (1994) Antibiotic-associated haemorrhagic colitis. *J. Clin. Gastroenterol.*, 18, 227–31.

Mulholland, M.W., Delaney, J.P. (1983) Neutropenic colitis and aplastic anaemia. *Ann. Surg.*, 197, 84–90.

Muller-Lissner, S. (1996) What has happened to cathartic colon. *Gut*, 39, 486–8.

Newbold, K.M., Lord, M.G., Baglin, T.P. (1987) Role of clostridial organisms in neutropenic enterocolitis. *J. Clin. Pathol.*, 40, 471.

Pardi, D.S., Tremaine, W.J., Rothenberg, H.J., Batts, K.P. (1998) Melanosis coli in inflammatory bowel disease. *J. Clin. Gastroenterol.*, 26, 167–70.

Pawel, B.R., de Chaderavian, J.P., Franco, M.E. (1997) The pathology of fibrosing colopathy of cystic fibrosis: a study of 12 cases and review of the literature. *Hum. Pathol.*, 28, 395–9.

Price, A.B. (2003) Pathology of drug-associated gastrointestinal disease. *Br. J. Clin. Pharmacol.*, 56. 477–82.

Puspok, A., Kiener, H.P., Oberhuber, G. (2000) Clinical, endoscopic and histologic spectrum of nonsteroidal anti-inflammatory drug-induced lesions in the colon. *Dis. Colon Rectum*, 43, 685–91.

Read, N.W., Krejs, G.J., Read, M.G., Santa Ana, C.A., Morawski, S.G., Fordtran, J.S. (1980) Chronic diarrhoea of unknown origin. *Gastroenterology*, 78, 264–71.

Reinhart, W.H., Kapppeler, M., Halter, F. (1983) Severe pseudomembranous colitis and ulcerative colitis during gold therapy. *Endoscopy*, 17, 70–1.

Riddell, R.H., Tanaka, M., Mazzoleni, G. (1992) Non-steroidal anti-inflammatory drugs as a possible cause of collagenous colitis: a case control study. *Gut*, 33, 683–7.

Roe, A.M., Warren, B.F., Brodribb, A.J.M., Brown, C. (1993) Diversion colitis and the involution of the defunctioned rectum. *Gut*, 34, 382–5.

Roy, J., Snover, D., Weisdorf, S., Mulvahill, A., Filipovich, A., Weisdorf, D. (1991) Simultaneous upper and lower endoscopic biopy in the diagnosis of graft-versus-host disease. *Transplantation*, 51, 642–6.

Ryan, C.K., Potter, G.D. (1995) Disinfectant colitis. Rinse as well as you wash. *J. Clin. Gastroenterol.*, 21, 6–9.

Sale, G.E., McDonald, G.B., Shulman, H.M., Thomas, E.D. (1979) Gastrointestinal graft-versus-host disease in man. A clinico-pathologic study of the rectal biopsy. *Am. J. Surg. Pathol.*, 3, 291–9.

Shidham, V.B., Chang, C-C., Shidham, G. *et al.* (2003) Colon biopsies for evaluation of acute graft-versus-host disease (A-GVHD) in allogeneic bone marrow transplantation patients. *BMC Gastroenterol.*, 3, 5.

Shulman, H.M., Sullivan, K.M., Weiden, P.L. *et al.* (1980) Chronic graft-versus-host syndrome in man. A long-term clinicopathologic study of 20 Seattle patients. *Am. J. Med.*, 69, 204–17.

Snover, D.C. (1985) Mucosal damage simulating graft-versus-host reaction in cytomegalovirus colitis. *Transplantation*, 39, 669–70.

Snover, D.C. (1990) Graft-versus-host disease of the gastrointestinal tract. *Am. J. Surg. Pathol.*, 14 (Suppl. 1), 101–8.

Sondheimer, J.M., Sokol, R.J., Narkewicz, M.R., Tyson, R.W. (1995) Anastomotic ulceration: a late complication of ileocolonic anastomosis. *J. Pediatr.*, 127, 225–30.

Stein, B.L., Lamoureux, E., Miller, M., Vasilevsky, C.A., Julien, L., Gordon, P.H. (2001) Glutaraldehyde-induced colitis. *Can. J. Surg.*, 44, 113–16.

Subramanyan, K., Rajan, R.T., Hearn, C.D. (1988) Barium granuloma of the sigmoid colon. *J. Clin. Gastroenterol.*, 10, 98–100.

Tamai, O., Nozato, E., Miyazato, H. *et al.* (1999) Radiation-associated rectal cancer: report of four cases. *Dig. Surg.*, 16, 238–43.

Tanner, A.S.R., Raghunath, A.S. (1988) Colonic inflammation and nonsteroidal anti-inflammatory drug administration. An assessment of the frequency of the problem. *Digestion*, 41, 116–20.

Taverner, D., Talbot, I.C., Carr-Locke, D.L., Wicks, A.C.B. (1982) Massive bleeding from the ileum: a late complication of pelvic radiotherapy. *Am. J. Gastroenterol.*, 77, 29–31.

Teodorescu, V., Bauer, J., Lichtiger, S., Chapman, M. (1993) Gold-induced colitis: a case report and review of the literature. *Mt Sinai J. Med.*, 60, 238–41.

Tokar, B., Aydoglu, S., Pasaoglu, O., Ilhan, H., Kasapoglu, E. (2003) Neutropenic enterocolitis: is it possible to break vicious circle between neutropenia and the bowel wall inflammation by surgery? *Int. J. Colorerctal Dis.*, 18, 455–8.

Tomori, H., Yasuda, T., Shiraishi, M., Isa, T., Muto, T., Egawa, H. (1999) Radiation-associated ischaemic coloproctitis: report of two cases. *Surg. Today*, 29, 1088–92.

Volk, E.E., Shapiro, B.D., Easley, K.A., Goldblum, J.R. (1998) The clinical significance of a biopsy-based diagnosis of focal active colitis: a clinicopathologic study of 31 cases. *Mod. Pathol.*, 11, 789–94.

Warren, B.F., Shepherd, N.A. (1992) Diversion proctocolitis. *Histopathology*, 21, 91–3.

Warren, B.F., Shepherd, N.A., Bartolo, D.C., Bradfield, J.W. (1993) Pathology of the defunctioned rectum in ulcerative colitis. *Gut*, 34, 514–16.

Watts, D.A., Lessells, A.M., Penman, I.D., Ghosh, S. (2002) Endoscopic and histologic features of sodium phosphate bowel preparation-induced colonic ulceration: case report and review. *Gastrointest. Endosc.*, 55, 584–7.

West, A.B., Kuan, S.F., Bennick, M., Lagarde, S. (1995) Glutaraldehyde colitis following endoscopy: clinical and pathological features and investigation of an outbreak. *Gastroenterology*, 108, 1250–5.

White, R.F., Major, G.A. (1983) Gold colitis. *Med. J. Aust.*, 1, 174–5.

Willems, M., van Buuren, H.R., de Krijger, R. (2003) Anthranoid self-medication causing rapid development of melanosis coli. *Neth. J. Med.*, 61, 22–4.

Wong, N.A., Penman, I.D., Campbell, S., Lessells, A.M. (2000) Microscopic focal cryptitis associated with sodium phosphate bowel preparation. *Histopathology*, 36, 476–8.

Wong, V., Wyatt, J., Lewis, F., Howdle, P. (1993) Gold-induced enterocolitis complicated by cytomegalovirus infection: a previously unrecognised association. *Gut*, 34, 1002–5.

Yeong, M.L., Bethwaite, P.B., Prasad, J., Ibister, W.H. (1991) Lymphoid follicular hyperplasia – a distinctive feature of diversion colitis. *Histopathology*, 19, 55–61.

Zwas, F.R., Cirillo, N.W., el-Serag, H.B., Eisen, R.N. (1996) Colonic mucosal abnormalities associated with oral sodium phosphate solution. *Gastrointest. Endosc.*, 43, 463–6.

CHAPTER 12

THE DIFFERENTIAL DIAGNOSIS OF INFLAMMATORY BOWEL DISEASE

12.1 General principles   203
12.2 Significance of the normal
     biopsy   203
12.3 Minor abnormalities   204
   12.3.1 Non-specific inflammation,
     acute   205
   12.3.2 Non-specific inflammation,
     chronic   206
   12.3.3 Terminology for non-diagnostic
     biopsies, biopsy series and
     indeterminate colitis   206
12.4 Major disease entities: ulcerative
     colitis vs. Crohn's disease vs.
     infection   209
   12.4.1 Histopathology   209
   12.4.2 Mucosal immunology   210
   12.4.3 Natural history   211
   12.4.4 Diagnostic reliability   211
   12.4.5 Serological markers   212
12.5 Other forms of colitis   212
   12.5.1 Antibiotic-associated colitis 213
   12.5.2 Ischaemic colitis   213
   12.5.3 The solitary ulcer   214
   12.5.4 Diverticulitis   215
   12.5.5 Microscopic colitis – collagenous,
     lymphocytic and non-collagenous
     non-lymphocytic varieties   216

12.5.6 Minimal change colitis   216
12.5.7 Acute self-limiting colitis
     (transient colitis)   216
12.5.8 Cathartic colon   217
12.5.9 Irritable bowel syndrome   217
12.5.10 Eosinophilic or allergic colitis 217
12.5.11 Radiation-induced colitis   218
12.5.12 Immunodeficiency states   218
12.5.13 Graft-versus-host disease   219
12.5.14 Drug-induced disease
     (excluding antibiotics)   219
12.5.15 Connective tissue disorders   219
12.6 The terminal ileal biopsy   219
   12.6.1 The normal biopsy   219
   12.6.2 The inflamed biopsy   220
   12.6.3 Interpretation of the inflamed
     ileal biopsy   221
12.7 Backwash ileitis and ileal
     complications of ulcerative
     colitis   224
   12.7.1 Backwash ileitis   224
   12.7.2 Ileal pathology following
     colectomy   224
12.8 Ileal nodular lymphoid
     hyperplasia   225
12.9 Conclusions   226
References   226

12.1 GENERAL PRINCIPLES

In previous chapters the diagnostic pictures of individual entities have been described. Here, the differential diagnoses are considered in the form of a problem on the pathologist's desk. This is usually a rectal biopsy accompanied by a clinical request form which queries inflammatory bowel disease, simply states that the patient has diarrhoea or is devoid of all information. However, it is important to know whether one is looking at a first biopsy or a follow-up as this influences the interpretation. Colonoscopic series are seldom the first challenge and are more likely to follow an initial rectal biopsy.

Awareness on the part of the pathologist of the diagnostic possibilities is crucial. Other conditions such as ischaemic colitis and solitary ulcer, for example, may masquerade clinically as chronic inflammatory bowel disease (Rickert, 1984; Goldman, 1994; Jenkins *et al.*, 1997b). The diagnostic difficulties revolve around the question of specificity of histological features for any one disease, and the converse, the overlapping features across the spectrum of inflammatory bowel diseases. As so few histological features are diagnostic, it is important to appreciate the predictive probability of the various histological signs. The sum of these determines the degree of diagnostic confidence which is put into the biopsy report. At all times the biopsies need to be placed in clinical context and this is often best achieved at multidisciplinary team meetings.

An initial glance at low power shows whether the biopsy is adequate or requires sectioning at deeper levels, being curled or not deep enough. A second decision is the recognition of a normal biopsy, described in Chapter 2. Perhaps surprisingly, in an observer variation study by Giard *et al.* (1985) there was considerable variation in the recognition of normality. Normal colonoscopic biopsies often show minor changes, such as a slight focal infiltrate of neutrophils due to the often vigorous manipulation entailed in the procedure or a consequence of bowel preparation (Rejchrt *et al.*, 2004). Furthermore, the lamina propria of the right colon is more cellular than the left (Fig. 12.1) and this must not be misinterpreted as inflammation. The cellularity of the mucosal lamina propria throughout the colon

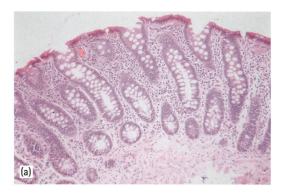
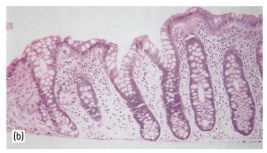

Figure 12.1 These two biopsies from the right colon (a) and descending colon (b) illustrate the difference in cellularity of the lamina propria between the proximal right colon and the remainder of the colon and rectum. The unwary, especially with a thick section, could misinterpret this as proximal inflammation.

shows a gradient of diminishing density from superficial to deep layers. In a normal biopsy the loose areolar connective tissue of the lower half of the lamina propria is easily visible (Fig. 12.2). When obscured by the inflammatory cell component, it is a useful sign that genuine inflammation is present. Mild depletion of goblet cells is acceptable as within the normal range and some increased mitotic activity for this can be induced by purgation and enemas given in the course of bowel preparation (Driman and Preiksaitis, 1998).

12.2 SIGNIFICANCE OF THE NORMAL BIOPSY

Even when the biopsy is normal some diagnostic comments can be helpful to the clinician over and

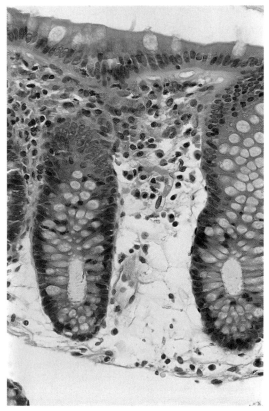

Figure 12.2 The normal cellular gradient in the lamina propria showing the normal complement of inflammatory cells in the upper half and the loose areolar connective tissue of the lower half. The loss of this demarcation can be a useful clue in appreciating minor degrees of inflammation.

above stating 'This is a normal biopsy'. For example, given certain caveats, the diagnosis is unlikely to be ulcerative colitis and this can be stated, if clinically relevant. The rectum nearly always shows some residual abnormality in ulcerative colitis. The first caveat, as described in Section 5.1, is rectal sparing and a return to normality, in particular as a response to drug therapy such as steroids (Price, 1977) and 5-aminosalicylic acid (Odze et al., 1993a). Second, children may not show the expected rectal pathology (Markovitz et al., 1993; Glickman et al., 2004). Naturally, the interpretative remarks on any abnormality must reflect the clinical situation. Virtually any of the conditions listed at the beginning of this chapter may coexist with a normal biopsy, on the basis of sampling error or disease distribution;

thus, in florid pseudomembranous colitis the mucosa between lesions is often normal (Price and Davis, 1977). A normal biopsy within any inflamed colonoscopic series, or taken from the rectum, in the clinical context of Crohn's disease is evidence in its favour and suitable comment can be made. A normal biopsy may be seen in proven infective diarrhoeas (Dickinson et al., 1979), a point that may not be appreciated by the examining clinician, especially if not a gastroenterologist. A normal follow-up biopsy, taken a few weeks after one showing severe acute colitis, is also evidence in favour of an infection (Dickinson et al., 1979) and warrants such a comment.

Some pathologists may argue that such comment is unnecessary, even insulting, to clinicians. Admittedly, as the relationship between gastroenterologist and pathologist develops, via regular multidisciplinary team meetings, a bland statement of normality is probably adequate. However, in most hospitals, rectal biopsies are also taken by other specialist teams who do not attend such meetings and will still appreciate useful diagnostic interpretation, as do the junior clinicians needing to learn.

12.3 MINOR ABNORMALITIES

Abnormalities under this heading seldom lead to a diagnosis in their own right but may contribute to the combined clinical picture and overall diagnostic decision. Many of the individual features have been dealt with in Chapter 3. In busy routine practice it is tempting to look quickly at a biopsy, observe minimal abnormality at low power and dismiss the biopsy as of no diagnostic value. However, minor inflammatory changes may constitute a diagnostic sign in certain clinical situations. For example, a microgranuloma (Fig. 3.42) (caused by Crohn's disease) may be present in normal or only mildly abnormal mucosa and it behoves one to cut through a biopsy where this is a serious clinical possibility (Rotterdam et al., 1977; Seldenrijk et al., 1991). The early changes of the solitary ulcer (Section 15.10), the presence of spirochaetosis (Section 4.5) or the subtle connective tissue alterations in the lamina propria in mild radiation proctocolitis (Section 11.1) all have diagnostic appearances and are easily over-looked, in what at low power, may seem a normal or only mildly abnormal, biopsy. Amoebiasis (Section 4.7.1), cytomegalovirus infection and amyloid (Section 20.8) are further examples of conditions that can be associated with minimal histological abnormalities.

Perhaps the commonest abnormality under this heading is a cellular infiltrate seen against a back-ground of regular cryptal architecture and variable goblet cell depletion. In the absence of clinical details Geboes and Villanacci (2005) suggest this is a rare occasion when the term 'non-specific colitis' may be justifiable. Appreciating a minor increase in cellularity of this type that warrants classification as abnormal requires careful judgement (Giard *et al.*, 1985) and, as just mentioned (Section 12.1), the gradient of inflammatory cells in the lamina propria

is a useful guide. A thick section can also appear hypercellular and is easily misinterpreted. The abnor-mal infiltrative pattern can be divided into two. In one, polymorphs are present, infiltrating the cryptal or surface epithelium and, in the other, the infiltrate is mainly plasma cells and lymphocytes with no epithelial invasion by polymorphs. It is convenient to consider these as acute and chronic varieties of 'non-specific' inflammation.

12.3.1 Non-specific inflammation, acute

For this label, polymorphs should be found infiltrat-ing crypts and surface epithelium with an arbitrary minimum involvement of three or four crypts, not necessarily contiguously. A few may be dilated (Figs 12.3 and 12.4). The significance of finding only

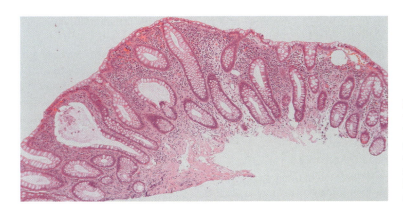

Figure 12.3 This is an example of focal acute non-specific inflammation that has been referred to as 'focal active colitis'. Some dilated crypts containing neutrophil polymorphs are present along with a minor increase in lymphocytes and plasma cells in the lamina propria.

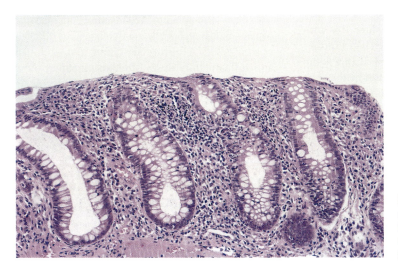

Figure 12.4 A more florid example of focal acute non-specific inflammation than in Fig. 12.3; there is a limited cryptitis and slight goblet cell depletion.

one affected crypt has been considered in Section 3.6.7. An obvious question is whether such a minor degree of cryptitis may simply be a consequence of coexistent diarrhoea from any cause. Deductions from the literature make it unlikely that diarrhoea itself, irrespective of cause, produces histological abnormalities. The mucosa is normal in many cases of severe infective diarrhoea (Price, 1977; Dickinson et al., 1979; Mandal et al., 1982). In severe Crohn's disease a normal rectal mucosa is a frequent finding. There are many similar pointers to the conclusion that the histopathologist need not consider diarrhoea, per se, a primary cause of histological abnormality.

The acute element of the inflammation is usually accompanied by a mild focal increase in plasma cells and lymphocytes. The crypts remain straight or may be dilated and a few crypt abscesses are common. Mild goblet cell depletion can occur and the changes can be focal or diffuse (Fig. 12.4). By the time there is extensive destruction of the crypts or florid crypt abscess formation, other diagnostic clues can usually be found in the biopsy and a more definitive diagnosis offered. The pattern is one of definite mucosal inflammation manifesting as a cryptitis, perhaps with some cryptal dilatation, but with insufficient other signs to classify it further. By definition, the abnormalities are of mild degree.

How should such a biopsy be reported? The report must emphasize that this is a definite, though mild, acute proctitis or colitis. It is helpful to state that there are no well-developed signs of ulcerative colitis, infection or Crohn's disease and that any inflammatory condition might produce this picture at some stage. To interpret the changes further the clinical data must be considered. If this is the first biopsy from a patient with a short history, the disease is most likely to resolve and be a presumed bout of infection. If, however, there is good evidence of bowel disease at another site, Crohn's disease can be suggested on the grounds of disease distribution. A diagnosis of ulcerative colitis would have to await follow-up biopsies. Any one of the rarer causes of colitis listed at the beginning of the chapter might be considered if the history is relevant and a drug history should always be taken. On biopsies from patients with pertinent clinical history multiple levels should be examined in the search for granulomas, parasites and lesions of

pseudomembranous colitis. Some authors have looked at the outcome of this pattern of focal acute inflammation referring to it as focal active colitis (Section 12.3.3a) (Greenson et al., 1997).

12.3.2 Non-specific inflammation, chronic

In this second pattern of 'non-specific' inflammation, polymorphs may be seen in the lamina propria, but few within the epithelium. There may also be eosinophils and their numbers may show considerable geographical variation (Goldman, 1994). There is an increase in plasma cells and lymphocytes, often marked, which can be focal or diffuse and is beginning to extend into the basal one-third of the lamina propria (Fig. 12.5). Except for minor derangement the crypts remain intact and aligned, with or without some goblet cell depletion. The picture is of definite chronic inflammatory changes but does not conform to a diagnostic pattern. In a colonoscopic series some normal areas may remain. It is our experience that resolving infection or the resolving initial attack of ulcerative colitis are the most likely diagnoses. On occasions there may also be an increase in intra-epithelial lymphocytes, above the normal of 5 per 100 epithelial cells but well below the 20 per 100 epithelial cells required for a confident diagnosis of microscopic colitis – lymphocytic variety (Sections 9.3.2 and 9.3.6). In such circumstances the differential needs to include paucicellular lymphocytic colitis as described by Goldstein and Bhanot (2004) and microscopic colitis – non-lymphocytic, non-collagenous (Kitchen et al., 2002). A history of taking non-steroidal anti-inflammatory drugs often accompanies these abnormalities. In a small number of patients a chronic inflammatory cell infiltrate following infection can persist for a long time and accompany post-infection irritable bowel syndrome (Spiller et al., 2000; Spiller, 2003).

12.3.3 Terminology for non-diagnostic biopsies, biopsy series and indeterminate colitis

It is important to have a consistent and understandable reporting style for these areas of diagnostic

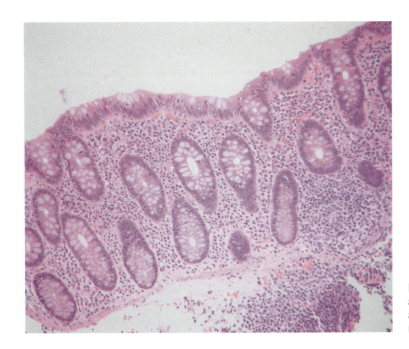

Figure 12.5 In this biopsy there is a chronic inflammatory cell infiltrate across the lamina propria but with no other diagnostic clues present.

uncertainty, the implications of which are understood by clinicians and on which they can base their management. In our opinion and that of others, merely to conclude 'non-specific colitis' is unhelpful (Geboes *et al.*, 2003). The clinician, excluding the normal colonoscopic picture associated with microscopic colitis, is usually aware of this from the endoscopic appearances. It is more helpful to be descriptive and evaluate the diagnostic possibilities. Terms used in the literature to group the mild acute features and the chronic, but still non-diagnostic picture, have been focal active colitis (Greenson *et al.*, 1997) and variations of colitis – unclassified, colitis indeterminate and colitis – not yet categorized (Price, 1978; Jenkins *et al.*, 1997b; Guindi and Riddell, 2004; Geboes and Villanacci, 2005).

12.3.3a Focal active colitis

This term has been used to classify patients with no history of inflammatory bowel disease or endoscopic abnormality in whom there are foci of predominantly acute inflammation, as described above (Greenson *et al.*, 1997; Volk *et al.*, 1998). If restricted

to a solitary focus in a rectal biopsy or merely an occasional crypt in a colonoscopic series focal active cryptitis may be a more appropriate term (Greenson *et al.*, 1998) (Figs 12.3 and 12.4). Greenson *et al.* (1997) followed 42 cases of focal active colitis. None developed chronic inflammatory bowel disease but 19 had an acute self-limiting colitis-like illness, 11 were incidental findings during polyp follow-up protocols, six had irritable bowel syndrome, four had been on antibiotics and two developed ischaemic colitis. Significantly, clinical data revealed that 20 patients were immunocompromised and 19 were taking non-steroidal anti-inflammatory drugs. Similar studies on a paediatric population with focal active colitis (Volk *et al.*, 1998) showed that 31 per cent of the 31 patients developed Crohn's disease, once again demonstrating that morphological patterns of chronic inflammatory bowel disease in children may be different from adults (Glickman *et al.*, 2004; Markovicz *et al.*, 1993). Acute self-limiting colitis was, however, still the commonest putative diagnosis. The results of Xin *et al.* (2003) were similar.

Focal active colitis can be a useful category for encompassing minor inflammatory abnormalities, provided that the clinician is aware of the diagnostic implications. In adults the data suggest that chronic inflammatory bowel disease is unlikely to develop.

12.3.3b Indeterminate colitis

It is our practice, and recommended by others (Guindi and Riddell, 2004), to limit the use of the term indeterminate colitis to surgical excision specimens for the following reasons. Colitis indeterminate as originally described (Price, 1978) conforms to the defined clinical picture of ulcerative colitis and Crohn's disease in an acute fulminant stage. This corresponds to a morphological pattern of extensive mucosal loss with ulceration, surviving intervening polypoid mucosal islands, transmural inflammation, extensive deep fissuring ulceration and myocytolysis (Price, 1978; Lee *et al.*, 1979; Guindi and Riddell, 2004) (Fig. 12.6a). Some of these features would normally indicate Crohn's disease but in the fulminant state they can be seen as the morphological end-stage in ulcerative colitis (Yantiss *et al.*, 2006) and some enteric infections. There are no biopsy features from which such a diagnosis can be made. Indeed, in the typical case colonoscopy is contraindicated for fear of perforation. The fulminant attack is commonly centred on the transverse colon so that while a rectosigmoid biopsy may be taken it generally shows minimal abnormality. On the rare occasions biopsies are obtained from an involved area they comprise granulation tissue with ulcer slough if from a denuded area, or if from a polypoid area, surviving mucosa with surprisingly limited inflammation and crypt damage (Fig. 12.6b). This might be a picture obtainable at biopsy from a large range of inflammatory bowel diseases at some stage in their evolution. Thus, we believe the term indeterminate colitis should not be diluted and should remain restricted to the surgical specimen for which the clinical outcomes have been well documented (Wells *et al.*, 1991; Yu *et al.*, 2000; Dayton *et al.*, 2002).

What then might be appropriate terminology for unclassifiable cases in biopsy practice? There are many reasons for failure to reach a diagnosis. First, there may be the simple technical reason that the

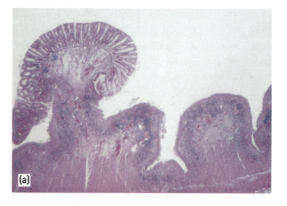
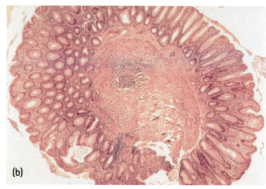

Figure 12.6 (a) Detail from an emergency colectomy specimen showing the typical features to be found in indeterminate colitis, namely full-thickness damage, fissuring ulceration and surviving mucosal islands that can be remarkably free of inflammation despite the severe adjacent pathology. (b) This is a rectal biopsy that preceded an urgent colectomy for colitis classified as indeterminate. It emphasizes the misleading relatively normal appearance of residual mucosa in such cases.

biopsies are of poor quality. Second, they may be insufficient or not representative in location or time. The latter is among the most common of reasons. Biopsies are merely a snapshot, a single point in time, during the natural history of what is usually a life-long disease process, the biopsies having been taken when the characteristic features of the disease were not evident. The third and final reason for diagnostic difficulty is that, because of overlapping morphological patterns of disease, more clinical and/or radiological information is essential for diagnosis. The role of the evolving diagnostic process can be appreciated from data in a comparative study on the incidence of chronic inflammatory bowel disease between 20 centres in northern and southern Europe (Price, 1996). This involved biopsies from 2200 cases. Use of the term indeterminate colitis was unrestricted. Under these circumstances, on solely histological criteria, the incidence of indeterminate colitis in the Northern centres, for example, was 16 per cent but fell to 9 per cent when the clinical data were considered. Moreover, this had fallen to 5 per cent after 2 years of follow-up. In the prospective studies of Moum *et al.* (1997) indeterminate colitis formed 13 per cent of the cohort of patients with chronic inflammatory bowel disease and 50 per cent had been reclassified as Crohn's disease or ulcerative colitis within 2 years. Meucci *et al.* (1999) found that 80 per cent of cases given an initial diagnosis of indeterminate colitis could be confidently classified within 8 years. Whatever terminology is used to describe patients in whom a confident diagnosis cannot be given at the time of biopsy, these studies show that it is a temporary state, with a confident diagnosis being built up over the follow-up period. This is the rationale behind asking that biopsies are repeated at intervals to accrue a set of criteria from which a final confident diagnosis can be made.

12.3.3c Conclusions

For minor inflammatory abnormalities in which there is no history of chronic inflammatory bowel disease and no endoscopic abnormality, focal active colitis is a succinct summary term if the clinicians are aware of its implications (Greenson *et al.*, 1997). Where the changes are more florid and it is clear chronic inflammatory bowel disease of some description is likely to be present it is our practice to conclude 'inflammatory bowel disease – currently type uncertain', the term 'currently' conveying the dynamic concept for the role of follow-up in determining the final diagnosis. However, there is clearly a need for a national and international consensus on terminology. Non-specific colitis we believe is unhelpful and, as explained above, we recommend indeterminate colitis be restricted to the surgical excision with its specific clinicopathological profile.

12.4 MAJOR DISEASE ENTITIES: ULCERATIVE COLITIS VS. CROHN'S DISEASE VS. INFECTION

The commonest question is, 'Which main type of inflammatory bowel disease; ulcerative colitis, Crohn's disease or infection, is present?' Other conditions are usually considered after this and are prompted by the clinical data. For example, ischaemia must be seriously considered in a 75-year-old patient but will be low down the diagnostic list when looking at a biopsy from a 20-year-old. A constant problem is the absence of one specific histological feature that is invariably present in any one condition and invariably absent from the others. Even a granuloma does not necessarily mean Crohn's disease if crypt-related ulcerative colitis can still be a possibility (Mahadeva *et al.*, 2002) (Fig. 5.8). If the patient is of Indian or African origin, tuberculosis or parasitic disease need careful exclusion. Equally, when reporting an initial biopsy with the features of acute infection it is sensible to draw attention to the possibility of acute ulcerative colitis mimicking infection and the value of a second biopsy after an appropriate interval (Therkilsdjen *et al.*, 1989; Schumacher *et al.*, 1994a).

12.4.1 Histopathology

Crypt distortion (branching glands), a villous surface, goblet cell depletion, prominent crypt abscesses and a diffuse, predominantly plasma cell infiltrate extending into the lower third of the lamina propria are key attributes for ulcerative colitis (Section 5.2.1). When all these features are present this diagnosis is unlikely to be wrong (Surawicz and Belic, 1984; Schumacher *et al.*, 1994b; Jenkins *et al.*, 1997a) (Figs 5.1–5.3).

By contrast, in infection, the crypts remain aligned but show characteristic degeneration (Section 4.2.1). Polymorphs are the most conspicuous inflammatory cells, clustered in the lamina propria and migrating between the cryptal epithelial cells. The plasma cell infiltrate is light to moderate and oedema, by thinning out the inflammatory component, dilutes the impact of inflammation as seen under the low-power lens (Price *et al.*, 1979; Schumacher *et al.*, 1994a,b; Jenkins *et al.*, 1997a) (Figs 4.1–4.4).

With the caveats mentioned above and in Section 5.2.1d the cardinal sign of Crohn's disease is the granuloma (Section 6.3.3) (Fig. 3.43). However, in routine practice it is present in 25–30 per cent of biopsies (Petri *et al.*, 1982; Heresbach *et al.*, 2005), so has limited value. The yield increases over the course of multiple examinations and if serial sections are cut on any one particular biopsy (Seldenrijk *et al.*, 1991; Heresbach *et al.*, 2005). In Crohn's colitis, in the face of a moderate inflammatory cell infiltrate, the crypts remain aligned with little mucin depletion. The plasma cell and mononuclear cell infiltrate is typically discontinuous and basal lymphoid aggregates or basal plasmacytosis are a useful sign (McGovern and Goulston, 1968; Schumacher *et al.*, 1994b). Polymorphs can form crypt abscesses or remain as a 'cryptitis' but neither feature arrests the eye as in ulcerative colitis or infection. Microgranulomas (focal collections of inflammatory cells which include histiocytes), are useful pointers to Crohn's disease (Rotterdam *et al.*, 1977) (Fig. 3.42). They are easily overlooked sited between relatively normal crypts and are poorly delineated from any accompanying inflammation. The presence of giant cells should prompt a search for granulomas but giant cells alone have little discriminatory significance. In the absence of granulomas, clusters of histiocytes (Seldenrijk *et al.*, 1991) and definite patchy inflammation are more suggestive of Crohn's disease than the other common inflammatory conditions (Section 6.3.2). However, patchy inflammation can be a feature of ulcerative colitis (Kleer and Appelman, 1998) once treatment has commenced, if the biopsy is taken as disease goes into remission, or if taken from the proximal limits of inflammation (Fig. 12.7).

12.4.2 Mucosal immunology

In routine practice there is little diagnostic value in determining the immunological profile and distribution of plasma cells within the mucosa in patients with inflammatory bowel disease in the hope of distinguishing the major forms. There are many studies that have attempted this (Balkien and Brandtzaeg, 1975; O'Donoghue and Kumar, 1979; Keren *et al.*, 1984). The variable outcomes of such studies are largely the result of differing methodologies of staining and quantification plus a failure to control for disease activity. Scott *et al.* (1983), in a careful study of plasma cells in rectal biopsies, claimed that there was no significant

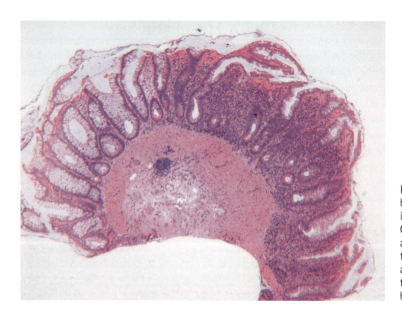

Figure 12.7 In chronic inflammatory bowel disease patchy inflammation is taken as a pointer towards Crohn's disease. However, it can be a feature of ulcerative colitis once treatment has commenced, or appear to be present, as here, when the proximal limit of disease has been biopsied.

difference in plasma cell populations between the various types of inflammatory bowel disease if account was taken of disease activity.

Some trends have been apparent in the literature in certain circumstances and may have a role as an adjunct to diagnosis. Rosekrans *et al.* (1980a) demonstrated that a raised mucosal plasma cell immunoglobulin M (IgM) in inactive disease is a feature specific to Crohn's disease in the context of inflammatory bowel disease. This would seem a readily appreciated finding and therefore of potential diagnostic use. This finding was also present in the study of Seldenrijk *et al.* (1991), helping to distinguish patients with Crohn's disease. van Spreeuwel *et al.* (1985) noted that in infective colitis the plasma cell immunoglobulin E (IgE) levels remain low compared with active Crohn's disease or ulcerative colitis (O'Donoghue and Kumar, 1979). Again, this is a feature that would be easy to appreciate without complex morphometry and one of diagnostic value. It is claimed that high levels of IgE-containing plasma cells may delineate a group of colitics with limited distal disease who have an allergic basis and respond to anti-allergic preparations (Heatley *et al.*, 1975; Rosekrans *et al.*, 1980b).

While T- and B-cell responses in inflammatory bowel disease are becoming better understood, at present detailed investigations of their profiles have no diagnostic place in an individual case.

12.4.3 Natural history

Attention should be given to the time a biopsy or biopsy series was taken relative to the onset of symptoms or start of therapy. This can modify interpretation and the issues are dealt with in Sections 5.5.4 and 12.3.3b. The key attributes of ulcerative colitis and infection (Sections 4.2.1 and 5.2) correspond to biopsies taken at the optimum times after symptoms develop. This is within the first week in infectious colitis but from 2 to 5 weeks or longer in ulcerative colitis (Surawicz and Belic, 1984; Schumacher *et al.*, 1994a). Time and therapy alter the pathology considerably (Odze *et al.*, 1993a; Bernstein *et al.*, 1995; Kim *et al.*, 1999; Geboes and Dalle, 2002) and the necessary details to take account of this are seldom stated on the clinical request form. This information is less critical in Crohn's

disease as the pathology is thought to maintain a more constant pattern.

Similar interpretative problems occur in the resolving phase of both ulcerative colitis and infection. In infective colitis the inflammation takes on a more chronic and patchy distribution (Sections 4.2.2c and 4.2.3). In ulcerative colitis goblet cells recover and the inflammatory infiltrate becomes less dense and is commonly focal (Section 5.2.2). These features make a distinction from Crohn's disease more difficult (Price, 1977). As a general rule, within 4–6 weeks any infection will have resolved to leave normal mucosa, whereas in typical ulcerative colitis, evidence of permanent damage is accruing (Schumacher *et al.*, 1994a,b). Sequential biopsies may be the only way of establishing the diagnostic pattern, while the addition of a colonoscopic series, if only rectal biopsies were available, adds not only more microscopic data but the appreciation of the macroscopic picture. This is especially valuable when the histological details are equivocal. Thus, the biopsy conclusion might be 'colitis – currently type uncertain' yet the colonoscopic picture shows linear serpiginous ulceration with skip lesions typical of Crohn's disease. This also emphasizes the need to collate all the available data.

12.4.4 Diagnostic reliability

There have been many studies of both the reliability of histological signs and their observer agreement believed to yield a distinction between the major forms of inflammatory bowel disease (Cook and Dixon, 1973; Lessels *et al.*, 1994; Theodossi *et al.*, 1994; Dundas *et al.*, 1997; Farmer *et al.*, 2000; Tanaka *et al.*, 2001; Bentley *et al.*, 2002). A useful synthesis of this literature is gained from the diagnostic guidelines for the diagnosis of inflammatory bowel disease compiled by Jenkins *et al.* (1997b) derived from a Medline analysis of the pertinent data. The acceptable criterion for reliability of a particular microscopic feature was that it had been shown, in more than one valid study, to have a minimum κ value of 0.4 or a percentage observer agreement of at least 80 per cent. The specificity and sensitivity of a sign had to exceed 50 per cent. The clinical setting had to be relevant, with the feature being shown as objective and reproducible. For a diagnosis of ulcerative colitis crypt architectural distortion, decreased crypt density, a villous mucosal surface and transmucosal inflammation emerged as the most reliable. For a diagnosis of Crohn's disease the most reliable parameters were granulomas, discontinuous crypt distortion and discontinuous mucosal inflammation. To diagnose infectious colitis only normal crypt architecture and superficial mucosal inflammation satisfied the criteria.

Another problem for the histopathologists is to appreciate how often the biopsy in ulcerative colitis or Crohn's disease mimics infection, or vice versa. It is well known that, clinically, both ulcerative colitis and Crohn's disease may present as infection (Dronfield et al., 1974) or be precipitated by it (Harries et al., 1985; Schumacher et al., 1994b). Again, few hard data exist on such problems. Reports suggest that between 7 and 30 per cent of biopsies from patients who are culture-positive, or carry a confident clinical diagnosis of infectious diarrhoea, have a biopsy more in keeping with ulcerative colitis or Crohn's disease (Day et al., 1978; Dickinson et al., 1979; Lambert et al., 1979; McGovern and Slavutin, 1979; Price et al., 1979; Jewkes et al., 1981; Mandal et al., 1982). Figures for the converse, that is, patients with ulcerative colitis or Crohn's disease with biopsies typical of infection, culled from the same authors, are also few but seem to be around 5–7 per cent. Where infection and idiopathic inflammatory bowel disease coexist, biopsies usually reflect the ulcerative colitis or Crohn's disease (Day et al., 1978). Comparing the data is plagued by the problem of the timing of the biopsy, as discussed in Section 12.4.3.

Several papers quote figures for the percentage of occasions in which diagnoses are changed. This also reflects the problem of timing as well as the problem of observer variation and the related issue of diagnostic experience. Therkilsden et al. (1989) claim at least one-third of their 32 cases in which index biopsies had no initial pointers to chronic inflammatory bowel disease developed it on follow-up. In their population-based study of 830 patients Moum et al. (1997) found that 10 per cent on follow-up 2 years later had to be reclassified. The role of experience is seen in the biopsy study of Farmer et al. (2000) in which the opinion of gastrointestinal expert pathologists differed from general pathologists in as many as 54 per cent of cases. However, in the study by Bentley et al. (2002) only a small difference was found between expert and non-expert pathologists. While all such data may be interesting, none are strictly comparable because of differences in design of the studies, in particular sampling and the data made available to the participants. For any individual patient to have the optimum chance of an accurate diagnosis the pathologist must be equipped with good-quality biopsies, adequate sampling, adequate clinical details and the opportunity for clinical liaison. In the correct context it should be possible to make a confident diagnosis in the large majority of cases.

12.4.5 Serological markers

Although outside the remit of biopsy interpretation the pathologist should be aware of the potential value of the serological markers, perinuclear anti-neutrophilic cytoplasmic antibody (pANCA) and anti-*Saccharomyces cerevisiae* antibody (ASCA), in particular when having to resort to a classification of 'colitis – currently type uncertain'. In a follow-up study (Joossens et al., 2002) of 97 cases in which, at the outset, no distinction between ulcerative colitis and Crohn's disease could be made, ASCA +ve/pANCA −ve serology correctly predicted a follow-up diagnosis of Crohn's disease in 80 per cent of cases and ASCA −ve/pANCA +ve serology identified ulcerative colitis in 63 per cent. Of interest was that the majority of patients who were negative for both markers (40 of 47) remained unclassified during a mean follow-up period of 10.7 years. Those in whom a definitive diagnosis was reached had a mean disease follow-up time of 6 years.

12.5 OTHER FORMS OF COLITIS

Discussion, so far, has centred on the commonest differential problem, ulcerative colitis vs. Crohn's disease vs. infection. The salient points of other conditions in the differential diagnosis are now considered.

12.5.1 Antibiotic-associated colitis

In terms of the differential diagnosis of ulcerative colitis/Crohn's disease and infection the recognition of the Type I and Type II lesions of pseudomembranous colitis is not a problem. The difficulty of distinguishing patterns of pseudomembranous colitis from ischaemia is considered in Sections 8.3, 10.6.1, 10.6.2, 10.6.3 and 10.6.4. A problem exists, however, when typical pseudomembranous lesions are absent. Thus, antibiotic-associated colitis, whether *Clostridium difficile* is present or not, may show a pattern of inflammation similar to that of infective colitis of mild degree (Section 8.2.2). The biopsy is often oedematous, with a definite patchy increase in neutrophil polymorphs. The surface epithelium is infiltrated and small surface knots of epithelial cells may give a clue (Fig. 8.10). When these features are seen, multiple levels should be cut through the specimen to attempt to detect a 'summit lesion' (Section 8.2.1a). However, it is worth re-emphasizing the pitfall of misinterpreting surface intercryptal erosion (Fig. 8.4). This only indicates early pseudomembranous colitis when seen against a background of normal or minimally inflamed mucosa. The presence of a significant plasma cell infiltrate is strongly against the diagnosis of any pattern of antibiotic-associated colitis, as is crypt irregularity. A careful drug history should be obtained when the diagnostic conclusion seems to be non-specific and in the category of focal active colitis (Section 12.3.3a).

12.5.2 Ischaemic colitis

Time since the onset of symptoms and rate of onset of disease determine how closely the biopsy pattern of ischaemic colitis resembles the patterns of ulcerative colitis, Crohn's disease or infection. The distribution of disease is also important, making colonoscopic examination and biopsy essential in a difficult case. It is unusual to diagnose ischaemia from a rectal biopsy, except in the context of the 'mucosal prolapse syndrome' (Section 15.10).

Unlike ulcerative colitis and Crohn's disease, when attention is usually focused on the inflammatory element, in ischaemia the eye is first drawn to degenerative changes in the crypt cells and their impact on crypt pattern plus the staining quality of the lamina propria. The crypt changes may cause differential problems with pseudomembranous colitis when it is the upper halves of the crypts that are dilated and show epithelial loss (Fig. 8.9a). Confusion with other bacterial infections may occur when the whole crypt length is degenerate (Section 4.2.1). Coupled with damage to the crypts, there is also an increased eosinophilia and opacity within the lamina propria (Figs 8.9b and 12.8). This can be appreciated before the fibrosis of more

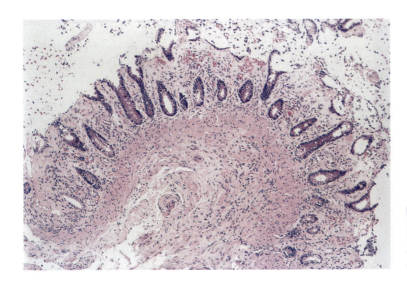

Figure 12.8 Ischaemic colitis illustrating the cryptal damage, limited inflammatory infiltrate and characteristic eosinophilic opacity of the background lamina propria.

chronic ischaemic damage. Although there is an increase in both acute and chronic inflammatory cells in ischaemia this is not a striking feature. Nuclear debris may be present and, of course, when the ischaemic damage is severe and acute, the mucosa becomes necrotic and replaced by a layer of debris and acute inflammatory cells. The differential here has already been discussed in relation to the Type III pattern of pseudomembranous colitis (Section 8.3).

It is rare to see a florid vasculitis in a biopsy, as it is usually too superficial. Capillary thrombi should be looked for but given guarded significance as a primary event if the mucosa is ulcerated (Section 10.8).

Overall, the acute ischaemic lesion is more likely to be confused with infective colitis and pseudomembranous colitis than ulcerative colitis or Crohn's disease.

In long-standing ischaemia, fibrosis of the lamina propria is the prominent feature. However, the re-epithelialization and healing of ischaemic ulceration often results in crypt distortion (Section 10.6.3), a point of potential confusion with ulcerative colitis. Inflammation will be muted in ischaemia at this stage, though of course this is also true of

ulcerative colitis in remission. Differentiation is helped by examination of the lamina propria which, in chronic ulcerative colitis, will only exceptionally be fibrotic and limited to a band immediately above the muscularis mucosae (Section 5.2.3b) (Fig. 5.14). Iron pigment in macrophages, when present, is an additional pointer to a diagnosis of ischaemia.

12.5.3 The solitary ulcer

In the differential diagnosis of an ischaemic biopsy, solitary ulcer, or the mucosal prolapse syndrome (Section 15.10), needs consideration (accepting that the pathogenesis of the solitary ulcer is prolapse, with consequential ischaemia). In addition to the points already made above, the presence of ramification of the muscularis mucosae within the lamina propria is a key feature in solitary ulcer (Figs 3.51 and 12.9). Superficial ectatic capillaries are also observed. Neither of these last two are diagnostic features of ulcerative colitis, Crohn's disease or infection. When seen, they suggest that the aetiology of any ischaemic biopsy is mucosal prolapse rather than a primary vascular event. Inflammation, if present, is seldom dominant, even adjacent to

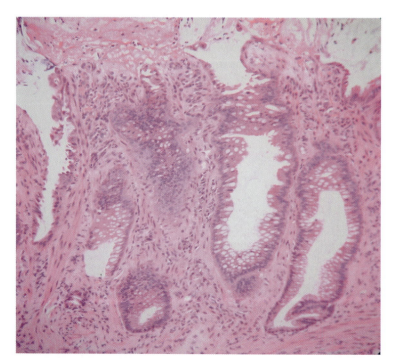

Figure 12.9 Part of a biopsy illustrating the solitary ulcer syndrome to show the ramification of muscle fibres from the muscularis mucosae into the lamina propria. They are seen alongside the degenerate crypt to the left of the picture. There is also surface erosion that could cause confusion with the early lesions of pseudomembranous colitis.

ulceration. It should be remembered that the clinical details may suggest a polyp, one form of presentation of mucosal prolapse (Sections 15.10 and 19.2.7), or even an obstructing carcinoma.

12.5.4 Diverticulitis

There is no one diagnostic biopsy picture that will allow an unequivocal conclusion of diverticular disease. On the other hand, there are several pitfalls

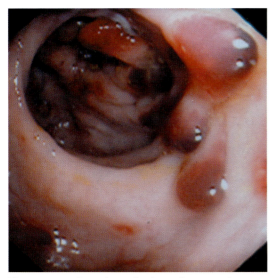

Figure 12.10 An endoscopic picture from a patient with florid diverticular disease demonstrating the redundant mucosa thrown up into polypoid projections, the histology from which can show features of prolapse and ischaemic change.

in attempting to make that diagnosis in biopsy practice. It was originally thought that only the mucosa of the diverticulum in diverticular disease becomes inflamed. However, it is now appreciated that a segmental colitis can exist, i.e. there is inflammation of the luminal mucosa between diverticula (Cawthorn *et al.*, 1983; Sladen and Filipe, 1984; Makapugay and Dean, 1996). Gore *et al.* (1992) draw attention to polypoid mucosa and prominent crescentic folds seen at endoscopy in the majority of cases (Fig. 12.10) and point out that biopsies from these areas can show a large range of appearances from merely mucosal congestion or features of mucosal prolapse to florid active inflammation that mimics ulcerative colitis. Ischaemia may be mimicked if there has been an element of prolapse while the occurrence of granulomatous cryptitis from crypt disruption can lead to a mistaken diagnosis of Crohn's disease (Makapugay and Dean, 1996). Indeed, in surgical excisions diverticulitis can show most of the hallmarks of Crohn's disease with granulomas, fissures and transmural inflammation (Gledhill and Dixon, 1998). To complicate the issue further genuine ulcerative colitis and Crohn's disease may be associated with diverticulitis (Shepherd, 1996).

The pathologist has to be aware of all of the above possibilities in order to construct a report appropriate with all known relevant clinical and radiological data. Moreover, when considering the diagnosis of segmental colitis (Fig. 12.11) caused by diverticular disease it is crucial to have received

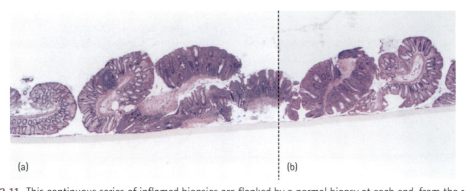

(a)   (b)

Figure 12.11 This continuous series of inflamed biopsies are flanked by a normal biopsy at each end, from the rectum in (a) and splenic flexure (b), respectively. For a diagnosis of segmental colitis the endoscopist must provide biopsies from above and below the affected area.

biopsies from above and below the colonoscopically documented segment. In the typical case this will mean biopsies from the rectum and the splenic flexure area.

12.5.5 Microscopic colitis – collagenous, lymphocytic and non-collagenous non-lymphocytic varieties

These entities are extensively described in Chapter 9. Only certain points are mentioned that impinge on the differential diagnosis with chronic inflammatory bowel disease.

There are now well documented cases of collagenous colitis and lymphocytic colitis predating and postdating a diagnosis of Crohn's disease or ulcerative colitis (Sections 9.3.1c and 9.3.2a) (Goldstein and Gyorfi, 1999; Pokorny *et al.*, 2001). The aetiopathogenesis of these relationships is unclear. Pseudomembranous and granulomatous patterns as variants of both main types of microscopic colitis have also been described (Yuan *et al.*, 2003; Saurine *et al.*, 2004). A further pitfall is that increased intra-epithelial lymphocytes can be an accompaniment of typical cases of both ulcerative colitis and Crohn's disease as well as a feature of drug-induced colitis, in particular non-steroidal anti-inflammatory drugs (Lee, 1994; Kitchen *et al.*, 2002; Goldstein and Bhanot, 2004). Such occurrence highlights the dangers of reporting biopsies in the absence of clinical information and out of context.

In the majority of cases there should be no difficulty in diagnosing either collagenous colitis or lymphocytic colitis. In both there will have been a history of watery diarrhoea and a normal colonoscopic examination and in both there will a comparatively mild colitis with regular crypt architecture. Collagenous colitis will show the characteristic thickened subepithelial collagen plate (Fig. 9.1) and lymphocytic colitis (Fig. 9.2) the characteristic increase in intra-epithelial lymphocytes. A diagnosis of non-collagenous non-lymphocytic colitis is more problematic (Section 9.3.6). The clinical criteria for microscopic colitis (Sections 9.2.1 and 9.2.5) must be met, otherwise the picture would warrant the label of colitis – currently type uncertain (Section 12.3.3b)

with the microscopy showing intact architecture, focal cryptitis and mild or moderate diffuse chronic inflammation. Non-steroidal anti-inflammatory drugs are frequently implicated (Lee, 1994; Kitchen *et al.*, 2002; Goldstein and Bhanot, 2004).

12.5.6 Minimal change colitis

To add to the confusion of similar-sounding terms, this is used to describe patients with biopsy features of ulcerative colitis or Crohn's disease, who have normal barium studies and sigmoidoscopy (Elliott *et al.*, 1982). Colonoscopic abnormalities are mild. The term's value is to remind clinicians that biopsies should be done despite normal radiology and sigmoidoscopy.

12.5.7 Acute self-limiting colitis (transient colitis)

This term is common in North America and in this book is synonymous with bacterial infectious colitis (Section 4.1) whether culture–positive or culture negative (Kumar *et al.*, 1982). It has also been termed 'transient colitis' by Mandal *et al.* (1982). By definition, in acute self-limiting colitis (ASLC) the mucosa returns swiftly to normal, with regression of symptoms. In addition to the classical infective picture (discussed in Chapter 4), the term has also been employed to cover unexplained, spontaneously resolving diarrhoeas in which the biopsy shows only non-specific inflammatory features (Section 12. 3.1) (Nostram *et al.*, 1987; Therkildsen *et al.*, 1989; Schumacher *et al.*, 1994a,b).

The problem of differentiation from chronic inflammatory bowel disease is covered in Section 4.2.5. While certain features such as cryptitis, crypt withering and a predominantly neutrophilic infiltrate in the lamina propria are positive pointers to the diagnosis of ASLC, the diagnosis is more frequently derived by noting the absence of findings that characterize chronic inflammatory bowel disease, in particular the absence of crypt architectural distortion. Part of the explanation for this relates to the speed with which the typical features of infection resolve and the time interval between the onset of symptoms and the patient presenting for biopsy.

12.5.8 Cathartic colon

Melanosis coli is the best clue to this diagnosis (Section 11.10) and in a classical case is accompanied by a thickened muscularis mucosae. Small numbers of inflammatory cells may be present, representing minor obstructive colitis (Section 13.6.2). Cathartic colon can only be diagnosed by exclusion following discussion with the clinician. However, it is doubtful whether this should still be considered a specific entity (Muller-Lissner, 1996; Muller-Lissner *et al.*, 2005).

12.5.9 Irritable bowel syndrome

A succinct '?IBS' is a frequent clinical history to accompany what is usually a 'succinct' rectal biopsy specimen, though practice is gradually changing to the provision of colonoscopic series in order to be able to exclude microscopic colitis. Biopsies are nearly always normal in this syndrome (Jenkins *et al.*, 1997a), but where there might be a post-infectious component a persisting minor increase in chronic inflammatory cells may be present (Spiller *et al.*, 2000).

12.5.10 Eosinophilic or allergic colitis

A pathologist's attention is drawn to this diagnosis by noting a dominance of eosinophils in the biopsies (Fig. 12.12). In very young infants, nearly always less than 1 year of age, allergic proctocolitis is a well-recognized entity and among the commonest causes of diarrhoea and rectal bleeding in this age group (Goldman and Proujansky, 1986; Odze *et al.*, 1993b). It is related to intolerance to human or cow's milk protein. Apart from infiltration of the mucosa by eosinophils there are no other significant histological abnormalities. Eosinophils should be seen in the lamina propria, infiltrating crypts and surface epithelium, plus penetrating the muscularis mucosae. The eosinophil count (Winter *et al.*, 1990) should be at least six per high-power field (HPF) and in the study by Odze *et al.* (1993b) the average was 15.6 eosinophils per HPF. These

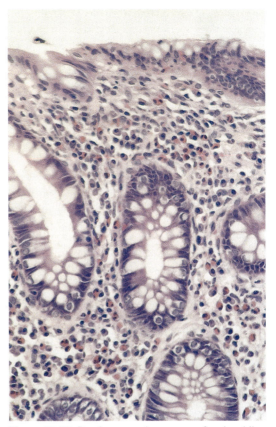

Figure 12.12 Dominance and an excess of eosinophils infiltrating the lamina propria are required for a diagnosis of eosinophilic colitis. This biopsy is from a child with allergic eosinophilic colitis. (Courtesy of Professor P. Domizio.)

authors stress the patchy nature of the infiltrate within and between biopsies. The condition resolves following exclusion of the offending milk protein.

In adults, infiltration of the gastrointestinal tract by eosinophils, and eosinophilic colitis in particular, is part of the spectrum of eosinophilic gastroenteritis. As a disease, eosinophilic gastroenteritis is most common in the third and sixth decades. Only between 50 and 70 per cent of patients will give a history of allergy (Blackshaw and Levison, 1986; Tally *et al.*, 1990) and a peripheral eosinophilia is so variable that Tally *et al.* (1990) did not include it in their criteria for the diagnosis. Any region or layer of the gut may be involved, together or separately, forming the basis for a classification (Klein *et al.*, 1970). Naturally, a biopsy will detect those with mucosal involvement and, where deep enough, submucosal disease. The commonest sites of involvement are the stomach and small intestine. Colonic involvement is rare such that in 1985 Naylor and Pollett could only identify 22 cases in the literature. In the 40 cases reported by Tally *et al.* (1990) two of the five patients in whom colonic biopsies were taken had infiltration, while five of six in whom ileal surgical material was examined showed infiltration. When the colon is involved it is mainly the right side (Naylor and Pollett, 1985). The diagnosis on biopsy is made purely by observing a large number of eosinophils in the mucosa and submucosa, including oedema of the latter, if included. Because eosinophils can be increased in several inflammatory bowel diseases, such as Crohn's disease, ulcerative colitis, drug-induced colitis and parasitic diseases, a confident diagnosis can only be made if the increase in eosinophils is florid. It must also be appreciated that the normal complement of eosinophils in the lamina propria can show considerable geographical variation (Pascal and Gramlich, 1993). There should be infiltration of the epithelium, eosinophilic cryptitis and crypt abscess formation along with infiltration of the muscularis mucosae and submucosa. It may also be possible to demonstrate an increase in mast cells (Al-Haddad and Riddell, 2005) and IgE-containing plasma cells (Rosekrans *et al.*, 1980b). The eosinophilic infiltrate dominates the picture and signs of other inflammatory diseases are absent, in particular the crypt architecture remains intact, no worms are identified and no eggs or larvae seen. It is important to appreciate that eosinophilic gastroenteritis is a patchy disease and normal mucosa can be seen alongside infiltrated mucosa. Moreover, the mucosal layer may not be involved at all, in which case biopsy will fail to establish the diagnosis.

An interesting variant called pericryptal eosinophilic gastroenteritis has been described by Clouse *et al.* (1992) in which a clinical picture resembling microscopic colitis (Section 9.2.1) is present: that is, watery diarrhoea and normal colonoscopy. The biopsies reveal a pericryptal excess of eosinophils limited to the base of crypts and the area between the crypt bases and the muscularis mucosae. 50 per cent of these cases had an accompanying connective tissue disorder.

12.5.11 Radiation-induced colitis

Clinicians frequently omit the key piece of information, that there has been previous radiotherapy. One possible reason for this might be the gap between the therapy and the onset of colitis. This can be many years. Without recognizing some telangiectasia, hyalinization of the lamina propria, thickened vessels or atypical fibroblasts the diagnosis cannot be made, as the inflammatory component is not characteristic (Fig. 11.1). Crypt irregularity may mimic ulcerative colitis (Fig. 11.2) and be misinterpreted if the connective tissue abnormalities are minimal (Section 11.1).

12.5.12 Immunodeficiency states

12.5.12a Acquired immunodeficiency syndrome

The best clue to the syndrome is to identify an opportunistic pathogen in the biopsy such as cytomegalovirus, cryptosporidia species, *Mycobacterium avium-intracellulare* or adenovirus, though cytomegalovirus and cryptosporidia can occur in non-acquired immune-deficiency syndrome (AIDS), immunocompetent individuals (Chapter 4). Diarrhoea and colitis also occur in patients who are human immunodeficiency-virus (HIV) positive but do not yet fulfil the criteria for AIDS. Organisms may be absent (Kotler *et al.*, 1984). The biopsy, although it may be normal, often shows a nonspecific infiltrate of chronic inflammatory cells, some neutrophils and with the architecture still well maintained. Clues to considering such a diagnosis can be a slight increase in intra-epithelial lymphocytes, apoptotic bodies in the bases of crypts and increased numbers of mast cells (Section 4.4.4) (Kotler *et al.*, 1986). The picture has some resemblance to graft-versus-host disease (Section 11.6).

12.5.12b Common variable immunodeficiency

In patients with hypogammaglobulinaemia diminished numbers of plasma cells in the presence of mild acute inflammation and a few incipient crypt abscesses should draw attention to the diagnosis. There can also be an increase in apoptotic bodies and a mild increase in intraepithelial lymphocytes, though well below the numbers seen in lympho-cytic colitis (Washington *et al.*, 1996; personal observations). The picture must be interpreted in context, as drug-induced colitis, graft-versus-host disease and HIV infection result in similar abnormalities.

12.5.13 Graft-versus-host disease

The history and the diagnostic focal 'exploding crypt' are the pointers to this diagnosis (Sections 3.6.3 and 11.6). The main problem for pathologists is during the first 20 days post-graft when the biopsy features cannot be distinguished from the proctitis produced by the drugs given to produce immunological tolerance (Section 11.6).

12.5.14 Drug-induced disease (excluding antibiotics)

The principal biopsy clues that might initiate con-sideration of a primary drug-induced colitis, while by no means specific, are increased apoptosis, increased intra-epithelial lymphocytes, an increase in eosinophils (Section 11.4.3) and melanosis. In clinical context this combination of features should raise the possibility of drug-induced pathology. The relevant information is not always easily obtained, partly owing to widespread 'over-counter' sales, especially of drugs such as the non-steroidal anti-inflammatory agents (NSAIDs). Patients might not even consider these as drugs. As described in Section 11.4 a wide variety of intestinal patholo-gies can be precipitated by drugs, among these are all the varieties of microscopic colitis, occlusive ischaemia, vasculitides and focal patterns of inflammation that are readily misinterpreted as Crohn's disease. The chemotherapeutic and anti-mitotic drugs can result in bizarre epithelial cell nuclear changes in the crypts, which in the absence of clinical details, may be confused with the regen-erative mucosa of ulcerative colitis and even with dysplasia. They may also precipitate neutropenic colitis. Immunosuppressive agents can be the basis

for infectious colitis. Indeed, whenever confronted with difficulties in what should be a straightfor-ward diagnostic problem the modifying role of drugs should be carefully considered.

12.5.15 Connective tissue disorders

The colitis seen in the course of systemic lupus erythematosus, rheumatoid arthritis, scleroderma or polyarteritis is related to vascular pathology and attention should be directed to the changes of ischaemia, care being taken to examine small ves-sels in the submucosa (Sections 10.8 and 20.1.2). An ileocaecitis has been documented in patients with reactive arthritis. Some of these cases are indistinguishable from Crohn's disease (Sections 12.6.3c and 20.1.2).

12.6 THE TERMINAL ILEAL BIOPSY

In the investigation of chronic inflammatory bowel disease an ileal biopsy usually accompanies a colonoscopic biopsy series. Its main purpose is to provide evidence to help in the distinction of Crohn's disease from ulcerative colitis. The prin-ciples, appreciation and interpretation of the micro-scopic features are little different from those outlined for the colonic mucosa throughout the book (Cuvelier *et al.*, 2001). There are very few conditions in which an ileal biopsy would be the primary investigative procedure.

12.6.1 The normal biopsy

Normal ileal mucosa has well-formed villi that are shorter than those in the proximal small intestine and often bent. The villus epithelium comprises absorptive cells and goblet cells while in the crypts there are Paneth cells and a variety of enterochro-maffin cells. The lamina propria, like that of the colonic mucosa, has a background 'physiological' infiltrate of inflammatory cells which are mainly plasma cells and lymphocytes, with some mast cells, macrophages, occasional neutrophils and

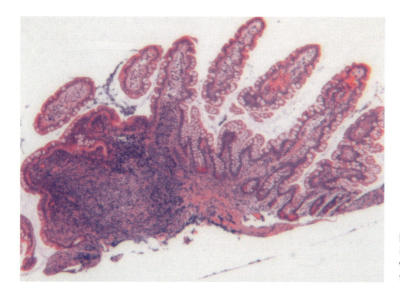

Figure 12.13 A normal terminal ileal biopsy with tall, well-formed villi and a prominent lymphoid follicle.

small numbers of eosinophils. Major components of the ileal mucosa are the lymphoid follicles (Peyer's patches) and the overlying follicle-associated epithelium (Fig. 12.13). The latter include M-cells (membranous or microfold cells) (Cuvelier *et al.*, 2001) that play an important role in antigen uptake. The follicles may straddle the muscularis mucosae. A small number of CD8-positive intraepithelial lymphocytes are present in the villi with quoted means ranging from 2 to 8 per cent (Sapp *et al.*, 2002; Padmanabhan *et al.*, 2003). This is well below the number found in the proximal small intestine.

12.6.2 The inflamed biopsy

12.6.2a Acute ileitis

In acute ileitis polymorphonuclear leukocytes and eosinophils dominate, infiltrating the villous epithelium and crypts. There may also be oedema causing some swelling of the villi (Fig. 12.14). Plasma cells may be increased in the lamina propria especially as the acute phase subsides. The cryptal architecture remains intact but ulceration can occur and follicular hyperplasia is common. The most frequent causes of acute ileitis are the intestinal bacterial pathogens such as *Salmonella* spp., *Shigella* spp. and *Campylobacter* spp. Common causes in some countries, in which the primary disease can be the terminal ileum, are yersiniosis (Section 4.2.7a)

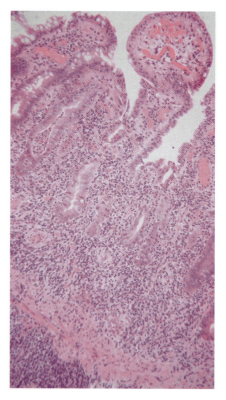

Figure 12.14 Acute ileitis from a case of shigellosis. The villi are blunted and oedematous with acute inflammatory cells infiltrating the lamina propria. Crypt abscesses and reactive epithelial changes are also seen in the villi.

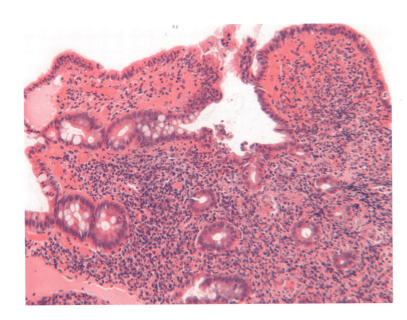

Figure 12.15 Chronic ileitis showing a heavy chronic inflammatory cell infiltrate in the lamina propria and some villous blunting.

and tuberculosis (Section 4.2.7b). The picture of acute ileitis *per se* is non-specific and must be interpreted alongside the pathology elsewhere in the gastrointestinal tract and in the clinical context.

12.6.2b Chronic ileitis

In chronic ileitis the ileal biopsy shows crypt architectural damage, such as villous atrophy and crypt branching. The lamina propria is expanded by increased numbers of plasma cells and lymphocytes (Fig. 12.15). Ulcer-associated lineage cells can be prominent reflecting the healing of prior ulceration. An acute inflammatory component may still be evident along with current ulceration, the former signifying active chronic disease. As Crohn's disease is one of the commonest causes of chronic ileitis a careful search for granulomas, microgranulomas and giant cells should be made with yields being improved by cutting additional levels into the biopsy as for colonic biopsies (Section 6.3.3).

12.6.2c Aphthous and 'incidental' ulceration

Aphthoid ulcers are small erosions visible on endoscopy (Fig. 12.16) and are small breaks in the epithelium usually in M-cell areas (Cuvelier *et al.*, 1994) over lymphoid follicles. They are associated with a fibrinous exudate and a superficial infiltrate

of neutrophil polymorphs. They were originally believed to be a diagnostic sign of early Crohn's disease (Rickert and Carter, 1980) (Section 6.3.4) but it is now appreciated that small foci of terminal ileal ulceration can be associated with some drugs, in particular non-steroidal anti-inflammatory agents (Lee, 1994; Schneider *et al.*, 1999) (Section 11.4.4).

Terminal ileal isolated aphthoid ulceration is now also an increasingly recognized incidental finding during colonoscopic investigation of non-inflammatory conditions such as polyp follow-up protocols, in the course of which the ileum is inspected as part of the routine. Our experience with biopsies from these lesions is that the actual erosion is seldom apparent (Fig. 12.17) but represented by small clusters of neutrophil polymorphs infiltrating the epithelium, either over follicles or towards the tips of adjacent villi. There have been few formal studies of these incidental isolated aphthoid lesions but the likelihood is that the majority reflect subclinical infections or are drug-related. Goldstein (2005) found that 29 per cent developed ileocolonic Crohn's disease and 14 per cent were ingesting NSAIDs.

12.6.3 Interpretation of the inflamed ileal biopsy

The preceding descriptions of acute and chronic ileitis are non-diagnostic and the role of ileal biopsy,

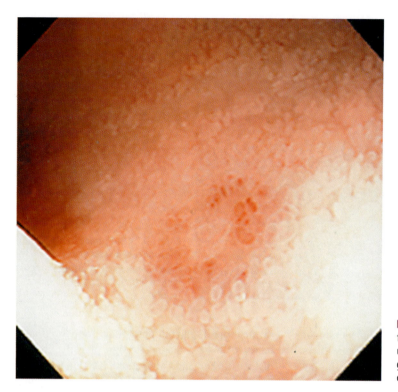

Figure 12.16 The endoscopic features of incidental aphthoid ulceration. The adjacent mucosa gave no suggestion of any more extensive or specific disease process.

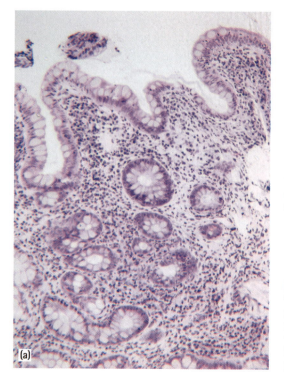

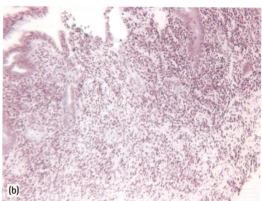

Figure 12.17 These two biopsies illustrate what can be found in biopsies taken from aphthoid ulcers such as those seen in Fig. 12.16. (a) There is minimal damage represented by some cryptitis with neutrophils infiltrating the crypts in the centre of the field. (b) There is a more obvious acute inflammatory cell infiltrate in the superficial half of the mucosa with disruption of the surface.

for the most part, is very much an adjunct to the interpretation of any coexisting colonic pathology. Some perspective of its value can be gained from two studies which looked at slightly different cohorts of patients. Geboes *et al.* (1998) report on a series of 257 patients thought to have chronic inflammatory bowel disease. Ileal biopsy was considered essential to the diagnosis in 15 and contributory in 53. Of 123 in whom the colon was normal ileal disease was found in 44. The authors concluded that the main indication for ileal biopsy in this clinical group was if the colon was normal and in the differential diagnosis of a pancolitis or predominantly left-sided colitis. In the broader based study by Shah *et al.* (2001) of patients with chronic diarrhoea 83 ileal biopsies were available from a cohort of 168 patients. The biopsy was helpful in five (6 per cent) and diagnostic in two (one was a case of Crohn's disease and the other a case of cytomegalovirus). A careful drug history should be taken whenever ileal inflammation or ulceration is present and the clinical data do not indicate chronic inflammatory bowel disease or infection.

12.6.3a Crohn's disease and ulcerative colitis

In the limited context of chronic inflammatory bowel disease inflammation in a mucosal biopsy from the distal 10–15 cm of terminal ileum may represent Crohn's disease or backwash ileitis in ulcerative colitis (Section 12.7). In clinical practice, post-colectomy cases apart (Section 12.7.2), this is seldom a problem faced in isolation as there will be an accompanying series of colonic biopsies that provide additional clues. Thus, a normal colonic series, or one with rectosigmoid disease only and a biopsy showing active chronic ileitis, is evidence to support Crohn's disease. The same biopsy in the presence of diffuse pancolitis with crypt architectural distortion would be reported as backwash ileitis in support of a diagnosis of ulcerative colitis. In less obvious circumstances a confident diagnosis of Crohn's disease has to depend on identifying a granuloma and the same caveats apply as in the colon (Section 6.3.3), in particular appreciating that inflammatory crypt damage, of whatever cause, can result in crypt-associated granulomas

(Mahadeva *et al.*, 2002) (Fig. 5.8). Furthermore, the less well-delineated clusters of epithelioid histiocytes referred to as microgranulomas (Rotterdam *et al.*, 1997) occur in a large proportion of biopsies from patients with spondyloarthropathy and ileitis (Cuvelier *et al.*, 1987). Well-formed granulomas are seen in cases of *Yersinia pseudotuberculosis* though not in *Yersinia enterocolitica* (Section 4.2.7a) and of course in tuberculosis (Section 4.2.7b). In tuberculosis caseation may be present and the granulomas can be confluent while in Crohn's disease they remain discrete. In yersiniosis a diagnostic clue can be found in any follicles in the biopsy which may contain a central microabscess. A pitfall to be wary of in limited distal left-sided disease is the presence of a skip lesion in ulcerative colitis in which there is associated ileocaecal inflammation (Section 5.5.2a).

As mentioned above, the inflammatory picture of the backwash ileitis of ulcerative colitis is nonspecific and can only be interpreted in the clinical context. A related problem is the inflammatory pathology to be found in the neoterminal ileum after surgery, be it for ulcerative colitis, proximal to an ileostomy for whatever cause (Section 12.7.2) or in an ileal pouch (Section 7.5).

12.6.3b Microscopic colitis – lymphocytic colitis and collagenous colitis – ileal villous mucosal atrophy

The terminal ileum can occasionally be involved as part of lymphocytic and collagenous colitis (Section 9.3.4a), an abnormal intra-epithelial lymphocyte count or a thickened collagen plate being recognized according to the variety of microscopic colitis present.

A pattern of total ileal villous mucosal atrophy has been described (Marteau *et al.*, 1997) as a primary defect and also in association with both main forms of microscopic colitis (Fig. 12.18). Its aetiopathogenesis is unclear but bile salt malabsorption is not responsible as an ileal biopsy is usually normal in this situation (Sciarretta *et al.*, 1994; Fernandez-Banares *et al.*, 2001).

12.6.3c Reactive arthritis

The features of chronic ileitis may be found in terminal ileal biopsies from patients with reactive

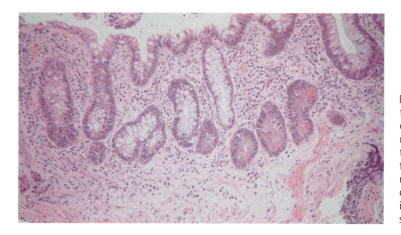

Figure 12.18 A flat ileal biopsy from a patient with microscopic colitis (lymphocytic variety). It is a rare occurrence and, in this case, the biopsy could easily be mistaken for colonic mucosa. It is only the number of Paneth cells and the clinician's conviction that the ileum was biopsied that allows such a conclusion.

arthritis and ankylosing spondylitis (Cuvelier *et al.*, 1987) but not in those with rheumatoid arthritis. Ill-defined granulomas may be seen leading to difficulty in totally excluding Crohn's disease, which itself is associated with an increased incidence of arthropathy. In the series of Cuvelier *et al.* (1987) only 27 per cent of patients with spondyloarthropathy and ileal inflammation had gastrointestinal symptoms.

12.7 BACKWASH ILEITIS AND ILEAL COMPLICATIONS OF ULCERATIVE COLITIS

12.7.1 Backwash ileitis

Backwash ileitis is the term given to inflammation of the terminal ileum found in 10–20 per cent of patients with ulcerative colitis and believed to be due to reflux of colonic contents through a dilated and incompetent ileocaecal valve. Thus, it is more commonly seen in total colitis, though Haskell *et al.* (2005) document it in a small number of cases with subtotal and left-sided colitis, while in other studies it is documented without contiguous ileocaecal involvement (Geboes *et al.*, 1998). This might infer that backwash was not the sole pathogenesis. It often involves up to 25 cm of the terminal ileum. A biopsy will show the features of active chronic ileitis with a combination of villous blunting, crypt distortion and a mixed inflammatory cell infiltrate

in the lamina propria. There are no diagnostic features and, in general, the severity mirrors that of the accompanying colitis (Haskell *et al.*, 2005).

The importance of backwash ileitis is to avoid making a mistaken diagnosis of Crohn's disease. Whether or not it is also an indicator of the risk of developing pouchitis is disputed, with some series showing a correlation (Schimdt *et al.*, 1998; Abdelrazeq *et al.*, 2005), others not (Gustavsson *et al.*, 1987; Haskell *et al.*, 2005). There is one claim of an association of backwash ileitis with cancer in colitis but this too is contentious (Heuschen *et al.*, 2001; Kaiser, 2002; Rutter *et al.*, 2004; Haskell *et al.*, 2005).

12.7.2 Ileal pathology following colectomy

It is now appreciated that the ileum, in patients with undisputed ulcerative colitis be it in an ileoanal pouch (Goldstein *et al.*, 1997), in the neoterminal ileum proximal to a pouch (Bell *et al.*, 2006), in the ileum proximal to a stoma or to an ileoanal anastomosis (Hallak *et al.*, 1994), can show a range of inflammatory features closely resembling Crohn's disease. The pathology of pouchitis is covered in Section 7.5. Several authors (Romero, 2004; Rubenstein *et al.*, 2004) document such changes in up to 80 cm of ileum in these post-colectomy situations. Endoscopically nodular mucosa and even serpiginous ulceration can be seen closely mimicking Crohn's disease. Biopsies reveal active chronic ileitis but granulomas are not reported. However close might be the resemblance to Crohn's disease it is important to review the original pathology of the excised colon and not to change the diagnosis solely on the basis of the post-surgical ileal pathology.

12.8 ILEAL NODULAR LYMPHOID HYPERPLASIA

Lymphoid nodules (Peyer's patches) are a normal component of the terminal ileal mucosa (Fig. 12.13; Section 12.6.1) and are most prominent in childhood. Nodular lymphoid hyperplasia is therefore predominantly a diagnostic problem of paediatric biopsy practice. The basis for such hyperplasia is poorly understood, but given the role of Peyer's patches in antigen uptake from the gut lumen, it is likely an antigenic response has a major role (Kokkonen and Karttunen, 2002).

As lymphoid nodules are frequently part of a normal ileal biopsy it is a difficult judgement for a pathologist to decide on mild degrees of hyperplasia in any individual biopsy specimen (Fig. 12.19). This is probably best appreciated macroscopically by the endoscopist. Normal lymphoid nodules appear yellow-white and up to 2 mm in diameter. At the extreme end of the spectrum, with florid hyperplasia present, the ileal lumen can become occluded by mucosal polypoid projections with the accompanying risks of intussusception and obstruction (Atwell et al., 1985; Hasegawa et al., 1998). Such a picture can occasionally occur in adults (Rubin and Isaacson, 1990).

The hyperplastic nodules show prominent germinal centres and tingible body macrophages but it is inadvisable to make a diagnosis of nodular hyperplasia on microscopy if only a single nodule is seen in a biopsy. At least two or three are required, preferably becoming confluent, to suggest such a diagnosis. This should also be backed up by the appropriate endoscopic appearances. In the majority of instances of nodular lymphoid hyperplasia there are no other mucosal abnormalities present and it is assumed that most cases are the response to infection. In children food allergy also plays an important role (Kokkonen and Karttunen, 2002), in which case mucosal eosinophils can be prominent (Machida et al., 1994). Lymphoid nodular hyperplasia is also a feature of immunodeficiency disorders (Washington et al., 1996; Webster et al., 1997).

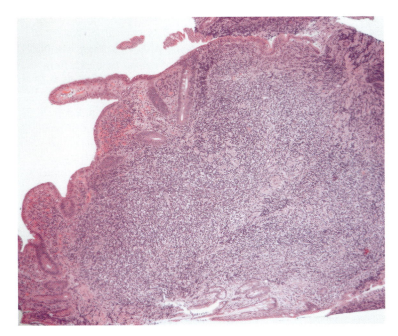

Figure 12.19 Prominent lymphoid follicles distorting the mucosa in a terminal ileal biopsy. However, deciding whether this represents true hyperplasia or merely part of the normal spectrum can only be done in conjunction with the endoscopic features.

In adults the presence of any associated inflammation brings the many causes of inflammatory bowel disease covered in this chapter into the differential diagnosis.

There has been considerable recent debate concerning the relationship of ileal lymphoid nodular hyperplasia, accompanying intestinal tract pathology and the autistic spectrum disorder. Such association originated with the suggestion that the measles/mumps/rubella triple vaccine played a role in the aetiology of the autism (Wakefield *et al.*, 1998) but most of the epidemiological data have so far failed to support this (Taylor *et al.*, 2002). However, it is still claimed that children with autistic spectrum disorder do have ileal lymphoid nodular hyperplasia and accompanying low-grade ileocolonic inflammatory changes. Indeed, Wakefield *et al.* (2005) report that isolated lymphoid nodular hyperplasia in the absence of any other inflammatory abnormalities in the intestine is very rare, being present in less than 3 per cent of their 178 children with autistic spectrum disorder. If these findings are confirmed by others, then identifying the additional changes in suspected cases will be an important part of deciding whether any apparent lymphoid nodular hyperplasia is pathological or not. However, many of these children suffer coexisting dietary problems. This, alongside the difficulties in obtaining suitable paediatric control material for the necessary studies and the problem of observer variation when considering minor alterations in mucosal inflammatory cell numbers, has ensured that the part played by nodular lymphoid hyperplasia and any ileo-colitis in the autistic spectrum disorder remains a contentious issue (Jass, 2005).

12.9 CONCLUSIONS

Careful study of a biopsy yields a list of histological signs. Some attempt has been made in this chapter to evaluate their relevance to allow a diagnostic statement about their sum. On many occasions this will not get beyond a 'non-specific proctitis/colitis'. This term is of little clinical value and alternative nomenclature is suggested. However, semantics aside, in all cases an attempt should be made to inform the clinician of the possibilities and probabilities having first taken account of the clinical context of the case.

REFERENCES

Abdelrazeq, A.S., Wilson, T.R., Leitch, D.L., Lund, J.N., Leveson, S.H. (2005) Ileitis in ulcerative colitis: is it backwash? *Dis. Colon Rectum*, 48, 2038–46.

Al-Haddad, S., Riddell, R.H. (2005) The role of eosinophils in inflammatory bowel disease. *Gut*, 54, 1674–5.

Atwell, J.D., Burge, D., Wright, D. (1985) Nodular lymphoid hyperplasia of the intestinal tract in infancy and childhood. *J. Pediatr. Surg.*, 20, 25–9.

Balkien, K., Brandtzaeg, P. (1975) Comparative mapping of the local distribution of immunoglobulin-containing cells in ulcerative colitis and Crohn's disease of the colon. *Clin. Exp. Immunol.*, 22, 197–209.

Bell, A., Price, A.B., Forbes, A., Ciclititra, P.J., Groves, C., Nicholls, R.J. (2006) Pre-pouch ileitis: a disease of the ileum in ulcerative colitis after restorative proctocolectomy. *Colorectal Dis.*, 8, 402–10.

Bentley, E., Jenkins, D., Campbell, F., Warren, B. (2002) How could pathologists improve the initial diagnosis of colitis? Evidence from an international workshop. *J. Clin. Pathol.*, 56, 955–60.

Bernstein, C.N., Shanahan, F., Anton, P.A., Weinstein, W.M. (1995) Patchiness of mucosal inflammation in treated ulcerative colitis: a prospective study. *Gastrointest. Endosc.*, 42, 232–7.

Blackshaw, A.W., Levison, D.A. (1986) Eosinophilic infiltrates of the gastrointestinal tract. *J. Clin. Pathol.*, 39, 1–7.

Cawthorn, S.J., Gibbs, N.M., Marks, C.G. (1983) Segmental colitis: a new complication of diverticular disease. *Gut*, 24, A500 (Abstract).

Clouse, R.E., Alpers, D.H., Hockenbery, D.M., DeSchryver-Keeskemeti, K. (1992) Pericrypt eosinophilic enterocolitis and chronic diarrhoea. *Gastroenterology*, 103, 168–76.

Cook, M.G., Dixon, M.F. (1973) An analysis of the reliability of detection and diagnostic value of various pathological features in Crohn's disease and ulcerative colitis. *Gut*, 14, 255–62.

Cuvelier, C., Barbatis, C., Mielants, H., De Vos, M., Roels, H., Veys, E. (1987) Histopathology of intestinal inflammation related to reactive arthritis. *Gut*, 394, 401.

Cuvelier, C.A., Quatacker, J., Mielants, H., De Vos, M., Veys, E., Roels, H.L. (1994) M-cells are damaged and increased in numbers in inflamed human ileal mucosa. *Histopathology*, 24, 417–26.

Cuvelier, C., Demetter, P., Mielants, H., Veys, E.M., De Vos, M. (2001) Interpretation of ileal biopsies: morphological features in normal and diseased mucosa. *Histopathology*, 38, 1–12.

Day, D.W., Mandal, B.K., Morson, B.C. (1978) The rectal biopsy appearances in *Salmonella* colitis. *Histopathology*, 2, 117–31.

Dayton, M.T., Larsen, K.R., Christianson, D.D. (2002) Similar functional results and complications after ileal pouch anastomosis in patients with indeterminate colitis vs. ulcerative colitis. *Arch. Surg.*, 137, 690–4.

Dickinson, R.J., Gilmour, H.M., McClelland, D.B.L. (1979) Rectal biopsy in patients presenting to an infectious disease unit with diarrhoeal disease. *Gut*, 20, 141–8.

Driman, D.K., Preiksaitis, H.G. (1998) Colorectal inflammation and increased cell proliferation associated with oral sodium phosphate bowel preparation. *Hum. Pathol.*, 29, 972–8.

Dronfield, M.W., Fletcher, J., Langman, M.J.S. (1974) Coincident *Salmonella* infections and ulcerative colitis: problems of recognition and management. *Br. Med. J.*, 1, 99–100.

Dundas, S.A., Dutton, J., Skipworth, P. (1997) Reliability of rectal biopsy in distinguishing between chronic inflammatory bowel disease and acute self-limiting colitis. *Histopathology*, 331, 60–6.

Elliott, P.R., Williams, C.B., Lennard-Jones, J.E. *et al.* (1982) Colonoscopic diagnosis of minimal change colitis in patients with a normal sigmoidoscopy and normal air–contrast barium enema. *Lancet*, i, 650–1.

Farmer, M., Petras, R.E., Hunter, L.E., Janosky, J.E., Galandiuk, S. (2000) The importance of diagnostic accuracy in colonic inflammatory bowel disease. *Am. J. Gastroenterol.*, 95, 3184–8.

Fernandez-Banares, F., Esteve, M., Salas, A., Forne, M., Espinos, J.C., Martin-Comin, J., Viver, J.M. (2001) Bile acid malabsorption in microscopic colitis and in unexplained functional chronic diarrhoea. *Dig. Dis. Sci.*, 46, 2231–38.

Geboes, K., Dalle, I. (2002) Influence of treatment on morphological features of mucosal inflammation. *Gut*, 50 (Suppl. 3), III 37–42.

Geboes, K., Villanacci, V. (2005) Terminology for the diagnosis of colitis. *J. Clin. Pathol.*, 58, 1133–4.

Geboes, K., Ectors, N., D'Haens, G., Rutgeerts, P. (1998) Is ileoscopy with biopsy worthwhile in patients presenting with symptoms of inflammatory bowel disease. *Am. J. Gastroenterol.*, 93, 201–6.

Geboes, K., Joossens, S., Prantera, C., Rutgeerts, P. (2003) Indeterminate colitis in clinical practice. *Curr. Diagn. Pathol.*, 9, 179–87.

Giard, R.W.M., Hermans, J., Rutter, D.J., Hoedemaeker, P.J. (1985) Variations in histopathological evaluation of non-neoplastic colonic mucosal abnormalities; assessment and clinical significance. *Histopathology*, 9, 535–41.

Gledhill, A., Dixon, M.F. (1998) Crohn's-like reaction in diverticular disease. *Gut*, 42, 392–5.

Glickman, J.N., Bousvaros, A., Farraye, F.A. *et al.* (2004) Pediatric patients with untreated ulcerative colitis may present initially with unusual morphological findings. *Am. J. Surg. Pathol.*, 28, 190–7.

Goldman, H. (1994) Interpretation of large intestinal mucosal biopsy specimens. *Hum. Pathol.*, 25, 1150–9.

Goldman, H., Proujansky, R. (1986) Allergic proctitis and gastroenteritis in children. *Am. J. Surg. Pathol.*, 10, 75–86.

Goldstein, N.S. (2005) Clinicopathologic significance of isolated aphthous erosions, a long-term follow-up study. *Mod. Pathol.*, 18 (Suppl. 1), 104A.

Goldstein, N.S., Bhanot, P. (2004) Paucicellular and asymptomatic lymphocytic colitis; Expanding the clinicopathologic spectrum of lymphocytic colitis. *Am. J. Clin. Pathol.*, 122, 405–11.

Goldstein, N.S., Gyorfi, T. (1999) Focal lymphocytic colitis and collagenous colitis: patterns of Crohn's colitis. *Am. J. Surg. Pathol.*, 23, 1075–81.

Goldstein, N.S., Sandford, W.W., Bodzin, J.H. (1997) Crohn's-like complications in patients with ulcerative colitis after total proctocolectomy and ileal pouch–anal anastomosis. *Am. J. Surg. Pathol.*, 21, 1343–53.

Gore, S., Shepherd, N.A., Wilkinson, S.P. (1992) Endoscopic crescentic fold disease of the sigmoid colon: the clinical and histopathological spectrum of a distinctive endoscopic appearance. *Int. J. Colorectal Dis.*, 7, 76–81.

Greenson, J.K., Stern, R.A., Carpenter, S.I., Barnett, J.L. (1997) The clinical significance of focal active colitis. *Hum. Pathol.*, 28, 729–33.

Greenson, J.K., Barnett, J.L., Stern, R.A. (1998) Active focal colitis. *Hum. Pathol.*, 29, 888 (Corr.).

Guindi, M., Riddell, R.H. (2004) Indeterminate colitis. *J. Clin. Pathol.*, 57, 1233–44.

Gustavsson, S., Weiland, L.H., Kelly, K.A. (1987) Relationship of backwash ileitis to ileal pouchitis after ileal pouch–anal anastomosis. *Dis. Colon Rectum*, 30, 25–8.

Hallak, A., Baratz, M., Santo, M., Halpern, Z., Rabau, M., Werbin, N., Gilat, T. (1994) Ileitis after colectomy for ulcerative colitis or carcinoma. *Gut*, 35, 373–6.

Harries, A.D., Myers, B., Cook, C.C. (1985) Inflammatory bowel disease: a common cause of bloody diarrhoea in visitors to the tropics. *Br. Med. J.*, 291, 1686–7.

Hasegawa, T., Ueda, S., Tazuke, Y. *et al.* (1998) Colonoscopic diagnosis of lymphoid hyperplasia causing recurrent intussusception: report of a case. *Surg. Today*, 28, 301–4.

Haskell, H., Andrews, C.W. Jr, Reddy, S.I. *et al.* (2005) Pathological features and clinical significance of 'backwash' ileitis in ulcerative colitis. *Am. J. Surg. Pathol.*, 29, 1472–81.

Heatley, R.V., Rhodes, J., Calcraft, B.J., Whitehead, R.H., Fifield, R., Newcombe, R.C. (1975) Immunoglobulin E in rectal mucosa of patients with proctitis. *Lancet*, ii, 1010–12.

Heresbach, D., Alexandre, J.L., Branger, B. *et al.* (2005) Frequency and significance of granulomas in a cohort of incident cases of Crohn's disease. *Gut*, 54, 215–22.

Heuschen, U.A., Hinz, U., Allemeyer, E.H. *et al.* (2001) Backwash ileitis is strongly associated with colorectal carcinoma in ulcerative colitis. *Gastroenterology*, 122, 245–6.

Jass, J.R. (2005) The intestinal lesion of autistic spectrum disorder. *Eur. J. Gastroenterol. Hepatol.*, 17, 821–2.

Jenkins, D., Goodall, A., Scott, B.B. (1997a) Simple objective criteria for diagnosis of causes of acute diarrhoea on rectal biopsy. *J. Clin. Pathol.*, 50, 580–5.

Jenkins, D., Balsitis, M., Gallivan, S. *et al.* (1997b) Guidelines for the initial biopsy diagnosis of suspected chronic inflammatory bowel disease. The British Society of Gastoenterology Initiative. *J. Clin. Pathol.*, 50, 93–105.

Jewkes, J., Larson, H.E., Price, A.B., Sanderson, P.J., Davies, H.A. (1981) Aetiology of acute diarrhoea in adults. *Gut*, 22, 388–92.

Joossens, S., Reinisch, W., Vermeire, S. *et al.* (2002) The value of serologic markers in indeterminate colitis: a prospective follow-up study. *Gastroenterology*, 122, 1242–7.

Kaiser, A.M. (2002) Discussion of 'Backwash ileitis is strongly associated with colorectal carcinoma in ulcerative colitis'. *Gastroenterology*, 120, 245–6.

Keren, D.F., Appelman, H.D., Dobbins, W.O. *et al.* (1984) Correlation of histopathologic evidence of disease activity with the presence of immunoglobulin-containing cells in the colons of patients with inflammatory bowel disease. *Hum. Pathol.*, 15, 757–63.

Kim, B., Barnett, J.L., Kleer, C.G., Appelman, H.D. (1999) Endoscopic and histological patchiness in treated ulcerative colitis. *Am. J. Gatsroenterol.*, 94, 3258–62.

Kitchen, P.A., Levi, A.J., Domizio, P., Talbot, I.C., Forbes, A., Price, A.B., London Inflammatory Bowel Disease Forum (2002) Microscopic colitis: the tip of the iceberg? *Eur. J. Gastroenterol. Hepatol.*, 14, 1199–204.

Kleer, C.G., Appelman, H.D. (1998) Ulcerative colitis: patterns of involvement in colorectal biopsies and changes with time. *Am. J. Surg. Pathol.*, 22, 983–9.

Klein, N.C., Hargrove, R.L., Sleisenger, M.H., Jeffries, G.H. (1970) Eosinophilic gastroenteritis. *Medicine*, 49, 299–319.

Kokkonen, J., Karttunen, T.J. (2002) Lymphoid nodular hyperplasia on the mucosa of the lower gastrointestinal tract in children: an indication of enhanced immune response? *J. Pediatr. Gastroenterol. Nutr.*, 34, 42–6.

Kotler, D.P., Caetz, H.P., Large, M., Klein, E.B., Holt, P.R. (1984) Enteropathy associated with the acquired immunodeficiency syndrome. *Ann. Intern. Med.*, 101, 421–8.

Kotler, D.P., Weaver, S.C., Terzakis, J.A. (1986) Ultrastructural features of epithelial cell degeneration in rectal crypts of patients with AIDS. *Am. J. Surg. Pathol.*, 10, 531–8.

Kumar, N.B., Nostrant, T.T., Appelman, H.D. (1982) The histopathologic spectrum of acute self-limited colitis (acute infectious-type colitis). *Am. J. Surg. Pathol.*, 6, 523–9.

Lambert, M.E., Schofield, P.F., Ironside, A.G., Mandal, B.K. (1979) *Campylobacter* colitis. *Br. Med. J.*, 1, 857–9.

Lee, F.D. (1994) Drug-related pathological lesions of the intestinal tract. *Histopathology*, 25, 303–8.

Lee, K.S., Medline, A., Shockey, S. (1979) Indeterminate colitis in the spectrum of inflammatory bowel disease. *Arch. Pathol. Lab. Med.*, 103, 173–6.

Lessels, A.M., Beck, J.S., Burnett, R.A. *et al.* (1994) Observer variability in the histopathological reporting of abnormal rectal biopsy specimens. *J. Clin. Pathol.*, 47, 48–52.

McGovern, V.J., Goulston, S.J. (1968) Crohn's disease of the colon. *Gut*, 9, 164–76.

McGovern, V., Slavutin, L.J. (1979) Pathology of salmonella colitis. *Am. J. Surg. Pathol.*, 3, 483–90.

Machida, H.M., Catto Smith, A.G., Gall, D.G., Trevenen, C., Scott, R.B. (1994) Allergic colitis in infancy: clinical and pathological aspects. *J. Pediatr. Gastroenterol. Nutr.*, 19, 22–6.

Makapugay, L.M., Dean, P.J. (1996) Diverticular disease-associated chronic colitis. *Am. J. Surg. Pathol.*, 20, 94–102.

Mahadeva, U., Martin, J.P., Patel, N.K., Price, A.B. (2002) Granulomatous ulcerative colitis: a reappraisal of the mucosal granuloma in the distinction of Crohn's disease from ulcerative colitis. *Histopathology*, 41, 166–8.

Mandal, B.K., Schofield, P.F., Morson, B.C. (1982) A clinicopathological study of acute colitis: The dilemma of transient colitis syndrome. *Scand. J. Gastroenterol.*, 17, 865–9.

Markowitz, J., Kahn, E., Grancher, K., Hyams, J., Treem, W., Daum, F. (1993) Atypical; rectosigmoid histology in children with newly diagnosed ulcerative colitis. *Am. J. Gastroenterol.*, 88, 2034–7.

Marteau, P., Lavergne-Slove, A., Lemann, M. *et al.* (1997) Primary villous atrophy is often associated with microscopic colitis. *Gut*, 41, 561–4.

Meucci, G., Bortoli, A., Riccioli, F.A., Girelli, C.M., Radaelli, F., Rivolta, R., Tatarella, M. (1999) Frequency and clinical evolution of indeterminate colitis: a retrospective multi-centre study in northern Italy. *Eur. J. Gastroenterol. Hepatol.*, 11, 809–13.

Moum, B., Ekbom, A., Vatn, M.H. *et al.* (1997) Inflammatory bowel disease: re-evaluation of the diagnosis in a prospective population based study in south eastern Norway. *Gut*, 40, 328–32.

Muller-Lissner, S.A. (1996) What has happened to the cathartic colon. *Gut*, 39, 486–8.

Muller-Lissner, S.A., Kamm, M.A., Scarpignato, C., Wald, A. (2005) Myths and misconceptions about chronic constipation. *Am. J. Gastroenterol.*, 100, 232–42.

Naylor, A.R., Pollet, J.E. (1985) Eosinophilic colitis. *Dis. Col. Rectum*, 28, 615–18.

Nostram, T.T., Kumar, N.B., Appelman, H.D. (1987) Histopathology differentiates acute self-limiting colitis from ulcerative colitis. *Gastroenterology*, 92, 318–28.

O'Donoghue, D.P., Kumar, P. (1979) Rectal IgE cells in inflammatory bowel disease. *Gut*, 20, 149–53.

Odze, R., Antonioli, D., Peppercorn, M., Goldman, H. (1993a) Effect of topical 5-aminosalicylic acid (5-ASA) therapy on rectal mucosal biopsy morphology in chronic ulcerative colitis. *Am. J. Surg. Pathol.*, 17, 869–75.

Odze, R.D., Bines, J., Leichtner, A.M., Goldman, H., Antonioli, D.A. (1993b) Allergic proctocolitis in infants: a prospective clinicopathologic biopsy study. *Hum. Pathol.*, 24, 668–74.

Padmanabhan, V., Callas, P.W., Li, S.C., Trainer, T.D. (2003) Histopathological features of the terminal ileum in lymphocytic and collagenous colitis: a study of 32 cases and review of the literature. *Mod. Pathol.*, 16, 115–19.

Pascal, R.R., Gramlich, T.L. (1993) Geographic variations in eosinophil concentration in normal colonic mucosa. *Mod. Pathol.*, 6, 51A.

Petri, M., Poulsen, S.S., Christensen, K., Jarnum, S. (1982) The incidence of granulomas in serial sections of rectal biopsies from patients with Crohn's disease. *Acta Pathol. Microbiol. Scand. (A)*, 90, 145–7.

Pokorny, C.S., Kneale, K.L., Henderson, C.J. (2001) Progression of collagenous colitis to ulcerative colitis. *J. Clin. Gastroenterol.*, 32, 435–8.

Price, A.B. (1977) Difficulties in the differential diagnosis of ulcerative colitis and Crohn's disease. In: Yardley, J.H., Morson, B.C., Abell, M.R. (eds) *The gastrointestinal tract, International Academy of Pathology monograph.* Baltimore: Williams and Wilkins, pp. 1–14.

Price, A.B. (1978) Overlap in the spectrum of non-specific inflammatory bowel disease: colitis indeterminate. *J. Clin. Pathol.*, 31, 567–77.

Price, A.B. (1996) Indeterminate colitis – broadening the perspective. *Curr. Diagn. Pathol.*, 3, 35–44.

Price, A.B., Davies, D.R. (1977) Pseudomembranous colitis. *J. Clin. Pathol.*, 30, 1–12.

Price, A.B., Jewkes, J., Sanderson, P.J. (1979) Acute diarrhoea: *Campylobacter* colitis and the role of rectal biopsy. *J. Clin. Pathol.*, 32, 990–7.

Rejchrt, S., Bures, J., Siroky, M., Kopacova, M., Slezak, L., Langer, F. (2004) A prospective observational study of colonic mucosal abnormalities associated with orally administered sodium phosphate for colon cleansing before colonoscopy. *Gastrointest. Endosc.*, 59, 651–4.

Rickert, R.R. (1984) The important 'imposters' in the differential diagnosis of inflammatory bowel disease. *J. Clin. Gastroenterol.*, 6, 153–64.

Rickert, R.R., Carter, H.W. (1980) The 'early' ulcerative lesion of Crohn's disease: correlative light- and scanning electron-microscopic studies. *J. Clin. Gastroenterol.*, 2, 11–19.

Romero, R. (2004) Postcolectomy ileitis. *J. Clin. Gastroenterol.*, 38 (Suppl. 1), S32.

Rosekrans, P.C.M., Meijer, C.J.L.M., van der Wal, A.M., Cornelisse, C.J., Lindeman, J. (1980a) Immunoglobulin containing cells in inflammatory bowel disease of the colon: a morphometric and immunohistochemical study. *Gut*, 21, 941–7.

Rosekrans, P.C.M., Meijer, C.J.L.M., van der Wal, A.M., Lindeman, J. (1980b) Allergic proctitis, a clinical and immuno-pathological entity. *Gut*, 21, 1017–23.

Rotterdam, H., Korelitz, B.I., Sommers, S.C. (1977) Microgranuloma in grossly normal rectal mucosa in Crohn's disease. *Am. J. Clin. Pathol.*, 67, 550–4.

Rubenstein, J., Sherif, A., Appelman, H., Chey, W.D. (2004) Ulcerative colitis associated enteritis: is ulcerative colitis always confined to the colon? *J. Clin. Gastroenterol.* 38, 46–51.

Rubin, A., Isaacson, P.G. (1990) Florid reactive lymphoid hyperplasia of the terminal ileum in adults: a condition bearing a close resemblance to low-grade malignant lymphoma. *Histopathology*, 17, 19–26.

Rutter, M.D., Saunders, B.P., Wilkinson, K.H. *et al.* (2004) Cancer surveillance in longstanding ulcerative colitis: endoscopic appearances help predict cancer risk. *Gut*, 53, 1724–5.

Sapp, H., Ithamukkala, S., Brien, T.P. *et al.* (2002) The terminal ileum is affected in patients with lymphocytic and collagenous colitis. *Am. J. Surg. Pathol.*, 236, 1484–92.

Saurine, T.J., Brewer, J.M., Eckstein, R.P. (2004) Microscopic colitis with granulomatous inflammation. *Histopathology*, 45, 82–6.

Schmidt, C.M., Lazenby, A.J., Hendrickson, R.J., Sitzmann, J.V. (1998) Preoperative terminal ileal and colonic resection histopathology predicts risk of pouchitis in patients after ileoanal pull-through procedure. *Ann. Surg.*, 227, 654–62.

Schneider, A.R., Benz, C., Riemann, J.F. (1999) Adverse effects of non-steroidal anti-inflammatory drugs on the small and large bowel. *Endoscopy*, 31, 761–7.

Schumacher, G., Sandstedt, B., Kollberg, B. (1994a) A prospective study of first attacks of inflammatory bowel disease and infectious colitis. Clinical findings and early diagnosis. *Scand. J. Gastroenterol.*, 29, 265–74.

Schumacher, G., Kollberg, B., Sandstedt, B. (1994b) A prospective study of first attacks of inflammatory bowel disease and infectious colitis. Histologic course during the 1st year after presentation. *Scand. J. Gastroenterol.*, 29, 318–32.

Sciarretta, G., Furno, A., Morrone, B., Malaguti, P. (1994) Absence of histopathological changes of ileum and colon in functional diarrhoea associated with bile acid malabsorption by SeHCAT test: a prospective study. *Am. J. Gastroenterol.*, 89, 1058–61.

Scott, B.B., Goodall, A., Stephenson, P., Jenkins, D. (1983) Rectal mucosal cells in inflammatory bowel disease. *Gut*, 24, 519–24.

Seldenrijk, C.A., Morson, B.C., Meuwissen, S.G., Schipper, N.W., Lindeman, J., Meijer, C.J. (1991) Histopathological evaluation of colonic mucosal biopsy specimens in chronic inflammatory bowel disease: diagnostic implications. *Gut*, 32, 1514–20.

Shah, R.J., Fenoglio-Preiser, C., Bleau, B.L., Giannella, R.A. (2001) Usefulness of colonoscopy with biopsy in the evaluation of patients with chronic diarrhoea. *Am. J. Gastroenterol.*, 96, 1091–5.

Shepherd, N.A. (1996) Diverticular disease and chronic inflammatory bowel disease: associations and masquerades. *Gut*, 38, 801–2.

Sladen, G.E., Filipe, M.I. (1984) Is segmental colitis a complication of diverticular disease. *Dis. Colon Rectum*, 27, 513–14.

Spiller, R.C. (2003) Postinfectious irritable bowel syndrome. *Gastroenterology*, 124, 1662–71.

Spiller, R.C., Jenkins, D., Thornley, J.P., Hebden, J.M., Wright, T., Skinner, M., Neal, K.R. (2000) Increased rectal mucosal enteroendocrine cells, T lymphocytes, and increased gut permeability following acute *Campylobacter* enteritis and in post-dysenteric irritable bowel syndrome. *Gut*, 47, 804–11.

Surawicz, C.M., Belic, L. (1984) Rectal biopsy helps to distinguish acute self limited colitis from idiopathic inflammatory bowel disease. *Gastroenterology*, 86, 104–13.

Tally, N.J., Shorter, R.G., Phillips, S.F., Zinsmeister, A.R. (1990) Eosinophilic gastroenteritis: a clinicopathological study of patients with disease of the mucosa, muscle layer, and subserosal tissues. *Gut*, 31, 54–8.

Tanaka, M., Masuda, T., Yao, T., Saito, H., Kusumi, T., Nagura, H., Kudo, H. (2001) Observer variation of diagnoses based on simple biopsy criteria differentiating among Crohn's disease, ulcerative colitis, and other forms of colitis. *J. Gastroenterol. Hepatol.*, 16, 1368–72.

Taylor, B., Lingam, R., Simmons, A., Stowe, J., Miller, E., Andrews, N. (2002) Autism and MMR vaccination in North London: no causal relationship. *Mol. Psychiatry*, 7 (Suppl. 2), S7–S8.

Theodossi, A., Spiegelhalter, D.J., Jass, J. *et al.* (1994) Observer variation and discriminatory value of biopsy features in inflammatory bowel disease. *Gut*, 35, 961–8.

Therkildsen, M.H., Jensen, B.N., Teglbjaerg, P.S., Rasmussen, S.N. (1989) The final outcome of patients presenting with their first episode of acute diarrhoea and an inflamed rectal mucosa with preserved crypt architecture. A clinicopathologic study. *Scand. J. Gastroenterol.*, 24, 158–64.

van Spreeuwel, J.P., Lindeman, J., Meijer, C.J.L.M. (1985) A quantitative study of immunoglobulin containing cells in the differential diagnosis of acute colitis. *J. Clin. Pathol.*, 38, 774–7.

Volk, E.E., Shapiro, B.D., Easley, K.A., Goldblum, J.R. (1998) The clinical significance of a biopsy-based diagnosis of focal active colitis: a clinicopathologic study of 31 cases. *Mod. Pathol.*, 11, 789–94.

Wakefield, A.J., Murch, S.H., Anthony, A. *et al.* (1998) Ileal–lymphoid–nodular hyperplasia, non-specific colitis, and pervasive developmental disorder in children. *Lancet*, 351, 637–41.

Wakefield, A.J., Ashwood, P., Limb, K., Anthony, A. (2005) The significance of ileo-colonic lymphoid nodular hyperplasia in children with autistic spectrum disorder. *Eur. J. Gastroenterol. Hepatol.*, 17, 827–36.

Washington, K., Stenzel, T.T., Buckley, R.H., Gottfried, M.R. (1996) Gastrointestinal pathology in patients with common variable immunodeficiency and X-linked agammaglobulinaemia. *Am. J. Surg. Pathol.*, 20, 1240–52.

Webster, A.D.B., Kenwright, S., Ballard, J. *et al.* (1977) Nodular lymphoid hyperplasia of the bowel in primary hypogammaglobulinaemia: study of *in vitro* lymphocyte function. *Gut*, 18, 364–72.

Wells, A.D., McMillan, I., Price, A.B., Ritchie, J.K., Nicholls, R.J. (1991) Natural history of indeterminate colitis. *Br. J. Surg.*, 78, 179–81.

Xin, W., Brown, P.I., Greenson, J.K. (2003) The clinical significance of focal active colitis in pediatric patients. *Am. J. Surg. Pathol.*, 27, 1134–8.

Winter, H.S., Antonioli, D.A., Fukagawa, N., Marcial, M., Goldman, H. (1990) Allergy-related proctocolitis in infants: diagnostic usefulness of rectal biopsy. *Mod. Pathol.*, 3, 5–10.

Yantiss, R.K., Farraye, F.A., O'Brien, M.J. *et al.* (2006) Prognostic significance of superficial fissuring ulceration in patients with severe 'indeterminate' colitis. *Am. J. Surg. Pathol.*, 30, 165–70.

Yu, C.S., Pemberton, J.H., Larson, D. (2000) Ileal pouch–anal anastomosis in patients with indeterminate colitis: long-term results. *Dis. Colon. Rectum*, 43, 1487–96.

Yuan, S., Reyes, V., Bronner, M.P. (2003) Pseudomembranous collagenous colitis. *Am. J. Surg. Pathol.*, 27, 1375–9.

CHAPTER 13

DISORDERS OF MOTILITY

13.1 Introduction   233
13.2 The normal innervation   233
13.3 Congenital megacolon:
     neuronal dysplasias, including
     Hirschsprung's disease   235
     13.3.1 The diagnostic biopsy   236
     13.3.2 The operative biopsy   236
     13.3.3 Aganglionosis   236
     13.3.4 Hypoganglionosis   239
     13.3.5 Hyperganglionosis   239

13.3.6 Biopsy policy in childhood
       constipation   241
13.4 Idiopathic megacolon of
     childhood   242
13.5 Acquired megacolon   242
13.6 Features associated with
     megacolon   244
     13.6.1 Melanosis coli   244
     13.6.2 Obstructive colitis   244
References   246

13.1 INTRODUCTION

Apart from irritable bowel syndrome, in which abdominal pain is the predominant symptom and biopsy histology is normal (MacIntosh *et al.*, 1992), patients with motility disorders present with a variety of manifestations, but the most frequent symptom is 'constipation'. Biopsy plays a part in the investigation of constipation in patients of all ages, but particularly in young babies and children. It is important to remember that a histological abnormality can be demonstrated in only a proportion of these cases (Barnes *et al.*, 1986). The abnormalities which may be present can be considered as either congenital (neuronal dysplasias) or acquired. Congenital abnormalities tend to present in early life, often displaying diagnostic morphological features. Acquired abnormalities often have little to show histologically and can be subdivided clinically into pseudo-obstruction and acquired megacolon.

In infancy, correct diagnosis of abnormal innervation as the cause of constipation is of critical importance because of the frequency with which necrotizing enterocolitis complicates aganglionosis in particular (Section 13.6.2).

Before interpretation of biopsies is possible from patients with neuronal dysplasia, it is necessary to appreciate the normal pattern of innervation of the large bowel, as revealed by acetylcholinesterase staining. Routine use of this technique and the management of motility disorders in infancy is limited to specialist centres but will be described here.

13.2 THE NORMAL INNERVATION

For a distance of up to 1 cm above the dentate line the submucosa and wall of the rectum are normally deficient in ganglia (the 'hypoganglionic zone'; Aldridge and Campbell, 1968). In this

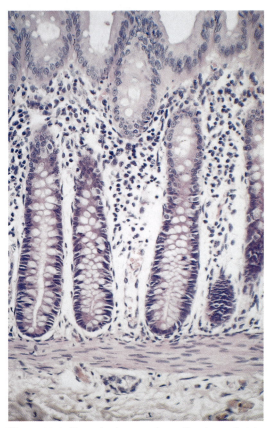

Figure 13.1 Normal submucosal ganglion, immediately beneath muscularis mucosae. Neonatal rectal mucosa.

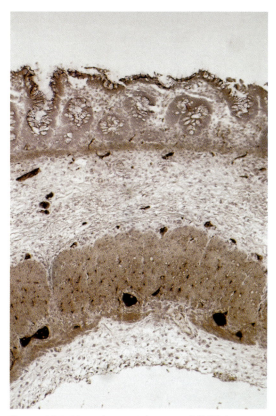

Figure 13.2 Normal neonatal rectum, full thickness biopsy, stained by Karnovsky and Roots method for acetylcholinesterase. Sparsely scattered fine nerve fibres are present in the lamina propria and muscularis mucosae. In the submucosa the ganglia are arranged in superficial and deep layers and nerve bundles are inconspicuous. The muscularis propria is only weakly stained but fine nerve fibres are scattered between the fibres of the circular muscle. The ganglia of the myenteric plexus lie close to the lower edge of this field. Cryostat section of unfixed tissue.

hypoganglionic zone there are reduced numbers of submucosal ganglia (an average of one for every 8 mm length of rectum, as seen in histological sections) and a small mucosal biopsy will often appear to be aganglionic. Examination of the myenteric plexus in this zone shows few ganglion cells but prominent nerve bundles. Above this level there are submucosal ganglia situated immediately beneath the muscularis mucosae (Fig. 13.1) and, rather more sparsely, immediately superficial to the circular muscle coat. Small, inconspicuous nerve bundles are scattered through the submucosa. These features can be recognized in haematoxylin and eosin-stained paraffin sections.

The normal appearance following staining for acetylcholinesterase is shown in Fig. 13.2. Quite apart from the submucosal ganglion cells and nerve bundles, which are positively stained for acetylcholinesterase, there are sparsely scattered, fine nerve fibres in the muscularis mucosae and in the lamina propria. The muscularis mucosae also stains diffusely, but only weakly. These features are seen in both the hypoganglionic zone and more proximally. Ganglion cells are not normally evident in the lamina propria.

In full-thickness biopsies from above the hypoganglionic zone the myenteric plexus (Auerbach) normally consists of clearly defined, easily identified

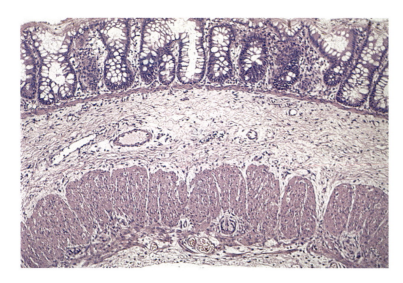

Figure 13.3 Full-thickness biopsy of infant's rectum, with normal myenteric plexus. Nerve bundles connecting the ganglia between the muscle layers are inconspicuous.

ganglia and their interconnecting nerve bundles, lying between the circular and longitudinal muscle layers (Fig. 13.3). Staining for acetylcholinesterase (Fig. 13.2) reveals, in addition, fine nerve fibres passing between weakly stained muscle cells, vertically in the circular muscle coat and horizontally in the longitudinal muscle coat.

13.3 CONGENITAL MEGACOLON: NEURONAL DYSPLASIAS, INCLUDING HIRSCHSPRUNG'S DISEASE

We use the term neuronal dysplasia to denote any congenital abnormality of the innervation of the rectum, with or without involvement of more proximal bowel. Three categories of abnormality are recognized (Garrett and Howard, 1981), any of which may present with a Hirschsprung-like syndrome, usually in infancy, but, in 18 per cent of cases, over the age of 5 years (Kleinhaus et al., 1979):

1. Aganglionosis (Hirschsprung's disease).
2. Hypoganglionosis.
3. Hyperganglionosis – 'neuronal intestinal dysplasia' (Meier-Ruge, 1974) or 'intestinal neuronal dysplasia' (IND).

Any of these abnormalities may be present alone or in combination but, common to all, there is invariably some degree of hypoganglionosis proximal to a segment of aganglionosis, the so-called transition zone (Garrett et al., 1969).

Although, in our experience, aganglionosis is by far the commonest variety of neuronal dysplasia, Howard et al. (1984) have encountered pure hypoganglionosis in 20 of 60 cases presenting with a Hirschsprung-like syndrome (i.e. more frequently than aganglionosis). Furthermore, Fadda et al. (1983) allege that 'neuronal intestinal dysplasia' (equivalent to hyperganglionosis, as defined in this chapter) is equal in incidence to Hirschsprung's disease. It is possible that the statistics presented by both of these groups of workers are biased by the large number of referred problems in their series. A further factor which may distort the incidence data is that hyperganglionosis is reported to resolve as a child grows older (Meier-Ruge et al., 1995; Cord-Udy et al., 1997).

The more obvious abnormalities, such as absence of ganglia, can be detected in routine paraffin sections, stained with haematoxylin and eosin but, for precise and reliable diagnosis, it is necessary to use specific staining methods for autonomic nerves and ganglia. These, unfortunately, still require fresh, unfixed tissue. We have found that the Karnovsky and Roots method for acetylcholinesterase (Bancroft, 2002) is the most useful for diagnostic purposes.

To identify ganglia in a frozen section, for per-operative guidance to the surgeon in siting a colostomy, a rapid non-specific esterase (Yam *et al.*, 1971) is useful. Meier-Ruge and Bruder (2005) rec-ommend a lactic dehydrogenase for this purpose. It is likely that, ultimately, large intestinal innerv-ation may be delineated by an immunohistochem-ical method (Klück *et al.*, 1984; Meyrat *et al.*, 2001) but there has been insufficient experience with candidate antibodies such as neurofilament or neural cell adhesion molecule (NCAM) antibodies to recommend them for routine use.

13.3.1 The diagnostic biopsy

The diagnostic biopsy must be clearly distinguished from the subsequent operative procedure, during which the pathologist may be called upon to give an immediate opinion on the normality, or other-wise, of the innervation of the bowel at the level at which the surgeon wishes to make a colostomy. The diagnostic biopsy may be initially, at least, a mucosal biopsy or series of biopsies, on the one hand from high enough in the rectum to be clear of the normal hypoganglionic zone (1.0 cm), but, on the other, low enough to avoid missing a short seg-ment abnormality, which may be only 1 cm long, or even less. This naturally requires careful biopsy technique, with a calibrated instrument, of the type developed by Noblett (1969). For this diagnostic biopsy a specific stain for acetylcholinesterase is required. In order to receive the biopsy tissue fresh, we make sure that it is transported dry, unfixed, to the laboratory, as if it were a standard rapid-frozen section specimen. The method is robust in practice; acetylcholinesterase staining has been shown to be satisfactory for diagnosis in rectal biopsy tissue kept moist at 4°C for up to 14 days and for up to 5 days at room temperature (Byard and Carli, 1998).

If, following the initial mucosal biopsy a diagno-sis of aganglionosis is made, the surgeon can, on a subsequent occasion, perform a colostomy, followed later by a definitive 'pull-through', sphincter-pre-serving operation. However, if hypoganglionosis or hyperganglionosis is suspected, further full-thick-ness biopsies should be taken from multiple sites along the bowel wall to determine the extent of the anatomical abnormality, which may not be grossly

apparent. This may be extensive, with extension, in rare cases, even proximal to the ileocaecal valve. Schmittenbecher *et al.* (2000) have shown that IND (hyperganglionosis) proximal to the aganglionic seg-ment is associated with long-standing persisting constipation unless adequately resected. In prac-tice, the surgeon may accept the possibility of a trial colostomy at this stage, with further more proxi-mal biopsies later, if colostomy function is not satisfactory.

13.3.2 The operative biopsy

At operation, in order to guide the surgeon where to fashion a colostomy, as previously mentioned, a rapid non-specific esterase technique or staining for lactate dehydrogenase (LDH) gives a clearer picture of the innervation of the bowel wall than haema-toxylin and eosin in a frozen section, and only takes 15 minutes. We find that a toluidine blue-stained section is also helpful for the rapid identification of ganglia. However, it must be stressed, diagnosis of hypo- and hyper-ganglionosis can only be reli-ably made from careful study of specific acetyl-cholinesterase staining followed up by good paraffin sections of biopsies. The diagnosis will be con-firmed from the examination of serial sections of the full thickness of the bowel wall, either from full-thickness biopsies or from the colorectal resection specimen itself. Meier-Ruge and Bruder (2005) rec-ommend enzyme histochemistry on a 'Swiss roll' of the entire length of the resected specimen.

It is important that there is full communication between surgeon and pathologist, so that the pathol-ogist knows the precise site of each biopsy and the surgeon is made aware of any difficulty or uncer-tainty on the part of the pathologist which make a further biopsy necessary. This may mean that a definitive operative procedure should be delayed until good sections, stained specifically for acetyl-cholinesterase, have been examined.

13.3.3 Aganglionosis

Ganglia are absent from both submucosal and myen-teric plexuses in the affected segment of bowel. In 80 per cent of cases the abnormality is confined to

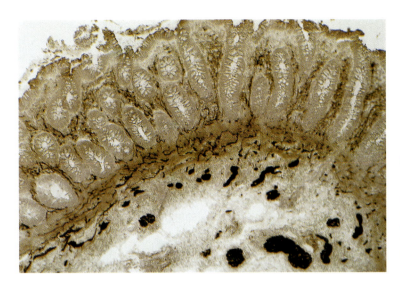

Figure 13.4 Aganglionosis. Mucosal biopsy of rectum from an infant, stained for acetylcholinesterase. Irregular coarse nerve fibres in the submucosa pass through the muscularis mucosae into the lamina propria. The mucosa also contains thick nerve fibres. Cryostat section of unfixed tissue.

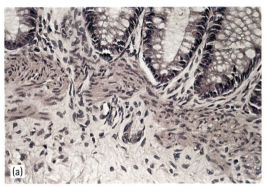

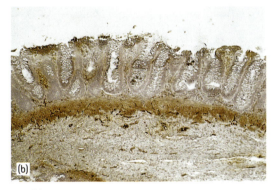

Figure 13.5 Immaturity of innervation in a premature neonate. (a) Submucosal ganglion of bizarre appearance. (Paraffin section.) (b) Staining for acetylcholine shows darkly stained muscularis mucosae but no abnormal nerve fibres within the mucosa. (Cryostat section of unfixed tissue.)

the rectum or rectum and sigmoid colon. Coarse and irregular acetylcholinesterase-positive nerve fibres are seen in the muscularis mucosae and in the lamina propria (Fig. 13.4). Irregular large submucosal nerve bundles and trunks are also typically present. This picture is so characteristic that a diagnosis can be confidently made from a mucosal biopsy in such circumstances. However, before issuing a definitive report, it is still advisable to process the tissue remaining after histochemistry for paraffin sections, for the following reasons. Occasionally, cases of aganglionosis may show a normal staining pattern (Garrett and Howard, 1981). Conversely, there may be equivocal staining of nerves in the muscularis mucosae (but not the lamina propria) (Barr

et al., 1985). It is then necessary to examine serial sections of paraffin-processed biopsies to establish the diagnosis of aganglionosis. In practice, we recommend that six slides, each bearing a ribbon of 6 to 10 serial sections, be screened. We have seen babies born prematurely, who have been constipated for the first 3–4 weeks of neonatal life, with equivocal staining for acetylcholinesterase and equivocal ganglia in paraffin sections who have subsequently had normal bowel function and normal biopsies (Fig. 13.5). It seems that in these circumstances there is both structural and functional immaturity of the autonomic ganglia, which results in a temporary Hirschsprung-like state (Bughaighis and Emery, 1971; Holschneider *et al.*, 1994).

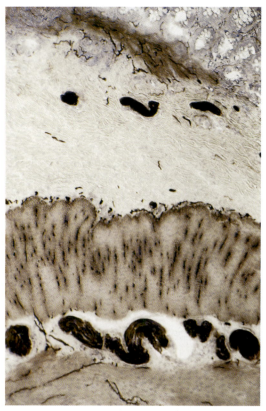

Figure 13.6 Aganglionosis. Full-thickness biopsy of rectum stained for acetylcholinesterase. There are thick nerve bundles in the submucosa and large irregular nerve trunks in place of the myenteric ganglia. The circular muscle coat is stained diffusely brown and contains unusually prominent, vertically orientated nerve fibres. (Cryostat section of unfixed tissue.)

If, after examination of the mucosal biopsy, doubt remains, examination of full-thickness biopsies is recommended. Staining of these for acetyl-cholinesterase shows irregular coarse nerve fibres, particularly in the circular muscle coat (Fig. 13.6) and there may also be abnormally prominent, thick nerve fibres diffusely arranged between the individual smooth muscle cells. Immediately above the affected segment there is typically a 'transition' zone with a mixed picture of hyperganglionosis and hypoganglionosis (Fig. 13.7). More proximally there is usually (normal) slight staining of smooth muscle and the normal complement of fine intramuscular nerve fibres (Fig. 13.2). If normal bowel function is to be achieved, it is important that the abnormal transitional zone bowel, whether hyperganglionic or hypoganglionic, is resected (Farrugia et al., 2003). Assessment of this is not easy, as, in our experience, there is frequently hypertrophy of myenteric ganglia and nerves proximal to any intestinal obstruction or pseudo-obstruction. Such neuronal hypertrophy may extend for a considerable distance along the length of the colon (Fig. 13.8). This may be a marker of increased neuromuscular activity resulting from the distal obstruction and should not be confused with hyperganglionosis, which is characterized by similar large ganglia and nerves, but in which there is also an increase in numbers and thickness of acetylcholinesterase-positive nerve fibres between myocytes (Section 13.3.5). To confirm complete excision, the most satisfactory procedure is to examine

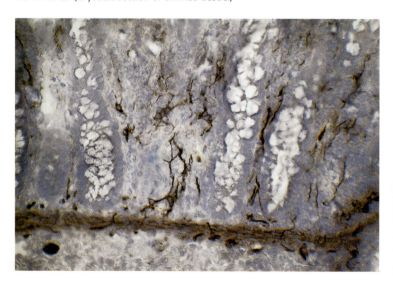

Figure 13.7 Transitional hypoganglionic zone, proximal to aganglionic segment in Hirschsprung's disease. The coarse nerve fibres are still present in the lamina propria, but not in the muscularis mucosae.

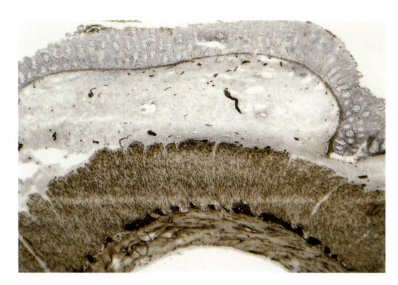

Figure 13.8 Transitional hyperganglionic zone, proximal to aganglionic and hypoganglionic zones of Hirschsprung's disease. Submucosal ganglia and nerves are randomly arranged rather than being placed in superficial and deep strata. The myenteric plexus is enlarged, with ganglia fused with large nerve trunks. Function in this type of large bowel is variable. (Cryostat section of unfixed biopsy, stained for acetylcholinesterase.)

by enzyme histochemistry and histology, a transverse circumferential section of the proximal resection margin of the resected bowel.

The distribution of the nerve staining for acetylcholinesterase in a typical case of aganglionosis is shown diagrammatically in Fig. 13.9.

13.3.4 Hypoganglionosis

Reduced number or size of ganglion cells, rather than their absence, may be the cause of constipation with overflow incontinence and tends to present for the first time in older children. The ganglion cells may be reduced to one-tenth their normal number. A rough guide to normality here is the figure of one submucosal ganglion per linear millimetre length of muscularis mucosae (Aldridge and Campbell, 1968). Despite this rule of thumb the condition is difficult to diagnose from haematoxylin and eosin stained sections of mucosal biopsies (Watanabe et al., 1999). When hypoganglionosis is suspected, full-thickness biopsies should be examined by histochemical methods. The biopsies should be taken from multiple sites, both to avoid confusion with the transition zone of aganglionosis and to delineate the extent of the abnormality, as a large proportion, if not all, of the colon can be involved (Fadda et al., 1983).

Rapid, non-specific esterase, LDH or, preferably, acetylcholinesterase staining shows only a few scattered myenteric ganglion cells and unusually prominent nerve trunks (Fig. 13.10). There is also a reduction in the fine intramuscular nerve fibres in both the muscularis mucosae and in the muscularis propria.

This condition tends to be associated with aganglionosis and is rarely found in isolation but the diagnosis is of importance, as although the large bowel may be extensively affected and the presenting symptoms severe, Howard et al. (1984) report that many of these cases are able to recover good function following a low rectal myotomy, rather than a resection.

13.3.5 Hyperganglionosis

This condition, also described as 'IND, type B' (Meier-Ruge, 1974; Puri et al., 1977; Munakata et al., 1985; Meier-Ruge et al., 1995) may accompany Hirschsprung's disease. Less frequently, it can occur in isolation or associated with other malformations (Berger et al., 1998) and has been implicated as a cause of constipation presenting after the age of 6 months. One important clinical difference is that only in Hirschsprung's disease is there a classical 'funnel-shaped' stricture seen at the junction between the normal proximal bowel and the distal abnormal bowel. Hyperganglionosis/IND is characterized by abnormally large submucosal

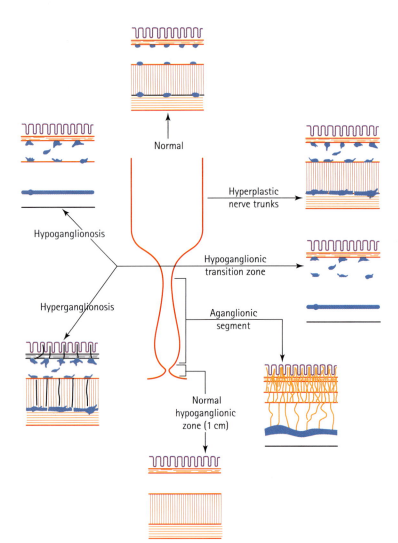

Figure 13.9 Diagram of patterns of innervation of the distal colon and rectum. The funnel-shaped deformity associated with aganglionosis is illustrated in the centre and the corresponding features in Hirschsprung's disease (sections stained for acetylcholinesterase) are shown on the right. On the left are the features seen in other neuronal dysplasias (including intestinal neuronal dysplasia).

and myenteric plexuses, with giant ganglia (containing at least eight neurones) (Fig. 13.11a). Smooth muscle fibres have also been described in the lamina propria of the mucosa. Staining for acetylcholinesterase reveals a moderate increase in the number of cholinergic nerve fibres in the lamina propria, muscularis mucosae and muscularis propria and isolated ganglion cells in the lamina propria (Fig. 13.11b). The pathologist should be aware that small numbers of ganglia can be found in the lamina propria of the mucosa in normal individuals and, even in adults, it is normal to find that up to 20 per cent of submucosal ganglia can be of 'giant' type (Wilder-Smith *et al.*, 2002). According

to Meier-Ruge and colleagues (1995), for reliable diagnosis, up to 30 serial sections need to be examined. Furthermore, it has been shown (Cord-Udy *et al.*, 1997) that hyperplasia of the submucosal plexus is often a manifestation of developmental immaturity, which spontaneously resolves, rather than a permanent malformation.

It is important to bear the possibility of hyperganglionosis in mind when plentiful ganglia are seen in a biopsy from a child with clinical Hirschsprung's disease. Schmittenbecher *et al.* (2000) found that when hyperganglionosis is present in the bowel proximal to aganglionosis, problems with constipation remain unless the abnormally innervated bowel

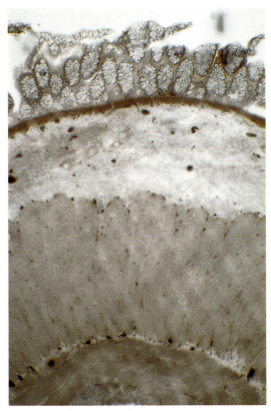

Figure 13.10 Hypoganglionosis. Acetylcholinesterase-stained full-thickness biopsy. Ganglia are reduced in size and number in both the submucosal and myenteric plexuses. Submucosal trunks are prominent but there are few intramuscular nerve fibres in the muscularis mucosae and muscularis propria.

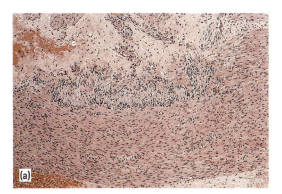

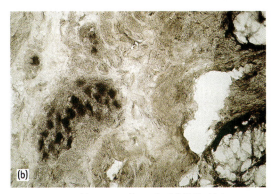

Figure 13.11 Hyperganglionosis. (a) Full-thickness biopsy. The ganglia of the myenteric plexus are increased in number and size. (b) Giant ganglia are a feature of hyperganglionosis (also called 'intestinal neuronal dysplasia'). Cryostat section of unfixed tissue, stained for acetylcholinesterase.

is adequately excised. This can involve as much as the transverse or even ascending colon (Fadda *et al.*, 1983). Ileal involvement is also recorded.

When hyperganglionosis is suspected, multiple full-thickness biopsies should be examined, not under the conditions of a rapid, per-operative, procedure.

13.3.6 Biopsy policy in childhood constipation

The ideal, towards which the pathologist should aim, is to be able, from biopsy tissue, to determine whether or not the innervation is normal and to define precisely which category of neuronal dysplasia is present. It is also necessary to define the extent of the disease, so that the surgeon knows how much bowel to resect, if any, at a definitive operation. Unfortunately, these aims are not always fulfilled because not every case can be simply placed into one category, and there may be combined features of both aganglionosis and hyperganglionosis, for example. The extent of the disease may not be determined until rapid frozen sections are available at the time of surgery.

Notwithstanding these difficulties, provided that biopsies have been taken from precisely the correct points along the colon and rectum, the average pathologist should be able to diagnose aganglionosis confidently, with the help of histochemical staining for acetylcholinesterase and careful examination of good paraffin sections. Hyperganglionosis should pose no problem. However, it is more difficult to be certain of hypoganglionosis because this is a quantitative deficiency and small biopsy fragments are not amenable to measurement. Fortunately, Garrett and Howard (1981) have shown that conservative surgery including anorectal myotomy and/or anal stretch are usually successful in the management of this condition and only if these measures fail does colorectal resection become necessary. There should have been ample opportunity for the pathologist to examine full-thickness biopsies by the time this stage is reached.

13.4 IDIOPATHIC MEGACOLON OF CHILDHOOD

This is a term which has been applied to the occasional case of late-onset intractable childhood constipation in whom no morphological abnormality of ganglia or nerves is seen in routine paraffin sections (Kapilla *et al.*, 1975; Puri *et al.*, 1977). The functional abnormality is evidently caused by a generalized large intestinal hypotonia. Radiologically and clinically there is no specifically localized funnel-shaped zone or distal spastic stricture.

We have no direct experience of such a case. According to Puri *et al.* (1977) the pathological basis of this condition is destruction of parasympathetic nerve axons, leading to a deficiency of fine intramuscular nerve fibres within the layers of the muscularis propria – the ganglia appearing normal. This situation is only appreciated in fresh cryostat sections stained for acetylcholinesterase.

13.5 ACQUIRED MEGACOLON

Over-dilatation of the colon (megacolon), associated with acquired constipation, with or without spurious diarrhoea, can have several distinct causes. Adults are more frequently affected than children. Biopsy is of value to identify those cases

Table 13.1 Pseudo-obstruction and acquired megacolon

With abnormal ganglia
Infective
Chagas disease, cytomegalovirus, Epstein–Barr virus infection

With normal ganglia
Obstructive
Proximal to stricture or tumour

Pseudo-obstruction
Myopathies: hollow visceral myopathies, systemic sclerosis, dermatomyositis
Endocrine disease: myxoedema, diabetes mellitus, hypoparathyroidism
Drug-induced: phenothiazines, tricyclic antidepressants, antiparkinsonian and ganglion-blocking agents, cloridine
Amyloidosis
Idiopathic/psychogenic

in which the nerve ganglia are abnormal (Table 13.1). Investigation of infective plexitis and muscle disease require full-thickness biopsy. It is helpful to know what the findings of barium enema studies have been, as acquired megarectum and megacolon are not associated with the tight 'funnel-neck'-type stricturing of the rectum which is characteristic of Hirschsprung's disease.

The infective plexitides are characterized by infiltration in and around the myenteric plexuses by lymphocytes (Fig. 13.12). Histologically, there are no features which distinguish the various infections from each other. Chagas' disease, caused by infection with *Trypanosoma cruzi*, from bites by the triatomine bug, occurs exclusively in South and Central America and usually presents after the fourth decade of life. The oesophagus and heart can also be affected. Damage to myenteric ganglia can be so severe that the affected bowel (commonly the rectum and left colon) can be effectively aganglionic. Distinction from Hirschsprung's disease must be made from the history and geographical context.

In visceral myopathy there is cytoplasmic vacuolation of muscle cells, with nuclear enlargement and hyperchromasia and fibrosis of one or both layers of the muscularis propria (Fig. 13.13).

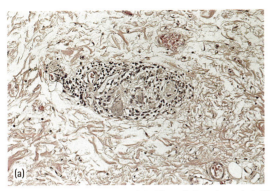 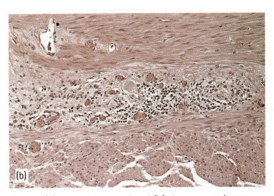

Figure 13.12 Infective plexitis. There is lymphocytic infiltration of (a) the submucosal and (b) the myenteric nerve plexuses. (Paraffin sections of biopsy and colon from patients with Chagas disease.)

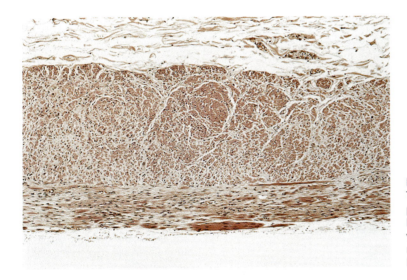

Figure 13.13 Visceral myopathy. There is fibrosis of the muscularis propria, in this case affecting both layers. There is cytoplasmic vacuolation of muscle cells, with nuclear enlargement and hyperchromasia. (Paraffin section.)

The diagnosis is best made from full thickness biopsies, as the abnormalities may be inconspicuous in the muscularis mucosae. Similar vacuolation of myocytes may be produced as an artefact, with the resulting danger of false positive diagnosis. Systemic sclerosis can cause a very similar picture (Fig. 13.14), although it may be more patchy and accompanied by characteristic changes in the submucosal blood vessels.

Amyloidosis affects the colon and rectum in different ways, depending on the type of amyloid disease (Tada *et al.*, 1993). The broad category of reactive ('secondary') amyloidosis (i.e. AA amyloidosis) (Section 20.8) tends to be associated with deposits in the autonomic plexuses, principally the myenteric plexus, and is therefore a potential cause

of autonomic neuropathy, whereas the primary amyloidoses (AL and AH amyloidosis) are associated with deposition in the muscularis mucosae and propria, leading to a myopathy.

Megacolon from other causes requires diagnosis by exclusion (Barnes *et al.*, 1986). Biopsy has little to contribute, as there is no specific abnormality of ganglia and any alteration in thickness of muscle coats will not be evident. Frequently, in megacolon, the myenteric ganglia are enlarged and prominent due to proliferation of Schwann cells (Fig. 13.15). This process of 'Schwannosis' is probably a variant of the neuronal hypertrophy frequently associated with aganglionosis, which seems to be a secondary phenomenon and is not specific to any particular disease.

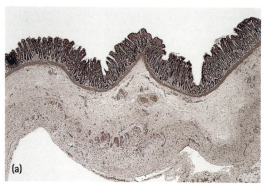 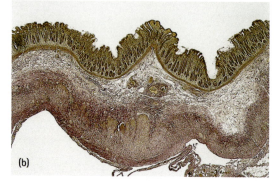

Figure 13.14 Systemic sclerosis. There is patchy replacement of the muscularis propria by collagen and elastic fibres, in this case particularly affecting the circular muscle layer. Typical vascular changes are not always seen. Resected colon. (a) Haematoxylin and eosin; (b) elastic van Gieson.

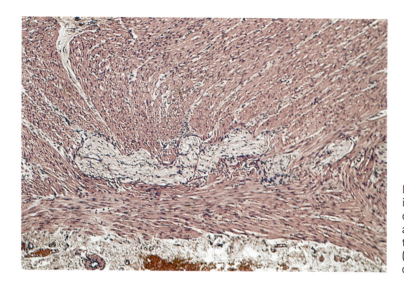

Figure 13.15 'Schwannosis'. Often in constipation and in chronic obstruction, the myenteric ganglia are enlarged and prominent owing to proliferation of Schwann cells. (Resected colon proximal to an obstruction.)

13.6 FEATURES ASSOCIATED WITH MEGACOLON

13.6.1 Melanosis coli

Melanosis coli (Section 11.10 and Fig. 3.38) is frequently found in mucosal biopsies from patients with motility disorders, as a result of self-medication with anthroquinone laxatives (Walker *et al.* 1988).

Apparently, as a consequence of chronic constipation with overdistension of the large bowel by faeces, obstructive colitis may develop.

13.6.2 Obstructive colitis

This is not a diagnosis which can be made from the biopsy appearances alone; information that the patient has an obstruction, neuronal dysplasia or one of the other conditions which may cause megacolon (Table 11.1), should alert the pathologist to the possibility. It is said to occur in up to 7 per cent of patients with colonic obstruction (Gratama *et al.*, 1995), most frequently caused by adenocarcinoma. Obstructive colitis can be associated with any form of diminished motility. It is not always appreciated that diverticular disease, by

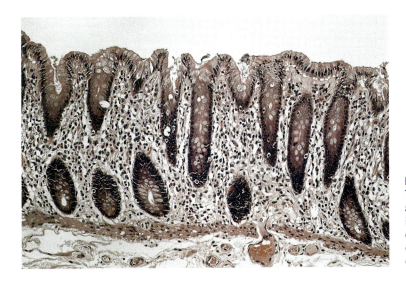

Figure 13.16 Obstructive colitis. There is depletion of goblet cells and the lamina propria is diffusely infiltrated by chronic inflammatory cells, masking oedema. (Resected colon mucosa, proximal to an obstructing carcinoma.)

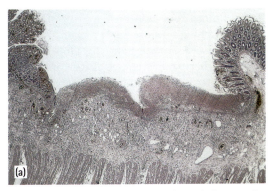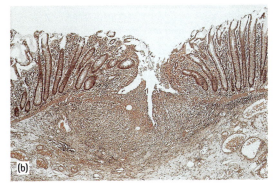

Figure 13.17 Stercoral ulceration. These lesions are from colons resected for obstruction associated with diverticular disease. The mucosa of the proximal colon was reddened and there were sharply defined ulcers. (a) A large ulcer lined by slough and granulation tissue; the adjacent mucosa is normal. (b) A smaller ulcer in a segment of acutely inflamed mucosa.

producing functional obstruction, is the second most frequent cause (Toner *et al.*, 1990) and can lead to quite severe obstructive colitis or entero-colitis (Feldman, 1975; Levene and Price, 1994).

The biopsy may merely show small superficial foci of polymorphs and mucosal or submucosal oedema (Fig. 13.16). Without relevant clinical information casual observation may result in a dismissive report of non-specific inflammation. It is the bowel proximal to the obstruction which is usually affected, often separated from the obstruction by an intervening zone of normal mucosa. The histology can be similar to the early stages of ischaemic bowel disease, and in advanced cases may be indistinguishable from inflammatory bowel disease (Gratama *et al.*, 1995). The diagnosis is important, as the more severely affected bowel may become extensively ulcerated ('stercoral' ulceration, Fig. 13.17; Feldman, 1975). Perforation can occur (Gekas and Schuster, 1981), especially in the elderly, in whom this can be sudden and massive (so-called 'blow-out'). Furthermore, a relatively mild inflammatory reaction of this nature in the rectal mucosa of an infant with Hirschsprung's disease or other neuronal dysplasia may be a marker for a more florid, necrotizing enterocolitis proximally (Elhalaby *et al.*, 1995a) or even within the aganglionic segment itself (Elhalaby *et al.*, 1995b). Despite the 'non-specific' appearance of the inflammation, obstructive colitis appears to be a result of impairment of the blood supply consequent on over-distension of the bowel (Saegesser and Sandblom, 1975; Levene and Price, 1994).

REFERENCES

Aldridge, R.T., Campbell, P.E. (1968) Ganglion cell distribution in the normal rectum and anal canal. A basis for the diagnosis of Hirschsprung's disease by anorectal biopsy. *J. Pediatr. Surg.*, 3, 475–89.

Bancroft, J.D. (2002) Enzyme histochemistry and its diagnostic applications – acetylcholinesterase. In: Bancroft, J.D., Gamble, M. (eds) *Theory and practice of histological techniques*, 5th edn. Edinburgh, London, New York: Churchill Livingstone, p. 605.

Barnes, P.R.H., Lennard-Jones, J.E., Hawley, P.R., Todd, I.P. (1986) Hirschsprung's disease and idiopathic megacolon in adults and adolescents. *Gut*, 27, 534–41.

Barr, L.C., Booth, J., Filipe, M.I., Lawson, J.O.N. (1985) Clinical evaluation of the histochemical diagnosis of Hirschprung's disease. *Gut*, 26, 393–9.

Berger, S., Ziebel, P., Offsler, M., Hofman-von Kap-herr, S. (1998) Congenital malformations and perinatal morbidity associated with intestinal neuronal dysplasia. *Pediatr. Sur. Int.*, 13, 474–9.

Bughaighis, A.C., Emery, J.L. (1971) Functional obstruction of the intestine due to neurological immaturity. *Prog. Pediatr. Surg.*, 3, 37–52.

Byard, R.W., Carli, M. (1998) Temporal stability of acetylcholinesterase staining in colonic and rectal neural tissue. *Pediatr. Surg. Int.*, 13, 29–31.

Cord-Udy, C.L., Smith, V.V., Ahmed, S., Risdon, R.A., Milla, P.J. (1997) An evaluation of the role of suction rectal biopsy in the diagnosis of intestinal neuronal dysplasia. *J. Pediatr. Gastroenterol. Nutr.*, 24, 1–6

Elhalaby, E.A., Coran, A.G., Blane, C.E., Hirschl, R.B., Teitelbaum, D.H. (1995a) Enterocolitis associated with Hirschsprung's disease: a clinical–radiological characterization based on 168 patients. *J. Pediatr. Surg.*, 30, 76–83.

Elhalaby, E.A., Teitelbaum, D.H., Coran, A.G., Heidelberger, K.P. (1995b) Enterocolitis associated with Hirschsprung's disease: a clinical histopathological correlative study. *J. Pediatr. Surg.*, 30, 1023–6.

Fadda, B., Maier, W.A., Meier-Ruge, W., Sharli, A., Daum, R. (1983) Neuronale intestinale Dysplasie. Eine kritische 10-Jahres-Analyse klinischer und bioptischer Diagnostik. *Kinderchirurgie*, 38, 305–11.

Farrugia, M.K., Alexander, N., Clarke, S., Nash, R., Nicholls, E.A., Holmes, K. (2003) Does transitional zone pull-through in Hirschsprung's disease imply a poor prognosis? *J. Pediatr. Surg.*, 38, 1766–9.

Feldman, P.S. (1975) Ulcerative disease of the colon proximal to partially obstructive lesions: report of two cases and review of the literature. *Dis. Col. Rectum*, 18, 601–12.

Garrett, J.R., Howard, E.R. (1981) Myenteric plexus of the hind-gut: developmental abnormalities in humans and experimental studies. In: *Development of the autonomic nervous system.* (Ciba Foundation Symposium 83). London: Pitman Medical, pp. 326–54.

Garrett, J.R., Howard, E.R., Nixon, H.H. (1969) Autonomic nerves in rectum and colon in Hirschsprung's disease. *Arch. Dis. Child.*, 44, 406–17.

Gekas, P., Schuster, M.M. (1981) Stercoral perforation of the colon; case report and review of the literature. *Gastroenterology*, 80, 1054–8.

Gratama, S., Smedts, F., Whitehead, R. (1995) Obstructive colitis: an analysis of 50 cases and a review of the literature. *Pathology* 27, 324–9.

Holschneider, A.M., Meier-Ruge, W., Ure, B.M. (1994) Hirschsprung's disease and allied disorders – a review. *Eur. J. Pediatr. Surg.*, 4, 260–6.

Howard, E.R., Garrett, J.R., Kidd, A. (1984) Constipation and congenital disorders of the myenteric plexus. *J. R. Soc. Med. Suppl.*, 3, 77, 13–19.

Kapilla, L., Haberkorn, S., Nixon, H.H. (1975) Chronic adynamic bowel simulating Hirschsprung's disease. *J. Pediatr. Surg.*, 10, 885–92.

Kleinhaus, S., Boley, S.J., Sheran, M., Sieber, W.K. (1979) Hirschsprung's disease. A survey of the members of the surgical section of the American Academy of Pediatrics. *J. Pediatr. Surg.*, 14, 588–97.

Klück, P., van Muijen, G.N.P., van der Kamp, A.W.M., Tibboel, D., van Hoorn, W.A., Warnaar, S.O., Molenaar, J.C. (1984) Hirschsprung's disease studied with monoclonal antineurofilament antibodies on tissue sections. *Lancet*, i, 652–3.

Levene, T.S., Price, A.B. (1994) Obstructive enterocolitis: a clinico-pathological discussion. *Histopathology*, 25, 57–64.

MacIntosh, D.G., Thompson, W.G., Patel, D.G., Barr, R., Guindi, M. (1992) Is rectal biopsy necessary in irritable bowel syndrome? *Am. J. Gastroenterol.* 87, 1407–9.

Meier-Ruge, W. (1974) Hirschsprung's disease: its aetiology, pathogenesis and differential diagnosis, In: Grundmann E., Kirsten, W.H. (eds) *Current topics in pathology*, vol. 59. Berlin: Springer Verlag, pp. 131–79.

Meier-Ruge, W.A., Bronnimann, P.B., Gambazzi, F., Schmid, P.C., Schmidt, C.P., Stoss, F. (1995) Histopathological criteria for intestinal neuronal dysplasia of the submucosal plexus (type B). *Virchows Arch.*, 426, 549–56.

Meier-Ruge, W.A., Bruder, E. (2005) *Pathology of chronic constipation in pediatric and adult coloproctology.* Basel, Freiburg, Paris, London, New York, Bangalore, Bangkok, Singapore, Tokyo, Sydney: Karger.

Meyrat, B.J., Lesbros, Y., Laurini, R.N. (2001) Assessment of the colon innervation with serial biopsies above the aganglionic zone before the pull-through procedure in Hirschsprung's disease. *Pediatr. Surg. Int.*, 17, 129–35.

Munakata, K., Morita K., Okabe, I., Sueoka, H. (1985) Clinical and histologic studies of neuronal intestinal dysplasia. *J. Pediatr. Surg.*, 20(3), 231–5.

Noblett, H.R. (1969) A rectal suction biopsy tube for use in the diagnosis of Hirschsprung's disease. *J. Pediatr. Surg.*, 4, 406–9.

Puri, P., Lake, B.D., Nixon, H.H., Mishalany, H., Claireaux, A.E. (1977) Neuronal colonic dysplasia: an unusual association of Hirschsprung's disease. *J. Pediatr. Surg.*, 12, 681–5.

Saegesser, F., Sandblom, P. (1975) Ischaemic lesions of the distended colon. A complication of obstructive colorectal cancer. *Am. J. Surg.*, 129, 309–15.

Schmittenbecher, P.P., Gluck, M., Wiebecke B., Meir-Ruge W. (2000) Clinical long-term follow-up results in intestinal neuronal dysplasia (IND). *Eur. J. Pediatr. Surg.*, 10, 17–22.

Tada, S., Iida, M., Yao, T., Kitamoto, T., Fujishima, M. (1993) Intestinal pseudo-obstruction in patients with amyloidosis: clinicopathologic differences between chemical types of amyloid protein. *Gut*, 34, 1412–17.

Toner, M., Condell, D., O'Briain, D.S. (1990) Obstructive colitis. Ulceroinflammatory lesions occurring proximal to colonic obstruction. *Am. J. Surg. Pathol.*, 14, 719–28.

Walker, N.I., Bennett, R.E., Axelsen, R.A. (1988) Melanosis coli. A consequence of anthraquinone-induced apoptosis of colonic epithelial cells. *Am. J. Pathol.* 131, 465–76.

Watanabe, Y., Ito, F., Ando, H., Seo, T., Kaneko, K., Harada, T., Iino, S. (1999) Morphological investigation of the enteric nervous system in Hirschsprung's disease and hypoganglionosis using whole-mount colon preparation. *J. Pediatr. Surg.* 34, 445–9.

Wilder-Smith, C.H., Talbot, I.C., Merki, H.S., Meier-Ruge, W.A. (2002). Morphometric quantification of normal submucous plexus in the distal rectum of adult healthy volunteers. *Eur. J. Gastroenterol. Hepatol.*, 14, 1339–42.

Yam, L.T., Li, C.Y., Crosby, W.H. (1971). Cytochemical identification of monocytes and granulocytes. *Am. J. Clin. Pathol.*, 55, 283–90.

CHAPTER 14

NEOPLASIA IN THE COLON AND RECTUM AND ITS CLASSIFICATION

14.1 Definitions   248   References   250

14.1 DEFINITIONS

Dysplasia of the colorectal epithelium is the series of architectural and cytological changes that represent unequivocal neoplastic transformation (Riddell *et al.*, 1983) and is a precancerous lesion. As defined by the World Health Organization (WHO) (Hamilton *et al.*, 2000) only when components of the abnormal epithelium have penetrated through the muscularis mucosae into the submucosa is the lesion considered as invasive adenocarcinoma.

The diagnosis of dysplasia in the gastrointestinal tract is a controversial matter on two counts.

1. There is poor intraobserver and interobserver reproducibility (Dixon *et al.*, 1988; Melville *et al.*, 1989).
2. There is a different approach between Western and Japanese pathologists (Schlemper *et al.*, 1998). As a consequence, apart from genuine geographical differences, the apparent prevalence of colorectal cancer and its treatment differ between East and West.

To try to overcome these differences and provide a unified framework for pathologists world-wide, the Vienna Classification of gastrointestinal epithelial neoplasia was introduced (Schlemper *et al.*, 2000). It is shown in Table 14.1 and although, for reasons to

Table 14.1 The Vienna classification of gastrointestinal epithelial neoplasia.

Category 1	Negative for neoplasia/dysplasia
Category 2	Indefinite for neoplasia/dysplasia
Category 3	Non-invasive low-grade neoplasia (low-grade adenoma/dysplasia)
Category 4	Non-invasive high-grade neoplasia
	4.1 High grade adenoma/dysplasia
	4.2 Non-invasive carcinoma (carcinoma *in situ*)
	4.3 Suspicious of invasive carcinoma
Category 5	Invasive neoplasia
	5.1 Intramucosal carcinoma
	5.2 Submucosal adenocarcinoma or beyond

be explained, it will not be adopted here we will cross-refer to it in the relevant sections.

A diagnosis of dysplasia has different connotations depending on the clinical context, for example, dysplasia in an adenoma (raised, flat or depressed), a serrated polyp, in a colon with long-standing inflammatory bowel disease, in a patient with past history of radiation or in a patient with a family history of inherited malignancy. In any of these situations, the diagnosis of dysplasia denotes differing chances of multifocality, concomitant cancer, or risk of future malignancy. For example, severe (high-grade) dysplasia in the context of a solitary adenoma will be treated by polypectomy, while high-grade dysplasia in a patient with long-standing ulcerative colitis is a strong indication for total proctocolectomy. These differing situations will be considered in greater detail in the appropriate chapters of the book.

In general, Vienna categories 4 and 5 (Table 14.1) represent the danger area by which a pathologist can signal something more may need to be done. The placing of intramucosal carcinoma in category 5, the category of invasive neoplasia, is in conflict with the WHO classification but, this aside, partial resolution of the East–West divide and improved intra- and inter-observer reproducibility is achieved by the scope of category 4 (non-invasive high-grade neoplasia). It is the subcategories that harbour the observational terminological difficulties but this has become a less critical issue since the advent of endomucosal endoscopic resection, as most of the treatment decisions are determined for the clinician by merely knowing the primary category.

The details of the classification still contain difficulties both for the individual diagnostic pathologist and for those interested in comparative data within and between countries. Category 2 (indefinite for dysplasia), as in the original Riddell classification (Riddell et al., 1983), is still included, acknowledging the dilemma, be one from the East or the West, in which the true nature of the patient's lesion remains uncertain and subsequent management is unresolved. Follow-up in such cases would seem mandatory (Bernstein et al., 1994), for these authors showed that at least 9 per cent can be associated with a future malignancy. Category 3, non-invasive low-grade neoplasia (low-grade adenoma/dysplasia), covers part of the biological spectrum of dysplasia in which there is least dispute, aside from its management in ulcerative colitis (Section 17.10.2). As already mentioned, the total remit of category 4, used as a danger signal to the clinician, improves diagnostic consistency and, with the advances in endoscopic surgery, allows 'lumpers' to negotiate the terminological minefield of its subcategories. Thus, much of the anxiety of decision making has shifted from the pathologist to the endoscopist. The subcategories of 4 and the definition of invasive neoplasia, category 5, are still controversial. At the fundamental level the WHO definition of colorectal 'invasive neoplasia' differs

from the Vienna classification. In the latter intramucosal carcinoma refers to 'invasion of the lamina propria or muscularis mucosae' and is placed in category 5, invasive neoplasia. However, the WHO definition is that only tumours that have 'penetrated through the muscularis mucosae into the submucosa are considered malignant'. In one respect this definition makes for simpler decision making if the guidelines and caveats about the completeness of excision and risks of nodal spread are obeyed (Section 16.4). The WHO rationale for this approach is that in the colorectum there is virtually no risk of metastasis for neoplastic lesions that are confined to the epithelium or invade only lamina propria, with no invasion through to the submucosa. We favour this approach and feel that high-grade intra-epithelial neoplasia is a more appropriate term than adenocarcinoma in situ, and intramucosal neoplasia more appropriate than intramucosal adenocarcinoma. This also effectively restricts use of the term carcinoma with its evocative overtones for the patient. This is not merely semantics since it has clinical implications and we have seen unnecessary extensive, radical surgery performed when the WHO definitions are ignored. Moreover, the histological separation of high-grade dysplasia, in-situ carcinoma and intramucosal carcinoma is the area of greatest difficulty and observational disagreement. We appreciate this is a very clinical approach to the problem and acknowledge that in the research field attempts to discover whether there are differences in natural history between these 'entities' is still important until proven otherwise.

The logic of accepting the WHO approach is to remove intramucosal carcinoma from category 5 and back into category 4. Given the difficulty of distinguishing high-grade dysplasia from carcinoma in situ and that such a distinction, in the current state of knowledge, has no clinical significance, category 4.1 could combine these two terms. This would allow intramucosal carcinoma to reside in category 4.2, one that has no treatment implications beyond complete endoscopic resection of the lesion. While such lesions are rare in the colorectum they are more often appreciated in gastric pathology and their macroscopic and microscopic assessment plus management are different. This is outside the scope of this book. Category 4.3 remains 'suspicious of invasive carcinoma'. Such a reorganization of the Vienna categories would place all the contentious high-grade nomenclature with its accompanying problems of inter- and intra-observer variation within category 4, simplifying matters for clinicians and leave category 5 for undisputed invasive carcinoma in WHO terms. This is an approach that future reviewers of the classification systems might consider. Here, in this predominantly clinically orientated book we prefer to follow the WHO definition of invasion but will make reference to the Vienna classification where relevant.

REFERENCES

Bernstein, C.N., Shanahan, F., Weinstein, W.M. (1994). Are we telling patients the truth about surveillance colonoscopy in ulcerative colitis? *Lancet*, 343, 71–4.

Dixon, M.F., Brown, L.J., Gilmour, H.M., Price A.B., Smeeton N.C., Talbot I.C., Williams G.T. (1988) Observer variation in the assessment of dysplasia in ulcerative colitis. *Histopathology*, 13(4), 385–97.

Hamilton, S.R., Vogelstein, B., Kudo, S. *et al.* (2000) Carcinoma of the colon and rectum. In: Hamilton, S.R., Aaltonen, L.A. (eds) *World Health Organization classification of tumours. Pathology and genetics. Tumours of the digestive system.* Lyon: IARC Press, p. 105.

Melville, D.M., Jass, J.R., Morson, B.C. *et al.* (1989). Observer study of the grading of dysplasia in ulcerative colitis: comparison with clinical outcome. *Hum. Pathol.*, 20(10):1008–14.

Riddell, R.H., Goldman, H., Ransohoff, D.F. *et al.* (1983) Dysplasia in inflammatory bowel disease: standardised classification with provisional clinical applications. *Hum. Pathol.*, 14, 931–68.

Schlemper, R.J., Itabashi, M., Kato, Y. *et al.* (1998) Difference in the diagnostic criteria used by Japanese and Western pathologists to diagnose colorectal carcinoma. *Cancer*, 82; 60–9.

Schlemper, R.J., Riddell, R.H., Kato, Y. *et al.* (2000) The Vienna classification of gastrointestinal epithelial neoplasia. *Gut*, 47, 251–55.

CHAPTER 15

POLYPS

15.1	Definition	251
15.2	Handling	251
15.3	Classification	252
15.4	Aberrant crypt foci	252
15.5	Adenomatous polyps	253
	15.5.1 Tubular adenoma	256
	15.5.2 Tubulovillous adenoma	256
	15.5.3 Villous adenoma	257
	15.5.4 Flat adenoma	258
15.6	Serrated polyps	260
	15.6.1 Metaplastic (hyperplastic) polyps	260
	15.6.2 Serrated adenomas	263
15.7	Juvenile polyps	264
15.8	Peutz–Jeghers polyps	266
15.9	Inflammatory polyps	268
	15.9.1 Post-inflammatory polyps – mucosal tags	269
	15.9.2 Granulation tissue and inflammatory 'cap' polyps	270
15.10	Mucosal prolapse syndrome, including inflammatory cap polyp and inflammatory myoglandular polyp	271
15.11	The Cronkhite–Canada syndrome	275
15.12	Problems in the diagnosis of mucosal polyps: differential diagnosis	275
	15.12.1 Adenomas – overdiagnosis of malignancy	275
	15.12.2 Adenomas – underdiagnosis of malignancy	275
	15.12.3 Adenomas – distinction from juvenile polyps	276
	15.12.4 Hamartomas	276
15.13	Lymphoid polyps	276
15.14	Leiomyomatous polyps	277
15.15	Lipomatous polyps	278
15.16	Vascular hamartoma	279
15.17	Neurofibroma	279
15.18	Ganglioneuroma	279
15.19	Cowden's (multiple hamartoma) syndrome	282
15.20	Granular cell tumour	282
15.21	Heterotopic gastric mucosa	282
15.22	Colonoscopic polypectomy	284
15.23	The reporting of polyps	285
References		286

15.1 DEFINITION

Any localized lesion projecting from the mucosa may be regarded as a polyp. Pedunculated polyps are usually less than 3 cm in diameter, but sessile polyps may be considerably larger.

15.2 HANDLING

The key to the handling of polyps is to provide a block that ensures a complete section through its stalk, base and head. Small polyps should be embedded whole, with instructions to cut well into

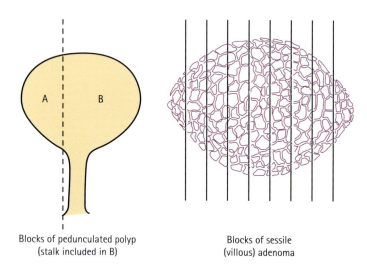

Blocks of pedunculated polyp
(stalk included in B)

Blocks of sessile
(villous) adenoma

Figure 15.1 Methods of cutting larger polyps into blocks for histological processing. Symmetrical bisection of pedunculated polyps should be avoided if a satisfactory section of stalk and base are to be achieved. Sessile lesions are most satisfactorily handled by pinning onto cork at the time of polypectomy to facilitate division entire into blocks orientated perpendicular to the base.

the stalk. The danger of bisecting small polyps through the stalk is that, during trimming of the block, the stalk is trimmed away. Polyps just too large to make one block may be sliced eccentrically (Fig. 15.1). The larger block will contain the complete stalk. Large polyps with an obvious thick stalk can be trimmed such that at least one block, or a composite, generates a complete view of head, stalk and base. All tissues must be embedded in order to detect focal areas of severe dysplasia, particularly at the base. It is useful to remember that carcinoma most frequently arises in the centre of adenomas.

Sessile polyps, are often large and tend to be removed piecemeal and present problems in orientation, which are only partly overcome by examination of sections at multiple levels in the blocks. They should, ideally, be surgically excised entire, together with a rim of normal mucosa. In any case, the whole of the tissue removed should be blocked for histology (Fig. 15.1), so that a focus of invasive tumour is not overlooked. This is best achieved if the surgeon or endoscopist pins the resected specimen onto a sheet of cork before fixation.

15.3 CLASSIFICATION

Polyps may arise from mucosal glands, and include lamina propria (i.e. mucosal polyps) or from connective tissue. They can be neoplastic, hamartomatous, inflammatory, the result of mechanical stress or of uncertain histogenetic origin (Table 15.1). The smallest and possibly earliest polypoid lesions are aberrant crypt foci.

15.4 ABERRANT CRYPT FOCI

First described in the colons of rodents exposed to carcinogens (Bird *et al.*, 1989), these tiny nodular lesions can be found endoscopically in humans, with the aid of magnification and/or dye spray (Nascimbeni *et al.*, 1999). They are not visible on routine inspection of the large bowel mucosa. They are defined endoscopically, rather than histologically, as small plaque-like foci and are histologically heterogeneous (Nucci *et al.*, 1997). Nascimbeni and colleagues found 720 aberrant crypt foci (ACF) in 103 colons resected either for adenocarcinoma or diverticular disease. In one series, one-third of lesions included only normal epithelium (Bouzourene *et al.*, 1999), whereas in another series, almost 90 per cent included hyperplastic, mucin-depleted epithelium, confined to the surface in small lesions and involving the crypts in larger lesions (Nascimbeni *et al.*, 1999). Focal dysplasia was present in 10.8 per cent of ACF in colons resected for adenocarcinoma and in only

Table 15.1 A classification of large intestinal polyps

Histogenesis	Single or few polyps	Polyposis
Mucosal		
Neoplastic	Adenoma	Familial adenomatous polyposis
Meta/hyperplastic, neoplastic	Serrated polyp; metaplastic/hyperplastic, adenomatous	Metaplastic/hyperplastic polyposis Serrated adenomatous polyposis
Hamartomatous	Juvenile polyp	Juvenile polyposis
	Peutz–Jeghers polyp	Peutz–Jeghers syndrome
Inflammatory	Inflammatory polyp	Inflammatory polyposis ('colitis polyposa')
	Benign lymphoid polyp	Benign lymphoid polyposis
Mechanical stress	Mucosal prolapse syndrome:	
	(a) inflammatory cap polyp	Inflammatory cap polyposis
	(b) inflammatory myoglandular polyp	
	(c) solitary rectal ulcer syndrome	
	(d) inflammatory cloacogenic polyp	
Uncertain		Cronkhite–Canada syndrome
Connective tissue		
Neoplastic	Leiomyomatous polyp	
	Lipomatous polyp	Lipomatous polyposis
Hamartomatous	Vascular hamartoma	
	Neurofibroma	Neurofibromatosis
	Ganglioneuroma	
	Cowden's syndrome	Cowden's syndrome

Patterns of colonic adenoma

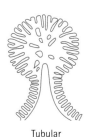
Tubular

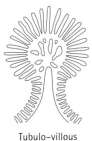
Tubulo–villous

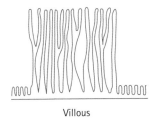
Villous

Figure 15.2 Adenomatous polyps: range of morphology. These lesions are all protuberant masses of dysplastic epithelium but show a variable tendency to exophytic (villous) growth.

2.8 per cent of ACF in colons resected for diverticular disease. Lymphoid follicles are frequently observed in the basal mucosa of both hyperplastic and dysplastic ACF (Shpitz *et al.*, 1998). ACF with dysplasia are characterized by larger size and elongated crypt orifices (Bouzourene *et al.*, 1999). These so-called microadenomas are related to mutations of the *APC* gene, the earliest morphological step in the chromosomal instability colorectal cancer sequence (Nascimbeni *et al.*, 1999). They are found frequently in the background mucosa in familial adenomatous polyposis.

15.5 ADENOMATOUS POLYPS

An adenoma consists of a circumscribed mass of dysplastic epithelium, and may have an exaggerated mucosal glandular arrangement (tubular adenoma), a predominantly villous or papillary configuration (villous adenoma) or a mixture of the two (tubulovillous adenoma) (Fig. 15.2). The last term is used when less than 80 per cent of the polyp conforms to either a tubular or villous pattern. The presence of dysplastic epithelium is an essential feature of all adenomatous polyps. The degree of dysplasia varies from lesion to lesion and from area to area within the same lesion. Pedunculated adenomatous polyps may fall into any of these categories; but villous adenomas are usually sessile. Occasionally, the dysplastic lesion may be virtually flat or even show a depression of the surface (Muto *et al.*, 1985), in which case the lesion hardly quali-fies as a polyp and should be classi-fied as a non-polypoid adenoma (flat adenoma) (Section 15.5.4).

There is a definite relationship between adenomas and carcinomas in the large intestine (the adenoma–carcinoma sequence). Hence, it is necessary to excise completely all polypoid lesions. It is not uncommon for invasive adenocarcinoma to be found arising in a polypoid adenoma. Before making such a diagnosis it is necessary to exclude the possibility of pseudocarcinomatous invasion. This pitfall is discussed in Chapter 16. The incidence of focal malignant change is greater in larger adenomas (46 per cent in adenomas over 2 cm in diameter) and in adenomas with severely dysplastic epithelium (Muto *et al.*, 1975). For this reason it is useful to classify the severity of dysplasia, using three grades: mild, moderate and severe (Day and Morson, 1978). The criteria for this assessment are subjective and are illustrated in Figs 15.3 and 15.4. The specific features which can be identified in

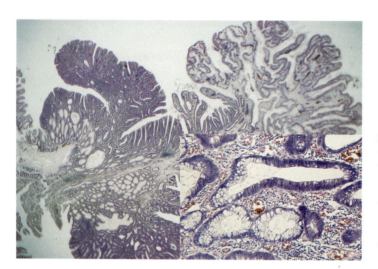

Figure 15.3 Tubular adenoma showing distinct areas of mild and moderate epithelial dysplasia (upper and lower halves, respectively). Inset is a magnified part of a gland, showing junction of the two grades of dysplasia. There is increased nuclear stratification in moderate dysplasia (on right) and more obvious goblet cell differentiation in mild dysplasia (on left).

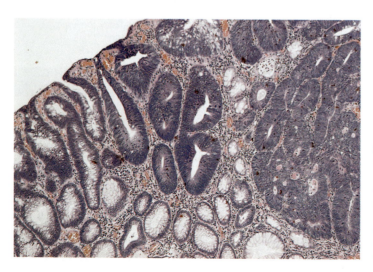

Figure 15.4 Moderate (left) and severe (right) epithelial dysplasia in a tubular adenoma. The severely dysplastic epithelium shows complete loss of cell polarity, with randomly placed nuclei. There is also a cribriform pattern caused by glandular budding present only to a minimal degree in the moderately dysplastic area.

dysplasia are shown in Table 15.2. Of these, only nuclear size and degree of nuclear stratification are consistently reliable diagnostic features (Brown *et al.*, 1985). Karyotypic analyses (Meijer *et al.*, 1998), as well as studies involving immunohistochemistry and mucin core protein expression (Ajioka *et al.*, 1997), show a progression parallel to the morphological continuum from mild to severe dysplasia, but this is of little practical use for the routine diagnostic pathologist.

While a three-tier classification is preferred in our institution, many endoscopists and surgeons use only two categories; low- and high-grade dysplasia (Table 15.3). Only the latter requires special attention for closer patient follow-up. Furthermore, some centres use the terms low- and high-grade colonic intraepithelial neoplasia (Park *et al.*, 2003), to fall into line with the general nomenclature in other epithelial-lined organs. An alternative term, intramucosal neoplasia, has been proposed (Talbot, 2001). Whatever the semantic value of the various terminologies, the crucial issue is for the reporting pathologist and their endoscopic and surgical colleagues to agree on a classification such that all parties understand the biological and clinical implications.

Foci of squamous epithelial differentiation are very occasionally present in large intestinal adenomas.

Cramer *et al.* (1986) consider that this feature is associated with increased malignant potential.

It has been shown that the larger adenomas (over 2 cm) and those with severe dysplasia, are concentrated in the left colon and rectum (Konishi and Morson, 1982). They parallel the anatomical distribution of colorectal cancer in high risk populations (Haenzel and Correa, 1971) and follow the commonest molecular pathway, that of chromosomal instability (de la Chapelle, 2003). Autopsy studies, on the other hand, have shown that small adenomas tend to be evenly distributed along the length of the large bowel (Williams *et al.*, 1982).

The results of a study of dysplasia in adenomas in the context of concurrent colorectal carcinoma are of importance. Morson *et al.* (1983) found that there was severe dysplasia in four of 38 adenomas removed at the same time as bowel resection for carcinoma. However, in another group of patients, who developed a second, metachronous adenocarcinoma, severe dysplasia was found in five out of 21 adenomas present in the original operation specimens. This suggests that, in a patient who has already had a colorectal carcinoma resected, the finding of severe dysplasia in an adenoma may be a marker for an increased risk of a second adenocarcinoma developing.

Table 15.2 Histological grading of dysplasia

	Mild	Moderate	Severe
Glandular pattern	Branched	Folded	Budded
Interglandular space	Minimally reduced	Reduced	Often obliterated
Nuclei			
Enlarged	+	++	+++
Hyperchromatic	+	++	+++ or chromatin clumped
Shape	Elongated	Elliptical	Pleomorphic
Position	Basal	Stratified	Random
Nucleoli	Not seen	Sometimes	Frequent
Mitotic rate	+	++	
Mucin droplets	Apical	Reduced	Absent
Goblet cells	Occasionally	Often dystrophic	Absent dystrophic

Table 15.3 Equivalence of dysplasia grading in three-tier and two-tier systems

Three-tier system	Two-tier system	Intraepithelial neoplasia (IEN)
Mild ⎫ Moderate ⎬	Low-grade dysplasia	Low-grade intraepithelial neoplasia
Severe	High-grade dysplasia	High-grade intraepithelial neoplasia

Multiple adenomatous polyps may be a signal that the patient has a polyposis syndrome. In familial adenomatous polyposis (FAP) there are typically over 100 and the polyps closely resemble single (sporadic) adenomas in both histology and behaviour, the majority being tubular in nature. Adenomas are also found in hereditary non-polyposis colon cancer (HNPCC) syndrome and despite its name, are often multiple. They tend to show a villous architectural pattern, as well as larger size and severe dysplasia and develop at a relatively earlier age. Furthermore, they almost always show loss of immunohistochemical expression of DNA mismatch repair protein (Iino *et al.*, 2000). Awareness of these features, in the appropriate clinical context and taking account of the relative preponderance of right-sided colonic lesions in HNPCC, may prompt the diagnostic pathologist to draw attention to a potentially inherited form of colorectal cancer. The pathologist should also be aware that in another rare polyposis syndrome, metaplastic/hyperplastic polyposis, many of the polyps can be dysplastic and are in reality serrated adenomas (Section 15.6.2).

15.5.1 Tubular adenoma

Tubular adenomas ('adenomatous polyps') are the type of polyp most frequently encountered by the histopathologist. They are characterized by a rounded but multilobulated shape, like miniature raspberries, well demonstrated by scanning electron microscopy (Elias *et al.*, 1981). They are often, but not invariably, pedunculated, with a stalk typically composed of normal mucosa and submucosa (Fig. 15.5). When sessile, they take the form of brownish nodules of variable thickness and size, but rarely exceed 4 cm in diameter.

Microscopically, these lesions vary from the mere presence of dysplastic epithelium in one or more crypts (microadenomas, Fig. 15.6) to masses of elongated and often irregular glands set in a thickened layer of lamina propria overlying a normal or thickened muscularis mucosae (Fig. 15.5). Sometimes, only the upper portions of the crypts are dysplastic, a feature seen most easily in small adenomas (Fig. 15.6). The epithelium is usually more darkly stained than in the normal mucosa and is

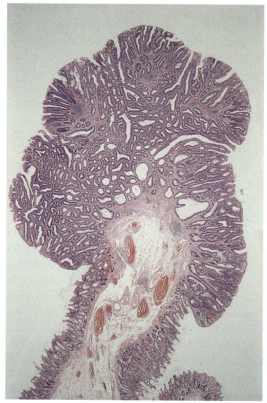

Figure 15.5 Pedunculated tubular adenoma, processed and sectioned entire. In these lesions the crypts, as well as being lined by dysplastic epithelium, are elongated. There is often cystic dilatation of some crypts, not necessarily dysplastic ones.

dysplastic to varying degree, the cells being tall columnar with eosinophilic, finely granular cytoplasm and relatively little mucin. Goblet cell differentiation is suppressed in tubular adenomas and, ultrastructurally, the columnar cells show features of partly differentiated 'absorptive cells' (Kaye *et al.*, 1973; Jass and Roberton, 1994). Paneth cells and enterochromaffin cells can usually be found scattered singly and in groups throughout the epithelium of adenomas (van den Ingh *et al.*, 1986), a feature not seen in non-neoplastic polyps.

15.5.2 Tubulovillous adenoma

Many adenomatous polyps, which otherwise show features of tubular adenoma, either sessile or pedunculated, also include some villous components

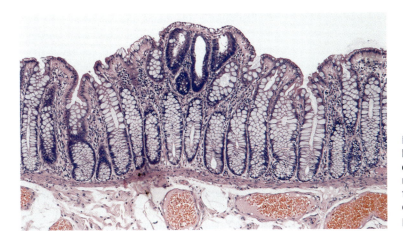

Figure 15.6 Microadenoma. Dysplastic epithelium here involves only a few crypts. Such lesions are not often seen at endoscopy but are found at histological examination of apparently normal colon, particularly in polyposis patients.

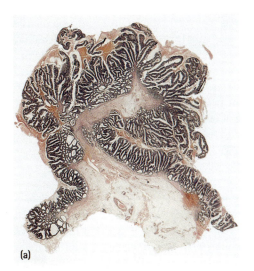

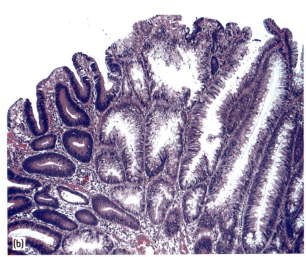

Figure 15.7 (a) Tubulovillous adenoma. This small pedunculated example shows a partly villous surface but there is still a tubular structure to the majority of the lesion. (b) Tubulovillous adenoma. This sessile lesion shows a sharp distinction between the tubular components on the left and the villous components on the right. Note that the latter is composed of villi which are almost devoid of lamina propria and are lined by tall epithelial cells which, although containing mucin vacuoles, possess large nuclei.

(Fig. 15.7). Study of serial sections suggests that apparently villous structures in adenomas are really flat folia separated by sulci (Wiebecke *et al.*, 1974). The dysplastic epithelium of such lesions resembles that of tubular adenomas and is usually monomorphic, despite the variable architecture. Tubulovillous adenoma is the term applied to those polyps in which less than 80 per cent of the lesion conforms to a single pattern (Konishi and Morson, 1982).

15.5.3 Villous adenoma

Villous adenomas are polyps composed principally of finger-like or leaf-like villous processes of lamina propria covered by dysplastic epithelium, and previously referred to as villous papillomas (Fig. 15.8). Although usually sessile and often very large, sometimes completely encircling the bowel, a stalk of normal mucosa and submucosa is occasionally present.

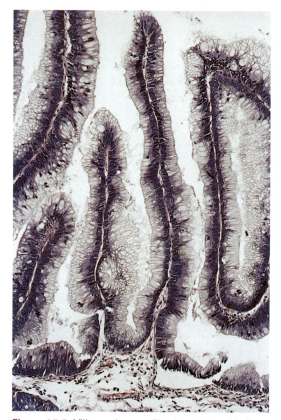

Figure 15.8 Villous adenoma. The dysplastic epithelium extends along elongated folia, which in this biopsy appear as villous processes, with thin cores of lamina propria. The bases of the villi lie immediately above the muscularis mucosae.

Unlike tubular adenomas, the epithelial cells frequently show goblet cell features, with varying degrees of differentiation. Severe epithelial dysplasia is relatively common in villous adenomas, being found in 20.6 per cent in one series, as compared with only 4.1 per cent in tubular adenomas (Konishi and Morson, 1982).

Diagnostic difficulty arises when, in a locally removed villous tumour, there are severely dysplastic glands closely related to muscularis mucosae at the base of the lesion (Fig. 15.9). The appearances can resemble those of adenocarcinoma but in the absence of definitive diagnostic features, may have to be classified as Vienna Category 4.3 (suspicious of invasive carcinoma). It is important not to underestimate such appearances; invasive adenocarcinoma has been shown to be present in the submucosa in 41 per cent of villous adenomas (Muto *et al.*, 1975). Surface ulceration, granulation tissue and stromal fibrosis are not typical features of adenomas and, if present, in association with apparent invasion of muscularis mucosae, should suggest a diagnosis of carcinoma. (For a fuller discussion of the diagnosis of malignancy see Chapter 16.)

15.5.4 Flat adenoma

A substantial minority of adenomas are not polypoid but are flat – as many as 38 per cent in one series (Fujii *et al.*, 1998). Nevertheless it is appropriate to

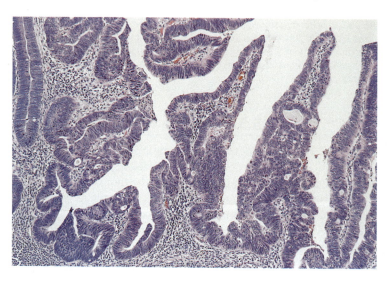

Figure 15.9 Severe dysplasia in villous adenoma. This focus of severely dysplastic epithelium lies in the centre of a locally excised villous adenoma. Although there is a granulation tissue reaction in this area, the glands still lie above the muscularis mucosae and the lesion should therefore not be regarded as malignant (Vienna category 4.3)

consider flat adenomas in this chapter, alongside adenomatous polyps. Muto *et al.* (1985) defined adenomas as flat when they measure less than twice the thickness of the surrounding normal mucosa.

When examining excision biopsies of small polyps orientation to the adjacent mucosa is distorted and it is unusual to be able to reliably classify a lesion in this way (Samowitz and Burt, 1995). Most flat adenomas are indistinguishable histologically from polypoid tubular adenomas in small excision biopsies. Fortunately, this rarely matters, as it appears that most flat adenomas have similar clinical significance to small polypoid tubular adenomas (O'Brien *et al.*, 2004). However, a subgroup of flat adenomas does show the distinctive features of straight unbranched crypts and a depressed centre (Fig. 15.10a). These have been classified as 'depressed' adenomas (Yao *et al.*, 1994), in contrast to 'flat-elevated' adenomas (Sakashita *et al.*, 2000). The latter authors found that 1.6 per cent of adenomas in a Japanese series were depressed and there is good reason to believe that the incidence is similar in Western populations (Fujii *et al.*, 1998). Depressed adenomas are composed of crypts of smaller diameter than polypoid adenomas and deficient in pericrypt sheath structures (Yao *et al.*, 1994). The dysplastic epithelium of the crypts comprises cells with enlarged nuclei but without enlarged cytoplasm, resulting in a high nucleo-cytoplasmic ratio but with little or no stratification (Fig. 15.10b). The dysplasia extends throughout the whole crypt length in the centre of the lesion but affects only the upper parts of the more peripheral crypts, giving a saucer-like shape to the whole lesion (Fig. 15.10a) (Masaki *et al.*, 1994; Yao *et al.*, 1994). These features can be recognized in biopsy material. It has been demonstrated that cell proliferation is preferentially increased in the upper crypts and postulated that, unlike polypoid adenomas, these lesions grow not by crypt fission (Wasan *et al.*, 1998) but by sideways spread of dysplasia along the surface epithelium (Kubota and Kino, 1995).

Apoptosis is relatively increased in flat and depressed adenomas, with a reduced proliferative: apoptotic ratio (Suzuki *et al.*, 2002; Watari *et al.*, 2002). K-ras mutations are relatively rare in flat adenomas (Minamoto *et al.*, 1994) and APC mutations are also reported to be unusual (Umetani *et al.*, 2000).

There is evidence that there is a distinct adenoma–carcinoma sequence, whereby flat and excavated adenocarcinoma arises from flat and especially depressed adenoma (Sakashita *et al.*, 2000). However, previous hypotheses that this was

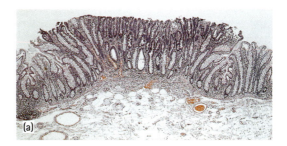

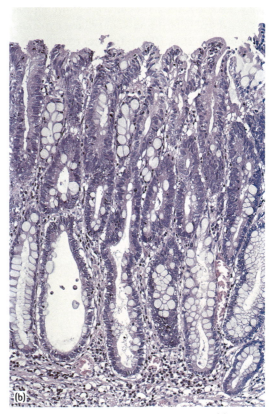

Figure 15.10 Flat adenoma, depressed type. (a) At low power, the dysplasia can be seen to involve the whole crypts in only the centre of the lesion, with progressively more superficial crypt dysplasia towards the periphery, giving a saucer-like shape. (b) At higher magnification the dysplastic epithelium is seen to show little nuclear stratification, despite obvious nuclear enlargement (so-called 'basal cell' dysplasia).

a particularly rapid pathway (Muto *et al.*, 1985) have not been confirmed (Kuramoto and Oohara, 1995) and the finding of flat adenomas is not an indication to alter surveillance protocols (Atkin and Saunders, 2002).

15.6 SERRATED POLYPS

The term 'serrated polyp' (Jass, 2001) embraces both metaplastic polyps, and serrated adenomas. They share the morphology of crowded, serrated epithelium composed of tall columnar cells containing gastric-type mucin (Jass, 1999), with relatively few goblet cells. The epithelial crowding was first suggested to be the result of cellular hypermaturity by Kaye *et al.* (1973). This has recently been confirmed and is caused by impaired apoptosis, found in all serrated polyps (Tateyama *et al.*, 2002). Such a pathogenesis contrasts with the growth of adenomatous polyps, which is the result of excess cell proliferation. The difference may result from mutation of genes in the mitogen-activated protein kinase signalling pathway, either *K-ras* or *BRAF*, present in many serrated polyps (Higuchi and Jass, 2004). It is likely that DNA hypermethylation, a feature of many metaplastic polyps and serrated adenomas, at least in hyperplastic polyposis (Chan

et al., 2002), also has a role in switching off apoptosis (Wynter *et al.*, 2004).

15.6.1 Metaplastic (hyperplastic) polyps

Metaplastic polyps are very common, pale nodules (Fig. 15.11), rarely measuring more than 3 mm in diameter, that increase in frequency with age (Williams *et al.*, 1980). However, occasional lesions measure up to 5 cm in diameter. They vary in morphology from flat lesions with a crypt pattern which differs only slightly from the normal (Fig. 15.12), to frankly pedunculated lesions with a considerably distorted glandular architecture (Fig. 15.13). The cardinal features are elongation of crypts in association with an apparent excess of tall columnar absorptive cells, giving the epithelium a crowded, tufted or crenated appearance (Fig. 15.12) (Wiebecke *et al.*, 1974). The epithelium in the basal portions of the crypts is usually more darkly stained and apparently hyperplastic. This should not be mistaken for dysplasia. For this reason the alternative name, hyperplastic polyp, has been applied to these lesions. Conversely, evidence to support the use of the term 'metaplastic' is provided by the observation that the epithelial cells of these polyps express growth factors such as epidermal growth factor (EGF) as well as trefoil peptides (Hanby *et al.*, 1993) – features of

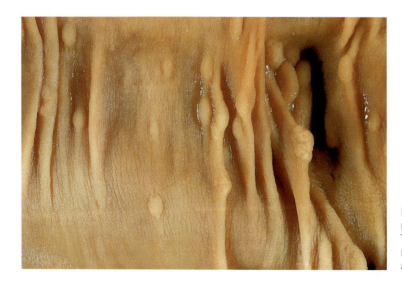

Figure 15.11 Gross appearance of metaplastic (hyperplastic) polyps. These polyps are pale sessile nodules, mostly situated at the apices of mucosal folds.

altered differentiation. Goblet cells are relatively sparse. The epithelial cells have no dysplastic features and the nuclei are small, uniform and basally situated. There is little mitotic activity, which is confined to the proliferative compartment at the base of the crypts.

Jass (1983) demonstrated similarities in the type of mucin in metaplastic polyps to that in dysplastic epithelium and suggested that metaplastic polyps may be induced by the same environmental stimuli that induce neoplastic polyps and carcinoma in a susceptible individual. The epithelium

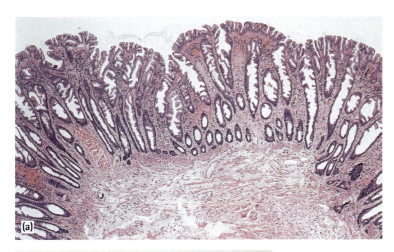

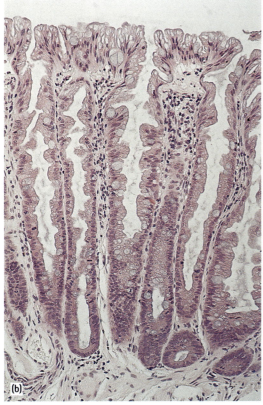

Figure 15.12 (a) Sessile metaplastic polyp. The epithelium at the crypt bases is hyperplastic and deficient in goblet cells. In the upper parts of the crypts the epithelium comprises excess numbers of tall columnar cells, aggregated into tufts, giving a serrated appearance.
(b) Portion of a metaplastic polyp showing the serrated epithelium. Although by usual criteria there is no dysplasia, the epithelium does show considerable irregularity.

of both metaplastic polyps and tubular adenomas belongs to the tall columnar cell rather than the goblet cell lineage (Jass and Roberton, 1994) and the associated mucin is chemically related to

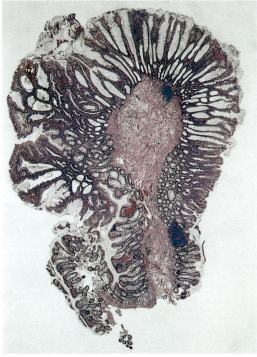

Figure 15.13 Pedunculated metaplastic polyp. The glands of this polyp are lined by typically serrated epithelium. There is considerable irregularity of architecture but there is no dysplasia.

gastric mucin. However, these observations do not mean that metaplastic polyps are, in themselves, pre-malignant (Jass, 1983). Thus, metaplastic polyps are common; remnants of metaplastic polyps associated with adenocarcinoma are seen only very rarely.

However, there is an increased risk of colorectal carcinoma in the condition of metaplastic/ hyperplastic polyposis (Leggett *et al.*, 2001). Here, the risk of neoplasia is in a subtly different serrated polyp, the so-called 'sessile serrated adenoma' found in this condition (Torlakovic and Snover, 1996). This lesion may show little or no dysplasia but differs from the generality of metaplastic polyps in its large size, location in the right colon, crypt dilatation, increased serration, greater irregularity of architecture with horizontal crypts and excess goblet cells (Torlakovic *et al.*, 2003) (Fig. 15.14) Unequivocal dysplasia develops in these polyps and correlates with mutation of the *BRAF* gene and hypermethylation of DNA (Higuchi and Jass, 2004). These lesions seem to be the specific precursor of the subset of MSI-H/ DNA hypermethylated colorectal cancers (Jass *et al.*, 2002), often right-sided. The diagnosis of metaplastic polyposis is not made merely from the presence of multiple metaplastic polyps, The World Health Organization (WHO) classification requires the following criteria (Burt and Jass, 2000):

● at least 30 metaplastic polyps throughout the colorectum, or

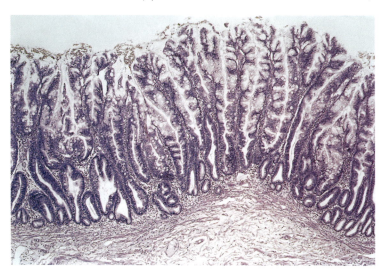

Figure 15.14 'Sessile hyperplastic-like polyp' of rectum. The crypts are dilated, with serrated epithelium extending down to the basal part of the mucosa. The basal parts of the crypts in these lesions tend to bend sideways to run parallel with the muscularis mucosae. Large sessile metaplastic polyps of this nature in the caecum and right colon have been identified as being potential precursors of sporadic microsatellite unstable adenocarcinoma (Torlakovic *et al.*, 2003).

- at least five metaplastic polyps proximal to the sigmoid colon, two of which measure more than 10 mm, or
- any metaplastic polyps in an individual with a first-degree relative with metaplastic polyposis.

15.6.2 Serrated adenomas

Serrated adenomas, as originally described (Longacre and Fenoglio-Preiser, 1990), architecturally appear as hyperplastic/metaplastic, but cytologically show the characteristic features of dysplasia, detailed in Table 15.3. Various combinations can occur; the whole lesion may be both serrated and dysplastic (Fig. 15.15), there may be focal dysplasia in a serrated polyp (so-called 'admixed' polyps) with well-defined hyperplastic and adenomatous areas (Estrada and Spjut, 1980; Longacre and Fenoglio-Preiser, 1990) (Fig. 15.16) or there may be focal serration in an otherwise ordinary tubular, tubulovillous or villous adenoma (Fig. 15.17). The significance of the various patterns is not yet clear. The glandular pattern of serrated adenomas is more complex than in metaplastic/hyperplastic polyps and the epithelium tends to be dense and eosinophilic (Fig. 15.15). Also, unlike metaplastic polyps, the subepithelial collagen layer is not thickened and endocrine cells are lacking (Torlakovic and Snover, 1996). The dysplasia is often confined to the superficial portion of the crypts.

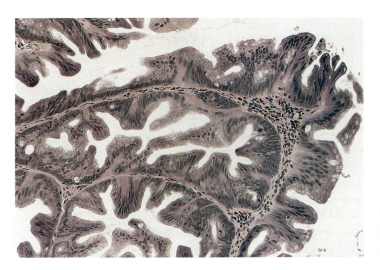

Figure 15.15 Serrated adenoma. This polyp is composed of crypts lined by epithelium which is dysplastic (low grade) and at the same time serrated.

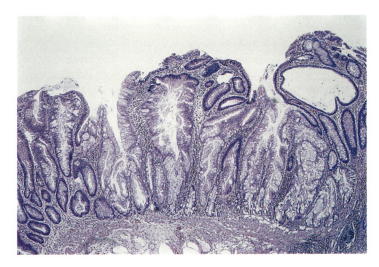

Figure 15.16 Admixed polyp. Collections of mildly dysplastic crypts, resembling tubular adenoma, lie within a metaplastic polyp. The architecture suggests that the adenoma arose in a pre-existing metaplastic polyp.

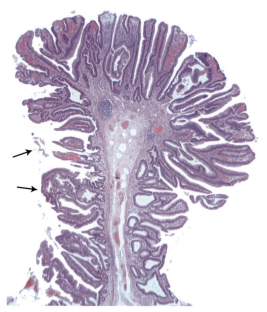

Figure 15.17 Admixed polyp. Serrated focus in tubulovillous adenoma. Most of this polyp is an adenoma of tubulovillous type but there are glands resembling the crypts of a metaplastic polyp. It is not possible with certainty to determine the sequence of development of this polyp.

By appropriate testing of DNA, Jass (1999) has found that some serrated adenomas show microsatellite instability (MSI) and has postulated that the MSI histogenetic pathway of colorectal cancer includes a serrated adenoma stage. Consistent with this is the finding that those serrated adenomas showing MSI with a high number of markers (MSI-H) showed loss of hMLH1 protein expression, as do most 'sporadic' MSI-H colorectal carcinomas (Jass *et al.*, 2000). Despite this interesting discovery, progression of serrated adenomas to malignancy is evidently rare and, unfortunately, there are no reliable histological markers of those serrated adenomas which carry this risk.

Serrated adenomas are usually small, no more than a few millimetres in diameter and occur singly or in clusters, in the distal colon or rectum. The majority are not associated with any specific genetic or pre-cancerous changes (Sawyer *et al.*, 2002) and seem to be of little clinical significance (Chandra *et al.*, 2006). It is the occasional, usually larger, lesion in the right colon which should be given more attention, as this is more specifically

associated with the MSI pathway to colorectal cancer (Higuchi and Jass, 2004). Serrated adenomas are also found among the polyps of metaplastic polyposis. Moreover, the variant 'serrated adenomatous polyposis' has been described (Torlakovic and Snover, 1996).

15.7 JUVENILE POLYPS

Juvenile polyps are rounded, commonly spherical masses of soft mucosal tissue, measuring anything up to several centimetres in diameter. They may occur anywhere in the large bowel but are commonest in the rectum. As the name implies, they occur most commonly in children, and are frequently multiple.

The polyps consist of normal columnar and goblet cell epithelium arranged in cystically dilated glands set in an often excessive oedematous lamina propria (Fig. 15.18). This abundant stroma is a helpful diagnostic feature and appreciated best at low-power microscopy. There is frequently an inflammatory cell exudate in both lamina propria and glands. The surface epithelium is also often inflamed or eroded.

These polyps contain no smooth muscle and usually have only a thin, easily twisted stalk. Ischaemic infarction, haemorrhage from the surface and auto-amputation are common, with haemosiderin-containing macrophages frequently observed in the stroma, reflecting this. The inflammatory reaction seen histologically is presumably a related phenomenon.

The epithelium that makes up the glands in juvenile polyps is usually of normal large intestinal crypt type, with a basal stem cell zone, in which there are occasional Paneth cells and argentaffin cells. It is extremely rare for a focus of dysplastic epithelium to be found in an otherwise typical (sporadic) juvenile polyp (Dajani and Kamal, 1984). This dysplasia is associated with mutations/inactivation of the APC/β-catenin molecular pathway and, as such, is similar to the genesis of sporadic adenomas (Wu *et al.*, 1997). It is important to appreciate that some inflammatory polyps can closely resemble juvenile polyps. This is relevant in the assessment of inflammatory polyps from adult patients (Section 15.9).

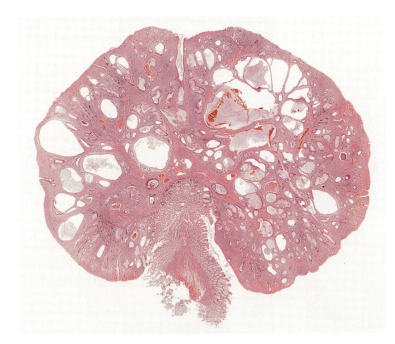

Figure 15.18 Juvenile polyp. These lesions have a smooth outline and are covered by a thin layer of flattened columnar cells. They are composed of a relative excess of lamina propria containing cystically dilated glands. The stalk is thin and delicate.

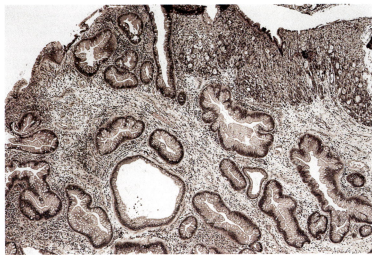

Figure 15.19 Juvenile polyp with focal severe dysplasia from a patient with juvenile polyposis. This unusual phenomenon does not occur in sporadic juvenile polyps.

Although isolated juvenile polyps can be regarded as hamartomatous and bear no relationship to colorectal neoplasia (Morson, 1962), juvenile polyposis is an autosomal dominant, familial cancer syndrome. The diagnostic criteria include: (a) more than five juvenile polyps in the colorectum, or (b) juvenile polyps throughout the gastrointestinal tract or (c) any number of polyps with a family history of juvenile polyposis (Jass *et al.*, 1988). Individuals usually develop 50–200 polyps, which are classically pedunculated and may adopt a multilobated appearance. While the smaller polyps are akin to the sporadic ones, the multilobated ones often take on a fronded and branched appearance, accompanied by a relative increase of epithelium versus stroma. Foci of dysplasia are identifiable in up to 50 per cent of atypical or multilobated juvenile polyps (Fig. 15.19), and the associated carcinomas are more likely to be poorly differentiated or mucinous (Jass *et al.*, 1988). A wide range of extra-intestinal manifestations are part of the syndrome in 11–20 per cent of cases. These are well described by Desai and colleagues (1995). Germline mutations of the SMAD4/DPC4 tumour suppressor genes are responsible for some of these cases (Hahn *et al.*, 1996) but many other genes have also been implicated.

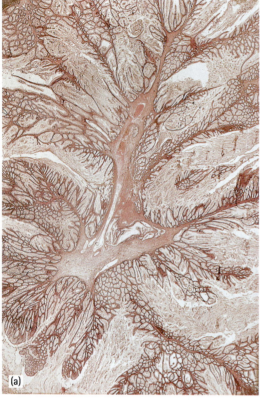

(a)

15.8 PEUTZ–JEGHERS POLYPS

Although these polyps are rarely seen unless associated with the Peutz–Jeghers syndrome, solitary lesions occasionally arise in the large bowel.

Peutz–Jeghers polyps can be either pedunculated or sessile and, characteristically, have a coarsely lobulated surface. The histological features are well described by Enterline (1976). Elongated and branched glands are lined by mature epithelial cells, which resemble normal crypt epithelium. Strands of smooth muscle extend upwards and divide the polyp into sectors. The epithelium is orientated to the smooth muscle as if the latter were muscularis mucosae (Fig. 15.20). Some degree of epithelial dysplasia is occasionally seen (Yaguchi *et al.*, 1982).

These lesions can be regarded as hamartomas. Peutz–Jeghers syndrome has been shown to be associated with and presumably caused by germline mutation of the *LKB1* gene on chromosome 19q (Hemminki *et al.*, 1998; Hemminki, 1999). *LKB1* belongs to the *PAR* family of genes which collectively govern cell polarity (Macara, 2004). Jansen and colleagues (2006) postulate that perturbation of LKB1 protein or other PAR protein results in epithelial prolapse, presumably at sites of mucosal prolapse and that the polyps in Peutz–Jeghers syndrome are a variant of the polyps that occur in

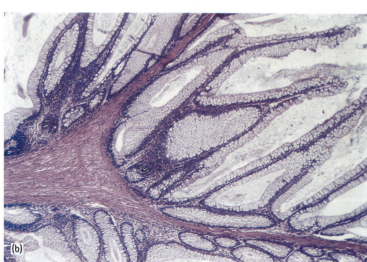

(b)

Figure 15.20 Peutz–Jeghers polyps. (a,b) Tree-like architecture, with normal colorectal epithelium resting on smooth muscle branches of the muscularis mucosae.

mucosal prolapse syndrome, with a particularly florid epithelial misplacement, responsible for the deep-seated mucin-filled cysts in Peutz–Jeghers polyps. The occasional finding of dysplasia in the epithelium of these polyps should be regarded as the result of secondary mucosal prolapse at the site of a pre-existing adenomatous polyp. Similarly, the few reported cases of adenocarcinomas occurring in the large intestine of people with Peutz–Jeghers syndrome (Dodds *et al.*, 1972; Tweedie and McCann, 1984) would be examples of the adenoma–carcinoma sequence, with polypoid mucosal prolapse occurring as an epiphenomenon,

rather than a hamartoma-carcinoma sequence, as had been suggested (Bosman, 1999; Wang *et al.*, 1999).

It is important to recognize the benign nature of the misplaced, mucin-filled, cystically dilated glands which lie in the smooth muscle of these polyps (Fig. 15.21). These cysts can be found in resection specimens in the deeper layers of the bowel wall (Shepherd *et al.*, 1987), even within the serosa. Such features should not be attributed to invasive carcinoma unless epithelial dysplasia and stromal desmoplasia are also seen (Sections 16.2 and 16.3).

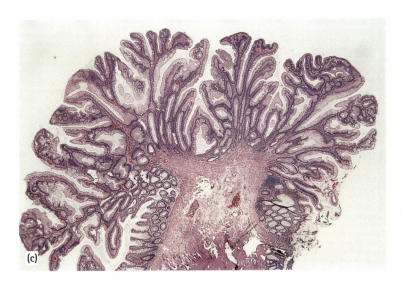

Figure 15.20 (c) Smaller, less developed Peutz–Jeghers polyp showing tree-like pattern but less conspicuous smooth muscle branching.

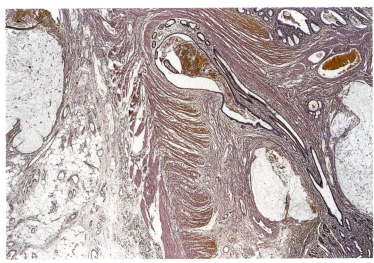

Figure 15.21 Resected colon at the site of a Peutz–Jeghers polyp, showing misplaced glands and pools of mucin within and external to the bowel wall.

15.9 INFLAMMATORY POLYPS

Inflammatory polyps are non-neoplastic prolifera-tions of mucosa and/or granulation tissue, which mark the site of previous severe mucosal ulcera-tion. Multiple inflammatory polyps (incorrectly called 'pseudopolyps') frequently develop in ulcer-ative colitis and are an important morphological feature of that condition (Section 5.6). Similar polyps are also often found in Crohn's disease and may occur in amoebiasis, bacillary dysentery and schistosomiasis (Fig. 15.22). In some inflammatory polyps the lamina propria may be oedematous, giving a rounded appearance which can resemble that of a juvenile polyp (Fig. 15.23). However, the lamina propria, although oedematous, may be more fibrous and chronically inflamed than in juvenile polyps (Fig. 15.18) and the glands may be less uniformly cystically dilated. A special, often

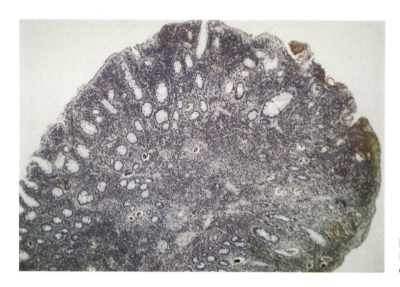

Figure 15.22 Inflammatory polyp in schistosomiasis. An inflamed tag of mucosa containing numerous ova.

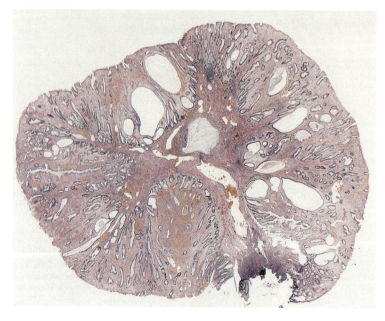

Figure 15.23 Inflammatory polyp resembling juvenile polyp. This polyp from the sigmoid colon in a patient with ulcerative colitis is composed of cystic glands and an excess of lamina propria similar to a juvenile polyp. In this particular inflammatory polyp, there is chronic inflammation and fibrosis.

giant, form of inflammatory polyp develops in the colon at the site of ureteric implantation (Fig. 15.24), where, presumably owing to chemical irritation, there is localized expansion of lamina propria and cystic dilatation of glands (Ansell and Vellacott, 1980; Ali *et al.*, 1984; Paterson *et al.*, 1985). Inflammatory polyps can also develop as part of the segmental colitis associated with diverticular disease; in this context, they have been described as myoglandular polyps (Nakamura *et al.*, 1992) or polypoid prolapsed folds (Kelly, 1991). The term 'eroded polypoid hyperplasia' would also be part of the inflammatory polyp spectrum (Burke and Sobin, 1990). Isolated, usually small, inflammatory polyps sometimes develop in the rectal mucosa in the absence of inflammatory bowel disease. In order to determine if there is underlying disease it is necessary to examine non-polypoid mucosa, which should be biopsied at the same time.

15.9.1 Post-inflammatory polyps – mucosal tags

In inflammatory bowel disease inflammatory polyps develop as islands of residual mucosa which protrude from areas of ulceration and are often undermined by it (Fig. 15.25). These features may not be appreciated in biopsy material as the polyps may consist of a tag or 'finger' of almost

normal mucosa with surprisingly normal crypt architecture. In contrast to adjacent diseased mucosa there may be very little inflammatory cell infiltration (Fig 15.26). The term 'post-inflammatory polyp' is appropriate for such polyps. They are also referred to as 'filiform' polyps or 'bizarre' or 'giant' polyps. They can be very numerous (Fig. 15.27).

Evidence of epithelial damage and regenerative atypia are often seen in inflammatory polyps, but genuine epithelial dysplasia, with elongation and stratification of nuclei is not found, except in rare cases of inflammatory bowel disease, when they are referred to as 'dysplasia-associated lesions or masses' (Section 17.11). It should also be remembered that sporadic adenomatous polyps can occur

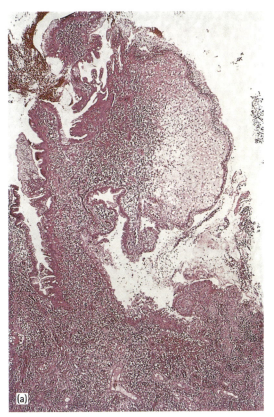

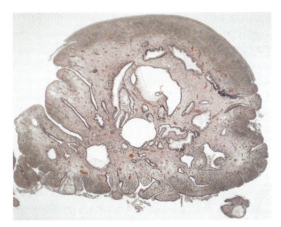

Figure 15.24 Polyp from uretero-sigmoidostomy site. This lesion, with abundant oedematous stroma, resembles a juvenile polyp, but has a broad base. There is also a cap of fibrin, betraying an inflammatory nature.

Figure 15.25 Inflammatory polyps in ulcerative colitis. These are really tags of mucosa which have been undermined by ulceration. In (a) the polyp is formed by swelling of the mucosal tissue by oedema, whereas in (b) the mucosa is chronically inflamed and shows reparative features, with glandular irregularity and epithelial hyperplasia.

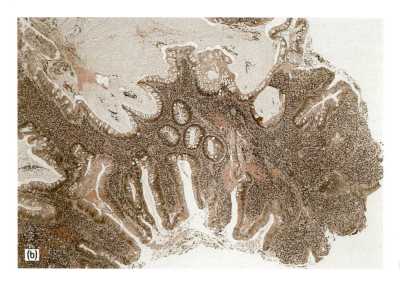

Figure 15.25 (*Continued*)

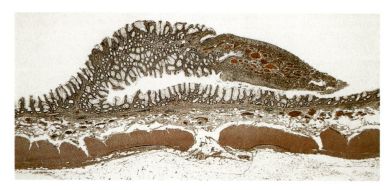

Figure 15.26 Post-inflammatory polyp in ulcerative colitis. This filiform polyp is composed of healed or healing mucosa with a cap of fibrin.

in patients with inflammatory bowel disease (Section 17.11).

15.9.2 Granulation tissue and inflammatory 'cap' polyps

Some inflammatory polyps consist of a rounded mass of granulation tissue with an attenuated or eroded epithelial covering and largely lack a crypt epithelial component. These polyps, which resemble pyogenic granulomas of the skin and mouth (Fig. 15.28), may sometimes arise in the absence of inflammatory bowel disease and may be the result of localized trauma, for example, at a colostomy. A variant of this type of polyp has been described as the inflammatory 'cap' polyp (Williams *et al.*, 1985)

and is considered in the next section (15.10). This is a polypoid thickening of mucosa, in which the glands are elongated and tortuous, the lamina propria contains smooth muscle fibres and there is surface erosion, often with a cap of fibrinous exudate. They may be sessile (Fig. 15.28) or pedunculated (Fig. 15.29). The histological features can resemble mucosal prolapse syndrome (Section 15.10) and it has therefore been postulated that these polyps, which may occur anywhere along the length of the large bowel, are the result of focal prolapse, possibly at the apices of mucosal folds. An occasional case with multiple cap polyps (Fig. 15.30) ('cap polyposis') has been reported (Campbell *et al.*, 1993) with presenting clinical features resembling inflammatory bowel disease. This is further considered in the next section (15.10).

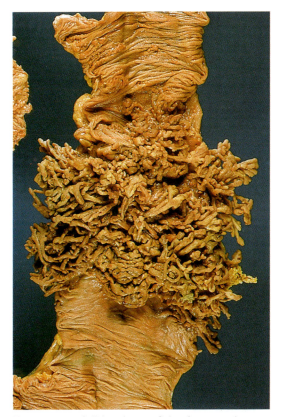

Figure 15.27 Colitis polyposa. Colon from a patient with long-standing ulcerative colitis. Multiple filiform, post-inflammatory polyps can present as a dramatic tumour-like mass. No tumour or dysplasia was found in this specimen.

15.10 MUCOSAL PROLAPSE SYNDROME, INCLUDING INFLAMMATORY CAP POLYP AND INFLAMMATORY MYOGLANDULAR POLYP

Mucosal prolapse syndrome, which develops in response to shearing stress of the mucosa is most commonly seen on the anterior rectal lining (solitary ulcer syndrome), but may be found at any site of prolapse (du Boulay *et al.*, 1983). At sigmoidoscopy, it may appear as a polyp (Fig. 15.31), but these lesions often grow to a large size and can resemble carcinomas (Madigan and Morson, 1969). In the rectum it may cause a mucous discharge, with or without bleeding. When on the anterior rectal wall, in the context of such symptoms, the lesion is referred to as a solitary rectal ulcer. This form of rectal mucosal prolapse occurs predominantly in young adults, as a result of excessive straining at stool (Womack *et al.*, 1987). Mucosal prolapse can also present at the anus, when it produces an 'inflammatory cloacogenic polyp' (Section 19.2.6).

In the typical case there is mucosal thickening with elongation, dilatation and tortuosity of glands (Fig. 15.32a,b). The glandular epithelial cells are

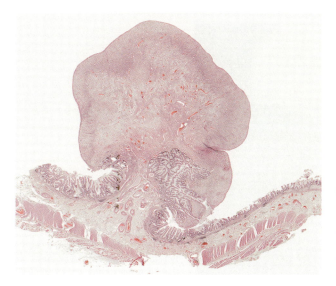

Figure 15.28 Inflammatory cap polyp. This example from a patient with ulcerative colitis shows how a cap of granulation tissue covers a mucosal defect at the edges of which there has been regenerative hyperplasia of mucosa. Such polyps can persist for a considerable time after ulcerative colitis has gone into remission.

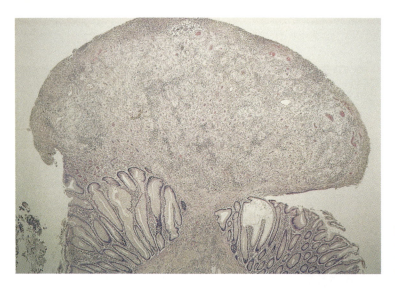

Figure 15.29 A small inflammatory cap polyp. As in Fig. 15.28, there is a central focus of hyperplastic mucosa.

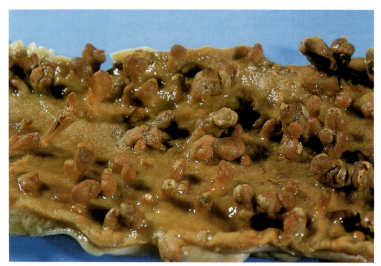

Figure 15.30 Gross appearance of multiple inflammatory cap polyps in the left colon in quiescent ulcerative colitis.

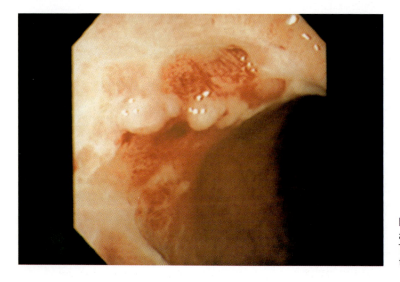

Figure 15.31 Endoscopic appearance of solitary rectal ulcer. Typically, around the ulcer edges there is polypoid mucosal thickening.

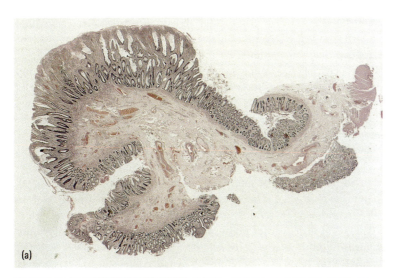

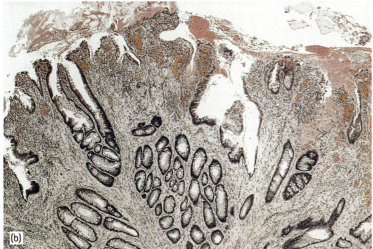

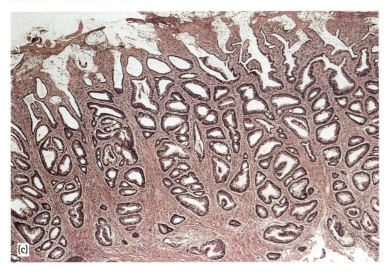

Figure 15.32 Mucosal prolapse/ solitary rectal ulcer. (a) The process of mucosal prolapse is causing mucosal thickening, crypt elongation and surface erosion. (b) The tip of a polypoid focus of prolapsed mucosa, forming an inflammatory cap polyp. As well as surface erosion, there is fibrosis of the lamina propria, elongation and tortuosity of crypts and hyperplasia of epithelium. (c) Glands can become so embedded in the hypertrophied muscularis mucosae that the picture can resemble invasive adenocarcinoma. This is a biopsy of solitary rectal ulcer.

commonly enlarged, the goblet cells appearing elongated. There may be loss of sulphated mucin seen by high iron diamine (HID) staining (Ehsanullah *et al.*, 1982). There is often, but not invariably, superficial erosion of the surface epithelium, with a little surface exudate of fibrin and polymorphs. This can resemble the Type I lesion of pseudomembranous colitis (Section 8.2.1a). In the lamina propria inflammatory cells are inconspicuous but small vessels are dilated (Fig. 3.54 on page 48). A characteristic and diagnostic feature is the presence, in the lamina propria, of vertically orientated smooth muscle fibres and bundles, in continuity with the muscularis mucosae, which is often thickened (Fig. 3.51 on page 46). The muscle fibres, together with fibrous tissue insinuate between the crypt bases, which become pointed and, on tangential and transverse sections, 'diamond-shaped' (Warren *et al.*, 1990). Sometimes the smooth muscle is so hypertrophic that the crypts appear to 'be embedded in the muscularis mucosae (Fig. 15.32c), giving an appearance which resembles colitis cystica profunda (Sections 3.11.3 and 20.11). This accounts for the use of the alternative name 'localized colitis cystica profunda' for solitary ulcer of the rectum (Epstein *et al.*, 1966).

Milder features of prolapse can be noted in many instances, such as the margin of a colostomy, in folds of redundant mucosa in the contracted colon of diverticular disease (so-called 'crescentic fold colitis'; Gore *et al.*, 1992), the apical aspect of a protruding haemorrhoid, in the vicinity of diverticula or in association with any polypoid lesion. In many of these instances the features are less clear-cut and this is probably one of the most frequently missed histological diagnoses. The mucosal surface may be only slightly distorted with slight widening of the crypts. The diagnosis is suggested when these features are accompanied by a few ectatic capillaries in the superficial lamina propria (Figs 3.54 and 15.32).

The two special forms of polyp which seem to result from mucosal prolapse are the *inflammatory cap polyp* and the *inflammatory myoglandular polyp* (Nakamura *et al.*, 1992). The latter does not have a fibrin-capped ulcerated surface, but in other respects resembles the inflammatory cap polyp, considered in the previous section. Both are composed of mucosa showing histological features similar to those of mucosal prolapse, with crypt elongation, irregularity and basal pointing, fibromuscular extension into the lamina propria and ectasia of superficial blood capillaries (Fig. 15.33). They are most frequently found in the left colon, particularly the sigmoid, where there are prominent transverse mucosal folds, muscle activity is maximal and the faeces are firmest, but may occur anywhere along the length of the large bowel.

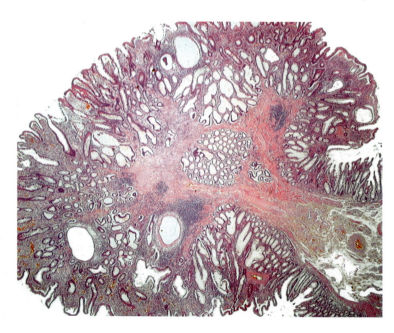

Figure 15.33 Inflammatory myoglandular polyp. This polyp is composed of hyperplastic elongated crypts set in a chronically inflamed lamina propria in which strands of smooth muscle extend upwards from the muscularis mucosae.

15.11 THE CRONKHITE–CANADA SYNDROME

Cronkhite–Canada syndrome is a rare, sporadic, diffusely polypoid condition of the mucosa of the stomach and small and large intestines, which may present as fulminant diarrhoea. The mucosa is thickened and there is oedema of the lamina propria with cystic dilatation of gland crypts (Fig. 15.34). The features are more fully discussed in Section 20.9.

15.12 PROBLEMS IN THE DIAGNOSIS OF MUCOSAL POLYPS: DIFFERENTIAL DIAGNOSIS

15.12.1 Adenomas – overdiagnosis of malignancy

The commonest and most important problem is to distinguish an adenoma from adenocarcinoma. This may be particularly difficult when only small and malorientated biopsies are available. The problem arises when the dysplastic glandular epithelium is seen surrounded by smooth muscle or lying in the submucosal tissue and is more worrisome if there is severe epithelial dysplasia. The difficulty is increased when there is tangential sectioning or when, through chronic stress to the head of an adenoma, there is extension of muscle bundles up into the polyp (Fig. 15.35). When in doubt, it is best to examine deeper sections from the block. Another, perhaps more disturbing cause of confusion with invasive carcinoma is the presence of pseudocarcinomatous invasion of the stalk of an adenoma. This is illustrated and described more fully in Section 16.2.2 but can be identified by the presence of an investing layer of lamina propria, often with haemorrhage and/or haemosiderin, around the misplaced glands (Fig. 16.2). Another pitfall is the stromal fibrosis in an adenoma which frequently develops following the taking of a small biopsy from a large polyp (Fig. 16.5 on page 296). This can closely resemble desmoplasia, one of the indicators of invasive malignancy. Knowledge that a biopsy has been taken within weeks of the polypectomy helps to avoid overdiagnosis and a Perl's stain, if positive, is helpful in indicating post-traumatic scarring.

15.12.2 Adenomas – underdiagnosis of malignancy

The surface of a relatively large colorectal lesion may be composed of severely dysplastic glands with a typical villous or tubular architectural pattern,

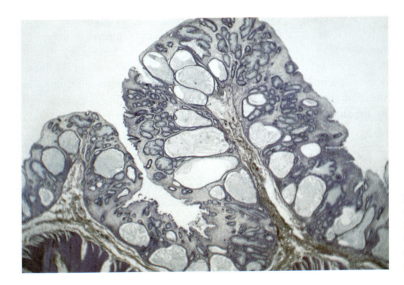

Figure 15.34 Cronkhite–Canada syndrome. A polypoid fold of thickened rectal mucosa. The cystically dilated glands and oedematous lamina propria resemble a juvenile polyp.

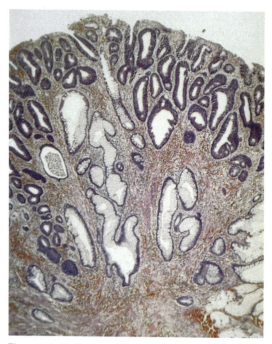

Figure 15.35 Hypertrophic smooth muscle in a tubular adenoma caused by chronic torsion. The muscle bundles are in continuity with the muscularis mucosae. The dysplastic glands retain an accompanying rim of lamina propria. The distension of crypt bases is caused by strangulation.

while the deep aspect of the lesion may already be showing invasion of submucosa. In this scenario, small superficial biopsies may look indistinguishable from a severely dysplastic adenoma, and a pathology report along those lines may not be representative of the invasiveness of the lesion. Thus, it is important to know the size of the polyp biopsied, and express a degree of caution in the report when the polyp is large or the endoscopic appearances are suspicious. Eventually, some of these biopsies may have to be considered as 'inadequate' for full diagnostic assessment.

15.12.3 Adenomas – distinction from juvenile polyps

In addition to the stromal excess, juvenile polyps ordinarily have a similar architectural pattern to tubular adenomas (Fig. 15.5), but lack epithelial dysplasia. Focal dysplasia is occasionally found in

the epithelium of a juvenile polyp (Fig. 15.19) and indicates the onset of neoplasia. The polyp then assumes the significance of an adenoma. This is rare outside the context of juvenile polyposis.

In rare instances, polyps in what appears to be a polyposis syndrome show mixed features of juvenile and adenomatous polyp, with some metaplastic features. These mixed polyps are found in only a few families, the condition showing Mendelian dominant inheritance and known as the 'hereditary mixed polyposis syndrome' (Whitelaw *et al.*, 1997). There is a high incidence of colorectal cancer among family members, although not at the 100 per cent level seen in FAP.

15.12.4 Hamartomas

Juvenile polyps and tubular adenomas can sometimes resemble Peutz–Jeghers polyps owing to an effect of chronic torsion, with resulting smooth muscle hypertrophy (Fig. 15.35). The interpretation of incomplete or crushed biopsies can be particularly difficult. However, a typical intact Peutz–Jeghers polyp contains an arborescent core of smooth muscle which is so well defined that confusion is unusual.

Distinction between juvenile and inflammatory polyps can also sometimes be difficult. This is particularly so when a juvenile polyp contains an inflammatory cell infiltrate following surface ulceration or torsion, which is apt to occur. Inflammatory cap polyps (Fig. 15.29) and myoglandular polyps (Fig. 15.33) may only differ from juvenile polyps in lacking cystic glands. The inflammatory polyps which develop at the ureteric orifices in those patients who still have uretero-sigmoidostomies in place have an abundant stroma, like juvenile polyps and have even been labelled as such (van Driel *et al.*, 1988) (Fig. 15.24).

15.13 LYMPHOID POLYPS

Polyps formed as a result of overgrowth of lymphoid tissue are rarities in the large intestine. They may result from reactive hyperplasia of the lymphoid

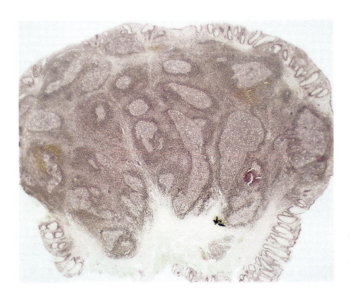

Figure 15.36 Benign lymphoid polyp. This is a rounded mass of hyperplastic lymphoid tissue with follicles and germinal centres, covered by mucosa, which is intact but focally thinned.

follicles normally present in the mucosa and submucosa and be benign, or they may be part of a lymphoma. Colorectal lymphomas are discussed in Chapter 18.

Benign lymphoid polyps may be single and measure up to 3 cm in diameter, or be present in very large numbers, particularly in the distal large bowel, and smaller, measuring between 3 mm and 6 mm. The solitary lesions are found in the rectum, anus and sigmoid colon, usually in young adults (Cornes *et al.*, 1961) or, rarely, in children (Byrne *et al.*, 1982).

Multiple benign lymphoid polyposis is found in adolescents with a familial immunodeficiency syndrome but may occasionally occur in children in its absence (Capitanio and Kirkpatrick, 1970), particularly in the right colon and terminal ileum. Cases have been reported in the families of patients with multiple adenomatous polyposis and can cause clinical confusion (Shull and Fitts, 1974). This suggests that these lesions may be at one end of the normal range of lymphoid hyperplasia found in young people. In adults, a diagnosis of benign lymphoid polyposis should only be made when mantle cell lymphoma is fully excluded, according to the parameters described in Chapter 18.

Histologically, benign lymphoid polyps show a sharply defined rounded mass of lymphoid tissue,

mainly in the submucosa. with stretching and thinning of the overlying mucosa (Fig. 15.36). There is a well-developed follicular structure, with germinal centres containing tingible body macrophages, reminiscent of a reactive lymph node. Benign lymphoid polyps have also been said to be distinguished by the presence of well-defined fibrous septa between the lymphoid follicles (Helwig and Hansen, 1951).

15.14 LEIOMYOMATOUS POLYPS

Small leiomyomas, arising from the muscularis mucosae, are occasional incidental findings, appearing as hard white nodules in the mucosa during colonoscopy for other disease (Walsh, 1984). These lesions are distinctive, circumscribed nodules of smooth muscle up to 1 cm in diameter and usually show no mitotic activity or other evidence of malignancy (Fig. 15.37). They are of no clinical consequence. They should not be confused with biopsy artefacts caused by bunching of the muscularis mucosae or of the muscularis propria. Recognition of Auerbach's plexus is a useful clue in the latter case.

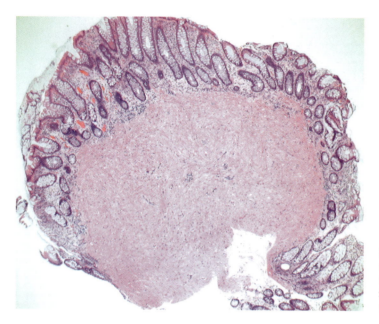

Figure 15.37 Polypoid leiomyoma of muscularis mucosae. These hard white nodules are composed of whorls of smooth muscle cells with little or no mitotic activity.

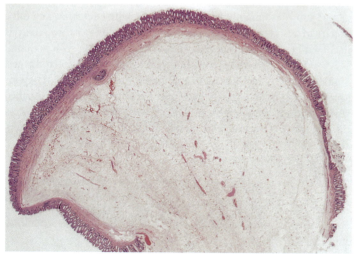

Figure 15.38 Polypoid lipoma. There is a rounded mass of mature adipose tissue in the submucosa.

15.15 LIPOMATOUS POLYPS

Submucosal nodules of mature adipose tissue (lipomas) are frequently seen endoscopically, and usually appear as smooth, polypoidal lesions (Fig. 15.38). They are usually symptomless, only being found incidental to other lesions, although in some instances lesions over 3 cm in diameter have been reported to cause intussusception and can become

infarcted (Creasy *et al.*, 1987; Ryan *et al.*, 1989). They are found more frequently in the caecum and ascending colon than in the distal large bowel (Castro and Stearns, 1972). In the caecum, a diffuse increase in submucosal fat is not infrequent and is known as 'lipohyperplasia of the ileocaecal valve' (Fig. 3.59). Lipomatous polyposis can involve both the small and large bowel (Ling *et al.*, 1959), and is presumed to be a hamartomatous phenomenon with no malignant association.

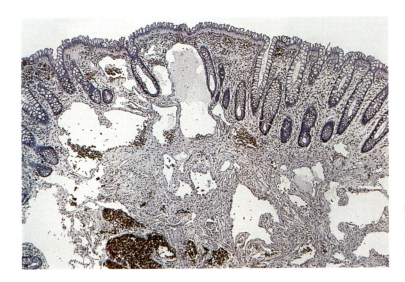

Figure 15.39 Vascular hamartoma. Biopsy of a localized rectal lesion. Multiple irregular sinusoidal channels are present in both mucosa and submucosa.

15.16 VASCULAR HAMARTOMA

Haemangiomatous malformations can involve any part of the small or large intestine and may be the cause of rectal bleeding. They may present to the endoscopist either as a discrete dark-red mucosal polyp or be more diffuse and extensively involve all coats of the bowel wall without a polypoid lesion. The former type can be excised at colonoscopy but the latter may require extensive surgical resection. Histologically, the features of a cavernous haemangioma are typically seen in the mucosa and submucosa (Fig. 15.39). In a biopsy, discrimination from angiodysplasia (Section 20.1.1) may not be possible and much will depend on the colonoscopic appearances.

15.17 NEUROFIBROMA

Multiple neurofibromatous polyps occasionally occur in the large intestine in von Recklinghausen's multiple neurofibromatosis. They may be symptomless or can cause rectal bleeding (Grodsky, 1958). The polyps are irregular in shape and firm in consistency. They are usually small (1–2 cm diameter). Sections show an ill-defined mass of spindle cells in the submucosa, which may extend into the mucosa (Fig. 15.40). The cells are arranged irregularly and are less eosinophilic than in a smooth muscle tumour, with which the lesion can be confused. They show expression of the S-100 antigen. It is excessively rare to find isolated neurofibromas in the large bowel in the absence of lesions elsewhere and enquiry about the clinical picture should confirm the diagnosis.

15.18 GANGLIONEUROMA

Mucosal polyps which contain nerve ganglion cells as well as proliferated Schwann cells and nerve bundles can be regarded as ganglioneuromatous and are rare in the large intestine. They can measure over 12 cm in diameter, but are usually only a few millimetres across and can arise anywhere along the large bowel. Histologically, they have a smooth surface and are characterized by atrophic crypts separated by sheets and bundles of spindle cells, resembling neurofibroma tissue, with, in addition, groups of large ganglion cells (Fig. 15.41). This tissue involves both the mucosa and submucosa.

These lesions are occasionally found in patients with von Recklinghausen's disease, who then also

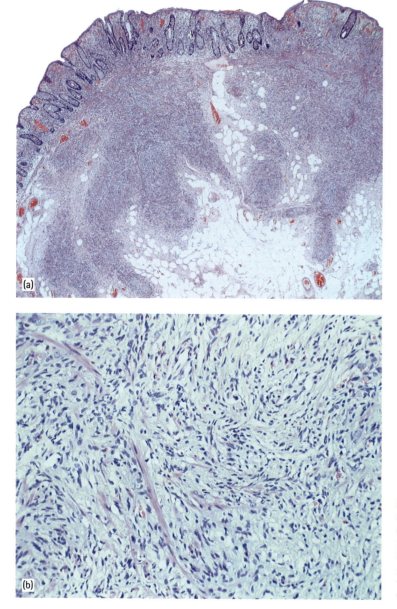

Figure 15.40 Neurofibroma. These are usually polypoid lesions and are composed of ill-defined masses of pale-staining spindle cells involving both submucosa and mucosa. The nuclei of the spindle cells are typically small and darkly stained, with pointed ends.

tend to have diffuse, non-polypoid, involvement of the mucosa by a similar process. An association with Cowden's syndrome has also been reported (see below). Symptoms akin to Hirschsprung's disease have been described in some of these patients, but it is likely that most are symptomless. Similar lesions may antedate the development of overt multiple endocrine neoplasia (MEN), type 2b (Carney and Hayles, 1977). Sporadic examples of ganglioneuromatous polyps of the large intestine have also been described in the absence of either von Recklinghausen's disease or the MEN syndrome, but in association with adenomatous and juvenile polyps (Weidner *et al.*, 1984).

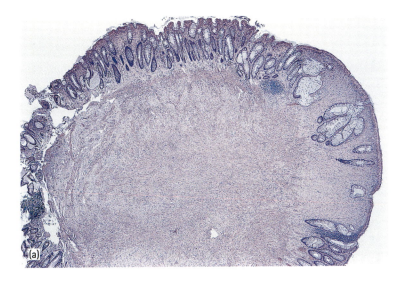

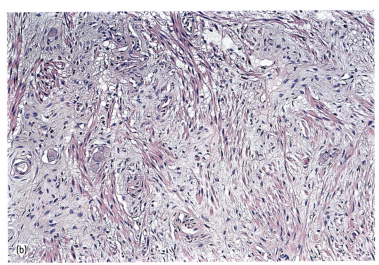

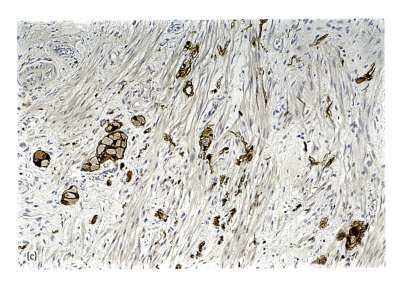

Figure 15.41 Ganglioneuroma. (a) These polypoid lesions resemble neurofibromas but, in addition, contain groups of large ganglion cells, seen at higher magnification in (b), and are highlighted by S100 staining (c).

15.19 COWDEN'S (MULTIPLE HAMARTOMA) SYNDROME

This is a rare familial syndrome characterized by multiple hamartomas of the skin, mouth and gastrointestinal tract, as well as lesions of the thyroid and breast (Carlson *et al.*, 1984). It is inherited as an autosomal dominant character and presents at around puberty. Families have a germline mutation of the *PTEN* gene in chromosome 10q21 (Nelen *et al.*, 1996). The colorectal polyps are small, measuring 1–2 cm in diameter, and have a variable composition of smooth muscle and fibrous tissue with or without adipose tissue, which projects upwards from the muscularis mucosae, forming an ill-defined mass in the lamina propria of the mucosa (Fig. 15.42). The mucosal glands are normal apart from distortion by the mesenchymal proliferation. Lashner *et al.* (1986) described the association with ganglioneuromatous lesions. Early reports of malignancy in the gastrointestinal tract in association with this syndrome have not been confirmed (Carlson *et al.*, 1984), although there does appear to be a high incidence of thyroid carcinoma and, in women, carcinoma of the breast (Salem and Steck, 1983).

15.20 GRANULAR CELL TUMOUR

This rare tumour, also known as granular cell myoblastoma (Weitzner *et al.*, 1976) may be found incidentally as a firm sessile polyp during colonoscopy but may occasionally cause symptoms. Johnston and Helwig (1981) collected 20 such lesions of large bowel from the files of the US Armed Forces Institute of Pathology. Three of the patients presented with rectal bleeding. Nine patients in their series had multiple lesions, including skin tumours.

Biopsy histology shows a submucosal mass of the characteristic large pale granular cells, typically in continuity with the muscularis mucosae (Fig. 15.43). The tumour cells are positively stained by the periodic acid–Schiff (PAS) method and by immunohistochemistry, using antibody to S-100 protein, the latter highlighting its nerve sheath origin.

15.21 HETEROTOPIC GASTRIC MUCOSA

This is a rare cause of polyp formation in the large bowel, typically in the rectum (Srinivasan *et al.*,

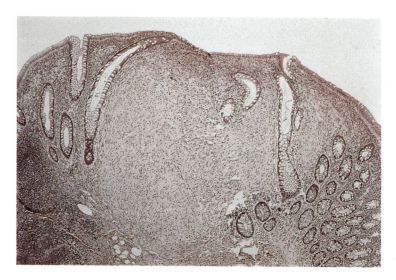

Figure 15.42 Cowden's syndrome. The hamartomatous polyps in this condition consist of a mixture of connective tissues, of which fibrous tissue is here the most prominent. There is also some adipose tissue.

1999). To the endoscopist the lesion is visible as a slightly raised nodule with a granular surface. Sometimes the patient presents with rectal bleeding and the lesion can be ulcerated. Colonization with

Helicobacter pylori has been observed (Kestemberg *et al.*, 1993). Histologically, the lesion is composed of normal gastric body mucosa (Fig. 15.44). This is no doubt a localized aberrant expression of a homeobox

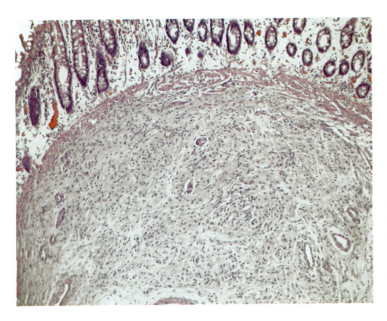

Figure 15.43 Polypoid granular cell tumour. A polyp removed at colonoscopy. There is a submucosal nodule of pale-staining cells with finely granular cytoplasm and uniform small nuclei. The lesion is closely associated with the muscularis mucosae.

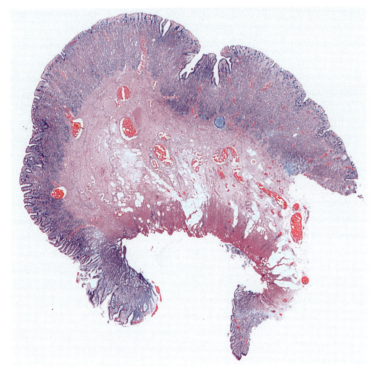

Figure 15.44 Gastric heterotopia. A rectal polyp found incidentally during investigation for diarrhoea. After excision, this lesion was seen to be a focus of complete replacement of the rectal mucosa by normal gastric body mucosa.

gene. Adenoma formation has been reported from the foveolar epithelium of the heterotopic mucosa (Vieth *et al.*, 2005).

15.22 COLONOSCOPIC POLYPECTOMY

The most frequent large intestinal polyps observed at colonoscopy are of metaplastic type. Although there is some evidence that metaplastic (serrated) polyps can be pre-neoplastic, it still holds true that adenomatous polyps have the greatest clinical significance.

Adenomas were present in the large bowel in 37 per cent of men and 29 per cent of women in a necropsy study in the UK (Williams *et al.*, 1982) and in 43 per cent of men and 32 per cent of women in a similar study in Norway (Eide and Stalsberg, 1978). The incidence of adenomatous polyps increases with age. In an autopsy study in the USA, such polyps were found in 58 per cent of men and 47 per cent of women over the age of 50 (Rickert *et al.*, 1979). Adenomas of large intestinal mucosa have been shown to be pre-cancerous lesions (Muto *et al.*, 1975), 46 per cent of adenomatous polyps over 2 cm in diameter already containing focal invasive carcinoma at the time of removal. Even adenomas between 1 cm and 2 cm in diameter contain invasive adenocarcinoma in 9.5 per cent of the lesions. Detractors will argue that there is little evidence that a single adenoma *per se* has a significant chance of developing malignancy (Jass, 2003). In one study (Hofstad *et al.*, 1996), although adenomas measuring less than 5 mm tended to grow, those between 5 mm and 9 mm sometimes spontaneously regressed. In UK and European randomized controlled trials of faecal occult blood screening, the removal of adenomas had little impact in the incidence of colorectal cancer (Hardcastle *et al.*, 1996; Mandel *et al.*, 2000), although in the USA, where a more sensitive occult blood test was used and colonoscopy was more frequently done, a 20 per cent reduction in incidence was recorded (Allison, 1998; Schnoll-Sussmann *et al.*, 2000). However, colorectal carcinoma is still the third most frequent cancer to cause death in the UK (Office of Population Censuses and Surveys, 1999) and, thus, the best hope of reducing the incidence of this problem is to undertake prophylactic colonoscopic polypectomy on all individuals in whom polyps can be identified (Williams *et al.*, 1974).

Current endoscopic technology and expertise should allow full colorectal visualization in the vast majority of procedures. Modern endoscopy, using snare polypectomy and mucosectomy (Kudo, 1993), is increasingly therapeutic, allowing for the full resection of protruding adenomas, flat/depressed adenomas, and even adenocarcinomas with minimal (superficial) invasion. Conventional optic colonoscopy, or the more modern chromoendoscopy (Eisen *et al.*, 2002) and magnifying colonoscopy with indigo carmine (Konishi *et al.*, 2003; Rutter *et al.*, 2004) can not only permit the removal of polyps ranging from 1–2 mm to several centimetres, but can also predict the morphology and degree of dysplasia with a significant degree of accuracy. However, this accuracy is not 100 per cent, and indeed the miss rates for detection of all types of polyps may reach 30 per cent in some series (Harrison *et al.*, 2004). It is best practice, whenever possible, to retain all excised polyps for histological examination and repeat colonoscopy may be advisable.

As was stated in Section 15.2, it is important that all polyps are entirely removed. The base or stalk should be clearly identified by a thread, tied in place by the colonoscopist or his assistant. This is necessary because, during fixation, there is a tendency for the stalk to retract into the lesion and disappear. The pathologist has to decide not only whether or not stalk invasion (i.e. adenocarcinoma) is present, but also, if it is, whether the line of excision is clear of the carcinoma. Large, sessile, often villous lesions are difficult to remove by snaring and frequently contain focal invasive carcinoma. When the endoscopist is confident that a large polyp is benign, piecemeal snare excision can be justified. However, piecemeal removal means that the orientation for microscopic examination may be jeopardized and when the endoscopist is in any doubt about the benign nature of a polyp, every attempt should be made to remove the polyp intact. The issue of local excision of malignant polyps is discussed in Section 16.4.

Colonoscopy and its attendant therapeutic polypectomy, including the histopathological examination of multiple pieces of tissue, are labour-intensive procedures which require significant clinical and laboratory resources. However, these efforts are worthwhile because of the benefit both to individual patients, who will avoid abdominal surgery, and to the community, which, provided that at-risk patients can be appropriately screened, will show a reduced incidence of colorectal cancer.

15.23 THE REPORTING OF POLYPS

Assuming that the type of polyp can be identified without difficulty this should be stated, together with a comment about completeness of excision, essential for clinical management. The British Society of Gastroenterology guidelines for surveillance, following discovery of an adenoma (Atkin and Saunders, 2002), recommend three alternative strategies, depending on whether the adenoma is 'low risk', 'intermediate risk' or 'high risk'. Low risk is when only one or two small adenomas (less than 1 cm in diameter) are present. Following removal of these, follow-up colonoscopy is only recommended, if at all, after 5 years. Intermediate risk is three or four small adenomas or at least one >1 cm. Repeat colonoscopy at 3 years is then recommended. High risk is >5 small adenomas or >3 adenomas, at least one of which >1 cm. Follow-up colonoscopy is then recommended after 1 year. Although with completely excised, isolated adenomas the degree of dysplasia does not matter, dysplasia does become important if only part of the lesion has been removed, as carcinoma is more likely to be present in adenomas with severe epithelial dysplasia (Day and Morson, 1978). It is not always possible to identify the excision line in histological sections of polyps, even after examination of sections from multiple levels. This can be due to malorientation, to tissue crushing or to distortion of the tissue by diathermy heat. If the excision line of an adenoma cannot be clearly identified and the epithelium of the lesion is more than mildly dysplastic, the report should include a note that it is not possible to confirm completeness of excision. The endoscopist can then decide whether a repeat excision is necessary. Repeat excision is assisted if, because of concern at the endoscopic appearance, the endoscopist tattoos the site of the polyp at the time of first excision. If an adenoma is only small, mildly dysplastic and appears endoscopically to have been excised, recurrence is unlikely.

There will always be some biopsies in which a firm diagnosis is not possible, even after examination of sections at intervals through the block. For example, a polyp seen endoscopically in the distal colon may prove to be only normal colonic mucosa, the result of a polyp-like tag of mucosa produced by eversion of a diverticulum (Fig. 15.45); perhaps

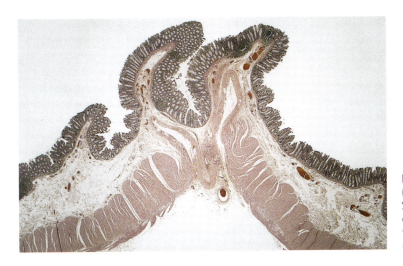

Figure 15.45 Everted diverticulum ('pseudopolyp') from sigmoid colon. Small mucosal diverticula frequently evert and confuse the endoscopist, who takes a biopsy of what is normal mucosa.

one situation in which the term 'pseudopolyp' is appropriate.

REFERENCES

Ajioka, Y., Watanabe, H., Jass, J.R. (1997) MUC1 and MUC2 mucins in flat and polypoid colorectal adenomas. *J. Clin. Pathol.*, 50, 417–21.

Ali, M.H., Satti, M.B., Al-Nafussi, A. (1984) Multiple benign colonic polyps at the site of ureterosigmoidostomy. *Cancer*, 53, 1006–10.

Allison, J.E. (1998) Review article: faecal occult blood testing for colorectal cancer. *Aliment. Pharmacol. Ther.*, 12, 1–10.

Ansell, I.D., Vellacott, K.D. (1980) Colonic polyps complicating ureterosigmoidostomy. *Histopathology*, 4, 429–36.

Atkin, W.S., Saunders, B.P. (2002) Surveillance guidelines after removal of colorectal adenomatous polyps. *Gut*, 51 (Suppl. 5), V6–9.

Bird, R.P., McLellan, E.A., Bruce, W.R. (1989) Aberrant crypts, putative precancerous lesions, in the study of the role of diet in the aetiology of colon cancer. *Cancer Surveys*, 8, 189–200.

Bosman, F.T. (1999) The hamartoma–adenoma–carcinoma sequence. *J. Pathol.*, 188, 1–2.

du Boulay, C.E.H., Fairbrother, J., Isaacson, P.C. (1983) Mucosal prolapse syndrome – a unifying concept for solitary ulcer syndrome and related disorders. *J. Clin. Pathol.*, 36, 1264–8.

Bouzourene, H., Chaubert, P., Seelentag, W., Bosman, F.T., Saraga, E. (1999) Aberrant crypt foci in patients with neoplastic and non-neoplastic colonic disease. *Hum. Pathol.*, 30, 66–71.

Brown, L.J.R., Smeeton, N.C., Dixon, M.F. (1985) Assessment of dysplasia in colorectal adenomas: an observer variation and morphometric study. *J. Clin. Pathol.*, 38, 174–9.

Burke, A.P., Sobin, L.H. (1990) Eroded polypoid hyperplasia of the rectosigmoid. *Am. J. Gastroenterol.*, 85, 975–80.

Burt, R.W., Jass, J.R. (2000) Hyperplastic polyposis. In: Hamilton, S.R., Aaltonen, L.A. (eds) *World Health Organization classification of tumours. Pathology and genetics. Tumours of the digestive system.* Berlin: Springer-Verlag, pp. 135–6.

Byrne, W.J., Jimenez, J.F., Euler, A.R., Golladay, E.S. (1982) Lymphoid polyps (focal lymphoid hyperplasia) of the colon in children. *Pediatrics*, 69, 598–600.

Campbell, A.P., Cobb, C.A., Chapman, R.W., Kettlewell, M., Hoang, P., Haot, B.J., Jewell, D.P. (1993) Cap polyposis – an unusual cause of diarrhoea. *Gut*, 34, 562–4.

Capitanio, M.A., Kirkpatrick, J.A. (1970) Lymphoid hyperplasia of the colon in children. *Radiology*, 94, 323–7.

Carlson, C.J., Nivatvongs, S., Snover, D.C. (1984) Colorectal polyps in Cowden's disease (multiple hamartoma syndrome). *Am. J. Surg. Pathol.*, 8, 763–70.

Carney, J.A., Hayles, A.B. (1977) Alimentary tract manifestations of multiple endocrine neoplasia, type 2b. *Mayo Clinic Proc.*, 52, 543–8.

Castro, E.B., Stearns, M.W. (1972) Lipoma of the large intestine. A review of 45 cases. *Dis. Col. Rectum*, 15, 441–4.

Chan, A.O., Issa, J.P., Morris, J.S., Hamilton, S.R., Rashid, A. (2002) Concordant CpG island methylation in hyperplastic polyposis. *Am. J. Pathol.* 160, 529–36.

Chandra, A., Sheikh, A.A., Cerar, A., Talbot, I.C. (2006) Clinico-pathological aspects of serrated adenomas. *World J. Gastroenterol.*, 12(17), 2770–2.

Cornes, J.S., Wallace, M.H., Morson, B.C. (1961) Benign lymphomas of the rectum and anal canal: a study of 100 cases. *J. Pathol. Bacteriol.*, 82, 371–82.

Cramer, S.F., Velasco, M.E., Whitlatch, S.P., Graney, M.F. (1986) Squamous differentiation in colorectal adenomas. Literature review, histogenesis and clinical significance. *Dis. Col. Rectum*, 29, 87–91.

Creasy, T.S., Baker, A.R., Talbot, I.C., Veitch, P.S. (1987) Symptomatic submucosal lipoma of the large bowel. *Br. J. Surg.*, 74, 984–6.

Dajani, Y.F., Kamal, M.F. (1984) Colorectal juvenile polyps: an epidemiological and histopathological study of 144 cases in Jordanians. *Histopathology*, 8, 765–79.

Day, D.W., Morson, B.C. (1978) The adenoma-carcinoma sequence. In: Morson, B.C. (ed.) *The pathogenesis of colorectal cancer, major problems in pathology*, vol. 10. Philadelphia, London and Toronto: W.B. Saunders, pp. 58–71.

de la Chapelle, A. (2003) Microsatellite instability. *N. Engl. J. Med.*, 349, 209–10.

Desai, D.C., Neale, K.F., Talbot, I.C., Hodgson, S.V., Phillips, R.K. (1995) Juvenile polyposis. *Br. J. Surg.*, 82, 14–17.

Dodds, W.J., Schulte, W.J., Hensley, G.T., Hogan, W.J. (1972) Peutz–Jeghers syndrome and gastrointestinal malignancy. *Am. J. Roentgenol.*, 115, 374–7.

Ehsanullah, M., Filipe, M.I., Gazzard, B. (1982) Morphological and mucus secretion criteria for differential diagnosis of solitary ulcer syndrome and non-specific proctitis. *J. Clin. Pathol.*, 35, 26–30.

Eide, T.J., Stalsberg, H. (1978) Polyps of the large intestine in northern Norway. *Cancer*, 42, 2839–48.

Eisen, G.M., Kim, C.Y., Fleischer, D.E. *et al.* (2002) High-resolution chromoendoscopy for classifying colonic polyps: a multicenter study. *Gastrointest. Endosc.*, 55, 687–94.

Elias, H., Hyde, D.M., Mullens, R.S., Lambert, F.C. (1981) Colonic adenomas: stereology and growth mechanisms. *Dis. Col. Rectum*, 24, 331–42.

Enterline, H.T. (1976) Polyps and cancer of the large bowel. In: Morson, B.C. (ed.) *Current topics in pathology, vol.* 63. *Pathology of the gastrointestinal tract*. Berlin, Heidelberg, New York: Springer Verlag, pp. 95–141.

Epstein, S.E., Ascari, W.Q., Ablaw, R.C., Seaman, W.B., Lattes, R. (1966) Colitis cystica profunda. *Am. J. Clin. Pathol.*, 45, 186–201.

Estrada, R.G., Spjut, H.J. (1980) Hyperplastic polyps of the large bowel. *Am. J. Surg. Pathol.*, 4, 127–33.

Fujii, T., Rembacken, B.J., Dixon, M.F., Yoshida, S., Axon, A.T. (1998) Flat adenomas in the United Kingdom: are treatable cancers being missed? *Endoscopy*, 30, 437–43.

Gore, S., Shepherd, N.A., Wilkinson, S.P. (1992) Endoscopic crescentic fold disease of the sigmoid colon: the clinical and histo-pathological spectrum of a distinctive endoscopic appearance. *Int. J. Colorectal Dis.*, 7, 76–81.

Grodsky, L. (1958) Neurofibroma of the rectum in a patient with von Recklinghausen's disease. *Am. J. Surg.*, 95, 474–6.

Haenzel, W., Correa, P. (1971) Cancer of the colon and rectum and adenomatous polyps. A review of epidemiologic findings. *Cancer*, 28, 14–24.

Hahn, S.A., Schutte, M., Hoque, A.T. *et al.* (1996) DPC4, a candidate tumor suppressor gene at human chromosome 18q21.1. *Science*, 271(5247), 350–3.

Hanby, A.M., Poulsom, S., Singh, R. *et al.* (1993) Hyperplastic polyps: a cell lineage which both synthesizes and secretes trefoil-peptides and has phenotypic similarity with the ulcer-associated cell lineage. *Am. J. Pathol.*, 142, 663–8.

Hardcastle, J.D., Chamberlain, J.O., Robinson, M.H. *et al.* (1996) Randomized controlled trial of faecal-occult-blood screening for colorectal cancer. *Lancet*, 348(9040), 1472–7.

Harrison, M., Singh, N., Rex, D.K. (2004) Impact of proximal colon retroflexion on adenoma miss rates. *Am. J. Gastroenterol.*, 99, 519–22.

Helwig, E.B., Hansen, J. (1951) Lymphoid polyps (benign lymphoma) and malignant lymphoma of the rectum and anus. *Surg. Gyn. Obstet.*, 92, 233–43.

Hemminki, A. (1999) The molecular basis and clinical aspects of Peutz–Jeghers syndrome. *Cell Mol. Life. Sci.*, 55, 735–50.

Hemminki, A., Markie, D., Tomlinson, I. *et al.* (1998) A serine/threonine kinase gene defective in Peutz–Jeghers syndrome. *Nature*, 391(6663), 184–7.

Higuchi, T., Jass, J.R. (2004) My approach to serrated polyps of the colorectum. *J. Clin. Pathol.*, 57, 682–6.

Hofstad, B., Vatn, M.H., Andersen, S.N., Huitfeldt, H.S., Rognum, T., Larsen, S., Osnes,

M. (1996). Growth of colorectal polyps: Redetection and evaluation of unresected polyps for a period of three years. *Gut*, 39, 449–56.

Iino, H., Simms, L., Young, J. *et al.* (2000) DNA microsatellite instability and mismatch repair protein loss in adenomas presenting in hereditary non-polyposis colorectal cancer. *Gut*, 47, 37–42.

Jansen, M., de Leng, W.W., Baas, A.F. *et al.* (2006) Mucosal prolapse in the pathogenesis of Peutz–Jeghers polyposis. *Gut*, 2006, 55, 1–5.

Jass, J.R. (1983) Relation between metaplastic polyp and carcinoma of the colorectum. *Lancet*, i, 28–30.

Jass, J.R. (1999) Serrated adenoma and colorectal cancer. *J. Pathol.*, 187, 499–502.

Jass, J.R. (2001) Serrated route to colorectal cancer: back street or super highway? *J. Pathol.*, 193, 283–5.

Jass, J.R. (2003) Serrated adenoma of the colorectum: a lesion with teeth. *Am. J. Pathol.*, 162, 705–8.

Jass, J.R., Roberton, A.M. (1994) Colorectal mucin histochemistry in health and disease: a critical review. *Pathol. Int.*, 44, 487–504.

Jass, J.R., Williams, C.B., Bussey, H.J., Morson, B.C. (1988) Juvenile polyposis – a precancerous condition. *Histopathology*, 13, 619–30.

Jass, J.R., Iino, H., Ruszkiewicz, A. *et al.* (2000) Neoplastic progression occurs through mutator pathways in hyperplastic polyposis of the colorectum. *Gut*, 47, 43–9.

Jass, J.R., Whitehall, V.L., Young, J., Leggett, B.A. (2002). Emerging concepts in colorectal neoplasia. *Gastroenterology*, 123, 862–76.

Johnston, J., Helwig, E.B. (1981) Granular cell tumors of the gastrointestinal tract and perianal region. A study of 74 cases. *Dig. Dis. Sci.*, 26, 807–16.

Kaye, G.I., Fenoglio, C.M., Pascal, R.R., Lane, N. (1973) Comparative electron microscopic features of normal, hyperplastic and adenomatous human colonic epithelium. Variations in cellular structure relative to the process of epithelial differentiation. *Gastroenterology*, 64, 926–45.

Kelly, J.K. (1991) Polypoid prolapsing mucosal folds in diverticular disease. *Am. J. Surg. Pathol.*, 15, 871–8.

Kestemberg, A., Marino, G., de-Lima, E., Garcia, F.T., Carrascal, E., Arredondo, J.L. (1993) Gastric heterotopic mucosa in the rectum with *Helicobacter pylori*-like organisms: a rare cause of rectal bleeding. *Int. J. Colorectal Dis.*, 8, 9–12.

Konishi, F., Morson, B.C. (1982) Pathology of colorectal adenomas: a colonoscopic survey. *J. Clin. Pathol.*, 35, 830–41.

Konishi, K., Kaneko, K., Kurahashi, T. *et al.* (2003) A comparison of magnifying and non-magnifying colonoscopy for diagnosis of colorectal polyps: a prospective study. *Gastrointest. Endosc.*, 57, 48–53.

Kubota, O., Kino, I. (1995) Depressed adenomas of the colon in familial adenomatous polyposis. Histology, immunohistochemical detection of proliferating cell nuclear antigen (PCNA), and analysis of the background mucosa. *Am. J. Surg. Pathol.*, 19, 318–27.

Kudo, S. (1993) Endoscopic mucosal resection of flat and depressed types of early colorectal cancer. *Endoscopy*, 25, 455–61.

Kuramoto, S., Oohara, T. (1995) How do colorectal cancers develop? *Cancer*, 75, 1534–8.

Lashner, B.A., Riddell, R.H., Winans, C.S. (1986) Ganglioneuromatosis of the colon and extensive glycogen acanthosis in Cowden's syndrome. *Dig. Dis. Sci.*, 31, 213–16.

Leggett, B.A., Devereaux, B., Biden, K., Searle, J., Young, J., Jass, J. (2001) Hyperplastic polyposis: association with colorectal cancer. *Am. J. Surg. Pathol.*, 25, 177–84.

Ling, C.S., Leagus, C., Stahlgren, L.H. (1959) Intestinal lipomatosis. *Surgery*, 46, 1054–9.

Longacre, T.A., Fenoglio-Preiser, C.M. (1990) Mixed hyperplastic adenomatous polyps/serrated adenomas. A distinct form of colorectal neoplasia. *Am. J. Surg. Pathol.*, 14, 524–37.

Macara, I.G. (2004) Parsing the polarity code. *Nat. Rev. Mol. Cell. Biol.*, 5, 220–31.

Madigan, M.R., Morson, B.C. (1969) Solitary ulcer of the rectum. *Gut*, 10, 871–81.

Mandel, J.S., Church, T.R., Bond, J.H. *et al.* (2000) The effect of fecal occult-blood screening on the incidence of colorectal cancer. *N. Engl. J. Med.*, 343, 1603–7.

Masaki, T., Sheffield, J.P., Talbot, I.C., Williams, C.B. (1994) Non-polypoid adenoma of the large intestine. *Int. J. Colorectal Dis.*, 9, 180–3.

Meijer, G.A., Hermsen, M.A., Baak, J.P. *et al.* (1998) Progression from colorectal adenoma to carcinoma is associated with non-random chromosomal gains as detected by comparative genomic hybridization. *J. Clin. Pathol.*, 51, 901–9.

Minamoto, T., Sawaguchi, K., Mai, M., Yamashita, N., Sugimura, T., Esumi, H. (1994) Infrequent K-ras activation in superficial-type (flat) colorectal adenomas and adenocarcinomas. *Cancer Res.*, 54, 2841–4.

Morson, B.C. (1962) Some peculiarities in the histology of intestinal polyps. *Dis. Col. Rectum*, 5, 337–44.

Morson, B.C., Bussey, H.J.R., Day, D.W., Hill, M.J. (1983) Adenomas of large bowel. *Cancer Surv.*, 2, 451–77.

Morson, B.C., Sobin, L.H. (1976) Histological typing of intestinal tumours. In: *International Histological Classification of Tumours, 15.* Geneva: WHO.

Muto, T., Bussey, H.J.R., Morson, B.C. (1975) The evolution of cancer of the colon and rectum. *Cancer*, 36, 2251–70.

Muto, T., Kamiya, J., Sawada, T. *et al.* (1985) Small 'flat adenoma' of the large bowel with special reference to its clinicopathologic features. *Dis. Col. Rectum*, 28, 847–51.

Nakamura, S., Kino, I., Akagi, T. (1992) Inflammatory myoglandular polyps of the colon and rectum. A clinicopathological study of 32 pedunculated polyps, distinct from other types of polyps. *Am. J. Surg. Pathol.*, 16, 772–9.

Nascimbeni, R., Villanacci, V., Mariani, P.P., Di Betta, E., Ghirardi, M., Donato, F., Salerni, B. (1999) Aberrant crypt foci in the human colon: frequency and histologic patterns in patients with colorectal cancer or diverticular disease. *Am. J. Surg. Pathol.*, 23, 1256–63.

Nelen, M.R., Padberg, G.W., Peeters, E.A. *et al.* (1996) Localization of the gene for Cowden disease to chromosome 10q22–23. *Nat. Genet.*, 13, 114–16.

Nucci, M.R., Robinson, C.R., Longo, P., Campbell, P., Hamilton, S.R. (1997) Phenotypic and genotypic characteristics of aberrant crypt foci in human colorectal mucosa. *Hum. Pathol.*, 28, 1396–407.

O'Brien, M.J., Winawer, S.J., Zauber, A.G. *et al.* (2004) Flat adenomas in the National Polyp Study: is there increased risk for high-grade dysplasia initially or during surveillance? *Clin. Gastroenterol. Hepatol.*, 2, 905–11.

Office of Population Censuses and Surveys (1999) *Mortality statistics 1999, England and Wales series DH2 no. 26*, London: HMSO.

Park, S.J., Rashid, A., Lee, J.H., Kim, S.G., Hamilton, S.R., Wu, T.T. (2003) Frequent CpG island methylation in serrated adenomas of the colorectum. *Am. J. Pathol.*, 162, 815–22.

Paterson, I.M., Logie, J.R.C., MePhie, J.L., Munro, A. (1985) Colonic polyps and ureterosigmoidostomy. *J. R. Coll. Surg. Edin.*, 30, 264–5.

Rickert, R.R., Auerbach, O., Garfinkal, L., Hammond, E.C., Frasca, J.M. (1979) Adenomatous lesions of the large bowel. An autopsy study. *Cancer*, 43, 1847–57.

Rutter, M.D., Saunders, B.P., Schofield, G., Forbes, A., Price, A.B., Talbot, I.C. (2004) Pancolonic indigo carmine dye spraying for the detection of dysplasia in ulcerative colitis. *Gut*, 53, 256–60.

Ryan, J., Martin, J.E., Pollock, D.J. (1989) Fatty tumours of the large intestine: a clinicopathological review of 13 cases. *Br. J. Surg.*, 76, 793–6.

Sakashita, M., Aoyama, N., Maekawa, S. *et al.* (2000) Flat-elevated and depressed, subtypes of flat early colorectal cancers, should be distinguished by their pathological features. *Int. J. Colorectal Dis.*, 15, 275–81.

Salem, O.S., Steck, W.D. (1983) Cowden's disease (multiple hamartoma and neoplasia syndrome). *J. Am. Acad. Dermatol.*, 8, 686–96.

Samowitz, W.S., Burt, R.L. (1995) The nonspecificity of histological findings reported for flat adenomas. *Hum. Pathol.*, 26, 571–3.

Sawyer, E.J., Cerar, A., Hanby, A.M., Gorman, P., Arends, M., Talbot, I.C., Tomlinson, I.P. (2002). Molecular characteristics of serrated adenomas of the colorectum. *Gut*, 51, 200–6.

Schnoll-Sussman, F., Markowitz, A.J., Winawer, S.J. (2000) Screening and surveillance for colorectal cancer. *Semin. Oncol.*, 27 (5 Suppl. 10), 10–21.

Shepherd, N.A., Bussey, H.J., Jass, J.R. (1987) Epithelial misplacement in Peutz–Jeghers polyps. A diagnostic pitfall. *Am. J. Surg. Pathol.*, 11, 743–9.

Shpitz, B., Bomstein, Y., Mekori, Y. *et al.* (1998) Aberrant crypt foci in human colons: distribution and histomorphologic characteristics. *Hum. Pathol.*, 29, 469–75.

Shull, L.N. Jr, Fitts, C.T. (1974) Lymphoid polyposis associated with familial polyposis and Gardner's syndrome. *Ann. Surg.*, 180, 319–22.

Srinivasan, R., Loewenstine, H., Mayle, J.E. (1999) Sessile polypoid gastric heterotopia of rectum: a report of 2 cases and review of the literature. *Arch. Pathol. Lab. Med.*, 123, 222–4.

Suzuki, Y., Honma, T., Hayashi, S., Ajioka, Y., Asakura, H. (2002) Bcl-2 expression and frequency of apoptosis correlate with morphogenesis of colorectal neoplasia. *J. Clin. Pathol.*, 55, 212–16.

Talbot, I.C. (2001) Dysplasia in the lower gastrointestinal tract. In: Lowe, D.G., Underwood, J.C.E. (eds) *Recent advances in histopathology*. 19th edn. Edinburgh: Churchill Livingstone, pp. 211–26.

Tateyama, H., Li, W., Takahashi, E., Miura, Y., Sugiura, H., Eimoto, T. (2002). Apoptosis index and apoptosis-related antigen expression in serrated adenoma of the colorectum: the saw-toothed structure may be related to inhibition of apoptosis. *Am. J. Surg. Pathol.*, 26, 249–56.

Torlakovic, A., Snover, D.C. (1996) Serrated adenomatous polyposis in humans. *Gastroenterology*, 110, 748–755.

Torlakovic, E., Skovlund, E., Snover, D.C., Torlakovic, G., Nesland, J.M. (2003). Morphologic reappraisal of serrated colorectal polyps. *Am. J. Surg. Pathol.*, 27, 65–81.

Tweedie, J.H., McCann, B.C. (1984) Peutz–Jeghers syndrome and metastasising colonic adenocarcinoma. *Gut*, 25, 1118–23.

Umetani, N., Sasaki, S., Masaki, T., Watanabe, T., Matsuda, K., Muto, T. (2000) Involvement of APC and K-ras mutation in non-polypoid colorectal tumorigenesis. *Br. J. Cancer*, 82, 9–15.

van den Ingh, H.F., van den Broek, L.J., Verhofstad, A.A.J. (1986) Neuroendocrine cells in colorectal adenomas. *J. Pathol.*, 148, 231–7.

van Driel, M.F., Zwiers, W., Grond, J., Verschueren, R.C., Mensink, H.J. (1988). Juvenile polyps at the site of a uretero-sigmoidostomy. Report of five cases. *Dis. Colon Rectum*, 31, 553–7.

Vieth, M., Kushima, R., de Jonge, J.P., Borchard, F., Oellig, F., Stolte, M. (2005) Adenoma with gastric differentiation (so-called pyloric gland adenoma) in a heterotopic gastric corpus mucosa in the rectum. *Virchows Arch.*, 446, 542–5.

Walsh, T.H. (1984) Smooth muscle neoplasms of the rectum and anal canal. *Br. J. Surg.*, 71, 597–9.

Wang, Z.J., Ellis, I., Zauber, P. *et al.* (1999) Allelic imbalance at the LKB1 (STK11) locus in tumours from patients with Peutz–Jeghers' syndrome provides evidence for a hamartoma–(adenoma)–carcinoma sequence. *J. Pathol.*, 188, 9–13.

Warren, B.F., Dankwa, E.K., Davies, J.D. (1990) 'Diamond-shaped' crypts and mucosal elastin: helpful diagnostic features in biopsies of rectal prolapse. *Histopathology*, 17, 129–34.

Wasan, H.S., Park, H.S., Liu, K.C. *et al.* (1998) APC in the regulation of intestinal crypt fission. *J. Pathol.*, 185, 246–55.

Watari, J., Saitoh, Y., Obara, T. *et al.* (2002) Natural history of colorectal nonpolypoid adenomas: a prospective colonoscopic study and relation with cell kinetics and K-ras mutations. *Am. J. Gastroenterol.*, 97, 2109–15.

Weidner, N., Flanders, D.J., Mitros, F.A. (1984) Mucosal ganglioneuromatosis associated with multiple colonic polyps. *Am. J. Surg. Pathol.*, 8, 779–86.

Weitzner, S., Lockard, V.G., Nascimento, A.G. (1976) Granular-cell myoblastoma of the cercum: report of a case. *Dis. Colon Rectum*, 19, 675–9.

Whitelaw, S.C., Murday, V.A., Tomlinson, I.P. *et al.* (1997) Clinical and molecular features of the hereditary mixed polyposis syndrome. *Gastroenterology*, 112, 327–34.

Wiebecke, B., Brandts, A., Eder, M. (1974) Epithelial proliferation and morphogenesis of hypoplastic adenomatous and villous polyps of the human colon. *Virchows Arch. Path. Anat. Hist.*, 364, 35–49.

Williams, A.R., Balgsooriya, B.A.W., Day, D.W. (1982) Polyps and cancer of the large bowel: a necropsy study in Liverpool. *Gut*, 23, 835–42.

Williams, C.B., Hunt, R.H., Loose, H., Riddell, R.H., Sakai, Y., Swarbrick, E.T. (1974) Colonoscopy in the management of colon polyps. *Br. J. Surg.*, 61, 673–82.

Williams, G.T., Arthur, J.F., Bussey, H.J.R., Morson, B.C. (1980) Metaplastic polyps and polyposis of the colorectum. *Histopathology*, 4, 155–170.

Williams, G.T., Bussey, H.J.R., Morson, B.C. (1985) Inflammatory 'cap' polyps of the large intestine. *Br. J. Surg.*, 72 (Suppl.), S133.

Womack, N.R., Williams, N.S., Holmfield, J.H., Morrison, J.F. (1987) Pressure and prolapse – the cause of solitary rectal ulceration. *Gut*, 28, 1228–33.

Wu, T.T., Rezai, B., Rashid, A. *et al.* (1997) Genetic alterations and epithelial dysplasia in juvenile polyposis syndrome and sporadic juvenile polyps. *Am. J. Pathol.*, 150, 939–47.

Wynter, C.V., Walsh, M.D., Higuchi, T., Leggett, B.A., Young, J., Jass, J.R. (2004) Methylation patterns define two types of hyperplastic polyp associated with colorectal cancer. *Gut*, 53, 573–80.

Yaguchi, T., Wen-Ying, L., Hasegawa, K., Sasaki, H., Nagasako, K. (1982) Peutz–Jegher's polyp with several foci of glandular dysplasia: report of a case. *Dis. Col. Rectum*, 25, 592–6.

Yao, T., Tada, S., Tsuneyoshi, M. (1994) Colorectal counterpart of gastric depressed adenoma. A comparison with flat and polypoid adenomas with special reference to the development of pericryptal fibroblasts. *Am. J. Surg. Pathol.*, 18, 559–68.

CHAPTER 16

THE DIAGNOSIS OF MALIGNANCY

16.1 Introduction   292
16.2 Overdiagnosis of malignancy   293
    16.2.1 Epithelial dysplasia in
        adenomas   293
    16.2.2 Misplaced epithelium
        (pseudoinvasion)   293
16.3 The stroma of invasive
    adenocarcinoma   293

16.4 Focal carcinoma in adenomatous
    polyps ('malignant polyps')   295
16.5 Decisions when reporting
    biopsies of neoplastic tissue   298
    16.5.1 Inadequate biopsies   298
References   300

16.1 INTRODUCTION

Most biopsies of large intestinal tumours, including polyps, will be either of adenocarcinomas or their benign, adenomatous precursors. Although the majority of adenocarcinomas of large bowel are believed to arise from adenomatous polyps, there is increasing evidence that adenocarcinoma may also develop via alternative pathways; namely from flat adenomas (Muto *et al.*, 1985) and from serrated polyps (Higuchi and Jass, 2004). In a study of nearly 2500 polyps, malignant change was found in 4.5 per cent of tubular adenomas, 22.5 per cent of tubulovillous adenomas and in 40.7 per cent of villous adenomas (Muto *et al.*, 1975). The relationships between size, grade of dysplasia and presence of malignancy in adenomas are discussed in Section 15.5. This chapter provides guidelines to assist the pathologist in deciding between adenoma and adenocarcinoma and to avoid certain pitfalls.

The most important principle to remember is that carcinoma, as defined in Chapter 14, can be said to be present when the neoplastic epithelium has extended into or through the muscularis mucosae (Morson and Sobin, 1976). To observe this in a biopsy requires an adequate sample and good orientation. These are not always achieved and, in practice, the features requiring scrutiny are:

1. The glandular epithelium and the degree of dysplasia.
2. The location of glandular elements relative to the muscularis mucosae (e.g. is there stalk invasion?).
3. The nature of the periglandular stroma.

Non-glandular tumours pose problems of identification as well as assessment of malignancy, but will be only briefly mentioned in this chapter.

In a biopsy from a neoplastic lesion there is potential for the overdiagnosis or underdiagnosis of malignancy. In some cases the biopsy may be inadequate for diagnosis, whatever the efforts of the pathologist.

16.2 OVERDIAGNOSIS OF MALIGNANCY

Two features instinctively raise the suspicion of malignancy in a polypoid lesion, whether pedunculated or sessile, and may lead to a false positive diagnosis. These are severe epithelial dysplasia and the presence of glandular epithelium inappropriately intermingled with muscle or within submucosa ('misplaced' epithelium). A further potential cause of diagnostic difficulty, the presence of plump endothelial cells in exuberant granulation tissue, is rarely a problem with polypoid lesions and has been discussed and illustrated in Section 3.9.7.

16.2.1 Epithelial dysplasia in adenomas

Adenomas, whether of tubular or villous configuration, are neoplastic lesions and some degree of epithelial dysplasia is invariable (Fig. 15.3). From a pathogenetic viewpoint, dysplastic epithelium is the hallmark of intramucosal neoplasia. When the dysplasia is severe there is often both marked cellular atypia and architectural distortion with glandular crowding and budding, forming a cribriform pattern of intraglandular acini. Caution should be exercised in this respect, when dealing with small biopsies which may be subject to crush artefact. In the absence of evidence of invasion even severe dysplasia cannot be relied on for the diagnosis of adenocarcinoma. Superficial biopsies of polypoid lesions are therefore inadequate for assessment of malignancy with but a few exceptions.

As discussed in Chapter 14, a diagnosis of malignancy should not be made merely because there is severe dysplasia of mucosal glands, whether in an adenoma or not.

16.2.2 Misplaced epithelium (pseudoinvasion)

It is also important to recognize the possibility of benign misplacement of epithelium and not make a false diagnosis of malignancy. This is a frequent cause of 'stalk invasion' in adenomatous polyps and must be distinguished from focal carcinoma (Section 15.12.1). Mucosal glands are found within or deep to the muscularis mucosae in an otherwise benign lesion as a result of reparative down-growth following damage to the main body of the polyp. In an adenoma this leads to the appearances which have been described as pseudocarcinomatous invasion (Muto *et al.*, 1973) or pseudoinvasion, observed in 3–10 per cent of benign adenomas (Greene, 1974; Qizilbash *et al.*, 1980), mostly from the sigmoid colon. The process is akin to endometriosis in the necessity to identify lamina propria around these misplaced glands (Figs 16.1 and 16.2). This is in contrast to the granulation tissue and collagen fibres (desmoplastic stroma) adjacent to frankly malignant epithelium (Section 16.3). There is often associated haemorrhage, which leads later to the deposition of refractile brown haemosiderin pigment within macrophages in the misplaced lamina propria. Muto *et al.* (1973) suggest that this is because the epithelium is misplaced during a reparative process following infarction caused by twisting of the polyp on its stalk.

The misplaced epithelium may be dysplastic, even severely so, normal, attenuated or destroyed owing to pressure atrophy (Fig. 16.1). However, because the incidence of invasion rises with the severity of dysplasia, the presence of the latter must alert the pathologist to a careful examination of the stalk of a polyp and to check the criteria of pseudoinvasion.

A similar, and misleading, picture is seen when there is hypertrophy of muscularis mucosae and extension of smooth muscle bundles upwards between the glands of an adenoma, due to torsion of the head of the polyp (Fig. 15.35) (Section 15.10).

16.3 THE STROMA OF INVASIVE ADENOCARCINOMA

An interesting and critical feature usually associated with the infiltrating glandular epithelium of an adenocarcinoma is the proliferation of fibroblasts, myofibroblasts and endothelial cells, apparently induced in the invaded tissue by the presence of the malignant tumour cells (Ohtani and Sasano, 1983). Sometimes this is associated with overt

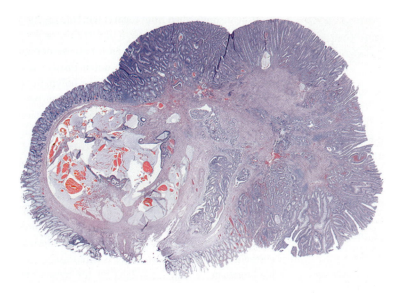

Figure 16.1 Pseudoinvasion in a tubular adenoma. There are multiple foci of adenomatous glands with lamina propria and pools of mucin within the submucosa of this polyp. The mucin pools are markers of sites of misplaced mucosa in which the epithelium has undergone degeneration and sloughing.

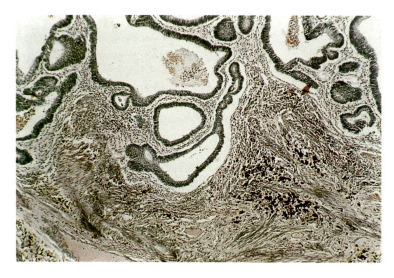

Figure 16.2 Misplaced glands in stalk of a polyp: sharply circumscribed nodules of aberrant adenomatous glands and lamina propria, with associated haemosiderin in the submucosa of the stalk of a polyp.

venous invasion (Talbot *et al.*, 1981). The resulting stroma often resembles granulation tissue (Fig. 16.3) and is different in appearance from the areolar tissue of the lamina propria.

Accompanying granulation tissue or a cellular fibrous stroma ('desmoplasia') (Fig. 16.4) is the single most important indication that atypical epithelium represents invasive adenocarcinoma, particularly in small biopsies which consist only of such dysplastic glands and connective tissue but no muscularis. The importance of this stromal reaction should be

remembered when evaluating the significance of 'misplacement' of dysplastic epithelium, in the stalk of a polyp. However, an important confounding factor is presented by fibrous scarring following previous biopsy of an adenoma, which sometimes happens with large sessile lesions (Fig. 16.5). It is necessary to know about the history of such an event if fibrosis is to be correctly interpreted. A molecular characterization of this peritumoral stroma has been postulated as useful in the distinction between pseudoinvasion in adenomas versus

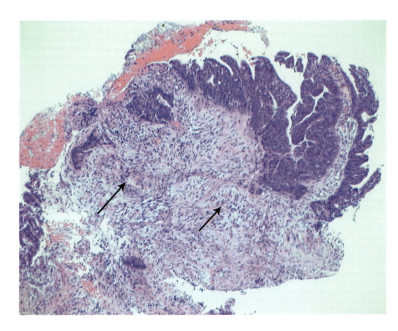

Figure 16.3 Granulation tissue stroma of adenocarcinoma. Biopsy of moderately differentiated adenocarcinoma showing a strip of abnormal epithelium surrounded by a granulation tissue-like stroma. It is the presence of such a stroma that is almost diagnostic of invasive malignancy. Close scrutiny reveals that small blood vessels within the granulation tissue are permeated by adenocarcinoma (arrowed), raising the possibility that the granulation tissue itself may have been derived from endothelial cells.

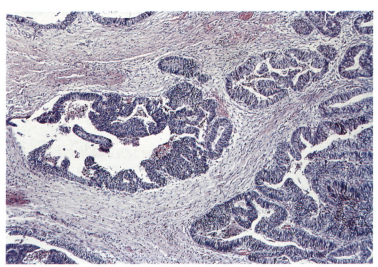

Figure 16.4 Desmoplastic stroma of adenocarcinoma. The invasive glands are surrounded by stroma composed of dense cellular fibrous tissue, comprising spindle cells and eosinophilic fibres, consistent with myofibroblasts and a collagenous reticular background.

truly invasive adenocarcinoma (Yantiss *et al.*, 2002), but in our opinion is insufficiently specific for routine diagnosis.

It should be noted that occasionally no desmoplastic stroma is seen around evidently invasive adenocarcinoma. This can pose a difficult diagnostic problem, particularly with well differentiated tumours (Fig. 16.6). The lack of lamina propria in such circumstances supports the diagnosis of malignancy.

16.4 FOCAL CARCINOMA IN ADENOMATOUS POLYPS ('MALIGNANT POLYPS')

If, having taken account of the above pitfalls, the pathologist is satisfied that neoplastic epithelium has infiltrated through the muscularis mucosae (Fig. 16.7) a diagnosis of focal carcinoma must

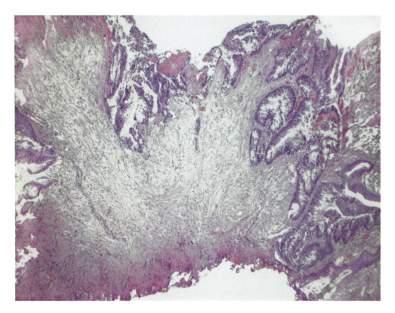

Figure 16.5 Fibrous scarring in adenoma resulting from previous biopsy, mimicking desmoplasia. This is one of a series of biopsies of a low rectal polyp (severely dysplastic tubulovillous adenoma), locally recurrent over several years but not malignant. There is so much distortion and dense fibrous scarring that the appearances mimic invasive adenocarcinoma with a desmoplastic stroma. Knowledge of the history is helpful in avoiding over-enthusiasm for a diagnosis of malignancy.

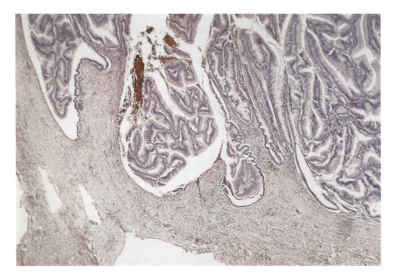

Figure 16.6 Well-differentiated adenocarcinoma invading smooth muscle of the rectal wall. There is little or no desmoplastic stroma. The only other feature which supports a diagnosis of malignancy here is the lack of lamina propria around the invading neoplastic papillary epithelium.

be made. The carcinomatous component will extend for a variable depth into the submucosa. The most important issue concerning malignant polyps is whether the polypectomy itself is adequate treatment or whether there is a significant risk of recurrent tumour, in which case radical surgery is required. Taking all malignant polyps together, there is a 10.4 per cent risk, overall, of metastasis (Wilcox *et al.*, 1986). A substantial factor in this

regard is the depth of submucosal penetration. When submucosal invasion is not extensive, and the adenocarcinoma is well or moderately differentiated, it is extremely unlikely that the tumour will have metastasized to lymph nodes (Morson *et al.*, 1984). This view was confirmed by the work of Haggitt *et al.* (1985), who reviewed 129 T1 colorectal cancers that originated in adenomas (i.e. where tumour invasion was not deeper than the

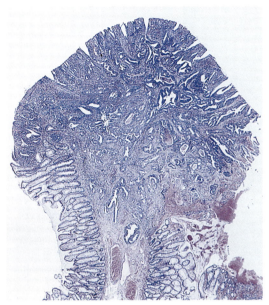

Figure 16.7 Polypoid adenocarcinoma. There is clearly infiltration of moderately differentiated tumour below the level of the muscularis mucosae. Without this feature, inspection of the mucosal part of the lesion alone, for example in a superficial biopsy, would not permit a definite decision on the malignant nature of this polyp.

submucosa). Four levels of invasion were proposed, namely:

0 – no invasion (confined to the mucosa)
1 – invasion of the head of the polyp
2 – invasion of the neck of the polyp
3 – invasion of the stalk of the polyp
4 – invasion of the adjacent submucosa.

In the study, metastases were present in 12.5 per cent of all invasive lesions, and were clearly related to level 4 invasion. Interestingly, most of these lesions were present in the rectum. Other subsequent studies have corroborated this idea, to the extent that further excision after polypectomy has only been recommended for level 4 patients (Kyzer *et al.*, 1992). Thus, only invasion of the lower third of the submucosa is shown to carry a significant risk of lymph node involvement (Nivatvongs, 2002). Unfortunately, in polypectomy specimens, it is rarely possible to assess precisely the depth of the submucosa and it can be uncertain as to whether the lower third of the submucosa is included in the specimen and whether or not tumour extends so

deeply. In an attempt to overcome this difficulty, the extent of submucosal invasion has been measured in millimetres (Sakuragi *et al.*, 2003), the normal submucosa being taken to be approximately 3-mm thick. In this study of surgically resected early cancers, 15.5 per cent of 278 malignant polyps in which the adenocarcinoma extended into the submucosa for at least 2 mm were associated with lymph node metastasis. This compared with lymph node involvement in only 0.7 per cent of cases in which submucosal extension was less than 2 mm. For most of the latter cases, therefore, provided that the excision line is clear of carcinoma, a further, more radical operation should not be necessary. However, in an attempt to avoid any risk of lymph node metastasis or recurrence, Ueno and colleagues (2004), following multivariate analysis, have identified further criteria as independent risk factors, namely, poor tumour differentiation, lympho-vascular invasion [using elastic-van Gieson (EVG) and immunocytochemistry for CD34], and tumour cell budding. Tumour cell budding (Fig. 16.8) in colectomy specimens was defined as at least 10 clusters of fewer than five cancer cells in a microscope field measuring $0.785 \, mm^2$ (using a $\times 20$ objective), counting a field showing maximum budding (Ueno *et al.*, 2002). They confirmed the importance of submucosal invasion at least as deep as 2 mm and also showed that a submucosal invasive front at least 4 mm wide was an adverse factor for lymph node metastases (Ueno *et al.*, 2004). Interestingly, they found that the most sensitive marker for completeness of excision, rather than a measurement in millimetres, was absence of tumour from the diathermy coagulation excision zone; lymph nodes were sometimes involved even when the excision line was over 2 mm from tumour, if tumour was present in the coagulation zone. In a series of 292 early (T1) invasive adenocarcinomas, given that there was complete excision, as defined by non-involvement of the diathermy zone, there were 138 patients without any adverse factors (tumour not poorly differentiated, no detectable lymphovascular invasion and, in biopsy tissue, less than five tumour cell buds per $\times 20$ objective field). Only one of these patients had positive lymph nodes, giving an identical nodal involvement rate to that of the Sakuragi study (0.7 per cent; Sakuragi *et al.*, 2003). When the quantitative criteria

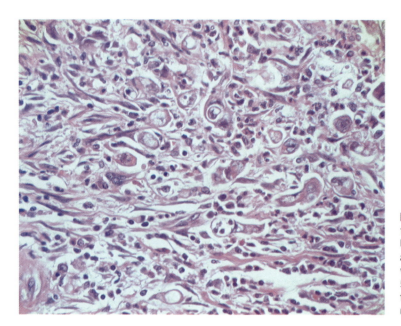

Figure 16.8 Adenocarcinoma with tumour cell budding. Tumour cell budding at the invasive margin of an adenocarcinoma is significant when at least 10 clusters of up to 5 tumour cells can be found in the field visible through a ×20 microscope objective.

were added (depth of submucosal invasion <2 mm and width of invasive front <4 mm), no patient had lymph node metastases or micrometastases. However, by imposing the latter strict criteria, the number of cases with meaningful data was reduced from 138 to 56. In practice, if a recurrence rate of 0.7 per cent is tolerable, the criteria proposed by Sakuragi *et al.* (2003) based on depth of invasion alone, seem acceptable and are relatively simple. We do, however, suggest that, in view of the Ueno findings, excision line involvement should be defined as tumour extending into the coagulation zone.

In any event, anticipation of this situation requires complete excision by the endoscopist of all polypoid lesions and correct orientation of each specimen, with identification of the stalk or base at the embedding stage in the laboratory (Section 15.2).

16.5 DECISIONS WHEN REPORTING BIOPSIES OF NEOPLASTIC TISSUE

Armed with the above information the following are the data which should be transmitted in the pathologist's report:

1. Severity of the dysplasia

2. Presence or absence of true carcinomatous invasion
3. Extent of any invasion (i.e. depth in mm)
4. Whether excision appears complete (i.e. no tumour in the coagulation rim)
5. Presence or absence of tumour cell budding.

In our experience, assessment of lympho-vascular invasion in adenocarcinomatous polypectomy specimens is of little practical value (Geraghty *et al.*, 1991).

When there is no glandular differentiation, other types of primary tumour may be present (Table 16.1). In the special situation of low rectal and anal tumours, the possibilities of basaloid carcinoma, melanoma or adenocarcinoma of anal gland should be considered (Section 19.3.5).

Finally, unusual histological appearances may suggest that the tumour is a metastasis from elsewhere. Those most frequently encountered are adenocarcinomas of ovary, prostate and transitional cell carcinoma of bladder (Figs 18.12–18.14).

16.5.1 Inadequate biopsies

Unfortunately, the pathologist is sometimes faced with small, irregular pieces of biopsied tumour tissue which consist of dysplastic (i.e. neoplastic)

Table 16.1 Procedures in making a diagnosis

Problem	Cause	Action
Adenoma or carcinoma?	Small irregular fragments of part of lesion	Request complete excision of a polyp or rebiopsy a tumour to find desmoplastic stroma
Primary or secondary?	Unusual history	Obtain adequate history Mucin stains Immunohistochemistry: specific markers
Carcinoma, carcinoid or lymphoma?	No glandular differentiation	Check location of tumour Immunohistochemistry: epithelial, endocrine and leucocyte markers Electron microscopy

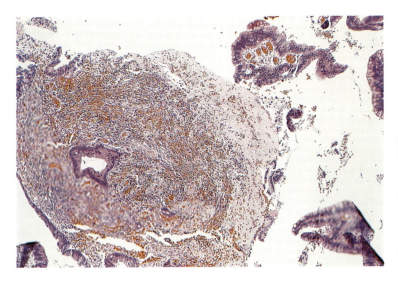

Figure 16.9 Inadequate biopsy. This biopsy of a rectal tumour includes atypical glands with a granulation tissue-like stroma, suspicious of malignancy. However, the stroma is not dense enough to be classified as desmoplastic and there is insufficient tissue to determine whether there is invasive malignancy.

glands, with stroma, but without smooth muscle from either the muscularis mucosae or muscularis propria. Three circumstances are then possible.

1. The biopsy may be too superficial to allow the necessary architectural assessment of its invasive potential (Fig. 16.9).
2. The biopsy may include only (benign) adenomatous tissue of either tubular or villous morphology but with no definite evidence of carcinoma. Although the patient may have a carcinoma the surgeon may have unluckily biopsied the remnant of a pre-existing adenoma at one edge of the malignant lesion. It should be remembered that the majority of colorectal carcinomas arise in pre-existing adenomas (Muto *et al.*, 1975) and that the occasional inclusion of adenomatous tissue in biopsies from the edge of carcinomas is inevitable.

3. The biopsy may consist, at least partly, of adenocarcinoma, but with a well-developed glandular or villous architecture, so that distinction from adenoma is difficult. The key to interpretation in this circumstance is the nature of the stroma; desmoplastic stroma between the glands of the lesion indicates that the epithelium is carcinomatous, whereas in the absence of abnormal connective tissue it is unwise to make a firm diagnosis of malignancy.

In situations (1) and (2), if the biopsy is inadequate the pathologist must say so, but he should have regard for the clinical impression and, if there is a strong suspicion of malignancy, another biopsy, which includes tissue from more than one area of the tumour and is of adequate depth, should be invited.

REFERENCES

Geraghty, J.M., Williams, C.B., Talbot, I.C. (1991) Malignant colorectal polyps: venous invasion and successful treatment by endoscopic polypectomy. *Gut*, 32, 774–8.

Greene, F.L. (1974) Epithelial misplacement in adenomatous polyps of the colon and rectum. *Cancer*, 33, 206–17.

Haggitt, R.C., Glotzbach, R.E., Soffer, E.E., Wruble, L.D. (1985) Prognostic factors in colorectal carcinomas arising in adenomas: implications for lesions removed by endoscopic polypectomy. *Gastroenterology*, 89, 328–36.

Higuchi, T., Jass, J.R. (2004) My approach to serrated polyps of the colorectum. *J. Clin. Pathol.*, 57, 682–6.

Kyzer, S., Begin, L.R., Gordon, P.H., Mitmaker, B. (1992) The care of patients with colorectal polyps that contain invasive adenocarcinoma. Endoscopic polypectomy or colectomy? *Cancer*, 70, 2044–50.

Morson, B.C., Sobin, L.H. (1976) Histological typing of intestinal tumours. In: *International classification of tumours No. 15*. Geneva: World Health Organization, p. 56.

Morson, B.C., Whiteway, J.E., Jones, E.A., Macrae, F.A., Williams, C.B. (1984) Histopathology and prognosis of malignant colorectal polyps treated by endoscopic polypectomy. *Gut*, 25, 437–44.

Muto, T., Bussey, H.J.R., Morson, B.C. (1973) Pseudo-carcinomatous invasion in adenomatous polyps of the colon and rectum. *J. Clin. Pathol.*, 26, 25–31.

Muto, T., Bussey, H.J.R., Morson, B.C. (1975) The evolution of cancer of the colon and rectum. *Cancer*, 36, 2251–70.

Muto, T., Kamiya, J., Sawada, T. *et al.* (1985) Small 'flat adenoma' of the large bowel with special reference to its clinicopathologic features. *Dis. Colon Rectum.*, 28, 847–51.

Nivatvongs, S. (2002) Surgical management of malignant colorectal polyps. *Surg. Clin. N. Am.*, 82, 959–66.

Ohtani, H., Sasano, N. (1983) Stromal cell changes in human colorectal adenomas and carcinomas. *Virchows Arch. Pathol. Anat.*, 401, 209–22.

Qizilbash, A.H., Meghji, M., Castelli, M. (1980) Pseudocarcinomatous invasion in adenomas of the colon and rectum. *Dis. Colon Rectum*, 23, 529–35.

Sakuragi, M., Togashi, K., Konishi, F., Koinuma, K., Kawamura, Y., Okada, M., Nagai, H. (2003). Predictive factors for lymph node metastasis in T1 stage colorectal carcinomas. *Dis. Colon Rectum*, 46, 1626–32.

Talbot, I.C., Ritchie, S., Leighton, M., Hughes, A.O., Bussey, H.J.R., Morson, B.C. (1981) Invasion of veins by carcinoma of rectum: method of detection, histological features and significance. *Histopathology*, 5, 141–63.

Ueno, H., Murphy, J., Jass, J.R., Mochizuki, H., Talbot, I.C. (2002). Tumour 'budding' as an index to estimate the potential of aggressiveness in rectal cancer. *Histopathology*, 40, 127–32.

Ueno, H., Mochizuki, H., Hashiguchi, Y. *et al.* (2004) Risk factors for an adverse outcome in early invasive colorectal carcinoma. *Gastroenterology*, 127, 385–94.

Wilcox, G.M., Anderson, P.B., Colacchio, T.A. (1986) Early invasive carcinoma in colonic polyps. *Cancer*, 57, 160–71.

Yantiss, R.K., Bosenberg, M.W., Antonioli, D.A., Odze, R.D. (2002) Utility of MMP-1, p53, E-cadherin, and collagen IV immunohisto-chemical stains in the differential diagnosis of adenomas with misplaced epithelium versus adenomas with invasive adenocarcinoma. *Am. J. Surg. Pathol.*, 26, 206–15.

CHAPTER 17

DYSPLASIA IN INFLAMMATORY BOWEL DISEASE

17.1 Introduction   301
17.2 Definitions   302
    17.2.1   Dysplasia   302
    17.2.2   Carcinoma *in-situ*   302
    17.2.3   Intramucosal carcinoma   302
    17.2.4   Precancer/premalignant   302
    17.2.5   Atypia   303
17.3 Patients at risk and cancer incidence   303
17.4 The reliability of dysplasia in cancer surveillance   305
17.5 The macroscopic lesion in dysplasia   306
17.6 Histological recognition and classification of dysplasia   307
    17.6.1   Cytological abnormalities   308
    17.6.2   Architectural abnormalities   309
    17.6.3   Degree of involvement   310
    17.6.4   Classification of dysplasia   311
    17.6.5   Degenerative features in colitic mucosa   311

17.6.6   Regenerative mucosa   312
17.6.7   Indefinite for dysplasia   312
17.6.8   Low-grade dysplasia   314
17.6.9   High-grade dysplasia   314
17.7 Observer variation   316
17.8 Other stains and methodologies   316
17.9 Molecular investigations   317
17.10 Implications of the pathologist's report   317
    17.10.1   Indefinite category   318
    17.10.2   Low-grade flat dysplasia   318
    17.10.3   High-grade dysplasia   319
17.11 The sporadic adenoma and dysplasia-associated lesion or mass in ulcerative colitis   319
17.12 Failure to find a lesion following recommendation for surgery   323
References   323

17.1   INTRODUCTION

Although carcinoma is now an accepted complication of both ulcerative colitis and Crohn's disease (de Dombal *et al.*, 1966; Greenstein *et al.*, 1979; Gyde *et al.*, 1980; Cooper *et al.*, 1984; Ekbom *et al.*, 1990; Eaden *et al.*, 2001a; Sharan and Schoen 2002), in routine diagnostic histopathology it is rare. Less than 1 per cent of deaths from colonic cancer are associated with ulcerative colitis. In the most recent 30-year analysis of the St Mark's Hospital colonoscopic surveillance programme only 30 cancers occurred within a surveillance cohort of 600 patients (Rutter *et al.*, 2006). Thus, the service pathologist working in a District General Hospital is unlikely to meet many cases during their career.

Apart from the confirmation of malignancy the pathologist's role in the colitis–carcinoma sequence is to recognize epithelial dysplasia. In a rectal biopsy it is a marker for the presence of a cancer or for its subsequent development, a concept introduced by Morson and Pang (1967). Screening for dysplasia in rectal and colonoscopic biopsies, with subsequent enrolment in a surveillance programme, is now part of the accepted cancer prevention programme in that cohort of the colitic population who are most at risk (Butt *et al.*, 1980).

The dysplasia–carcinoma relationship is not straightforward. Dysplasia does not invariably precede, or invariably accompany, cancer in colitis (Section 17.3) (Ransohoff *et al.*, 1985; Taylor *et al.*, 1992; Connell *et al.*, 1994a). It is a focal change and hence presents a problem of sampling in biopsy work (Cook and Goligher, 1975; Riddell and Morson, 1979). In addition, there is considerable observer variation between pathologists. Even when detected, a carcinoma may already be present (Lennard-Jones *et al.*, 1977; Blackstone *et al.*, 1981). Histologically, the milder degrees of dysplasia are difficult to distinguish from regenerative patterns and, because of the rarity of dysplasia, the pathologist has little experience in its recognition. The clinical problem is to decide on the course of action for the patient when a confident diagnosis of dysplasia has been made and no obvious cancer is detectable (Butt *et al.*, 1980; Lennard-Jones, 1995; Itzkowitz and Harpaz, 2004).

Notwithstanding these difficulties, histopathologists must be aware that they are dealing with patients at risk of developing malignancy, know how to interpret the biopsy and appreciate the significance of their report if a diagnosis of dysplasia is made. The clinician needs to appreciate how effective a rectal biopsy is as a marker of precancer, what might be gained by additional colonoscopic surveillance and the numbers of cancers likely to be missed, despite such careful monitoring.

17.2 DEFINITIONS

Discussion of dysplasia is dogged by difficulties in definition (Chapter 14) (Riddell, 1996).

17.2.1 Dysplasia

This has been defined, with respect to the large intestine, as unequivocal neoplastic transformation of the epithelium and the changes may be graded into degrees of severity (Riddell *et al.*, 1983) (Section 17.6). It is not known, for certain, if such changes can regress for subsequent negative biopsies might merely be sampling errors and there can be a long gap between one positive biopsy and another (Woolrich *et al.*, 1992). Neither is it known what determines their progression.

17.2.2 Carcinoma *in-situ*

This term implies a degree of cytological and architectural abnormality more severe than that seen in high-grade dysplasia but still with the basement membrane intact. In practice the distinction between the two has poor reproducibility (Schlemper *et al.*, 2000). In the Vienna classification (Chapter 14) both terms are in category 4 under the umbrella of non-invasive high-grade neoplasia. In colonic biopsy work the distinction has no clinical significance and to avoid confusion we do not use the term *in-situ* carcinoma (Fig. 17.1).

17.2.3 Intramucosal carcinoma

Although we believe that in clinical practice this category is not appropriate for neoplastic polyps, there are rare instances in ulcerative colitis when such a term is relevant, though we prefer to use 'high-grade intramucosal neoplasia'. A clear breakdown of the basement membrane is implied, with invasion of the lamina propria by cords and tubules of malignant epithelium or by diffuse sheets of single cells (Fig. 17.2). The muscularis mucosae is intact but the cryptal basement membrane is not.

17.2.4 Precancer/premalignant

Care must be taken to distinguish precancerous *conditions* from pre-cancerous *lesions*. We take precancerous lesions to be synonymous with dysplastic change. Precancerous conditions have much wider meaning and are usually non-morphological (i.e. disease states associated with a higher than normal risk of developing carcinoma).

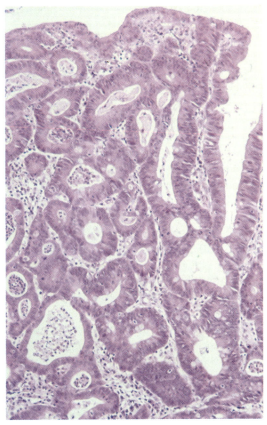

Figure 17.1 An example of the difficulty in distinguishing *in-situ* carcinoma from high-grade dysplasia. Here the basement is intact and non-invasive high-grade neoplasia (Vienna classification category 4) seems the safest opinion.

17.2.5 Atypia

Epithelial changes in which the cytological or architectural abnormality is more severe than expected given an observed degree of inflammation, yet falls short of those required for dysplasia, are best described as atypical. This therefore overlaps the 'indefinite' category in the widely used classification proposed by Riddell *et al.* (1983) (Section 17.6.7). In our opinion, 'atypical' transmits appropriate anxiety to the clinician, without the malignant overtones that are attached to dysplasia (Fig. 17.3). It is a useful term when interpreting mucosal changes in the presence of significant inflammation. In our experience the term triggers the clinical reflex for more careful short-term follow-up, in particular after the inflammation has settled.

17.3 PATIENTS AT RISK AND CANCER INCIDENCE

Several factors increase the risk of developing dysplasia and/or carcinoma in ulcerative colitis (Edwards and Truelove, 1964). The two most important are the durations of the colitis and its anatomical extent.

It is uncommon for any type of neoplasia to develop within 8 years of the onset of disease,

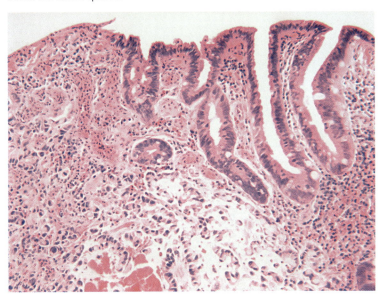

Figure 17.2 Intramucosal carcinoma in long-standing ulcerative colitis: dysplastic mucosa is seen on the right while on the left glandular architecture and basement membrane are destroyed being replaced by irregular glandular tubules and infiltrating clusters of cells.

though such cases have been documented (Mayer *et al.*, 1999). There is considerable variation in the published figures for the cumulative risk (CR) and standard incidence ratio (SIR) of cancer in colitis, which are determined not only by geographical and racial factors but by the way the data are collected and the composition of the patient cohorts, for example population-based or tertiary referral centre-based statistics. As examples, in a follow-up of children in North America the CR after 35 years has been reported as 43 per cent (Devroede *et al.*, 1971), but only 1.4 per cent at 18 years in an adult Danish study (Hendriksen *et al.*, 1985) where a large number of patients undergo colectomy in the presence of a total colitis. The CR calculated from 19 studies in a meta-analysis by Eaden *et al.* (2001a) was 2 per cent at 10 years, 8 per cent at 20 years and 18 per cent at 30 years. The variation in statistical data is again evident from the low CR figures quoted in the most recent St Mark's Hospital surveillance data (Rutter *et al.*, 2006) of 0 per cent at 10 years, 2.5 per cent at 20 years, 7.6 per cent at 30 years and 10.8 per cent at 40 years.

The second major risk factor is the anatomical extent of the colitis, the risk increasing with proximal extension of the disease. The anatomical limits on which calculations are based are usually proctitis and proctosigmoiditis, left-sided disease delineated as distal to the splenic flexure and pancolitis in which disease is proximal to the hepatic flexure.

For historical reasons the majority of the figures are based on barium studies for defining the limits of disease, but more recent knowledge from colonoscopic and pathology data show that such studies underestimate extent. In a study of colectomy specimens from patients with colitis-associated cancer Mathy *et al.* (2003) point out tumours were found in grossly normal bowel but in all cases there was microscopic pancolitis. Ekbom *et al.* (1990) report a SIR of 1.7 for proctitis, 2.8 for left-sided disease and 14.8 for pancolitis. Occasional studies have found patients with extensive and left-sided disease have a similar risk of dysplasia (Nugent *et al.*, 1991). There is one study in which backwash ileitis is shown to be an independent risk factor (Heuschen *et al.*, 2001) (Section 12.7). Because of the long follow-up period required before neoplasia becomes evident it will be many years before the data on the cancer risk in colitis are based on the more recent colonoscopic and microscopic data.

Other risk factors include a family history of colorectal cancer, in particular a first-degree relative (Askling *et al.*, 2001), primary sclerosing cholangitis (Jayaram *et al.*, 2001), the severity of inflammation both colonoscopic and microscopic (Rutter *et al.*, 2004c) and an early age of onset (Ekbom *et al.*, 1990). However, early age of onset has not been found to be a risk in all studies (Gilat *et al.*, 1988). The risk can be reduced by a policy advocating a high colectomy rate (Hendriksen *et al.*, 1985),

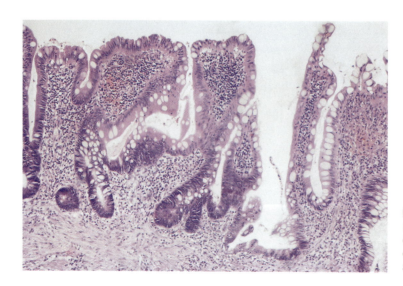

Figure 17.3 Chronic long-standing ulcerative colitis with distorted cryptal architecture and atypical cytological abnormalities but not amounting to dysplasia.

surveillance programmes (Section 17.10), regular visits to the general practitioner (Eaden *et al.*, 2000) and chemoprevention, in particular aminosalicylates (van Staa *et al.*, 2005).

17.4 THE RELIABILITY OF DYSPLASIA IN CANCER SURVEILLANCE

That dysplasia is considered a precancerous lesion, a suitable marker for cancer surveillance and an indicator for radical surgery has come about by a series of clinicopathological studies following on from the initial observation by Morson and Pang (1967). In marked contrast to sporadic colorectal carcinoma in which the majority of preceding dysplastic lesions are easily visible polypoid tubular, tubulovillous or villous adenomas, the majority of dysplastic lesions in ulcerative colitis have a flat or low elevated profile. Until the recent advent of improved endoscopic technology (Kiesslich *et al.*, 2003; Rutter *et al.*, 2004a) a significant proportion of lesions were also considered grossly invisible and only detectable by microscopy. Identification therefore depended on taking large numbers of nontargeted biopsies. It is interesting that gastric dysplasia, a complication of longstanding *Helicobacter*

pylori-associated chronic gastritis, is also predominantly flat and one may speculate that flat dysplasia, in contrast to the precancerous polypoid adenomas of sporadic colorectal cancer, is a complication of longstanding chronic inflammation. In the older literature the presence of an endoscopic raised lesion or mass – dysplasia-associated lesion or mass (DALM) – implied that the lesion was locally unresectable and the data indicated that between 43 and 68 per cent of such lesions already contained a focus of invasive carcinoma (Blackstone *et al.*, 1981; Butt *et al.*, 1983a; Rosenstock *et al.*, 1985; Bernstein *et al.*, 1994) (Fig. 17.4). This is in contrast to flat dysplasia where less than 4 per cent contained such a focus. A DALM was therefore an indicator for immediate colectomy. It is now appreciated that there is a morphological heterogeneity in elevated lesions and that local resection may be preferential for the pattern referred to as an 'adenoma-like DALM' (Section 17.11).

Undoubtedly, cancer can develop in the absence of any detectable dysplasia. This occurs in up to 25 per cent of cases (Ransohoff *et al.*, 1985; Taylor *et al.*, 1992; Connell *et al.*, 1994a) based on inspection of the surgical specimen and 17 of the 30 cancers in the study of Rutter *et al.* (2006) which had no preceding dysplasia identified in the surveillance biopsies. It is difficult to exclude sampling errors in biopsy data but this is discussed further below. In surveillance programmes the incidence of highgrade dysplasia, DALM or cancer developing is low

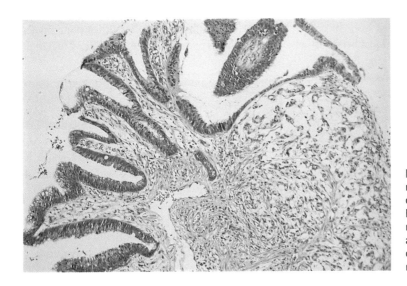

Figure 17.4 Severely dysplastic mucosa adjacent to signet ring cell carcinoma in a patient with a long history of ulcerative colitis. The mucosa has a villous architecture and the hyperchromatic epithelial cells showing complete loss of nuclear polarity.

if the index biopsy is negative, the figures being 0–2.4 per cent (Nugent et al., 1991; Woolrich et al., 1992; Bernstein et al., 1994). The focal nature of dysplasia and the fact that it can occur distant from the tumour create sampling problems that undermine the efficacy of many surveillance programmes. The chances of detecting dysplasia therefore depend both on its extent and the extent of the mucosal sampling (Riddell and Morson, 1979; Kewenter et al., 1982; Allen et al., 1985; Taylor et al., 1992; Connell et al., 1994a).

Early quantitative work by Riddell and Morson (1979) on 63 patients with rectal carcinoma, colonic cancer or dysplasia alone, showed that, in 65 per cent of the cases, more than 50 per cent of the rectal mucosa was dysplastic. In only three cases was rectal dysplasia absent and all their rectal cancers had accompanying dysplasia. These data are, however, biased in favour of rectal dysplasia, because of the referral pattern at St Mark's Hospital. However, since about 50 per cent of cancers in colitis occur in the rectosigmoid region (Mayer et al., 1999; Connell et al., 1994a; Rutter et al., 2006) there is a case for targeting this region. Butt et al. (1983b) reviewed data from other published series and showed that the maximum diagnostic yield of cancer based on the presence of severe dysplasia is 62 per cent. The likelihood of a rectal biopsy showing severe dysplasia when a cancer was subsequently resected was between 73 per cent and 87 per cent. De Dombal and Softley (1985) interpret the data of Butt et al. (1983b) and claim a sensitivity of severe dysplasia for cancer, using rectal biopsy, of just over 50 per cent and a positive predictive value of just below 50 per cent. These early data, especially the figures of Riddell and Morson (1979) contrast sharply with the recent data from the same centre (Rutter et al., 2006) in which 57 per cent of the 30 cancers detected in the surveillance programme failed to show preceding dysplastic biopsies and this despite 17 of the 30 cancers being in the rectosigmoid region. One explanation is that prior to 1983, when the classification of dysplasia was revised (Riddell et al., 1983), dysplasia was evidently overdiagnosed (Connell et al., 1994b).

A review of 10 prospective surveillance programmes since 1980 (Bernstein et al., 1994) found 42 per cent of patients with high-grade dysplasia and 16 per cent of those with low-grade dysplasia had a synchronous carcinoma when an immediate colectomy was carried out. The role of sampling is put in perspective when it is realized that a biopsy looks at less than 0.05 per cent of the colorectal mucosal surface. Rubin et al. (1992) calculated that to detect the highest grade of dysplasia with 90–95 per cent sensitivity 33–64 biopsies are required. Riddell (1995) claims that to be certain to detect a 2-cm patch of dysplasia in a 100-cm length of colon 300 biopsies would be necessary. It is a relief to know that 77.3 per cent of dysplastic lesions were visible endoscopically in the study of Rutter et al. (2004b). When they excluded obvious sporadic adenomas 89.3 per cent of their cohort of 50 patients had visible dysplasia. Targeted biopsy protocols, helped by chromoendoscopy (Kiesslich et al., 2003; Rutter et al., 2004a) considerably reduce the clinical and laboratory workload and ensure reliable surveillance. Thus, Rutter et al. (2004a) failed to detect any dysplasia in a series of 2904 non-targeted biopsies from 100 colitic patients in a surveillance programme. Immediate subsequent targeted re-examination after dye spray detected nine dysplastic lesions from only 157 biopsies.

Attention is drawn by Rubio et al. (1982) to another difficulty, which is the tendency, where dysplasia is predominantly in the base of villiform crypts, for it to be missed if only the surface is sampled at biopsy. This type of sampling error, one based on the depth of the biopsy, also accounts for the high cancer incidence found on resection in original descriptions of DALMs (Blackstone et al., 1981) which were not present in the biopsy material.

17.5 THE MACROSCOPIC LESION IN DYSPLASIA

In everyday histological practice the pathologist is frequently reporting the biopsy with little clue of the colonoscopic or radiological appearances. The macroscopic appearances, however, are vital for overall interpretation and management. Dysplasia in the non-colitic is almost invariably polypoid (the adenoma), and is the basis of the polyp–cancer sequence (Muto et al., 1975; Riddell, 1980) (Section

15.5). In contrast, the gross morphological patterns of dysplasia in colitis are flat, have a low elevated profile and, until recently (Rutter *et al.*, 2004b), believed to be grossly invisible. Butt *et al.* (1983a) describes the flat lesions as having a velvety mucosal surface and the elevated lesions as nodular, plaque-like or low-papillary (Fig. 17.5). Occasionally strictures and ulcers are to be found but such lesions are usually already malignant (Blackstone *et al.*, 1981). The background colitic mucosa is often irregular and nodular as a consequence of the disease, which creates difficulty for the colonoscopist in recognizing the subtle changes of focal flat dysplasia. In addition to targeting any obvious lesion the recommendations are that surveillance programme protocols should include at least four quadrantic biopsies every 10 cm throughout the colon and sample every 5 cm in the rectosigmoid region where dysplasia and cancer occur most frequently (Itzkowitz and Harpaz, 2004).

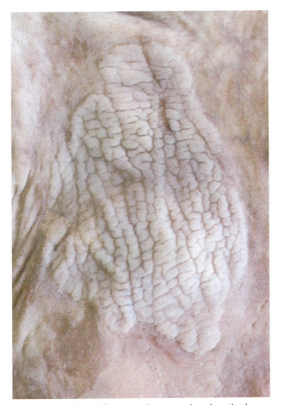

Figure 17.5 Detail from a colectomy showing the low elevated velvet-like nodular mucosal appearance of a common pattern of dysplasia in colitis.

The advent of modern endoscopic techniques, such as magnifying endoscopy and dye spray now allow appreciation of macroscopic detail down to the level of the pit pattern (Sada *et al.*, 2004). It is apparent that few dysplastic lesions can truly be described as flat to the point of being indistinguishable from normal mucosa (Rutter *et al.*, 2004b).

However such techniques are still mainly limited to specialist centres. The current management regimens are therefore still based on the old dictum that dysplastic lesions which were believed endoscopically invisible or only minimally elevated (Butt *et al.*, 1983a) carry a low cancer incidence, while cancer can be present in between 40 and 60 per cent of macroscopically raised lesions (Blackstone *et al.*, 1981; Butt *et al.*, 1983a; Bernstein *et al.*, 1994; Rutter *et al.*, 2004b).

As already mentioned, it was the study of Blackstone *et al.* in 1981 that coined the term DALM and because of the high association of such lesions with an existing cancer immediate colectomy became the standard management. It is now appreciated that DALMs have a heterogeneous morphology and that for some patterns endoscopic resection and continued surveillance, rather than colectomy, is the management of choice. This is discussed in more detail in Section 17.11.

Thus, the range of macroscopic appearances of dysplasia carry with them difficult management decisions focused on endoscopic resectability and further complicated by the problems of histological grading (Section 17.6). This contrasts with the relatively straightforward management by endoscopic resection of the large majority of adenomatous polyps, the dominant precursor lesion of sporadic colorectal carcinoma.

17.6 HISTOLOGICAL RECOGNITION AND CLASSIFICATION OF DYSPLASIA

The recognition of dysplasia depends on the appreciation of cytological and architectural abnormalities. Dysplasia was originally classified as mild, moderate or severe (Yardley and Keren, 1974;

Riddell, 1976) but following the paper of Riddell *et al.* (1983) the widely adopted classification of the grades of dysplasia in colitis is now simply the two tiers of high and low grade with an indefinite category (Table 17.1). When proposed the indefinite category was subclassified further into probably positive, unknown and probably negative. This is no longer thought to be useful (Riddell, 1996) and accredited to a better appreciation of the reparative and regenerative features in the colitic mucosa, which accounted for most of the indefinite probably negative group. The distinction between indefinite (unknown) and probably positive has also been dropped for it merely complicates matters when both have the same clinical implications, namely to repeat the biopsy.

The need for an indefinite group reflects the difficulty that pathologists experience in recognizing dysplasia. This is for three main reasons. First the colitis–dysplasia–carcinoma sequence is a biological continuum. A spectrum in which each stage evolves imperceptibly from the previous one. Second as a consequence of severe inflammation epithelial abnormalities arise that are very similar to dysplastic changes. Third, and as discussed earlier, dysplasia complicating colitis does not usually form a distinct epithelial mass (polyp) and may occasionally only involve isolated or small numbers of crypts interspersed among normal or reactive ones. Thus, the contrast between dysplasia and non-dysplasia in small biopsies is less clear cut than in the diagnosis of adenomas.

While it is possible to enumerate the cytological and architectural changes (Riddell *et al.*, 1978), no one of these is diagnostic of the presence or degree of dysplasia. Diagnosis is based on combinations of histological signs (much like the diagnosis of inflammatory bowel disease itself) onto which is superimposed the opinion of the pathologist. This,

and the biological continuum referred to above, results in inevitable inter- and intra-observer variation (Dundas *et al.*, 1987; Dixon *et al.*, 1988; Melville *et al.*, 1989; Guindi and Riddell, 2001) (see Section 17.7). In the evaluation of any particular local change much depends on the surrounding mucosa. Changes that might indicate dysplasia in intact non-inflamed mucosa have a different interpretation if there is obvious evidence of healing ulceration and/or severe inflammation.

17.6.1 Cytological abnormalities

The cell nuclei vary in size, shape and position. The variation in nuclear position causes the appearance of stratification of cells within a crypt (Fig. 17.6). The nuclear chromatin is coarse and results in

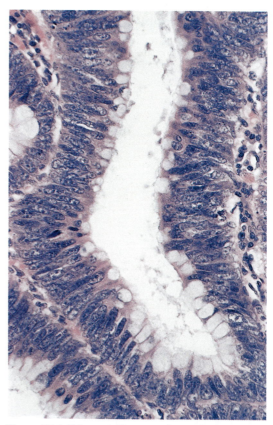

Figure 17.6 This crypt illustrates the cytological features of high-grade dysplasia. There is pseudostratification, mucin is reduced and the nuclei are markedly enlarged with hyperchromatic nuclei and coarse chromatin.

Table 17.1 Classification of colorectal epithelial dysplasia in colitis*

Dysplasia	High grade
	Low grade
Indefinite	
Regenerative	Clearly related to active disease
Normal	

*Based on Riddell *et al.* (1983) and Riddell (1996).

hyperchromatism (Riddell *et al.*, 1983). Mitoses are increased and their presence in the upper third of the crypt is a warning to search for other dysplastic signs.

Generally, the crypt epithelium fails to mature, so that the crypt contains undifferentiated cells and goblet cells are reduced. Mucin droplets may be limited to the cell apices. Alternatively, the goblet cells take on a rounded appearance, often with mucin displaced to the basal side of the nucleus – 'dystrophic' goblet cells (Fig. 17.7). A general reduction in mucin often leaves the cytoplasm markedly eosinophilic (Riddell, 1976).

Unfortunately, none of these features is unique to dysplasia, and each may be seen in isolation in inflamed or regenerating epithelium (Sections 17.6.5 and 17.6.6). Many of the discrepancies between Japanese and Western pathologists (Chapter 14) result from the emphasis placed on the cytological appearances by the former (Schlemper *et al.*, 2000).

17.6.2 Architectural abnormalities

The main architectural abnormalities often result in a thickened mucosa, either by elongation of crypts producing a villous pattern or by budding in a tubular adenomatous pattern (Figs 17.4, 17.8 and 17.9) (Lennard-Jones *et al.*, 1977). A thickened mucosa in long-standing ulcerative colitis should always arouse suspicion. The cytological changes may also be superimposed on the usual distorted architecture of a colitic or on the atrophic pattern of long-standing quiescent disease. In our experience in biopsy work it is not uncommon to see serrated changes in the mucosa as an accompaniment to dysplasia and also in non-dysplastic reactive epithelium. There is often an accompanying

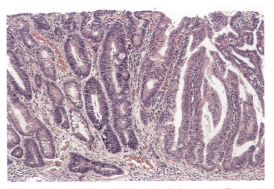

Figure 17.8 High-grade dysplasia in long-standing ulcerative colitis. There are florid architectural abnormalities as well as nuclear pseudostratification and pleomorphism throughout the deranged crypts.

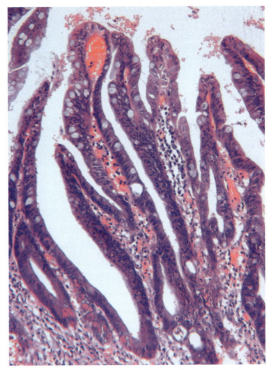

Figure 17.9 This illustrates high-grade dysplasia in which the crypts have a villiform configuration accompanying the typical cytological abnormalities.

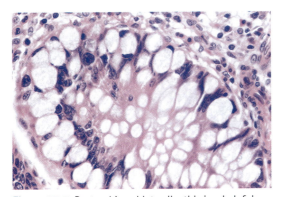

Figure 17.7 Dystrophic goblet cells: this is a helpful feature when interpreted in conjunction with other features in the diagnosis of dysplasia. Alone it is not diagnostic. The mucin is located on the basement side of the nucleus.

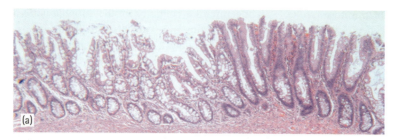

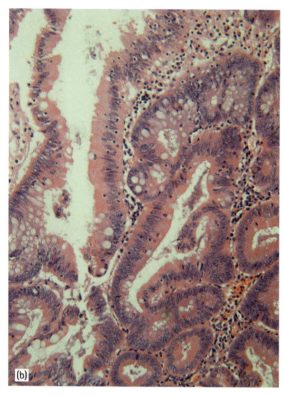

Figure 17.10 (a,b). These two figures show two adjacent fields demonstrating the serration and cytoplasmic eosinophilia that can occur alongside more obvious dysplastic features present in the right half of (b). The eosinophilia if accompanied by nuclear atypicality is an interpretative problem, when seen in isolation and may warrant a label of indefinite for dysplasia.

eosinophilia of the cell cytoplasm. The significance of this is unclear but Rubio *et al.* (2000) found, in their study of 50 colitics, that almost 30 per cent of dysplastic lesions juxtaposed to carcinomas showed serrated features (Fig. 17.10). This may be relevant to the molecular pathogenesis of the dysplasia–carcinoma pathway in ulcerative colitis (Jass *et al.*, 2002) (Section 17.9).

17.6.3 Degree of involvement

In a typical area of dysplasia immature and atypical cells will line the crypts from the base to the surface epithelium. If the cryptal lining cells seem to be maturing towards the surface caution is required before a dysplastic label is applied. Guindi and Riddell (2001) point out that while dysplasia is often maximal on the surface there are rare occasions when the changes are limited to either the luminal surface or the crypt base (Fig. 17.11) (Riddell, 1980; Riddell *et al.*, 1983; Rubio *et al.*, 1984). The fewer the crypts involved the more difficult the diagnosis (Fig. 17.12). In the extreme case only a cytological abnormality may exist. Notice must be taken of the adjacent mucosa but, when changes are restricted to one crypt, it is unlikely that

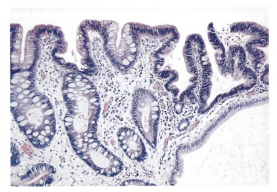

Figure 17.11 Low-grade dysplasia confined to the upper crypts and surface epithelium in a biopsy from a patient with a 10-year history of disease.

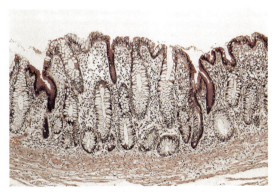

Figure 17.12 Dysplasia involving selected crypts highlighting how easily sampling errors might occur not only in choice of biopsy site but also within an individual biopsy.

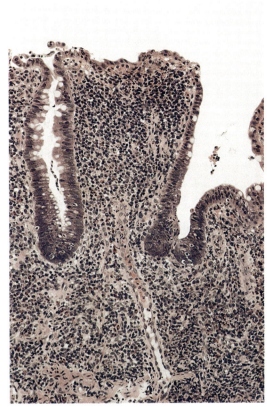

Figure 17.13 Obviously inflamed mucosa in which degenerative features are seen in the surface epithelium. In the upper half of the cryptal epithelium to the right atypicality due to the inflammation is observed and easily misinterpreted as dysplasia.

a confident diagnosis of dysplasia can be made. Riddell (1983) suggests that when less than four crypts are affected the category 'indefinite' ('atypical') should be used.

17.6.4 Classification of dysplasia

The need to classify dysplasia (Table 17.1) is based on the belief that increasingly severe degrees of dysplasia have increasing malignant potential (Lennard-Jones *et al.*, 1977). However, as pointed out earlier, this is probably only the case in flat lesions; in raised lesions carcinoma commonly coexists with low-grade dysplasia (Blackstone *et al.*, 1981). Thus, clinical experience has led to the realization that the

concept that dysplasia must evolve through increasing degrees of severity prior to frank carcinoma is incorrect (Isaacson, 1982; Riddell, 1984; Morson and Jass, 1985; Riddell 1996).

17.6.5 Degenerative features in colitic mucosa

In active colitis there are degenerative changes in the crypt epithelium, comprising goblet cell discharge, cytoplasmic swelling and epithelial sloughing away from the basement membrane. When these features are seen, signs of active inflammation should be sought in the lamina propria (Fig. 17.13). The presence of even a few neutrophils confirms that the epithelium is damaged by active colitis. Extreme caution is necessary before a diagnosis of dysplasia is made in such circumstances (Allen *et al.*, 1985). Irrespective of this Rutter *et al.* (2004c) found that severity of inflammation was a risk factor for the eventual occurrence of a carcinoma.

Good-quality sections are essential. An important artefact, which can lead to a mistaken diagnosis of dysplasia, is the irregularity and nuclear hyperchromatism which is often induced in crypt epithelium at the edge of a biopsy by shearing or crushing as the biopsy is taken (Fig. 3.29). Again, it is unwise to base a diagnosis of dysplasia on only one or two crypts confined to the edge of a biopsy.

17.6.6 Regenerative mucosa

As previously mentioned the presence of active colitis is a warning sign to interpret epithelial changes with caution (Riddell *et al.*, 1983). The resolving and regenerating phase of active disease, when inflammation is less obvious, causes the greatest problems of interpretation. Epithelial cells are of variable shapes, often cuboidal or low columnar. The nuclei are large, usually vesicular with prominent eosinophilic nucleoli. Polarity can be lost, to give some degree of pseudostratification, but the number of cells is usually not increased and the epithelium does not look crowded. There is absence of mucin or it is restricted to the luminal aspect of the crypts. The cuboidal cells are often eosinophilic (Fig. 17.14). Architecture is clearly distorted, the epithelium being flat over a healing ulcer or the crypt pattern is much simplified. The irregularity of healing can produce a villous appearance, causing confusion with a similar pattern in dysplastic mucosa.

As the mucosa recovers, the cells become more columnar, the nuclei larger, the chromatin more coarse and the picture more closely resembles low-grade dysplasia (Fig. 17.15). Usually, residual inflammation provides a clue to its regenerative nature. However, uncertainty at this stage warrants a diagnosis of indefinite for dysplasia and the recommendation to repeat the biopsy after a short interval.

17.6.7 Indefinite for dysplasia

The need for this category emphasizes the limitations of light microscopy and routine staining in

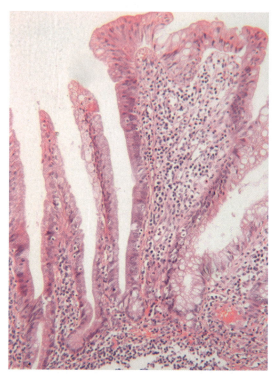

Figure 17.14 Regenerating villiform epithelium with underlying inflammation in the lamina propria. There is stratification of nuclei and cytoplasmic eosinophilia but the nuclei tend to be vesicular rather than hyperchromatic and polymorphic; cf. Fig. 17.9.

the diagnosis of dysplasia. Riddell *et al.* (1983) had originally divided the category 'indefinite' into 'probably negative', 'unknown' and 'probably positive', but these have fallen into disuse (Riddell, 1996) (see Section 17.6, pages 307–08).

The crypts in the mucosa are usually distorted, and fail to mature in an orderly fashion. The nuclei are enlarged, tending to hyperchromatism and pseudostratification. Mucin is diminished. While any one feature of genuine dysplasia may be present, the difficulty is that insufficient are seen together to warrant a firm opinion (Figs 17.16 and 17.17). Confidence in making a diagnosis of dysplasia is most frequently undermined by the presence of inflammatory cells and, when there is doubt, it is customary to request a repeat biopsy after a period of treatment.

Particular problems may occur in children with their exuberant reparative changes (Riddell, 1976)

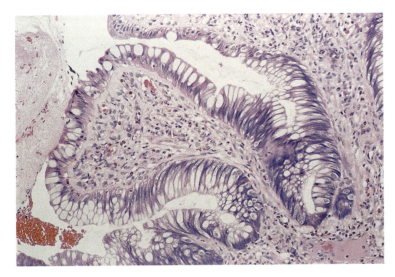

Figure 17.15 Regenerating epithelium with large cells lining the crypts but without the other nuclear changes associated with dysplasia. On first impression this is easily misinterpreted as dysplasia.

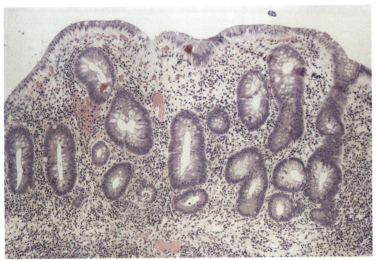

Figure 17.16 Indefinite for dysplasia. Although there is some hyperchromasia and pseudostratification it is mainly in the lower half of the crypts, with maturation towards the surface. There is also inflammation present with a small crypt abscess seen in the deep lamina propria.

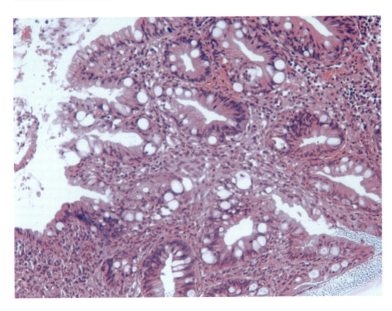

Figure 17.17 In this example of 'indefinite for dysplasia' inflammation is present; there is surface maturation but also some dystrophic goblet cells.

or from technical effects that alter staining, e.g. fixatives that enhance nuclear staining (Riddell *et al.*, 1983).

17.6.8 Low-grade dysplasia

In low-grade dysplasia the cytological and architectural changes outlined earlier should be confidently recognized, though not all will be present (Figs 17.18 and 17.19). The pattern can be adenomatous, as in polyps, or small groups of crypts may be enlarged, with moderate nuclear pleomorphism, hyperchromatism and loss of polarity. A serrated outline may give the epithelium an appearance

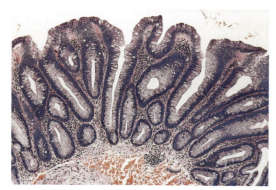

Figure 17.18 Low-grade dysplasia with hyperchromatic nuclei throughout the crypts and surface along with loss of mucin resulting in increased cytoplasmic staining. There is no inflammation.

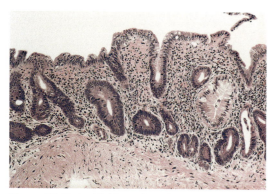

Figure 17.19 In this illustration of low-grade dysplasia there is marked nuclear pleomorphism that involves the surface epithelium and minimal inflammation.

akin to a metaplastic polyp (Riddell, 1983; Rubio *et al.*, 2000; Jass *et al.*, 2002). The changes can be along the crypt length, or limited to either the base or tip (Giundi and Riddell, 2001).

Where the superficial aspect of the crypt matures the surface epithelium often becomes villiform. The most severely dysplastic areas determine the final classification but, to upgrade a biopsy from low to high grade, more than two crypts must show the deterioration. There will clearly be difficulties at either end of the spectrum, i.e. whether to classify epithelial features as indefinite, rather than low-grade dysplasia on the one hand, or whether a biopsy qualifies as high grade on the other. It is in these areas that observer variation is the most disparate (Section 17.7). Experience is the most valuable tool but, because dysplasia is so rare, it is hard to come by and a second opinion has now become part of routine management as a way of overcoming observer variation.

17.6.9 High-grade dysplasia

The initial reaction to obvious high-grade dysplasia is to liken it to carcinoma *in-situ* seen at any other site. The majority of the cytological and architectural abnormalities of dysplasia are found. Loss of nuclear polarity is extreme, the nuclei being randomly located in the cell. The nuclei stain deeply and mitoses may be seen throughout the crypt (Figs 17.20 and 17.21). Crypt branching is often complex, with foci of glands closely crowded 'back to back'. Such is the severity of the features that they are obvious, even if there is accompanying inflammation. There is one exception to the general pattern of high-grade dysplasia, that known as 'basal cell proliferation' (Riddell, 1976) (Fig. 17.22). Attempts have been made to put the cytological and architectural patterns in dysplasia on a quantitative basis (Riddell, 1976; Lennard-Jones *et al.*, 1977; Allen *et al.*, 1987). As would be expected, in high-grade dysplasia a 'full house' of criteria is usually present, in contrast to the smaller number of abnormalities seen in low-grade dysplasia, but the above reported works also illustrate the poor specificity of any one of the morphological attributes.

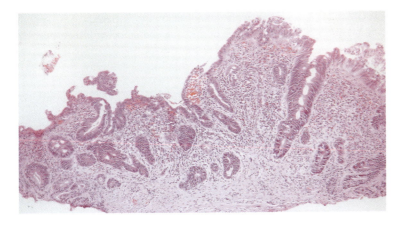

Figure 17.20 This is an example of high-grade dysplasia with a severe architectural distortion, crypt budding and nuclear polymorphism. There is some inflammation but it is insufficient to account for the severity of the epithelial abnormalities.

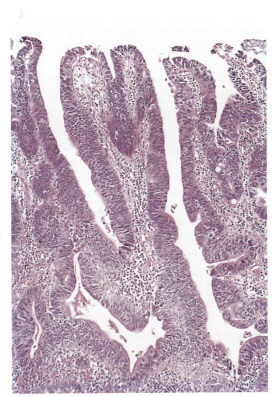

Figure 17.21 High-grade dysplasia with florid nuclear pseudostratification along the entire villiform crypt lengths.

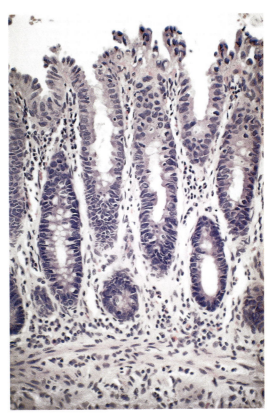

Figure 17.22 High dysplasia but in this pattern, in contrast to Fig. 17.21, the nuclei, while hyperchromatic and polymorphic, remain in a predominantly basal position.

17.7 OBSERVER VARIATION

The diagnosis and grading of dysplasia is a synthesis of several imprecise observations, e.g. nuclear size, nuclear position, architectural derangement, etc. Any group of pathologists will produce a curve around a mean when asked to carry out a grading exercise. Moreover the variation will be less at the tails of the curve, e.g. high-grade dysplasia and negative for dysplasia and most in the blurred areas between high and low grade and to either side of indefinite for dysplasia (Melville *et al.*, 1988; Connell *et al.*, 1994b; Riddell, 1996). When the current classification was drawn up the authors (Riddell *et al.*, 1983) carried out an observer variation study among themselves claiming a correct diagnosis of 77 per cent for high-grade dysplasia, 63 per cent for low grade dysplasia, 49 per cent for indefinite and 74 per cent for no dysplasia. Since then there have been several observer variation studies each with differing methodologies and a range of results (Dundas *et al.*, 1987; Dixon *et al.*, 1988; Melville *et al.*, 1989). In the study of Dixon *et al.* (1988) pairwise agreements over grades of dysplasia ranged from 49–72 per cent, κ values from fair to moderate (0.292– 0.584) and pairwise agreement improved to 68–84 per cent when only dysplasia versus no dysplasia was considered. Perhaps a startling result was that if one pathologist diagnosed high-grade dysplasia pairwise agreement ranged from 100 per cent down to 33 per cent. However, the disagreement was mostly of low-grade dysplasia. Melville *et al.* (1989) concluded that the diagnosis of dysplasia was unreliable. The common conclusions of these and other studies, bar one that concluded gastrointestinal expert pathologists performed no better than generalists (Eaden *et al.*, 2001b), was that before any management decision based on a diagnosis of dysplasia or indefinite for dysplasia is undertaken two experienced gastrointestinal pathologists should review the material.

It is worth reiterating the comments made by Dixon *et al.* (1988) that observer variation studies are artificial and in clinical practice the large majority of decisions about dysplasia and any course of action are made over a period time, after a review of several biopsies, with all the clinical details available and with multidisciplinary discussion. Few serious management mistakes should occur if this approach is followed.

17.8 OTHER STAINS AND METHODOLOGIES

There is an ongoing search for new markers of precancer or adjuncts to improve the recognition and consistency of the diagnosis of dysplasia. A range of special stains have been tried (Isaacson, 1976; Boland *et al.*, 1984; Ehsanullah *et al.*, 1985; Allen *et al.*, 1985; Jass *et al.*, 1986) from basic mucin stains such as the PAS reaction and high iron diamine Alcian blue to the more complex demonstration of the mucin-associated carbohydrate antigen Sialyl-Tn (Karlen *et al.*, 1998b). Other studies have looked at lectins (Ahnen *et al.*, 1987; Fozard *et al.*, 1987) and deoxyribonucleic acid (DNA) analysis by flow cytometry (Fozard *et al.*, 1986; Melville *et al.*, 1988; Lofberg *et al.*, 1992; Rubin *et al.*, 1992; Befrits *et al.*, 1994). Of these the most promising, if used in conjunction with routine haematoxylin and eosin staining, has been the detection of DNA aneuploidy by flow cytometry. Several studies show a correlation between aneuploidy and dysplasia. It can precede the appearance of dysplasia by several years and appears to be a relatively constant finding once detected. In their prospective 8-year follow-up study of 59 patients with long-standing ulcerative colitis Lofberg *et al.* (1992) found 15 (25 per cent) with DNA aneuploidy. In six it preceded dysplasia, in six it appeared concurrently with dysplasia, in one it post-dated dysplasia and in two it was detected on only one occasion. The study of Rubin *et al.* (1992) also showed aneuploidy to have prognostic value for the development of dysplasia. Melville *et al.* (1988) suggest the most effective role for aneuploidy would be as a guide in the indefinite group or to provide additional evaluation of negative biopsies following a positive biopsy of low grade dysplasia.

At the current time, with improving endoscopic techniques for the recognition of dysplastic lesions, the ease with which biopsies can be targeted or repeated and the increasing trend to ensure that two gastrointestinal orientated pathologists confirm any diagnosis of dysplasia, none of the above methods can justifiably be incorporated into routine laboratory procedures.

17.9 MOLECULAR INVESTIGATIONS

There are data to show that the molecular pathway of ulcerative colitis-associated cancer differs from that of sporadic colorectal carcinoma and, as is discussed in Section 17.11, stains that reflect over- or under-expression of gene products may come to have a diagnostic role. The most commonly identified mutations in sporadic colorectal carcinoma are of the three tumour suppressor genes, APC, p53 and DCC, plus one oncogene, K-ras (Brentnall *et al.*, 1994; Harpaz *et al.*, 1994; Nixon *et al.*, 1995; Fogt *et al.*, 1998; Itzkowitz, 2000; Wong and Harrison, 2001; Itzkowitz and Harpaz, 2004). In the development of dysplasia and ulcerative colitis-associated carcinoma, unlike sporadic cancers, mutation of the APC gene is a late event while mutations and loss of heterozygosity of the p53 gene are relatively early. There is also correlation between the overexpression of p53, the presence of aneuploidy and the severity of dysplasia (Brentnall *et al.*, 1994; Nixon *et al.*, 1995). Because overexpression of p53 is relatively easily demonstrated by immunohistochemical staining it has a use as an adjunct to some of the problems in identifying dysplasia and in defining important dysplasia-associated morphological variants (Section 17.11).

Data on the position in the colitis-associated cancer pathway of the K-ras gene and DCC gene are conflicting but their identification does not currently have a specific part to play in routine biopsy practice (Nixon *et al.*, 1995).

Because carcinoma in colitis can occur in a young age group, can be multifocal, shows a significant number of right-sided lesions and is often mucinous it has been suggested that, like hereditary non-polyposis colon cancer, the molecular pathogenesis may also involve defects in mismatch repair genes. In patients with dysplasia and cancer Suzuki *et al.* (1994) found evidence of microsatellite instability in 27 per cent of 63 patients while Brentnall *et al.* (1996) found similar evidence in 46 per cent of colitis patients with high-grade dysplasia and 40 per cent of those with cancer. However, Cawkwell *et al.* (2000) report an incidence of only 15 per cent for a single marker of microsatellite instability and only 2.4 per cent for two or more markers. Much of the discrepancy in this field of investigation is related to the markers chosen for investigation which need be standardized if comparisons are to be made (Itzkowitz, 2000). Jass *et al.* (2002) propose that one pathway to carcinoma might be the silencing of gene expression via methylation of DNA repair genes rather than mutations. They suggest the precancerous lesions in this pathway manifest a serrated morphology. Our own observations and those of Rubio *et al.* (2000) are of interest in this respect (Section 17.6.2).

17.10 IMPLICATIONS OF THE PATHOLOGIST'S REPORT

In most centres patients with long-standing ulcerative colitis (in excess of 8–10 years) are entered into a cancer surveillance programme. This involves annual colonoscopy or biennial colonoscopy with an annual intervening flexible sigmoidoscopy. There is considerable argument in the literature, outside the scope of this chapter (Lynch *et al.*, 1993; Axon, 1995, 1997; Lennard-Jones, 1995), as to whether such programmes are effective in preventing cancer but there are no randomized controlled trials and, for ethical reasons, unlikely to be any. However, several papers show that patients whose cancers are identified via a surveillance programme have a better outcome (Choi *et al.*, 1993; Connell *et al.*, 1994b; Lennard-Jones, 1995; Karlen *et al.*, 1998a). There is also an advantage if negative for dysplasia on entry to the programme (Nugent *et al.*, 1991; Connell *et al.*, 1994b). The pathologist's role is to make an accurate diagnosis on whether such surveillance biopsies are negative for dysplasia, are indefinite or, if dysplasia is present, whether it is high or low grade. One of the common outcomes of the observer variation studies (Section 17.7) has been the recommendation that for safe practice a second expert opinion should be sought, because the report might make the difference between colectomy and conservative management.

An overall perspective of the significance of the pathologist's opinion is gained from the paper by Bernstein *et al.* (1994). This analysed 10 prospective studies (1225 patients) aimed at questioning the assumption that surveillance can detect dysplasia prior to the development of cancer. In patients that had colectomy immediately following biopsy, out of 40 with a dysplasia-associated lesion or mass, cancer was already present in 43 per cent of the resected colons; out of 26 with high-grade flat dysplasia, cancer was already present in 42 per cent of the colons and out of 16 patients with flat low-grade dysplasia 19 per cent of the colons contained a carcinoma. In that analysis the risk of progression to dysplasia, for those with long-standing ulcerative colitis but index biopsy negative for dysplasia, was only 2.4 per cent. The mean follow up was 11 years.

When assessing the surveillance data in the literature it is important to be aware not only of the problems of observer variation (Section 17.7), especially in the categories of indefinite for dysplasia and low-grade dysplasia but also that many diagnoses of dysplasia were made prior to the impact of the classification proposed by Riddell *et al.* (1983) (Table 17.1).

17.10.1 Indefinite category

Much of the difficulty within this group results from the potential for inflammatory changes to mimic dysplasia. It is a sensible short-term approach, therefore, to shorten the interval of follow-up, while active medical treatment is instigated. The repeat biopsy needs to be targeted to the original area and ought to resolve the distinction between an exuberant inflammatory response or definite dysplasia. In one study in up to half the cases the changes resolved (Brostrom *et al.*, 1986). It is no surprise that with the existence of an indefinite category, and it being an area of maximum observer variation (Section 17.7), analysis of the clinical outcome suggests that patients in this category still require careful monitoring. In the survey of Bernstein *et al.* (1994), of 51 patients with an index biopsy indefinite for dysplasia, 18 per cent went on to develop high-grade dysplasia, a DALM or carcinoma. Of 95 patients whom, at some point, had a biopsy labelled indefinite 28 per cent eventually developed high-grade dysplasia, a

DALM or carcinoma. These figures are similar to the data on the outcome of the indefinite category which can be extracted from other studies (Connell *et al.*, 1994b; Jani *et al.*, 2003; Rutter *et al.*, 2006).

In routine clinical practice a sensible approach before signing out a biopsy as indefinite is to seek a second opinion. If there is agreement then recommend that the biopsy is repeated but targeted to the original site and perhaps with colonoscopic enhancement techniques, such as dye spray, employed. If not resolved and there are additional management difficulties in an individual patient's case, access to DNA ploidy studies may be contributory (Section 17.8).

17.10.2 Low-grade flat dysplasia

Since the last edition the management of a confirmed diagnosis of low-grade dysplasia has moved towards consideration of immediate colectomy, though there are still dissenters and conflicting data to this policy (Befrits *et al.*, 2002). Much of the dissent revolves around the reliability of the histological diagnosis, the grey area whether the lesion was truly flat or not and statistical interpretation of the patient cohort and follow-up details. As already mentioned interpreting the older data must take account of diagnoses made pre- or post-publication of the updated classification of dysplasia (Riddell *et al.*, 1983). A striking example of the effect of this publication is illustrated by the paper of Connell *et al.* (1994b). This documents that of 73 biopsies reported as low-grade dysplasia prior to 1983 only five were considered dysplastic on review by two experienced gastrointestinal pathologists using the new criteria. However, of 34 biopsies diagnosed as low-grade dysplasia after 1983 50 per cent were still considered dysplastic on review. This changed the predictive value for the 5-year progression of low-grade lesions to high-grade dysplasia or carcinoma from 16 per cent to 54 per cent. This paper and others (Bernstein *et al.*, 1994; Linberg *et al.*, 1996; Ullman *et al.*, 2002) were key to the recommendation that colectomy should be considered for a confident diagnosis of low-grade dysplasia if the clinical circumstances are appropriate. The arguments against this policy are that the diagnosis of low-grade dysplasia is unreliable (Lim *et al.*, 2003), it may only be present once (Befrits *et al.*, 2002), calculations purporting to show that the incidence of carcinoma in low-grade dysplasia is no greater than in colitics without a low-grade lesion and allegations that nearly all colitics will develop low-grade dysplasia if followed for long enough. As examples of these difficulties in the study of Befrits *et al.* (2002) 73 per cent of 60 patients with low-grade dysplasia followed for 10 years remained free of progression. Ullman *et al.* (2002), however, on an actuarial basis reported that the rate of progression to a higher grade lesion was 53 per cent at 5 years, while Linberg *et al.* (1996) found that low-grade dysplasia had a predictive value for high-grade dysplasia or carcinoma of 41 per cent. In the 10-study survey of Bernstein *et al.* (1994), of 798 patients with an index biopsy of low-grade dysplasia the available follow-up data for 55 showed 29 per cent progressed to high-grade dysplasia or cancer. Furthermore, of 16 coming to immediate colectomy, 19 per cent already had a cancer present. In the latest study from St Mark's Hospital (Rutter *et al.*, 2006) 40 per cent of 46 patients with low-grade dysplasia developed more advanced lesions. Bernstein (2004) gives the following reasons for favouring colectomy for low-grade dysplasia: nearly 20 per cent will already have a cancer present, there is documented evidence of progression to high-grade dysplasia or cancer in up to 50 per cent of cases within 5 years; since low-grade dysplasia is the only form of dysplasia found close to, or distant from, a carcinoma in nearly 50 per cent of cases (Connell *et al.*, 1994a) one cannot that assume progression is a monitorable biological continuum via lesions of increasing neoplastic severity.

Pathologists need to be aware of these arguments and differences but they are of primary concern to physicians and surgeons. The primary concern for the pathologist is to be certain that the diagnosis of low-grade dysplasia is a confident one and that it carries the backing of at least two expert opinions.

17.10.3 High-grade dysplasia

Following a diagnosis of high-grade dysplasia, with its concomitant risk of cancer, which is quoted as between 42 and 67 per cent (Taylor *et al.*, 1992; Bernstein *et al.*, 1994; Connell *et al.*, 1994b),

immediate proctocolectomy must be considered. If this is not the policy, there seems little point in pursuing an intense screening procedure. Nevertheless, the pathologist can only make recommendations; clinical decisions must take account of the operative risks and lifestyle of each patient.

Certain safeguards should be observed and a diagnosis of high-grade dysplasia confirmed in one of the following ways:

1. Document high-grade dysplasia in other biopsies taken during the same colonoscopy.
2. Document high-grade dysplasia in the same area at a repeat examination.
3. Have the diagnosis confirmed by a second pathologist.

17.11 THE SPORADIC ADENOMA AND DYSPLASIA-ASSOCIATED LESION OR MASS IN ULCERATIVE COLITIS

The term 'DALM' (dysplasia-associated lesion or mass) was coined by Blackstone *et al.* (1981) to indicate a macroscopically identifiable elevated dysplastic area, in contrast to flat dysplasia (Figs 17.23 and 17.24). Because, in 58 per cent of their 12 cases, carcinoma was found in the colectomy specimen deep to the biopsy site, even though only low-grade dysplasia was present, it became standard practice to regard DALM as an automatic indication for colectomy. This rationale has recently been overturned, as it has become apparent that the term DALM embraces a heterogeneous morphological spectrum and that certain patterns can be safely removed endoscopically. The undeserved infamy of DALM may have resulted from the unrepresentative and superficial nature of a biopsy taken from an elevated or mass lesion. It also highlights the issue discussed earlier (Section 17.10.2) that some low-grade lesions can progress to cancer without invariably evolving via a high-grade stage.

With improving endoscopic optics and technology that allows removal of lesions several centimetres in diameter it has become evident that if careful rules are followed, local excision of some patterns of DALM are warranted. In the original description (Blackstone *et al.*, 1981) as well as plaque-like lesions, polypoid lesions were described. It is this latter group that has become much better defined. Three patterns are recognized on the basis of endoscopy and histology. In the first the lesion is within the area of colitis, is polypoid, grossly discrete, sessile or pedunculated and virtually indistinguishable from a sporadic adenoma. It is not associated with any flat dysplasia in the surrounding mucosa or with an underlying carcinoma and is adjudged endoscopically resectable. It is best referred to as an adenoma-like DALM. The second pattern can be similar but crucially the adjacent mucosa contains one or more foci of flat dysplasia. Also included in this group are the lesions that do harbour an underlying carcinoma akin to the original description of Blackstone *et al.* (1981). This has been given the cumbersome title of a colitis-associated polypoid dysplastic lesion or non-adenoma-like DALM (Odze, 1999). The third pattern is the true sporadic adenoma. These, as one would expect, occur in patients with ulcerative colitis but unlike adenoma-like DALMs are outside the diseased segment of bowel, thus by definition excluded from patients who have a pancolitis.

There are now a considerable number of papers with follow-up data that have evaluated the validity of endoscopic resection of adenoma-like DALMs both in specific studies and as part of larger surveillance studies. All conclude that, provided that the criteria (see earlier) are followed, endoscopic resection with continued careful surveillance is safe and avoids immediate colectomy. This includes lesions with high-grade dysplasia (Engelsgjerd *et al.*, 1999; Rubin *et al.*, 1999). These adenoma-like DALMs can recur with almost the same frequency as sporadic adenomas.

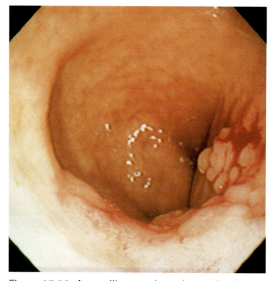

Figure 17.23 A surveillance endoscopic examination showing an elevated lesion. Low-grade dysplasia was identified. This localized abnormality contrasts with the more widespread dysplastic abnormality seen in Fig. 17.5.

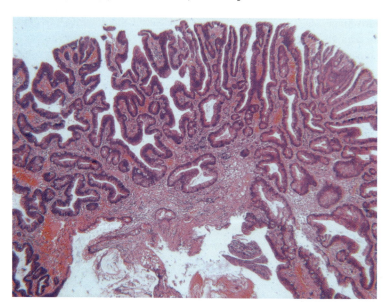

Figure 17.24 Low-grade dysplasia found in the dysplasia-associated lesion or mass (DALM) shown in Fig. 17.23.

Does the pathologist have a contribution to make in distinguishing these lesions either by morphological differences or by the use of special stains? Schneider and Stolte (1993) claimed to be able to show morphological differences between what they termed adenoma and non-adenomatous dysplastic lesions. Adenomas showed a more regular glandular pattern with less intervening stroma than the non-adenomatous lesions. They had a sharply delineated edge between the proliferating glands and the normal adjacent mucosa, the non-adenomatous lesions having ill-defined margins. Torres *et al.* (1998) reported a careful study of adenoma-like DALMs and non-adenoma-like DALMS, or what they termed ulcerative colitis-associated polypoid dysplastic lesions, in which both groups fulfilled the criteria listed above. They found the latter more often showed a tubulovillous or villous pattern, an admixture of normal and dysplastic epithelium on the surface and more mononuclear cell infiltration in the lamina propria. In routine biopsy reporting of small and often imperfect biopsy material, our own experience is that none of the characteristics in these two papers are reliable enough to form of a confident opinion upon which to base a management decision that could mean the difference between colectomy and endoscopic mucosal resection. It is our view, expressed in the paper by Rutter *et al.* (2004b), that the endoscopist is in the most favourable position for this decision. The paper states 'resectability is more important than whether a lesion is defined as a sporadic adenoma (adenoma-like DALM) or (non-adenoma-like) DALM'. However, essential to the decision-making is information on the presence or absence of flat dysplasia in the mucosa surrounding the lesion. Endoscopists must provide the appropriate biopsy material.

The pathologist may have a contribution to make with interpretation of special stains. Several studies purport to show that the molecular biology of adenoma-like DALMs has more in common with the sporadic adenoma than with the molecular biology of cancer in colitis (Odze, 1999; Fogt *et al.*, 2000; Odze *et al.*, 2000). This reinforces the validity of distinguishing the entities. The most useful stains in routine reporting are for p53, bcl-2 and β-catenin (Mueller *et al.*, 1999; Walsh *et al.*, 1999). β-Catenin staining becomes nuclear rather than cytoplasmic and membranous in association with adenomas that carry the adenomatous polyposis gene (*APC*). The combination of strong nuclear staining for p53, weak cytoplasmic staining for bcl-2 and negative nuclear staining for β-catenin favours a DALM (non-adenomatous polypoid dysplastic lesion), the reverse favours an adenoma-like DALM. The differences with all three immunostains are more easily appreciated when moderate or severe dysplasia is present.

Clearly, the presence of a DALM is not necessarily an indication for immediate colectomy and management depends on further subclassification (Medlicott *et al.*, 1997; Rubin *et al.*, 1999; Odze *et al.*, 2004). While the pathologist can attempt, from the characteristics mentioned above, to distinguish an adenoma-like DALM from a non-adenoma-like DALM or polypoid dysplastic lesion, in our view, even with the help of special stains this is unreliable (Figs 17.25 and 17.26; this series of illustrations

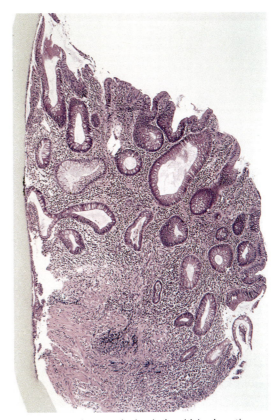

Figure 17.25 Low-grade dysplasia which, given the irregularity of the glands and the intervening stroma, might be classified as a non-adenomatous dysplastic lesion according to the criteria in the literature.

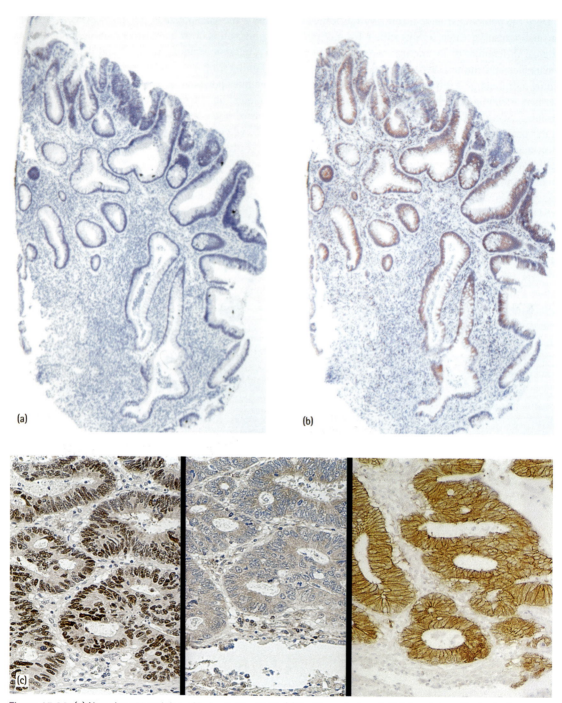

Figure 17.26 (a) Negative p53 staining of lesion in Fig. 17.25. (b) Positive cytoplasmic Bcl-2 staining of lesion in Fig. 17.25. This combination is the reverse of what might have been expected from the interpretation of appearances in Fig. 17.25. (c) This illustrates the expected immunostaining of a non-adenoma-like dysplasia-associated lesion or mass (DALM) being p53-positive (left frame), Bcl-2 negative (middle frame) and membranous β-catenin staining, not nuclear (right frame).

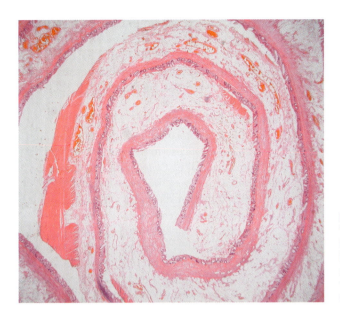

Figure 17.27 A mucosal strip wound into a 'Swiss roll' dissected from a colectomy specimen in a patient with long-standing ulcerative colitis in whom dysplasia was found on a biopsy but no macroscopic lesion was immediately identified on the colectomy. This technique allows examination of large areas of the mucosa.

demonstrate the difficulty in making a confident morphological distinction between adenomatous and non-adenomatous dysplastic lesions). The management decisions are more safely based on the endoscopic findings. If the lesion is endoscopically resectable and is unaccompanied by any surrounding flat dysplasia or overt malignancy in the lesion itself, local resection and careful continued surveillance is appropriate. Where this decision is difficult the histological findings and special stains may have some influence.

17.12 FAILURE TO FIND A LESION FOLLOWING RECOMMENDATION FOR SURGERY

Every pathologist will have to face the situation in which, after a biopsy diagnosis of dysplasia, no carcinoma is found in the resection. Between one-third and one-half of patients will not have a cancer despite the presence of dysplasia (Dobbins, 1977; Yardley *et al.*, 1979). However, this is the purpose of a surveillance programme and, in these patients, cancer has been prevented. Until better precancerous markers are developed this situation cannot be avoided since, unfortunately, it is not possible to judge which patient with dysplasia will progress to cancer and at what rate. A department, however, with large numbers of such instances needs to re-examine the criteria on which the diagnosis of dysplasia is based, or the care with which the surgical specimens are examined. Occasionally, the colectomy is not only negative for a cancer but also for more widespread dysplasia. While it is possible that a single, small area of dysplasia may have been removed by the biopsy, errors of judgement apart, the explanation is likely to be inadequate sampling. It is in such cases that the technique of dissecting and coiling long narrow strips of mucosa ('Swiss rolls') should be used (Fig. 17.27). This allows extensive microscopy of the excision specimen with limited impact on the laboratory workload. Although such situations require explanation to the clinician, the reassuring fact remains that long-standing colitics have an increased risk of cancer and proctocolectomy will always be the ultimate prophylactic procedure.

REFERENCES

Ahnen, D.J., Warren, G.H., Greene, L.J., Singleton, J.W., Brown, W.R. (1987) Search for a specific marker of mucosal dysplasia in chronic ulcerative colitis. *Gastroenterology*, 93, 1346–55.

Allen, D.C., Biggart, J.D., Pyper, P.C. (1985) Large bowel mucosal dysplasia and carcinoma in ulcerative colitis. *J. Clin. Pathol.*, 38, 30–43.

Allen, D.C., Hamilton, P.W., Watt, P.C., Biggart, J.D. (1987) Morphometrical analysis in ulcerative colitis with dysplasia and carcinoma. *Histopathology*, 11, 913–26.

Askling, J., Dickman, P.W., Karlen P., Brostrom, O., Lapidus, A., Lofberg R., Ekbom, A. (2001) Family history as a risk factor for colorectal cancer in inflammatory bowel disease. *Gastroenterology*, 120, 1356–62.

Axon, A.T.R. (1995) Colonic cancer surveillance in ulcerative colitis is not essential for every patient. *Eur. J. Cancer*, 31A, 1183–86.

Axon A.T. (1997) Screening and surveillance in ulcerative colitis. *Gastrointest. Endosc. Clin. N. Am.*, 7, 129–45.

Befrits, R., Hammarberg, C., Rubio, C., Jaramillo, E., Tribukait, B. (1994) DNA aneuploidy and histologic dysplasia in long-standing ulcerative colitis. A 10-year follow-up study. *Dis. Colon Rectum.*, 37, 313–19.

Befrits, R,. Ljung, T., Jaramillo, E., Rubio, C. (2002) Low-grade dysplasia in extensive, long-standing inflammatory bowel disease: a follow-up study. *Dis. Colon Rectum*, 45, 615–20.

Bernstein, C.H. (2004) Ulcerative colitis with low-grade dysplasia. *Gastroenterology*, 127, 950–6.

Bernstein, C.N., Shanahan, F., Weinstein, W.M. (1994) Are we telling patients the truth about surveillance colonoscopy in ulcerative colitis. *Lancet*, 343, 71–4.

Blackstone, M.O., Riddell, R.H., Rogers, B.H.G., Levin, B. (1981) Dysplasia-associated lesion or mass (DALM) detected by colonoscopy in long-standing ulcerative colitis: an indication for colectomy. *Gastroenterology*, 80, 366–74.

Boland, C.R., Lance, P., Levin, B., Riddell, R.H., Kim, Y.S. (1984) Abnormal goblet cell glycoconjugates in rectal biopsies associated with an increased risk of neoplasia in patients with ulcerative colitis: early results of a prospective study. *Gut*, 25, 1364–71.

Brentnall, T.A., Crispin, D.A.M., Rabinovitch, P.S., Haggitt, R.C., Rubin, C.E., Stevens, A.C., Burmer, G.C. (1994) Mutation in the p53 gene: an early marker of neoplastic progression in ulcerative colitis. *Gatroenterology*, 107, 369–78.

Brentnall, T.A., Crispin, D.A., Bronner, M.P. *et al.* (1996) Microsatellite instability in non-neoplastic mucosa from patients with chronic ulcerative colitis. *Cancer Res.*, 56, 1237–40.

Brostrom, O., Lofberg, R., Ost, A., Reichard, H. (1986) Cancer surveillance of patients with longstanding ulcerative colitis: a clinical, endoscopical, and histological study. *Gut*, 27, 1408–13.

Butt, J.H., Lennard-Jones, J.E., Ritchie, J.K. (1980) A practical approach to the risk of cancer in inflammatory bowel disease. *Med. Clin. N. Am.*, 64(6), 1203–20.

Butt, J.H., Konishi, F., Morson, B.C., Lennard-Jones, J.E., Ritchie, J.K. (1983a) Macroscopic lesions in dysplasia and carcinoma complicating ulcerative colitis. *Dig. Dis. Sci.*, 28, 18–26.

Butt, J.H., Price, A., Williams, C.B. (1983b) Dysplasia and cancer in ulcerative colitis. In: Allen, R.N., Keighley, M.R.B., Alexander-Williams, J., Hawkins C. (eds) *Inflammatory bowel disease.* Edinburgh: Churchill Livingstone, pp. 140–53.

Cawkwell, L., Sutherland F., Murgatroyd, H. *et al.* (2000) Defective hMSH2/hMLH1 protein expression is seen infrequently in ulcerative colitis-associated colorectal cancers. *Gut*, 46, 367–9.

Choi, P.M., Nugent, F.W., Schoetz, D.J. Jr., Silverman, M.L., Haggitt, R.C. (1993) Colonoscopic surveillance reduces mortality from colorectal cancer in ulcerative colitis. *Gastroenterology*, 105, 418–24.

Connell, W.R., Talbot, I.C., Harpaz, N., Britto, N., Wilkinson, K.H., Kamm, M.A., Lennard-Jones, J.E. (1994a) Clinicopathological characteristics of colorectal carcinoma complicating ulcerative colitis. *Gut*, 35, 1419–23.

Connell, W.R., Lennard-Jones, J.E., Williams, C.B., Talbot, I.C., Price, A.B., Wilkinson, K.H. (1994b) Factors affecting the outcome of endoscopic surveillance for cancer in ulcerative colitis. *Gastroenterology*, 1078, 934–44.

Cook, M.G., Goligher, J.C. (1975) Carcinoma and epithelial dysplasia complicating ulcerative colitis. *Gastroenterology*, 68, 1127–36.

Cooper, D.J., Weinstein, M.A., Korelitz, B.I. (1984) Complications of Crohn's disease predisposing to dysplasia and cancer of the intestinal tract: considerations of a surveillance program. *J. Clin. Gastroenterol.*, 6, 217–24.

Devroede, G., Taylor, W.F., Saver, W.G., Jackman, R.J., Stickler, G.B. (1971) Cancer risk and life expectancy of children with ulcerative colitis. *N. Engl. J. Med.*, 285, 17–21.

Dixon, M.F., Brown, L.J., Gilmour, H.M., Price, A.B., Smeeton, N.C., Talbot, I.C., Williams, G.T. (1988) Observer variation in the assessment of dysplasia in ulcerative colitis. *Histopathology*, 13, 385–97.

Dobbins, W.D. (1977) Editorial: Current status of pre-cancer lesions in ulcerative colitis. *Gastroenterology*, 73, 1431–3.

de Dombal, F.T., Softley, A. (1985) Cancer and inflammatory bowel disease – changing perspectives. In: de Dombal, F.T., Myran, J., Bouchier, I.A.D., Watkinson, G. (eds) *Inflammatory bowel disease, some international data and reflections*. Oxford: Oxford University Press, pp. 247–66.

de Dombal, F.T., Watts, J.McK., Watkinson, G., Goligher, J.C. (1966) Local complications of ulcerative colitis: stricture, pseudopolyposis and carcinoma of colon and rectum. *Br. Med. J.*, 1, 1442–7.

Dundas, S.A.C., Kay, R., Beck, S., Cotton, D.W.K., Coup, A.J., Slater, D.N., Underwood, J.C.E. (1987) Can histopathologists reliably assess dysplasia in chronic inflammatory bowel disease. *J. Clin. Pathol.*, 40, 1282–6.

Eaden, J., Abrams, K., Ekbom, A., Jackson, E., Mayberry, J. (2000) Colorectal cancer prevention in ulcerative colitis: a case-control study. *Aliment. Pharmacol. Ther.*, 14, 145–53.

Eaden, J.A., Abrams, K.R., Mayberry, J.F. (2001a) The risk of colorectal cancer in ulcerative colitis: a meta-analysis. *Gut*, 48, 526–35.

Eaden, J., Abrams, K., McKay, H., Denley, H., Mayberry, J. (2001b) Inter-observer variation between general and specialist gastrointestinal pathologists when grading dysplasia in ulcerative colitis. *J. Pathol.*, 194, 152–7.

Edwards, F.C., Truelove, S.C. (1964) The course and prognosis of ulcerative colitis, Part IV, Carcinoma of the colon. *Gut*, 5, 15–22.

Ehsanullah, M., Naunton-Morgan, M., Filipe, M.I., Gazzard, B. (1985) Sialomucins in the assessment of dysplasia and cancer risk patients with ulcerative colitis treated with colectomy and ileorectal anastomosis. *Histopathology*, 9, 223–36.

Ekbom, A., Helmick, C., Zack, M., Adami., H.O. (1990) Ulcerative colitis and colorectal cancer. A population-based study. *N. Engl. J. Med.*, 323, 1228–33.

Engelsgjerd, M., Farraye, F.A., Odze, R.D. (1999) Polypectomy may be adequate treatment for adenoma-like dysplastic lesions in chronic ulcerative colitis. *Gastroenterology*, 117, 1288–94.

Fogt, F., Vortmeyer, A.O., Goldman, H., Giordano, T.J., Merino, M.J., Zhuang, Z. (1998) Comparison of genetic alterations in colonic adenoma and ulcerative colitis-associated dysplasia and carcinoma. *Hum. Pathol.*, 29, 131–6.

Fogt, F., Urbanski, S.J., Sanders, M.E. *et al.* (2000) Distinction between dysplasia-associated lesions or mass (DALM) and adenomas in patients with ulcerative colitis. *Hum. Pathol.*, 31, 288–91.

Fozard, J.B.J., Quirke, P., Dixon, M.F., Giles, G.R., Bud, C.C. (1986) DNA aneuploidy in ulcerative colitis. *Gut*, 27, 1414–18.

Fozard, J.B.J., Dixon, M.F., Axon, A.T.R., Giles, G.R. (1987) Lectin and mucin histochemistry as an aid to cancer surveillance in ulcerative colitis. *Histopathology*, 11, 385–94.

Gilat, T., Fireman, Z., Grossman, A. *et al.* (1988) Colorectal cancer in patients with ulcerative colitis. A population study in central Israel. *Gastroenterology*, 94, 870–7.

Greenstein, A.J., Sacher, D.B., Smith, H. *et al.* (1979) Cancer in universal and left-sided ulcerative colitis: Factors determining risk. *Gastroenterology*, 77, 290–4.

Guindi, M., Riddell, R.H. (2001) The pathology of epithelial pre-malignancy of the gastrointestinal tract. *Best Pract. Res. Clin. Gastroenterol.*, 15, 191–210.

Gyde, S.N., Prior, P., Macartney, J.C., Thompson, H., Waterhouse, J.A.H., Allan, R.N. (1980) Malignancy in Crohn's disease. *Gut*, 21, 1024–9.

Harpaz, N., Peck, A.L., Yin, J. *et al.* (1994) p53 protein expression in ulcerative colitis-associated colorectal dysplasia and carcinoma. *Hum. Pathol.*, 25, 1069–74.

Hendriksen, C., Kreiner, S., Binder, V. (1985) Long term prognosis in ulcerative colitis – based on results from a regional patient group from the county of Copenhagen. *Gut*, 26, 158–63.

Heuschen, U.A., Hinz, U., Allemeyer, E.H. *et al.* (2001) Backwash ileitis is strongly associated with colorectal carcinoma in ulcerative colitis. *Gastroenterology*, 122, 245–6.

Isaacson, P. (1976) Tissue demonstration of carcinoembryonic antigen (CEA) in ulcerative colitis. *Gut*, 17, 561–7.

Isaacson, P. (1982) Immunoperoxidase study of the secretory immunoglobulin system in colonic neoplasia. *J. Clin. Pathol.*, 35, 14–25.

Itzkowitz, S.H. (2000) Microsatellite instability in colitis associated colorectal cancer. *Gut*, 46, 304–7.

Itzkowitz S.H., Harpaz, N. (2004) Diagnosis and management of dysplasia in patients with inflammatory bowel disease. *Gastroenterology*, 126, 1634–48.

Jani, N., Kornbluth,, A., Croog, V., Harpaz, N., Itzkowitz, S., Ullman, T. (2003) The fate of indefinite for dysplasia in ulcerative colitis. *Gastroenterology*, 124, A649.

Jass, J.R., England, J., Miller, K. (1986) Value of mucin histochemistry in follow up surveillance of patients with long-standing ulcerative colitis. *J. Clin. Pathol.*, 39, 393–8.

Jass, J.R., Whitehall, V.L., Young, J., Leggett, B.A. (2002) Emerging concepts in colorectal neoplasia. *Gastroenterology*, 123, 862–76.

Jayaram, H., Satsangi, J., Chapman, R.W. (2001) Increased colorectal neoplasia in chronic ulcerative colitis complicated by primary sclerosing cholangitis: fact or fiction. *Gut*, 48, 430–4.

Karlen. P., Kornfield, D., Brostrom, O., Lofberg, R., Persson, P.G., Ekbom, A. (1998a) Is colonoscopic surveillance reducing colorectal cancer mortality in ulcerative colitis? A population based case control study. *Gut*, 42, 711–14.

Karlen, P., Young, E., Brostrom, O. *et al.* (1998b) Sialyl-Tn antigen as a marker of colon cancer risk in ulcerative colitis: relation to dysplasia and DNA aneuploidy. *Gastroenterology*, 115, 1395–404.

Kewenter, J., Hulten, L., Ahren, C. (1982) The occurrence of severe epithelial dysplasia and its bearing on treatment of long-standing ulcerative colitis. *Ann. Surg.*, 195, 209–13.

Kiesslich, R., Fritsch, J., Holtmann, M. *et al.* (2003) Methylene blue-aided chromoendoscopy for the detection of intraepithelial neoplasia and colon cancer in ulcerative colitis. *Gastroenterology*, 124, 880–8.

Lennard-Jones, J.E. (1995) Is colonoscopic cancer surveillance in ulcerative colitis essential for every patient. *Eur. J. Cancer*, 31A, 1178–82.

Lennard-Jones, J.E., Morson, B.C., Ritchie, J.K., Shove, D.C., Williams, C.B. (1977) Cancer in colitis: assessment of the individual risk by clinical and histological criteria. *Gastroenterology*, 73, 1280–9.

Lim, C.H., Dixon, M.F., Vail, A., Forman, D., Lynch, D.A., Axon, A.T. (2003) Ten-year follow up of ulcerative colitis patients with and without low-grade dysplasia. *Gut*, 52, 1127–32.

Linberg, B., Persson, B., Veress, B., Ingelman-Sundberg, H., Granqvist S. (1996) Twenty years' colonoscopic surveillance of patients with ulcerative colitis. Detection of dysplastic and malignant transformation. *Scand. J. Gastroenterol.*, 31, 1195–204.

Lofberg, R., Brostrom, O., Karlen, P., Ost, A., Tribukait, B. (1992) DNA aneuploidy in ulcerative colitis: reproducibility, topographic distribution, and relation to dysplasia. *Gastroenterology*, 102, 1149–54.

Lynch, D.F., Lobo, A.J., Sobala, G.M., Dixon, M.F., Axon, A.T. (1993) Failure of colonoscopic surveillance in ulcerative colitis. *Gut*, 34, 1075–80.

Mathy, C., Schneider, K., Chen, Y.Y., Varma, M., Terdiman, J.P., Mahadevan, U. (2003) Gross versus microscopic pancolitis and the occurrence of neoplasia in ulcerative colitis. *Inflamm. Bowel Dis.*, 9, 351–5.

Mayer, R., Wong, W.D., Rothenberger, D.A., Goldberg, S.M., Madoff, R.D. (1999) Colorectal cancer in inflammatory bowel disease. *Dis. Colon Rectum*, 42, 343–7.

Medlicott, S.A., Jewell, J.D., Price, L., Fedorak, R.N., Sherbaniuk, R.W., Urbanski, S.J. (1997) Conservative management of small adenomata in ulcerative colitis. *Am. J. Gastroenterol.*, 92. 2094–8.

Melville, D.M., Jass, J.R., Shepherd, N.A. *et al.* (1988) Dysplasia and deoxyribonucleic acid aneuploidy in the assessment of precancerous changes in chronic ulcerative colitis. Observer variation and correlations. *Gastroenterology*, 95, 668–75.

Melville, D.M., Jass, J.R., Morson, B.C. *et al.* (1989) Observer study on the grading of dysplasia in ulcerative colitis: comparison with clinical outcome. *Hum. Pathol.*, 20, 1008–14.

Morson, B.C., Jass, J.R. (1985) *Precancerous lesions of the gastrointestinal tract. A histological classification*. London: Balliere Tindall.

Morson, B.C., Pang, L.S. (1967) Rectal biopsy as an aid to cancer control in ulcerative colitis. *Gut*, 8, 423–34.

Mueller, E., Vieth, M., Stolte, M., Mueller, J. (1999) The differentiation of true adenomas from colitis-associated dysplasia in ulcerative colitis: a comparative immunohistochemical study. *Hum. Pathol.*, 30, 898–905.

Muto, T., Bussey, H.J.R., Morson, B.C. (1975) The evolution of cancer of the colon and rectum. *Cancer*, 36, 2251–70.

Nixon, J.B., Burdick, S., Mirza, A.H. (1995) Premalignant changes in ulcerative colitis. *Semin. Surg. Oncol.*, 11, 386–93.

Nugent, F.W., Haggitt R.C., Gilpin, P.A. (1991) Cancer surveillance in ulcerative colitis. *Gastroenterology*, 100, 1241–8.

Odze, R.D. (1999) Adenomas and adenoma-like DALMs in chronic ulcerative colitis: a clinical, pathological, and molecular review. *Am. J. Gastroenterol.*, 94, 1746–50.

Odze, R.D., Brown, C.A., Hartmann, C.J., Noffsinger, A.E., Fogt, F. (2000) Genetic alterations in ulcerative colitis-associated adenoma-like DALMs and similar non-colitic sporadic adenomas. *Am. J. Surg. Pathol.*, 24, 1209–16.

Odze, R.D., Farraye, F.A., Hecht, J.L., Hornick, J.L. (2004) Long-term follow-up after polypectomy treatment for adenoma-like dysplasia lesions in ulcerative colitis. *Clin. Gastroenterol. Hepatol.*, 2, 534–41.

Ransohoff, D.F., Riddell, R.H., Levin, B. (1985) Ulcerative colitis and colonic cancer. Problems in assessing the diagnostic usefulness of mucosal dysplasia. *Dis. Col. Rectum*, 28, 383–8.

Riddell, R.H. (1976) The precarcinomatous phase of ulcerative colitis. In: Morson, B.C. (ed.) *Current topics in pathology: pathology of the gastrointestinal tract*. Berlin, Heidelberg and New York: Springer-Verlag, pp. 179–219.

Riddell, R.H. (1980) Dysplasia in inflammatory bowel disease. *Clin. Gastroenterol.*, 9, 439–58.

Riddell, R.H. (1983) Dysplasia in inflammatory bowel disease. In: Norris, H.T. (ed.) *Pathology of the colon, small intestine and anus*. New York, Edinburgh, London and Melbourne: Churchill Livingstone, pp. 77–107.

Riddell, R.H. (1984) Dysplasia and carcinoma in ulcerative colitis: a soluble problem? *Scand. J. Gastroenterol.*, 19 (Suppl. 104), 137–49.

Riddell, R.H. (1995) Grading of dysplasia. *Eur. J. Cancer*, 31A, 1169–70.

Riddell, R.H. (1996) Premalignant and early malignant lesions in the gastrointestinal tract: definitions, terminology, and problems. *Am. J Gastroenterol.*, 91, 864–72.

Riddell, R.H., Morson, B.C. (1979) Value of sigmoidoscopy and biopsy in detection of carcinoma and premalignant change in ulcerative colitis. *Gut*, 20, 575–80.

Riddell, R.H., Shove, D.C., Ritchie, J.K., Lennard-Jones, J.E., Morson, B.C. (1978) Pre-cancer in ulcerative colitis. In: Morson, B.C. (ed.) *Pathogenesis of colorectal cancer major problems in pathology.* London: W.B. Saunders, pp. 95–118.

Riddell, R.H., Goldman, H., Ransohoff, D.F. *et al.* (1983) Dysplasia in inflammatory bowel disease: standardized classification with provisional clinical applications. *Hum. Pathol.*, 14, 931–68.

Rosenstock, E., Farmer, R.G., Petras, R., Sivak, M.V. Jr, Rankin, G.B., Sullivan, B.H. (1985) Surveillance for colonic carcinoma in ulcerative colitis. *Gastroenterology*, 89, 1342–6.

Rubin, C.E., Haggitt, R.C., Burmer, G.C. *et al.* (1992) DNA aneuploidy in colonic biopsies predicts future development of dysplasia in ulcerative colitis. *Gastroenterology*, 103, 1611–20.

Rubin, P.H., Friedman, S., Harpaz, N. *et al.* (1999) Colonoscopic polypectomy in chronic colitis: conservative management after endoscopic resection of dysplastic polyps. *Gastroenterology*, 117, 1295–1300.

Rubio, C.A., Nylander, C., Johansson, C., Slezak, P. (1982) Non-dysplastic villous changes in endoscopic biopsies in ulcerative colitis with carcinoma. *Acta Pathol. Microbiol. Immunol. Scand. (A)*, 90, 277–82.

Rubio, C.A., Johannson, C., Slezak, P., Ohman, U., Hammarberg, C. (1984) Villous dysplasia: an ominous histologic sign in colitic patients. *Dis. Col. Rectum*, 27, 283–7.

Rubio, C.A., Befrits, R., Jaramillo, E., Nesi, G., Amorosi, A. (2000) Villous and serrated adenomatous growth bordering carcinomas in inflammatory bowel disease. *Anticancer Res.*, 20, 4761–4.

Rutter, M.D., Saunders, B., Schofield, G., Forbes, A., Price, A.B., Talbot, I.C. (2004a) Pancolonic indigo carmine dye spraying for the detection of dysplasia in ulcerative colitis. *Gut*, 53, 256–60.

Rutter, M.D., Saunders, B.P., Wilkinson, K,H., Kamm, M.A., Williams, C.B., Forbes, A. (2004b) Most dysplasia in ulcerative colitis is visible at colonoscopy. *Gastrointest. Endosc.*, 60, 334–9.

Rutter, M., Saunders, B., Wilkinson, K. *et al.* (2004c) Severity of inflammation is a risk factor for colorectal neoplasia in ulcerative colitis. *Gastroenterology*, 126, 451–9.

Rutter, M.D., Saunders, B.P., Wilkinson, K.H. *et al.* (2006) Thirty year analysis of a colonoscopic surveillance programme for neoplasia in ulcerative colitis. *Gastroenterology*, 304, 1030–8.

Sada, M., Igarashi, M., Yoshizawa, S. *et al.* (2004) Dye spraying and magnifying endoscopy for dysplasia and cancer surveillance in ulcerative colitids. *Dis. Colon Rectum*, 47, 1816–23.

Schlemper, R.J., Riddell, R.H., Kato, Y. *et al.* (2000) The Vienna classification of gastrointestinal epithelial neoplasia. *Gut*, 47, 251–5.

Schneider, A., Stolte, M. (1993) Differential diagnosis of adenomas and dysplastic lesions in patients with ulcerative colitis. *Z. Gastroenterol.*, 31, 653–6.

Sharan, R., Schoen, R.E (2002) Cancer in inflammatory bowel disease. An evidence-based analysis and guide for physicians and patients. *Gastroenterol. Clin. N. Am.*, 31, 237–54.

Suzuki, H., Harpaz, N., Tarmin, L. *et al.* (1994) Microsatellite instability in ulcerative colitis-associated colorectal dysplasias and cancers. *Cancer Res.*, 54, 4841–4.

Taylor, B.A., Pemberton, J.H., Carpenter, H.A. *et al.* (1992) Dysplasia in chronic ulcerative colitis: Implications for colonoscopic surveillance. *Dis. Colon Rectum*, 35, 950–6.

Torres, C., Antonioli, D., Odze, R.D. (1998) Polypoid dysplasia and adenomas in inflammatory bowel disease. A clinical, pathologic, and follow-up study of 89 polyps from 59 patients. *Am. J. Surg. Pathol.*, 22, 275–84.

Ullman, T.A., Loftus, E.V. Jr, Kakar, S., Burgart, L.J., Sandborn, W.J., Tremaine, W.J. (2002) The fate of low grade dysplasia in ulcerative colitis. *Am. J. Gastroenterol.*, 97, 922–7.

van Staa, T.P., Card, T., Logan, R.F., Leufkens, H.G. (2005) 5-Aminosalicylate use and colorectal cancer risk in inflammatory bowel disease: a large epidemiological study. *Gut*, 54, 1573–8.

Walsh, S.V., Loda, M., Torres, CV.M., Antonioli, D., Odze, R.D. (1999) p53 and β-catenin expression in chronic ulcerative colitis-associated polypoid dysplasia and sporadic adenomas. *Am. J. Surg. Pathol.*, 23, 963–9.

Wong, N.A.C.S., Harrison, D.J. (2001) Colorectal neoplasia in ulcerative colitis – recent advances. *Histopathology*, 39, 221–34.

Woolrich, A., DaSilva, M.D., Korelitz, B.I. (1992) Surveillance in the routine management of ulcerative colitis: The predictive value of low-grade dysplasia. *Gastroenterology*, 103, 431–8.

Yardley, J.H., Keren, D.F. (1974) Pre-cancer in lesions in ulcerative colitis: a retrospective study of rectal biopsy and colectomy specimens. *Cancer*, 34, 835–44.

Yardley, J.H., Bayless, T.M., Diamond, M.P. (1979) Cancer in ulcerative colitis. *Gastroenterology*, 76, 221–5.

CHAPTER 18

MALIGNANT TUMOURS

18.1 Carcinoma 330
    18.1.1 Definition, grading and features related to small biopsy interpretation 330
    18.1.2 Histological subtypes 332
    18.1.3 The concept of MSI-H colorectal adenocarcinoma and its relevance in biopsy diagnosis 334
    18.1.4 Local excision of adenocarcinoma 337
18.2 Endocrine cell (carcinoid) tumours 337
18.3 Lymphoma and leukaemia 340
    18.3.1 MALT lymphoma 340
18.3.2 Mantle cell lymphoma (malignant lymphomatous polyposis) 340
18.3.3 Other types of lymphoma 340
18.3.4 Diagnosis of colorectal lymphomas in small biopsies – diagnostic challenges 341
18.4 Mesenchymal tumours 342
    18.4.1 Gastrointestinal stromal tumours (GISTs) 342
    18.4.2 Kaposi sarcoma 344
18.5 Metastatic tumours 345
References 347

18.1 CARCINOMA

The majority of malignant tumours of the large intestine are adenocarcinomas. Other less common tumours with the same histogenesis, but with differing histological appearances, i.e. adenosquamous carcinoma and squamous carcinoma, resemble adenocarcinoma in clinical behaviour and may logically be grouped together with adenocarcinoma. With an adequate biopsy colonic carcinomas do not usually present any diagnostic difficulty, but problems may arise in deciding if small irregular fragments contain malignant glands or whether the tissue is part of an adenoma. Questions such as this and other diagnostic problems are discussed in Chapter 16.

18.1.1 Definition, grading and features related to small biopsy interpretation

Adenocarcinoma of large intestine has been defined by the World Health Organization as a malignant epithelial tumour of the colon and rectum which has already penetrated through muscularis mucosae into the submucosa (Hamilton *et al.*, 2000). Three grades are recognized (Morson and Sobin, 1976).

1. Well differentiated (low grade), when architecturally and cytologically the carcinoma resembles normal or only slightly dysplastic epithelium (Figs 16.6 and 18.1a).
2. Moderately differentiated (average grade), intermediate between (1) and (3) (Fig. 18.1b).
3. Poorly differentiated (high grade), when architecturally and cytologically the carcinoma only barely resembles the normal epithelium (Fig. 18.1c).

When such criteria are applied to histological sections of surgically excised tumours approximately 20 per cent are well differentiated, 60 per cent moderately differentiated and 20 per cent poorly differentiated (Day *et al.* 2003a). Following appropriate surgical treatment the crude 5-year survival rates are 80 per cent, 60 per cent and 25 per cent, respectively.

Alternatively, a two-tier system can be used, with low-grade and high-grade groups, the former

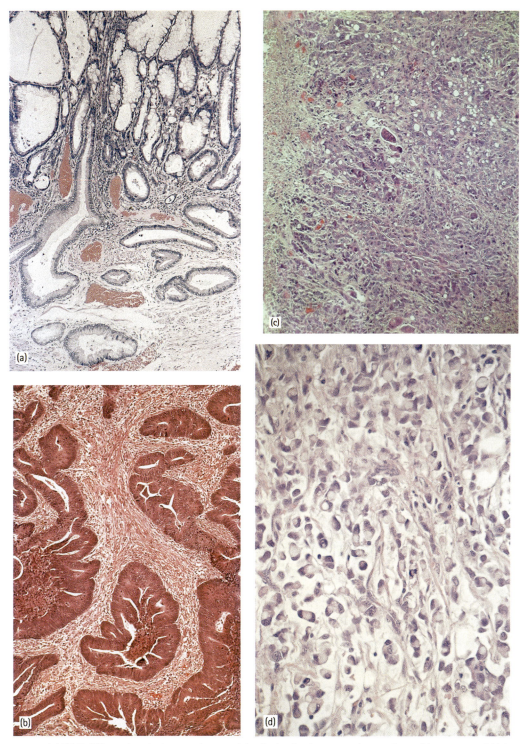

Figure 18.1 (a) Well-differentiated adenocarcinoma arising in dysplastic mucosa in a patient with many years' history of extensive ulcerative colitis. The adenocarcinoma, infiltrating through the muscularis mucosae into the submucosa is so well differentiated that the only feature distinguishing it from the non-invasive but dysplastic mucosa is the paradoxical greater cell pleomorphism of the latter. (b) Moderately differentiated invasive adenocarcinoma of rectum. Although the tumour is composed of well-defined glands, these deviate considerably from normal rectal mucosa. (c) Poorly differentiated adenocarcinoma of rectosigmoid colon. The tumour cells lie in sheets and are grouped in clumps and cords. Acini are not well defined. (d) Signet ring cell adenocarcinoma of colon.

including well differentiated and moderately differentiated.

Tumour heterogeneity may make grading difficult, particularly in small biopsies. In general, the grading should be based on the least differentiated component. However, it is important to remember that a small biopsy might not be representative of the whole tumour. In fact, it is not possible to make a reliable assessment of the histological grade of a whole tumour from a biopsy (Qualheim and Call, 1953). In a study of the subjective assessment of grade (i.e. degree of differentiation) of colorectal carcinoma by five experienced histopathologists, Thomas et al. (1983) found intra-observer agreement with that of the corresponding main tumours in only 56–69 per cent of all cases. Only 52 per cent of the important group of poorly differentiated tumours were correctly identified on biopsy, even by a particularly interested and experienced pathologist. Furthermore, there was considerable inter-observer variation in the grading of individual tumours, especially with biopsies of poorly differentiated carcinomas, on which there was agreement in only 33 per cent. Fortunately, it is seldom necessary to attempt to assess the grade of adenocarcinoma in a biopsy. The two exceptions to this are (a) when a surgeon contemplates treating a small, 'early' carcinoma by local excision, a procedure discussed in Section 16.4, and (b) in the context of the evaluation of high-frequency microsatellite instability (MSI-H) features (see below).

In addition to the neoplastic epithelial cells, whether they are arranged singly or in strips, biopsies usually include stromal tissue consisting of proliferating fibroblasts, type II collagen and blood capillaries. This pattern of granulation tissue-like or desmoplastic stroma is helpful in making a diagnosis of malignancy (Section 16.3). It should be noted that basement membrane is frequently present between the adenocarcinoma cells and the stromal connective tissue, although this is sometimes irregular and discontinuous (Forster et al., 1984).

18.1.2 Histological subtypes

In addition to conventional colorectal adenocarcinoma, other histological subtypes can be identified. Some of these subtypes are of importance,

as they may be related to the MSI-H phenotype. These are:

18.1.2a Mucinous adenocarcinoma

In about 15 per cent of large bowel adenocarcinomas, the tumour cells are dispersed among or stretched around pools of mucin, giving a highly characteristic mucinous or 'colloid' appearance to the tumour. At least 50 per cent of a tumour should comprise mucin to qualify for this label (Hamilton et al., 2000); this cannot be determined in small biopsy fragments. This pattern is present in many MSI-H adenocarcinomas (Alexander et al., 2001).

18.1.2b Signet ring carcinoma

This subtype, distinct from colloid carcinoma (Figs 18.1d and 17.4), is an extensively spreading tumour with a poor prognosis and is conventionally grouped with the poorly differentiated (high grade) category (Almagro, 1983). These tumours are often found to be of the diffusely infiltrating (linitis plastica) type, although signet ring cells are, in some respects, well differentiated and some workers have failed to confirm their invariably aggressive nature (Ciacchero et al., 1985; Sasaki et al., 1987). Some MSI-H tumours are of this type.

18.1.2c Medullary (large cell undifferentiated) carcinoma

Invariably associated with MSI-H status (Peltomaki et al., 2000), this is a rare variant of colorectal adenocarcinoma (Jessurun et al., 1999), characterized by sheets of loosely arranged large uniform cells with vesicular nuclei, prominent nucleoli and abundant, eosinophilic cytoplasm (Fig. 18.2). Acini are inconspicuous or absent. There is no keratin or melanin production. These tumours differ from adenocarcinomas in their cytokeratin profile, being both CK7 and CK20 negative (Table 18.1). Tumour cell apoptosis is prominent and the tumour parenchyma contains numerous single lymphocytes. A peritumoral lymphocytic infiltrate is sometimes conspicuous to the point of being 'Crohn's-like', but this is variable. These tumours are more frequent in the right colon than the left and are typically exophytic, large and bulky.

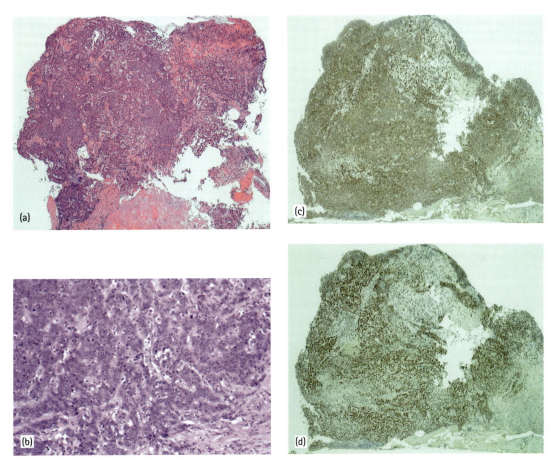

Figure 18.2 Medullary carcinoma. This biopsy (a–d) is of a large tumour of the ascending colon in a young man with a strong family history of colorectal cancer, probably hereditary non-polyposis colon cancer (HNPCC). This is a large-cell undifferentiated carcinoma with numerous apoptotic bodies and lymphocytes within the tumour [seen best at high power (b)]. (c) Negative staining by immunocytochemistry for the mismatch repair protein HML1, although there is rather a smudgy weak staining of the tumour cell cytoplasm, which is not specific. (d) Retention of nuclear staining for HMS2.

Table 18.1 Colorectal and anal tumours: immunoreactivity and mucin profile

	Cam 5.2	CK 7/20	Mucin	Vimentin	Chromogranin/ synaptophysin	S100/ HMB45	LCA	PSA	GCDFP
Adenocarcinoma	+	−/+	+	−	−	−	−	−	−
SCC	+	−/−	−	−	−	−	−	−	−
Undiff. carcinoma	+	−/−	−	−	−	−	−	−	−
Neuro-endocrine	±	−/−	−	−	+	−	−	−	−
Malig. melanoma	−	−/−	−	+	−	+	−	−	−
Paget's	+	+/−	+	+	−	−	−	−	+
Pagetoid spread	+	±/+	+	−	−	−	−	−	−
Prostate	+	−/−	−	−	−	−	−	+	−
Lymphoma	−	−/−	−	+	−	−	+	−	−

18.1.2d Small cell undifferentiated carcinoma

These are rare tumours, most having been reported in the rectum (Mills *et al.*, 1983). Biopsy fragments are usually bulky, irregular, white and friable, reflecting the gross appearances of the tumour. Schwartz and Orenstein (1985), however, do describe small examples, one of which was arising in a pedunculated polyp. Histologically, the sheets of tumour cells are tightly packed, with a trabecular arrangement (Fig. 18.3). There is extensive confluent necrosis and a tendency to perivascular pseudorosetting. The tumour cells are small, oval or fusiform, with very little cytoplasm and elongated hyperchromatic nuclei with small nucleoli. These tumours are analogous to oat cell carcinomas of lung and behave in a similar, highly malignant way. However, they appear to arise, like adenocarcinomas, in pre-existing adenomas. They also have a similar age incidence and topographical distribution to colorectal adenocarcinomas (Mills *et al.*, 1983). The tendency to trabecular and pseudorosetting patterns, as well as expression of neuroendocrine markers, are in keeping with a member of the 'oat cell' carcinoma family. Owing to its poor differentiation, a differential diagnosis with other entities (see Table 18.1) should be considered. Immunohistochemistry, showing expression of CD56 (Fig. 18.3c) or electron microscopy, demonstrating desmosomes and rather scanty, small, round neurosecretory granules are typical (Fig. 18.3d), and help in this regard. Immunocytochemistry for CK7 and CK20 is usually negative (Table 18.1).

18.1.2e Adenosquamous carcinoma

Such malignancies comprise distinct glandular components and malignant keratin-producing squamous areas (Fig. 18.4). Because a biopsy may not be representative, the distinction from focal squamous metaplasia in an otherwise typical adenocarcinoma ('adenoacanthoma') may be difficult and the diagnosis should be made with caution until the whole tumour is available. The degree of differentiation can be assessed from the glandular component, but these tumours have been found to behave in a rather more aggressive way than pure adenocarcinomas (Rubio *et al.*, 1981).

18.1.2f Squamous carcinoma

A purely squamous carcinoma is a rarity, but clinically and macroscopically it can present in an identical manner to adenocarcinoma. A biopsy of such a tumour may therefore take the pathologist by surprise as he looks down the microscope at tissue from a colorectal carcinoma which consists of sheets of squamous epithelial cells, with intercellular 'prickles' and keratin production (Fig. 18.5). It is worth seeking reassurance that the patient has no other possible primary tumour, for example in the lung, and a firm diagnosis can be reserved until surgical resection allows examination of the whole tumour. Nevertheless, metastatic squamous carcinoma in the large intestine is an even rarer event than a primary tumour of this type (Burgess *et al.*, 1979).

These tumours probably arise, like adenocarcinomas, from pre-existing adenomas (Williams *et al.*, 1979). They behave in a very similar way to adenocarcinomas, depending on the degree of differentiation. This should be assessed from the extent of keratinization. Clearly, squamous carcinoma in a low rectal biopsy is likely to have arisen in the anal canal (Section 19.3.2).

18.1.2g Other types

These include the stem cell carcinoma (Palvio *et al.*, 1985), crypt cell carcinoma or pleomorphic carcinoma. Diagnosis of these entities is almost exclusively from the full surgical resection specimen and is outside the scope of this book.

18.1.3 The concept of MSI-H colorectal adenocarcinoma and its relevance in biopsy diagnosis

Approximately 15 per cent of all colorectal cancers show marked accumulation of mutations throughout the genome, which are better detected in the

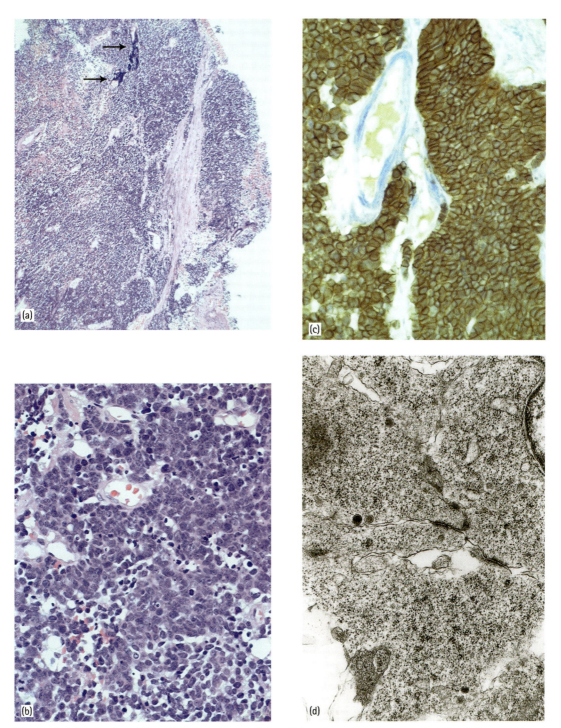

Figure 18.3 Small cell undifferentiated carcinoma – biopsy taken at proctoscopy from a large low-lying rectal tumour. (a) Low-power view showing a uniform pattern of sheets of small cells. There is a remnant of mucosa but the surface is mostly ulcerated. Perivascular DNA encrustation (arrowed) is present. (b) At higher magnification one can see ribbons of fusiform cells with large hyperchromatic nuclei. There is extensive necrosis and a tendency to form perivascular pseudo-rosettes. (c) By immunocytochemistry the tumour cells are shown to express the neuroendocrine marker CD56. (d) Electron microscopy shows desmosomes and small numbers of characteristic dense core granules.

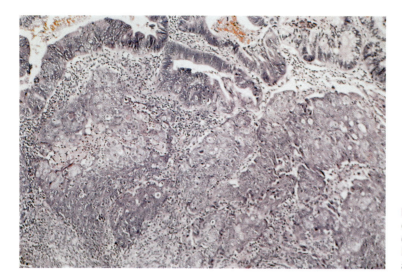

Figure 18.4 Adenosquamous carcinoma. Merging with well-developed glandular structures, lined by columnar epithelial cells, are solid sheets of squamous cells.

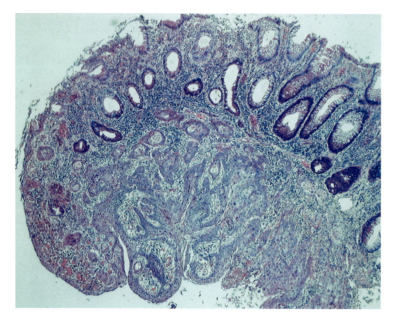

Figure 18.5 Squamous carcinoma. This biopsy of a well-differentiated keratinizing squamous carcinoma was taken via a sigmoidoscope from a large recto-sigmoid tumour.

so-called microsatellite regions. These are the high-frequency microsatellite instability (MSI-H) cancers (de la Chapelle, 2003). They are important because: (1) some are associated with the hereditary non-polyposis colorectal cancer syndrome; (2) in general, they have a more favourable prognosis (Lothe *et al.*, 1983); and (3) there is specific evidence that sporadic MSI-H cancers may show a favourable prognosis when treated with a conventional chemotherapy regime (Hemminki *et al.*,

2000; Ribic *et al.*, 2003). The MSI-H colorectal adenocarcinomas have a tendency to show specific histological features (Jass, 1998). Although the histopathologist cannot predict the H-MSI status of a neoplasm (Alexander *et al.*, 2001; Salto-Tellez *et al.*, 2004), awareness of these features should alert the pathologist to such a possibility. This would have positive implications for the management of the patient, as the appropriate molecular testing could be arranged before surgery and the patient then made aware of the possibility of a cancer subtype with hereditary and/or prognostic implications. Features that have been associated with MSI-H cases are (Shashidharan *et al.*, 1999; Alexander *et al.*, 2001): signet ring cells, mucinous histology, cribriform architecture, poor differentiation, medullary-type pattern, high apoptotic index, sponge-like mucinous growth, pushing invasive margin, Crohn's-like lymphoid response and tumour-infiltrating T lymphocytes (TILs). Particularly suggestive of MSI-H status are (1) mucinous adenocarcinomas of the caecum, ascending or transverse colon and (2) poorly differentiated adenocarcinomas of the caecum, ascending or transverse colon (Hamilton *et al.*, 2000).

When there is a high index of suspicion that a tumour may be MSI-H, immunocytochemistry for the mismatch repair proteins MLH1, MSH2 and MSH6 will confirm that the tumour is of so-called 'mutator type', if there is a loss of expression of one or other of these proteins (Cawkwell *et al.*, 1999).

18.1.4 Local excision of adenocarcinoma

Adenocarcinoma which has infiltrated the submucosa only ('early' rectal cancer; Morson *et al.*, 1977) and is well or moderately differentiated rarely spreads to lymph nodes. Hermanek and Gall (1985) found lymph node metastases in only 3 per cent of 131 surgically excised tumours of this type and Wilcox *et al.* (1986) found that metastases occurred following polypectomy for malignant polyps in 10.4 per cent of cases. It is therefore rational to consider limited local excision (i.e. from the mucosal aspect by a transanal approach) as a definitive method of treatment for some early rectal cancers. An important indicator of metastatic potential is the depth of submucosal invasion. Sakuragi *et al.* (2003) showed that submucosal invasion equal to or greater than 2000 μm was an accurate predictive factor for lymph node metastasis. They also showed that the finding of lymphovascular invasion correlated with increased risk of lymph node metastasis. However, it must be stressed that identification of lymphatic invasion, as well as accurate measurement of depth of invasion in the context of lesions that are commonly 'lifted-up' from the submucosal

layer, may be difficult and, thus, an accurate assessment of risk may not always be possible. The decision process and indications for radical surgery are considered in more detail in Chapter 16.

When the endoscopist embarks on polypectomy as possible definitive treatment of a polyp that he or she suspects of harbouring adenocarcinoma, it is important that both endoscopist and pathologist are aware that careful handling of the fresh tissue is essential, to avoid any distortion which may obscure the plane of excision (Morson, 1985). If sessile, the specimen is best pinned out on a flat piece of cork before fixation, so that well-orientated blocks can be cut from the entire tissue in the manner illustrated for sessile polyps in Fig. 15.1.

18.2 ENDOCRINE CELL (CARCINOID) TUMOURS

Carcinoid tumours in the large intestine arise predominantly in the rectum, followed by the caecum/right colon. The vast majority of the caecal/right-sided carcinoids are large masses (average diameter 5 cm) composed of enterochromaffin cells (EC-carcinoids) and have a so-called type A, or 'insular' histological pattern, which consists of a packetted or acinar arrangement of larger cells with clear or eosinophilic cytoplasm (Fig. 18.6). The tumour cells are usually argentaffin when stained by the Masson–Fontana method. These tumours behave as high-grade malignancies. In one series, Morgan *et al.* (1974) found that tumours measuring over 2 cm were invariably accompanied by lymph node metastases. Forty per cent of patients in a large series (Modlin and Sandor, 1997) had distant metastases at diagnosis and the 5-year survival rate of these was just 23 per cent.

Rectal carcinoids are usually smaller, predominantly less than 2 cm (Caldarota *et al.*, 1964) and are incidental findings, appearing as small sessile polyps. Rectal carcinoid may exhibit two histological types. The predominant type shows a trabecular or 'ribboned' arrangement, with uniform small oval or columnar cells (Fig. 18.7a), classified as type B (Soga and Tazawa, 1971; Dawson, 1976) or L-cell

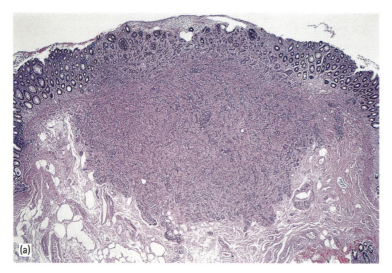

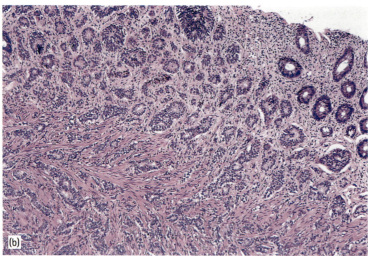

Figure 18.6 (a,b) Endocrine cell tumour (carcinoid tumour), insular pattern. This type of endocrine cell tumour, also known as 'Type A' or EC-cell carcinoid, tends to form rounded solid cell nests and acini.

tumours. This can be admixed with the type C, composed of tubuloacini or broad trabeculae with distinctive rosettes. Carcinoid tumours of the rectum are usually argentaffin negative (O'Briain *et al.*, 1982), but contain argyrophil cells which can be stained by the Grimelius method (in all cases, according to Wilander *et al.*, 1983). Immunocytochemistry is often negative for chromogranin A but positive for chromogranin B and synaptophysin (Riddell *et al.*, 2003). Neurosecretory granules seen on electron microscopy (Fig. 18.7d) are variable in morphology but may show glucagon ('H') features, or show the characteristic PP/PYY immunoreactivity

of the 'L' cell type (Solcia *et al.*, 1979). A wide range of other peptide hormones may be expressed (Riddell *et al.*, 2003). In contrast to right-sided carcinoids, the overall malignancy rate of rectal carcinoids is, at most, 14 per cent (Modlin and Sandor, 1997).

The diagnosis of malignancy in individual large intestinal endocrine cell tumours is problematic, especially from biopsy tissue, but a diameter of over 1 cm and numerous mitoses are indicators of aggressive potential. Another reliable indicator of malignancy would seem to be invasion of the muscularis propria (Burke *et al.*, 1987).

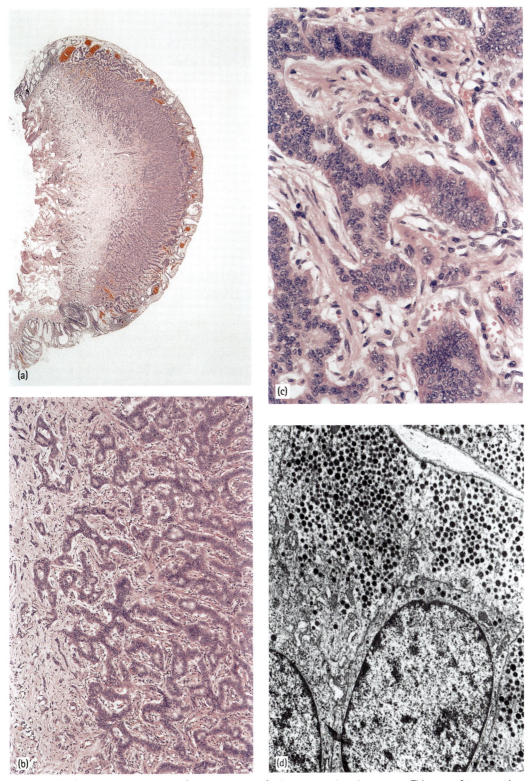

Figure 18.7 (a–c) Endocrine cell tumour (carcinoid tumour) of rectum, trabecular pattern. This type of tumour, also known as 'Type B' or L-cell carcinoid, has a characteristic ribboned pattern. These tumours often produce glucagon-like peptide or PP. (d) Electron micrograph: neurosecretory granules.

18.3 LYMPHOMA AND LEUKAEMIA

Most of the lymphomas in the colon and rectum are secondary; primary colorectal lymphomas account for only 0.2 per cent of the large intestinal malignancies (Shepherd *et al.*, 1988), although this overall frequency may have risen in the context of immunodeficiency patients (Müller-Hermelink *et al.*, 2000). Primary lymphoma of the colorectum is defined as a lymphoma arising in that region, with the bulk of the disease present in that organ, and the clinical presentation colorectal (Isaacson, 1999). An association with inflammatory bowel disease, particularly ulcerative colitis, is known (Shepherd *et al.*, 1989). Primary colorectal lymphomas are almost exclusively of B-cell nature, and two main types are recognized, namely mucosa-associated lymphoid tissue (MALT) lymphoma and mantle cell lymphoma. Burkitt-like lymphoma may occur in the context of acquired immune-deficiency syndrome (AIDS) patients, while the other types of lymphomas are very unusual. Primary T-cell lymphoma of the colon and rectum is extremely rare, and mostly confined to the Asian literature (Nagai *et al.*, 1991; Son *et al.*, 1997). Leukaemic involvement of the large intestine rarely presents in life. Gross lesions, often fleshy and bulky, were present in the colon in approximately 6 per cent of patients dying with leukaemia who were studied by Cornes and Jones (1962). However, microscopic evidence of infiltration of the gastrointestinal tract was demonstrated in over 50 per cent of cases, irrespective of the type of leukaemia (Prolla and Kirsner, 1964). When biopsy is performed, histology shows diffuse infiltration of the lamina propria, particularly in the basal half of the mucosa.

18.3.1 MALT lymphoma

The MALT lymphoma (extranodal marginal zone B-cell lymphoma) cells arise in the marginal zone of the pre-existing follicles, colonizing subsequently the whole follicle and eventually infiltrating and destroying the mucosal epithelium (so-called lymphoepithelial lesions) (Fig. 18.8). The cytology in the low-grade MALT lymphomas is very similar to centrocytes. However, if more than 20 per cent of the cells are blast cells, a high-grade MALT lymphoma diagnosis is in order (Day *et al.*, 2003b). The colorectal MALT lymphomas share the same immunohistochemical profile as the gastric ones, expressing CD20 and CD79a, but not CD10, CD5 or CD23. However, the characteristic t(11;18), described in MALT lymphomas in the stomach is not identifiable in the colorectal counterpart.

18.3.2 Mantle cell lymphoma (malignant lymphomatous polyposis)

This condition represents about 25 per cent of all colorectal lymphomas (Isaacson *et al.*, 1984; Lavergne *et al.*, 1994). Although clinically the symptomatology is related to the large intestinal disease, the lymphoma very commonly extends into the ileum. Macroscopically, it is characterized by numerous, well-circumscribed polypoid masses (Isaacson *et al.*, 1984), adopting an appearance not dissimilar to familial adenomatous polyposis (FAP) (Section 15.5). The neoplastic cells are small to medium, irregular lymphocytes. The disease appears to have a 'nodular' arrangement, with aggregates of cells in the mucosa and submucosa. However, within those 'nodules' (which are responsible for the polypoidal macroscopic impression), the infiltrate is usually diffuse (Fig. 18.9). Occasionally, reactive germinal centres are identified, with the neoplastic cells confined to the expanded mantle zones (Hamilton *et al.*, 2000). The malignant cells express CD20, CD5 and CD43. Immunohistochemical Bcl-1 expression is almost always identifiable; this is due to the characteristic t(11;14) and its effect in the *bcl-1* gene.

18.3.3 Other types of lymphoma

Although any B-cell lymphoma can arise in the colorectum, most of the non-MALT, non-mantle cell lymphomas are of Burkitt type (predominantly in the Middle East), Burkitt's-like and diffuse large B-cell lymphomas, usually in the context

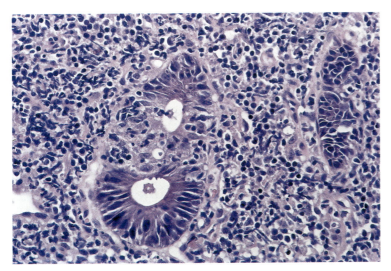

Figure 18.8 Mucosa-associated lymphoid tissue (MALT) lymphoma, low grade, of rectum. There is diffuse infiltration of the lamina propria by small lymphocytes, resembling centrocytes, with infiltration of the crypt epithelium ('lymphoepithelial lesions'). The latter feature is not seen in high-grade lymphomas, unfortunately the majority in the colon and rectum.

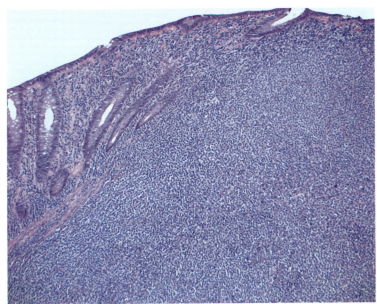

Figure 18.9 Malignant lymphomatous polyposis (mantle cell lymphoma). This condition typically presents to the endoscopist as a polyposis. The polyps, which are not confined to the large bowel, are composed of sheets of uniform small lymphoid cells (centrocytes). The infiltrating cells extend into the overlying mucosa, which is distorted but generally intact. Lymphoid follicles can be present but are indistinct.

of immunocompromised patients. Indeed, in AIDS patients the majority are Epstein–Barr virus (EBV)-associated high-grade B-cell lymphomas (Levine, 1992). Once it is established as a monoclonal population, AIDS-related intestinal lymphoma has the same poor prognosis as the extraintestinal ones (Cappell and Botros, 1994).

Primary follicular lymphoma is considered a rarity in the large bowel. However, Kodama *et al.* (2005) reported six cases of gastrointestinal polyposis with unequivocal colonic involvement, showing morphological, immunohistochemical and molecular features of follicular lymphoma. Only two of their cases were exclusively colorectal in origin.

18.3.4 Diagnosis of colorectal lymphomas in small biopsies – diagnostic challenges

A distinction between a MALT lymphoma and a mantle cell lymphoma may be difficult, particularly

Table 18.2 Differential diagnosis of the commoner B− cell lymphomas in the colon and rectum

	CD20	CD5	CD10	Rearrangements
MALT*	+	−	−	t(11;18) usually not detectable
Mantle (LP)	+	+	−	Commonly shows t(11;14)
Burkitt	+	−	+	Commonly shows t(8;14)
Follicular	+	−	+	Commonly shows t(14;18)

*MALT, mucosa-associated lymphoid tissue.

for those pathologists with no extensive exposure to lymphoproliferative disorders. A simplified diagnostic table (Table 18.2) is offered with the main immunohistochemical and molecular characteristics.

Another problem arises with large cell high-grade B-cell lymphomas, which occur as frequently in the colorectum as MALT lymphoma (Shepherd *et al.*, 1988). The clinical picture in extensive disease may not be definitive, and the pathologist faced with a small colonoscopic biopsy may not be able to indicate if the lymphoma is primarily colorectal with subsequent extension, or results from colonic involvement by a high-grade lymphoma originating elsewhere. However, it appears that the prognosis of the aggressive gastrointestinal lymphomas, stage for stage, is not dissimilar to those without gastrointestinal involvement (Salles *et al.*, 1991), and clinical staging after histological diagnosis is the most significant prognostic factor. In general, the pathologist should be prepared to ask for a repeat biopsy and, ultimately, to seek advice from a lymphoreticular specialist, if necessary.

18.4 MESENCHYMAL TUMOURS

Benign mesenchymal tumours can present as polyps and are dealt with more fully in Chapter 15. Primary malignant mesenchymal tumours of the colorectum are essentially of three types: gastrointestinal stromal tumour (GIST), leiomyosarcoma and Kaposi sarcoma. Other primary mesenchymal sarcomas are rarities.

18.4.1 Gastrointestinal stromal tumours (GISTs)

Colorectal GISTs are presumed to originate in the specialized Cajal cell of the gut wall (Sanders, 1996). They are composed almost entirely of spindle cells (Fig. 18.10a,b). Epithelioid cells are rare (Miettinen *et al.*, 2000). They are characterized immunohistochemically by CD117 (Fig. 18.10c), CD34 and vimentin positivity, and frequent negativity for muscle markers (Miettinen *et al.*, 1999). It is difficult to ascertain, now that we are in the 'GIST era', what percentage of malignant mesenchymal tumours are true leiomyosarcomas. In our review of 54 gastrointestinal mesenchymal tumours, 40 could be reclassified as GIST, 11 as leiomyomas, one as a neurofibroma and only one case could be labelled as a bona fide leiomyosarcoma (M. Salto-Tellez, personal observation). Hence, it is conceivable that the majority of malignant mesenchymal neoplasms of the colon and rectum belong to the GIST category. Genetically, there are specific mutations of different exons in the *c-kit* gene at chromosome 4q12 (Lasota *et al.*, 1999). GISTs can be treated with imatinib mesylate (Gleevec), a tyrosine kinase inhibitor and an effective anti-tumour agent (Heinrich *et al.*, 2003). Although the prognosis is notoriously unpredictable, as with their upper gastrointestinal tract counterparts, colorectal GISTs tend to have a worse prognosis than those arising in the stomach (Ueyama *et al.*, 1992), a fact that should be taken into account for therapeutic intervention after endoscopic biopsy. Finally, it has been suggested that small biopsies of GISTs may be misleading, because of their morphological heterogeneity and the possibility of atypical antibody expression

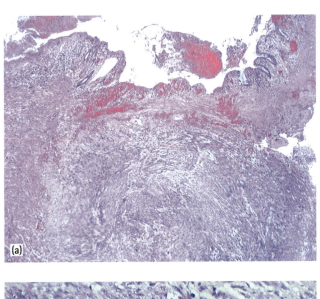

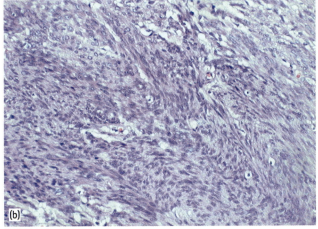

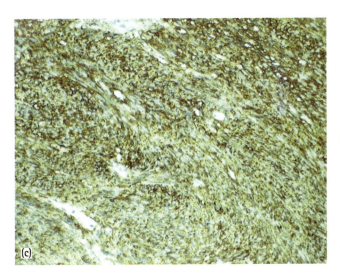

Figure 18.10 Biopsy of gastrointestinal stromal tumour (GIST) of rectum. (a) At low power it is an ulcerated spindle cell tumour. (b) At higher magnification, the spindle cells are arranged in palisades. Several mitoses per high-power field were present, indicating that this particular tumour was in the high-grade end of the spectrum. (c) Immunocytochemistry for CD117 (c-kit) shows tumour cell membrane staining.

(Nga *et al.*, 2002). The pathologist should be aware of this pitfall.

18.4.2 Kaposi sarcoma

Kaposi sarcoma of the colon and rectum is a common occurrence in AIDS patients: in these circumstances, almost 50 per cent of cases of Kaposi sarcoma involve the colon or rectum (Parente *et al.*, 1991). Occasional cases of Kaposi sarcoma related to inflammatory bowel disease or therapeutic immunosuppression are also reported (Miettinen *et al.*, 2000). The histological appearance is akin to that of Kaposi sarcomas elsewhere, with proliferation of irregular, often jagged vascular channels lined by rather inconspicuous endothelial cells and variable quantities of lymphocytes, plasma cells,

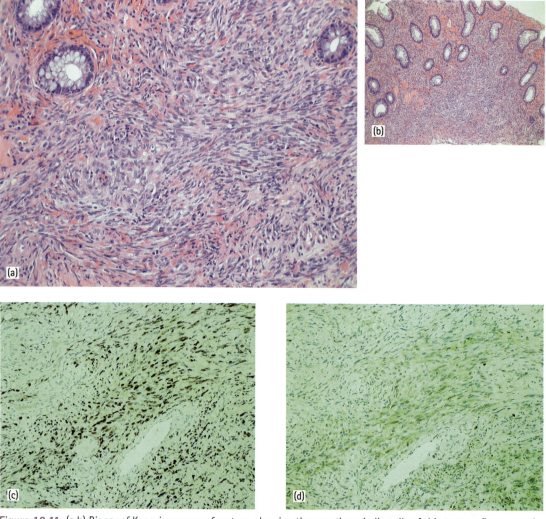

Figure 18.11 (a,b) Biopsy of Kaposi sarcoma of rectum, showing the way the spindle cells of this tumour flow around existing structures such as the mucosal crypts. Both between the spindle cells and sometimes within obvious small vascular channels, there are numerous red blood cells. (c) Immunocytochemistry for HSV-8 shows strong cytoplasmic staining. (d) Immunocytochemistry for CD117 shows some positive staining but this is located in the cell cytoplasm rather than the cell membrane; cf. the staining of a gastrointestinal stromal tumour (GIST) in Fig. 18.11.

haemosiderin deposition and eosinophilic, hyaline globules (Fig 18.11).

18.5 METASTATIC TUMOURS

Unusual or unexpected features in biopsy tissue from a colorectal tumour, ulcer or stricture suggest the possibility of metastatic tumour from another primary site. Apart from unusual histological features in the tumour tissue itself, which may be confined to the submucosa, the overlying mucosa is often intact (Fig. 18.15). Although not a diagnostic feature in biopsy tissue, lack of ulceration adds to the suspicion that a tumour may be metastatic.

The metastatic tumours most frequently encountered in biopsy material are from primary adenocarcinomas of ovary (Fig. 18.12), prostate (Fig. 18.13), stomach or elsewhere in the large bowel.

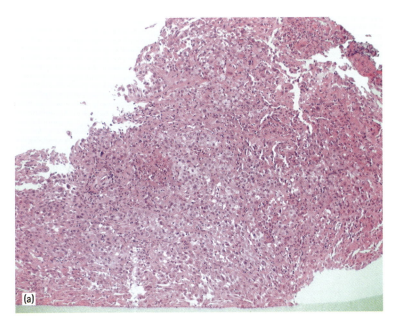

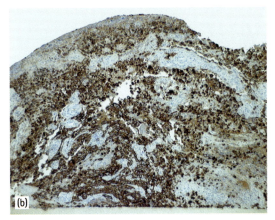

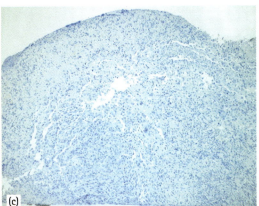

Figure 18.12 Metastatic adenocarcinoma from ovary. (a) No residual mucosa is visible in this biopsy of sigmoid colon, the normal structures being replaced by a diffuse infiltrate of large vacuolated epithelial cells. The cells of this ovarian metastasis characteristically express CK7 (b) but not CK20 (c).

Secondaries from lung, endometrium, kidney, bladder (Fig. 18.14), breast (Fig. 18.15) and cervix (Fig. 18.16) should also be considered, as well as metastatic malignant melanoma. Table 18.1 on page 333 summarizes the results to be expected, if mucin stains and a panel of antibodies are used to aid in the identification of a morphologically unusual tumour of the colon, rectum or anus.

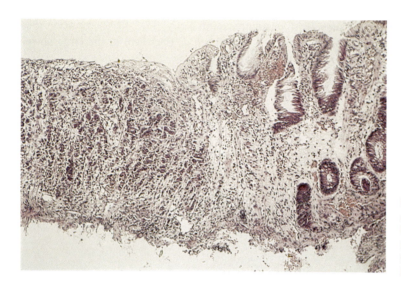

Figure 18.13 Metastatic adenocarcinoma from prostate in biopsy of rectal ulcer. The diffuse pattern, with small, ill-formed glands and flat ulceration, is unlike primary colorectal cancer.

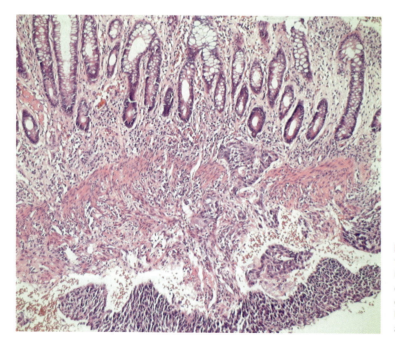

Figure 18.14 Metastatic transitional cell carcinoma of bladder in rectal biopsy. Note the oedematous mucosa, with crypt distortion, suggesting that this biopsy may be from the edge of an ulcer.

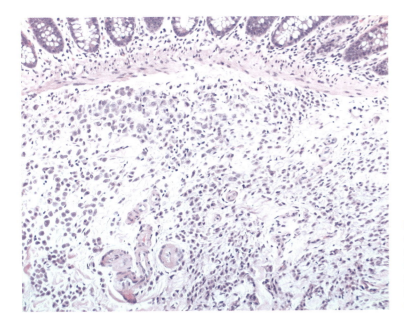

Figure 18.15 Metastatic lobular carcinoma of breast. Both the submucosal infiltration beneath an intact mucosa and the distinctive single cell pattern of infiltrating epithelial cells are clues to the nature of this tumour.

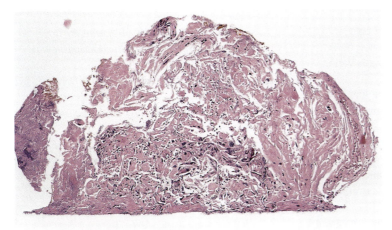

Figure 18.16 Squamous carcinoma of cervix metastatic to ascending colon. This colonoscopic biopsy consists almost entirely of heavily keratinized squamas.

REFERENCES

Alexander, J., Watanabe, T., Wu, T.T., Rashid, A., Li, S., Hamilton, S.R. (2001) Histopathological identification of colon cancer with microsatellite instability. *Am. J. Pathol.*, 158, 527–35

Almagro, U.A. (1983) Primary signet ring carcinoma of the colon. *Cancer*, 52, 1453–7.

Armitage, N.C., Robins, R.A., Evans, D.F., Turner, D.R., Baldwin, R.W., Hardcastle, J.D. (1985) The influence of tumour cell DNA abnormalities on survival in colorectal cancer. *Br. J. Surg.*, 72, 828–30.

Burgess, P.A., Lupton, E.W., Talbot, I.C. (1979) Squamous cell carcinoma of the proximal colon: report of a case and review of the literature. *Dis. Col. Rectum*, 22, 241–4.

Burke, M., Shepherd, N., Mann, C.V. (1987) Carcinoid tumours of the rectum and anus. *Br. J. Surg.*, 74, 358–61.

Caldarota, V.T., Jackman, J., Moertel, C.G., Dockerty, M.B. (1964) Carcinoid tumours of the rectum. *Am. J. Surg.*, 107, 844–9

Cappell, M.S., Botros, N. (1994) Predominantly gastrointestinal symptoms and signs in 11 consecutive AIDS patients with gastrointestinal lymphoma: a multicenter, multiyear study including 763 HIV-seropositive patients. *Am. J. Gastroenterol.*, 89, 545–9.

Cawkwell, L., Gray, S., Murgatroyd, H. *et al.* (1999) Choice of management strategy for colorectal cancer based on a diagnostic immunohistochemical test for defective mismatch repair. *Gut*, 45, 409–15.

Ciacchero, A., Aste, H., Baracch, P., Conio, M., Fulcheri, E., Lapertosa, G., Tanzi, R. (1985) Primary signet-ring carcinoma of the large bowel. *Cancer*, 56, 2723–6.

Cornes, J.S., Jones, T.C. (1962) Leukaemic lesions of the gastrointestinal tract. *J. Clin. Pathol.*, 15, 305–13.

Dawson, I.M.P. (1976) The endocrine cells of the gastrointestinal tract and the neoplasms which arise from them. In: Morson, B.C. (ed.) *Pathology of the gastrointestinal tract, current topics in pathology*, vol. 63. Berlin, Heidelberg and New York: Springer Verlag, pp. 221–58.

Day, D.W., Jass, J.R., Price, A.B., Shepherd, N.A., Talbot, I.C., Warren, B.F., Williams, G.T. (2003a) *Morson and Dawson's gastrointestinal pathology*. Oxford: Blackwell, p. 579.

Day, D.W., Jass, J.R., Price, A.B., Shepherd, N.A., Talbot, I.C., Warren, B.F., Williams, G.T. (2003b) *Morson and Dawson's gastrointestinal pathology*. Oxford: Blackwell, p. 612.

de la Chapelle A. (2003) Microsatellite instability. *N. Engl. J. Med.*, 349, 209–10.

Forster, S.J., Talbot, I.C., Critchley, D.R. (1984) Laminin and fibronectin in rectal adenocarcinoma: relationship to tumour grade, stage and metastasis. *Br. J. Cancer*, 50, 51–61.

Hamilton, S.R., Vogelstein, B., Kudo, S. *et al.* (2000) Carcinoma of the rectum and colon. In: Hamilton, S.R., Aaltonen, L.A. (eds) *Tumours of the digestive system, World Health Organization classification of tumours; pathology and genetics.* Lyon: IARC Press, p. 105–19.

Heinrich, M.C., Corless, C.L., Demetri, G.D. *et al.* (2003) Kinase mutations and imatinib response in patients with metastatic gastrointestinal stromal tumor. *J. Clin. Oncol.*, 21, 4342–49.

Hemminki, A., Mecklin, J.P., Jarvinen, H., Aaltonen, L.A., Joensuu, H. (2000) Microsatellite instability is a favourable prognostic indicator in patients with colorectal cancer receiving chemotherapy. *Gastroenterology*, 119, 921–8.

Hermanek, P., Gall, F.P. (1985) Early colorectal carcinoma. *Br. J. Surg.*, 72 (Suppl.), S134.

Isaacson, P.G. (1999) Gastrointestinal lymphomas of T- and B-cell types. *Mod. Pathol.*, 12, 151–8.

Isaacson, P., Wright, D.H. (1984) Extranodal malignant lymphoma arising from mucosa-associated lymphoid tissue. *Cancer*, 53, 2515–24.

Isaacson, P.G., MacLennan, K.A., Subbuswamy, S.G. (1984) Multiple lymphomatous polyposis of the gastrointestinal tract. *Histopathology*, 8, 641–56.

Jass, J.R. (1998) Diagnosis of hereditary non-polyposis colorectal cancer. *Histopathology*, 32, 491–7.

Jessurun, J., Romero-Guadarrama, M., Manivel, J.C. (1999) Medullary adenocarcinoma of the colon: clinicopathologic study of 11 cases. *Hum. Pathol.*, 30, 843–8.

Kodama, T., Ohshima, K., Nomura, K. *et al.* (2005) Lymphomatous polyposis of the gastrointestinal tract, including mantle cell lymphoma, follicular lymphoma and mucosa-associated lymphoid tissue lymphoma. *Histopathology*, 47, 467–78.

Lasota, J., Jasinski, M., Sarlomo-Rikala, M., Miettinen, M. (1999) Mutations in exon 11 of c-Kit occur preferentially in malignant versus benign gastrointestinal stromal tumors and do not occur in leiomyomas or leiomyosarcomas. *Am. J. Pathol.*, 154, 53–60.

Lavergne, A., Brouland, J.P., Launay, E., Nemeth, J., Ruskone-Fourmestraux, A., Galian, A. (1994) Multiple lymphomatous polyposis of the gastrointestinal tract. An extensive histopathologic and immunohistochemical study of 12 cases. *Cancer*, 74, 3042–50.

Levine, A.M. (1992) Acquired immunodeficiency syndrome-related lymphoma. *Blood*. 80, 8–20.

Lothe, R.A., Peltomaki, P., Meling, G.I. *et al.* (1983) Genomic instability in colorectal cancer: relationship to clinicopathological variables and family history. *Cancer Res.*, 53, 5849–52.

Miettinen, M., Sarlomo-Rikala, M., Lasota, J. (1999) Gastrointestinal stromal tumours: recent advances in understanding of their biology. *Hum. Pathol.*, 30, 1213–20.

Miettinen, M., Blay, J.Y., Kindblom, L.G., Sobin, L.H. (2000) Mesenchymal tumours of the colon and rectum. In: Hamilton, S.R., Aaltonen, L.A. (eds) *Tumours of the digestive system; World Health Organization classification of tumours, pathology and genetics.* Lyon: IARC Press, pp. 142–3.

Mills, S.E., Alien, M.S., Cohen, A.R. (1983) Small cell undifferentiated carcinoma of the colon. *Am. J. Surg. Pathol.*, 7, 643–51.

Modlin, I.M., Sandor, A. (1997) An analysis of 8305 cases of carcinoid tumors. *Cancer*, 79, 813–29.

Morgan, J.E., Marks, C., Hearn, D. (1974) Carcinoid tumors of the gastrointestinal tract. *Ann. Surg.*, 180, 720–7.

Morson, B.C. (1985) Histological criteria for local excision. *Br. J. Surg. Suppl.*, 72, S53–S58.

Morson, B.C., Sobin, L.H. (1976) Histological typing of intestinal tumours. *International histological classification of tumours, no. 15.* Geneva: World Health Organization.

Morson, B.C., Bussey, H.J.R., Samoorian, S. (1977) Policy of local excision for early cancer of the colorectum. *Gut*, 18, 1045–50.

Müller-Hermelink, H.K., Chott, A., Gascoyne, R.D., Wotherspoon, A. (2000) B-cell lymphoma of the colon and rectum. In: Hamilton, S.R., Aaltonen, L.A. (eds) *Tumours of the digestive system; World Health Organization classification of tumours, pathology and genetics.* Lyon: IARC Press, pp. 139–41.

Nagai, T., Koyama, R., Sasagawa, Y. *et al.* (1991) Diffuse infiltrating T-cell lymphoma of the colon associated with polyclonal hypergammaglobulinemia and hepatocellular carcinoma: report of a case. *Jpn. J. Med.*, 30, 57–63.

Nga, M.E., Wong, A.S., Wee, A., Salto-Tellez, M. (2002) Cytokeratin expression in gastrointestinal stromal tumours: a word of caution. *Histopathology*, 40, 480–1.

O'Briain, D.S., Dayal, Y., De Lellis, R.A., Tischler, A.S., Bendron, R., Wolfe, H.J. (1982) Rectal carcinoids as tumors of the hind-gut endocrine cells: a morphological and immunohistochemical analysis. *Am. J. Surg. Pathol.*, 6, 131–42.

Palvio, D.H.B., Sorensen, F.B., Klove-Mogensen, M. (1985) Stem cell carcinoma of the colon and rectum. Report of two cases and review of the literature. *Dis. Col. Rectum*, 28, 440–5.

Parente, F., Cernuschi, M., Orlando, G., Rizzardini, G., Lazzarin, A., Bianchi Porro, G. (1991) Kaposi's sarcoma and AIDS: frequency of gastrointestinal involvement and its effect on survival. A prospective study in a heterogeneous population. *Scand. J. Gastroenterol.*, 26, 1007–12.

Peltomaki, P., Vasen, H., Jass, J.R. (2000) Hereditary nonpolyposis colorectal cancer. In: Hamilton, S.R., Aaltonen, L.A. (eds) *Tumours of the digestive system; World Health Organization classification of tumours, pathology and genetics.* Lyon: IARC Press, p. 127.

Prolla, J.C., Kirsner, J.B. (1964) The gastro-intestinal lesions and complications of the leukaemias. *Ann. Intern. Med.*, 61, 1084–103.

Qualheim, R.E., Call, E.A. (1953) Is histologic grading of colon carcinoma a valid procedure? *Arch. Pathol.*, 56, 466–72.

Ribic, C.M., Sargent, D.J., Moore, M.J. *et al.* (2003) Tumor microsatellite-instability status as a predictor of benefit from fluorouracil-based adjuvant chemotherapy for colon cancer. *N. Engl. J. Med.*, 349, 247–57.

Riddell, R.H., Petras, R.E., Williams, G.T., Sobin, L.H. (2003). Endocrine cell tumors. In: *Tumors of the intestines.* Washington, DC: American Registry of Pathology, Armed Forces Institute of Pathology, pp. 279–323.

Rubio, C.A., Collins, V.P., Berg, C. (1981) Mixed adenosquamous carcinoma of the cecum; report of a case and review of the literature. *Dis. Col. Rectum*, 24, 301–4.

Sakuragi, M., Togashi, K., Konishi, F., Koinuma, K., Kawamura, Y., Okada, M., Nagai, H. (2003)

Predictive factors for lymph node metastasis in T1 stage colorectal carcinomas. *Dis. Colon Rectum*, 46, 1626–32.

Salles, G., Herbrecht, R., Tilly, H., Berger, F., Brousse, N., Gisselbrecht, C., Coiffier, B. (1991) Aggressive primary gastrointestinal lymphomas: review of 91 patients treated with the LNH-84 regimen. A study of the Groupe d'Etude des Lymphomes Agressifs. *Am. J. Med.*, 90, 77–84.

Salto-Tellez, M., Lee, S.C., Chiu, L.L., Lee, C.K., Yong, M.C., Koay, E.S. (2004) Microsatellite instability in colorectal cancer: considerations for molecular diagnosis and high-throughput screening of archival tissues. *Clin. Chem.*, 50, 1082–6.

Sanders, K.M. (1996) A case for interstitial cells of Cajal as pacemakers and mediators of neurotransmission in the gastrointestinal tract. *Gastroenterology*, 111, 492–515.

Sasaki, O., Atkin, W.S., Jass, J.R. (1987) Mucinous carcinoma of the rectum. *Histopathology*, 11, 259–72.

Schwartz, A.M., Orenstein, J.M. (1985) Small-cell undifferentiated carcinoma of the rectosigmoid colon. *Arch. Pathol. Lab. Med.*, 109, 629–32.

Shashidharan, M., Smyrk, T., Lin, K.M. *et al.* (1999) Histologic comparison of hereditary nonpolyposis colorectal cancer associated with MSH2 and MLH1 and colorectal cancer from the general population. *Dis. Colon Rectum*, 42, 722–26.

Shepherd, N.A., Hall, P.A., Coates, P.J., Levison, D.A. (1988) Primary malignant lymphoma of the colon and rectum. A histopathological and immunohistochemical analysis of 45 cases with clinicopathological correlations. *Histopathology*, 12, 235–52.

Shepherd, N.A., Hall, P.A., Williams, G.T., Codling, B.W., Jones, E.L., Levison, D.A., Morson, B.C. (1989) Primary malignant lymphoma of the large intestine complicating chronic inflammatory bowel disease. *Histopathology*, 15, 325–37.

Soga, J., Tazawa, K. (1971) Pathologic analysis of carcinoid. Histologic re-evaluation of 62 cases. *Cancer*, 28, 990–8.

Solcia, E., Capella, C., Buffa, R., Usellini, L., Frigerio, B., Fontana, P. (1979) Endocrine cells of the gastrointestinal tract and related tumors. In: Ioachim, H.L. (ed.) *Pathobiology annual*, vol. 9. New York: Raven Press, pp. 163–204.

Son, H.J., Rhee, P.L., Kim, J.J., Koh, K.C., Paik, S.W., Rhee, J.C., Koh, Y.H. (1997) Primary T-cell lymphoma of the colon. *Korean J. Intern. Med.*, 12, 238–41.

Thomas, E.D.H., Dixon, M.F., Smeeton, N.C., Williams, N.S. (1983) Observer variation in the histological grading of rectal carcinoma. *J. Clin. Pathol.*, 36, 385–91.

Ueyama, T., Guo, K.J., Hashimoto, H., Daimaru, Y., Enjoji, M. (1992) A clinicopathologic and immunohistochemical study of gastrointestinal stromal tumors. *Cancer*, 69, 947–55.

Wilander, E., El-Salky, M., Lundqvist, M. (1983) Argyrophil reaction in rectal carcinoids. *Acta Pathol. Microbiol. Immunol. Scand. (A)*, 91, 85–7.

Wilcox, G.M., Anderson, P.B., Colacchio, T.A. (1986) Early invasive carcinoma in colonic polyps. *Cancer*, 57, 160–71.

Williams, G.T., Blackshaw, A.J., Morson, B.C. (1979) Squamous carcinoma of the colorectum and its genesis. *J. Pathol.*, 129, 139–47.

CHAPTER 19

ANAL BIOPSY

19.1 Introduction	351	
19.1.1 Normal morphology	351	
19.1.2 Biopsy pathology	352	
19.2 Inflammatory lesions	352	
19.2.1 Fissures	352	
19.2.2 Fistulae	353	
19.2.3 Skin tags (fibroepithelial polyps)	357	
19.2.4 Venereal infections	357	
19.2.5 Haemorrhoids	358	
19.2.6 Fibrous polyp	358	
19.2.7 Prolapse	358	
19.2.8 Leucoplakia	358	
19.2.9 Warts (condyloma accuminatum)	358	
19.3 Tumours of the anal canal	361	
19.3.1 Anal intra-epithelial neoplasia	361	
19.3.2 Carcinoma of anal canal	363	

19.3.3 Verrucous carcinoma	365	
19.3.4 Malignant melanoma	366	
19.3.5 Adenocarcinoma of anal ducts	368	
19.3.6 Leukaemic infiltration	368	
19.3.7 Granular cell tumour	368	
19.4 Lesions of perianal skin	368	
19.4.1 Hidradenitis suppurativa	368	
19.4.2 Lichen sclerosus et atrophicus	369	
19.4.3 Bowen's disease	369	
19.4.4 Epidermodysplasia verruciformis (Bowenoid papulosis)	370	
19.4.5 Basal cell carcinoma	370	
19.4.6 Squamous carcinoma	371	
19.4.7 Keratoacanthoma	371	
19.4.8 Paget's disease	371	
19.4.9 Adenoma of apocrine gland	373	
References	374	

19.1 INTRODUCTION

Before biopsies from the anal region can be properly interpreted the anatomy and normal histology of the anal canal and the nature of the epithelium of the ano-rectal junction must be appreciated. These have been well described by Fenger (1997).

19.1.1 Normal morphology

The upper limit of the anal canal is defined surgically by the ano-rectal ring formed by the proximal border of the striated external sphincter (puborectalis) muscle. This part of the anal canal is lined by a short cuff of colorectal mucosa. Histologically, this is thinner than the mucosa of the main part of the rectum and the glands are slightly irregular in arrangement, simulating atrophy (Fig. 19.1). Below the colorectal mucosa there is usually a cuff of 'transitional' mucosa, forming the anal transitional zone (ATZ). The ATZ is lined by variable epithelium, including a unique stratified cuboidal epithelium (Fig. 19.2) resembling the transitional epithelium of the prostatic urethra, with intracellular mucin and 'umbrella' cells on the surface and sparsely scattered

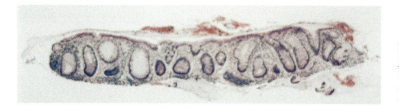

Figure 19.1 Mucosa from the junction of the rectum with the anal canal, showing morphology resembling rectal mucosa but thinner and with shorter glands.

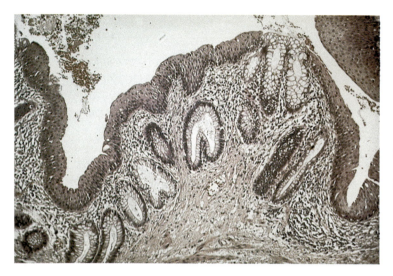

Figure 19.2 Normal anal mucosal types. The attenuated glands of the junctional rectal/upper anal mucosa underlie the transitional stratified cuboidal surface epithelium which, on the right, merges with the non keratinizing stratified squamous ('pecten') epithelium of the lower anal canal.

serotonin-producing endocrine cells (Fetissof *et al.*, 1984). The ATZ is, on average, 9 mm long and at approximately its lower edge is the dentate line (Helwig, 1983), the irregular line formed by the anal sinuses and valves at the upper limit of the anal columns of Morgagni (Fig. 19.3). The lowermost zone of the anal canal, or 'pecten', lies below the anal sinuses/valves and is 1 cm long. It is lined by thin stratified squamous epithelium which is usually non-keratinizing but may sometimes be keratinized (e.g. if there is some degree of mucosal prolapse) but does not typically contain skin appendages. The lower limit of the pecten lies at the 'anal verge': the anal orifice where the perianal skin begins, at the lower edge of the internal sphincter muscle.

19.1.2 Biopsy pathology

Biopsy specimens from the anal region fall into three categories:

1. Inflammatory lesions. (The biopsy tissue commonly consists of irregular fragments.)
2. Tumours of anal canal.

3. Lesions of perianal skin. (These are either incisional biopsies or more extensive local excisions.)

19.2 INFLAMMATORY LESIONS

19.2.1 Fissures

Anal fissures are small ulcers which, at the unique site of the anal verge, are slow to heal because of repeated stretching and trauma caused by passage of stool. These are rarely biopsied but, when they are excised, they are small, superficial skin ulcers (Fig. 19.4). The surrounding dermis may be chronically inflamed, sometimes severely, when there is ulcerative colitis but granulomas or other specific features are not seen unless there is underlying Crohn's disease or in the rare case of anal involvement by lymphogranuloma venereum (Section 19.2.4c). Underlying cytomegalovirus (CMV) infection should also be borne in mind when examining tissue from an anal fissure and granulation tissue should be scrutinized for inclusion bodies.

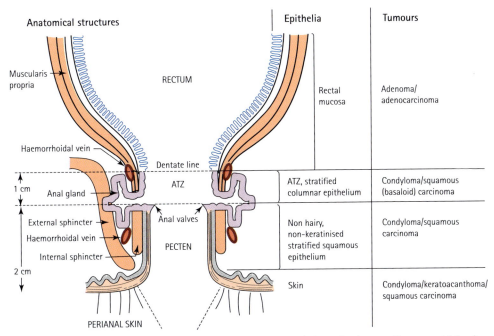

Anatomical structures	Epithelia	Tumours

Figure 19.3 The anatomy of the anus, showing the epithelial zones and the main classes of tumour which arise from them. (ATZ = anal transition zone).

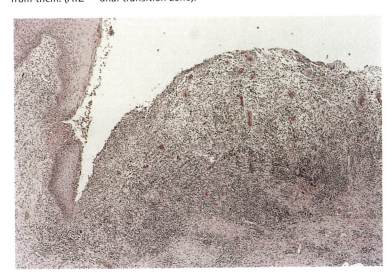

Figure 19.4 Excised anal fissure. This is an ulcer of anal verge (junction of anal canal with perianal skin). The ulcer is lined by granulation tissue and shows no specific features.

19.2.2 Fistulae

Surgical management of fistulae entails either curettage of the track or excision of a cylindrical core of the fistula itself, often several centimetres in length, with surrounding connective tissue. Such excision tends to be performed on intersphincteric fistulae, in which case, portions of striated as well as smooth muscle will be present within the core.

Careful examination of the excised tissue may reveal remnants of the anal gland from which the fistula arose (Fig. 19.5). In approximately one-third of cases there will be epithelialization of the fistula track (Bataille, 2004), in which case portions of stratified squamous epithelium (Fig. 19.6) or rectal-type mucosa can be found. It is believed that epithelialization may be responsible for failure of a fistula to heal. It is advisable to process and examine the

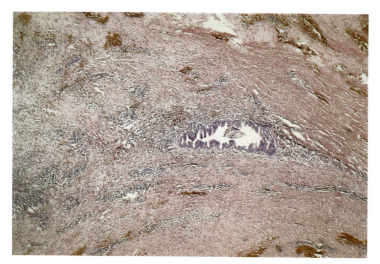

Figure 19.5 Inflamed anal gland in tissue removed along fistula track. This deep-seated anal gland lies in the plane between the smooth and striated muscle layers of the anal sphincter.

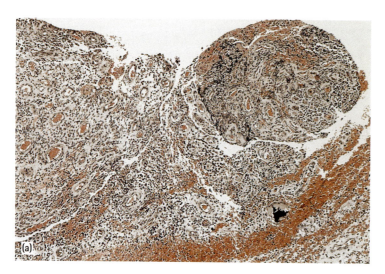

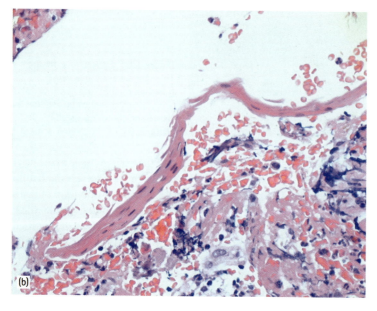

Figure 19.6 (a) Granulation tissue curetted from a fistula. Fragments of granulation tissue in these circumstances are often friable and oedematous. (b) Small strips of stratified squamous epithelium are often present and prevent healing but may be inconspicuous.

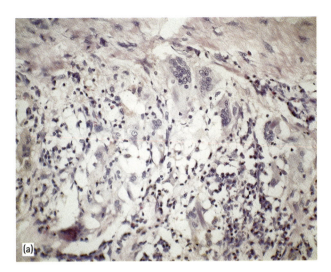

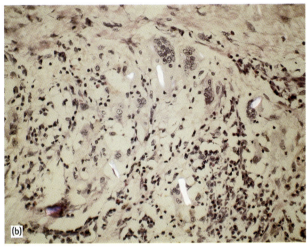

Figure 19.7 (a) Granulomatous reaction to faecally derived foreign material in perianal tissue removed during operation for fistula. The foreign body-type giant cells contain birefringent material. (b) Same field, with crossed polarized illumination.

whole of any curetted fragments of granulation tissue and it may be necessary to examine sections from the entire length of a core and at multiple levels to find the epithelium. To aid orientation it is helpful if the surgeon puts a stitch in the lower end of the excision specimen.

Fistulae and fissures are occasionally associated with underlying inflammatory bowel disease and as much of the available tissue as possible should be examined to avoid missing diagnostic features.

In addition to granulation tissue, three other features which should be sought are:

1. Scattered multinucleate giant cells of foreign body type. These accumulate in response to implanted faecal material, which may be birefringent (Fig. 19.7), or oil, possibly introduced therapeutically. This type of foreign body reaction does not exclude a diagnosis of inflammatory bowel disease, but makes it less likely. A foreign body reaction has been reported in association with threadworms which had invaded the perianal tissues, leading to an indurated tumour-like mass (Wafai and Mohit, 1983) and we have seen a similar case (Fig. 4.24).

2. Focal aggregates of lymphocytes and ill-defined granulomas composed of epithelioid cells, together with occasional Langhans giant cells (Fig. 19.8) indicate that the patient probably has Crohn's disease. Minor focal necrosis may be

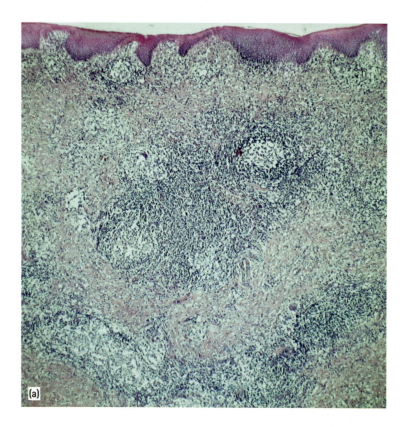

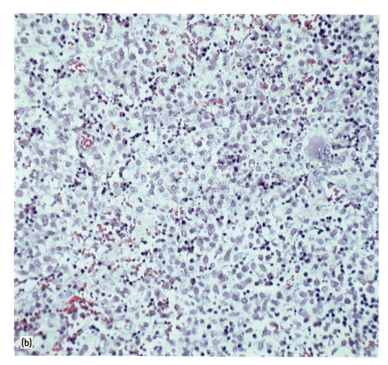

Figure 19.8 (a) Anal Crohn's disease. The subepithelial tissue is oedematous and contains lymphoid aggregates, ill-defined granulomas and Langhans cells. (b) Granulation tissue from a fistula in a patient with Crohn's disease may contain loosely arranged sheets of epithelioid cells that are not quite cohesive enough to be classically granulomatous.

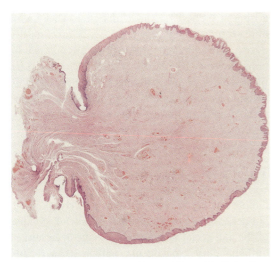

Figure 19.9 Anal skin tag. Tags or fibroepithelial polyps arise at the anal verge because of healing after previous trauma or ulceration. Inflammation is often inconspicuous or even absent. In the absence of skin appendages, keratinization of the epidermis is a clue to the origin of this polyp in skin rather than anal canal.

present, but not caseation. Birefringent material is not usually detected in these biopsies.

3. Confluent granuloma formation, with sheets of epithelioid cells and caseation necrosis is, of course, diagnostic of tuberculosis.

19.2.3 Skin tags (fibroepithelial polyps)

These are polypoid excrescences of redundant non-hairy stratified squamous epithelium which often form at the lower end of fissures and have a central core of fibrous tissue and smooth muscle (Fig. 19.9), which is not usually inflamed. A heavy infiltrate of lymphocytes and plasma cells in this situation should arouse suspicion of secondary syphilis (condyloma lata).

19.2.4 Venereal infections

Biopsies from anal lesions, usually from male homosexuals, can present as fissures or tags and it is easy to miss the underlying diagnosis unless the pathologist is alerted.

19.2.4a Syphilis

Occasionally mistaken clinically for a fissure, but notably painless, a chancre consists of granulation tissue heavily infiltrated by plasma cells, clustered around capillaries with swollen endothelium.

In secondary syphilis, condylomata lata are moist hypertrophic papules, which can be clinically confused with anal warts. Histologically, conspicuous sheets of plasma cells are the tell-tale sign.

The diagnosis of primary and secondary syphilis is more appropriately made in the clinic by examination of surface smears by dark-ground microscopy for the presence of spirochaetes.

19.2.4b Granuloma inguinale (Donovanosis)

This infection by *Klebsiella granulomatis* (Richens, 1992) is confined to Papua New Guinea, India, southern Africa and Brazil. However, it also occurs in Australian aborigines. It is occasionally seen in patients following travel to those areas. It is characterized by ano-genital ulcers which, on biopsy, consist of connective tissue and granulation tissue heavily infiltrated by plasma cells and polymorphs. Pseudocarcinomatous hyperplasia of stratified squamous epithelium at the external edge of the lesion is the rule. Large macrophages containing Leishman–Donovan bodies, best seen by Giemsa or Warthin–Starry staining, are diagnostic. Smears of swabs or scrapings are preferred to biopsy material for diagnosis.

19.2.4c Lymphogranuloma venereum

This may present as an anal fissure, but rectal disease generally dominates the clinical picture, patients presenting early with an active proctitis or later with a so-called 'ano-rectal syndrome' of painful fibrous anal stricturing (Section 4.4.3a). Biopsy tissue can resemble a 'non-specific' fissure, with granulation tissue, but there can also be prominent oedema, fibrous scar formation and, occasionally, granuloma formation. In addition, the presence of lymphocytic infiltration and neural

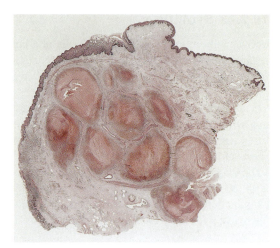

Figure 19.10 Thrombosed haemorrhoid. A few small bundles of anal sphincter muscle pass between distended sinusoidal veins. Excised haemorrhoids usually include rectal and anal mucosa (on the left of this field) as well as perianal skin (on the right).

hypertrophy may cause confusion with Crohn's disease (Day *et al.*, 2003a).

19.2.5   Haemorrhoids

On microscopy these consist of a mass of dilated tortuous sinusoidal veins set in a loose connective tissue (submucosal) stroma. The mucosa overlying is typically of transitional zone anal type, as haemorrhoids arise in this zone, but lower rectal mucosa, non-keratinized stratified squamous mucosa and skin are frequently also present in haemorrhoidectomy specimens. There is often thrombosis (Fig. 19.10). Occasionally there are atypical epithelial features and the pathologist should be alert to the possibility of dysplasia or carcinoma *in situ* (AIN) of this zone of the anus (Helwig, 1983). If the surgical procedure is a stapled haemorrhoidectomy, normal rectal mucosa is usually the only tissue excised.

19.2.6 Fibrous polyp

Fibrous polyps of anal canal form in relation to haemorrhoids and proximal to fissures, generally

arising at the level of the dentate line. They are of little diagnostic importance, usually being clinically overshadowed by one of these two primary conditions. However, it is necessary to be aware that these firm nodules of dense fibrous tissue may develop, whether by organization of thrombosis in a haemorrhoid or from fibrous scarring of the apex of a fissure.

19.2.7 Prolapse

Simple rectal and anal prolapse is rarely biopsied, but occasionally polyps arise at the site of prolapse of the ano-rectal mucosa. These have been termed 'inflammatory cloacogenic polyps' (Lobert and Appelman, 1981) and show features similar to the mucosal prolapse syndrome at more proximal sites (Section 15.10), with extension of smooth muscle and fibrous tissue between irregular elongated crypts and ectasia of superficial mucosal capillaries. They typically occur at the anal ring, at the junction of rectal and anal mucosa and often these two types of mucosa can be seen at either side of the polyp (Fig. 19.11).

19.2.8 Leucoplakia

Leucoplakia is a clinical appearance, in which the anal mucosa and/or perianal skin is white and thickened. This can simply be caused by acanthosis of the epithelium, usually with hyperkeratosis. Biopsies may sometimes show a lichen planus-like picture, with irregular exaggeration of rete processes, a band-like subepidermal lymphoid infiltrate and hyperkeratosis (Fig. 19.12). There may be parakeratosis. Squamous carcinoma has subsequently developed in some of these patients (Day *et al.*, 2003b).

19.2.9 Warts (condyloma accuminatum)

Warts around the anus are typically cauliflower-like lesions. Histologically, they show a papillary structure with a variable degree of acanthosis leading to

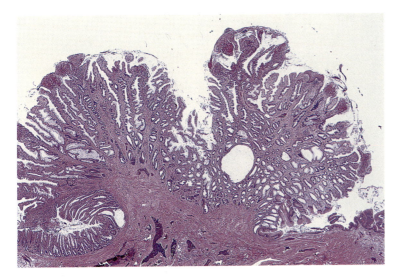

Figure 19.11 Prolapse of anorectal mucosa – inflammatory cloacogenic polyp. The mucosa of the lower rectum at the junction with the anal canal is thrown into folds. The crypts are hyperplastic, elongated and irregular. The lamina propria contains smooth muscle and fibrous tissue. The surface is eroded.

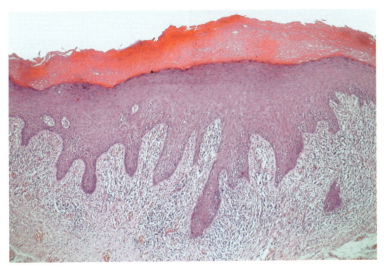

Figure 19.12 Biopsy of 'leucoplakia' of perianal skin. Although this is a clinical term, without precise pathological meaning, in our experience, when biopsied, this lichen planus-like picture can be seen. There is hyperkeratosis, with a band-like upper dermal infiltrate of lymphocytes, focal degeneration of the basal epidermis and a saw-tooth-like epidermal acanthosis. There may be parakeratosis.

broad, blunt rete processes (Fig. 19.13) and parakeratosis of the surface (Fig. 19.14a). There is normal maturation of the epithelium. A heavy infiltrate of plasma cells and lymphocytes is often present in the underlying connective tissue. Vacuolation of the more superficial keratinocytes is a variable feature, but can be quite striking (Fig. 19.14a) and resembles the koilocytosis associated, in the cervix, with papilloma virus infection (Dyson *et al.*, 1984) (Fig 19.14b). Occasionally, atypical cells are scattered through the epidermis and there may be individually keratinized cells, suggesting a relationship with

Bowenoid papulosis (Section 19.4.4). The presence of frequent mitotic figures is not indicative of malignancy and may be the result of podophyllin therapy, or may merely reflect the rapid growth of these lesions. The growth of condyloma accuminatum, as with common warts, is upwards.

19.2.9a Giant condyloma

The histological features of giant condyloma closely resemble those of condyloma accuminatum and distinction between these two lesions can

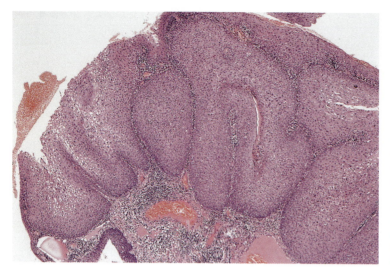

Figure 19.13 Anal wart (condyloma accuminatum). This lesion can be seen to lie at the junction of anal squamous and anal transition zone (ATZ) epithelium. Bulbous acanthosis gives the characteristic cauliflower-like papillomatous appearance to these lesions. Epithelial cell vacuolation (koilocytosis) can be seen.

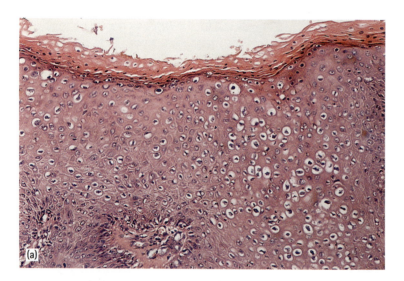

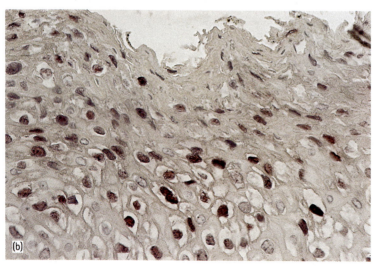

Figure 19.14 Anal wart (condyloma accuminatum). (a) At high magnification cell vacuolation with nuclear hyperchromatism and irregularity (koilocytosis) is seen in this haematoxylin and eosin preparation. (b) By *in-situ* hybridization the koilocytes can be seen to contain human papilloma virus DNA, in this case HPV6.

only be made on the basis of the large size and the more extensive and downward growth pattern of giant condyloma (Bogomoletz *et al.*, 1985). It is not possible, from biopsy material, to appreciate the pattern of growth and it is important to examine the whole lesion if at all possible.

Giant condylomas tend not to respond to podophyllin and are characterized by deep extension into the ischiorectal fossa. They spread laterally to involve the perianal skin and sometimes upwards to involve the lower rectum, whereas condyloma accuminatum rarely extends beyond the anal canal. Clinical information about these points is important when reporting the histopathology of anal warts.

The koilocytic vacuolation often found in these two lesions suggests that both are the result of human papilloma virus (HPV) infection. Both HPV types 6 and 11 have been specifically identified in condylomata accuminata (McCance *et al.*, 1986) (Fig 19.14b) and HPV has been found in squamous carcinoma of the anus (Hill and Coghill, 1986). Bogomoletz *et al.* (1985) consider that there is a continuum between condyloma accuminatum and giant condyloma and that the latter has a tendency to progress to verrucous carcinoma (Section 19.3.3) or, via a dysplastic phase, to conventional invasive squamous carcinoma. Indeed, most authorities now consider that giant condyloma and verrucous carcinoma are synonyms for the same lesion (Prioleau *et al.*, 1980; Fenger *et al.*, 2000). It would seem logical to follow the hypothesis of Bogomoletz *et al.* and regard giant condyloma as the least aggressive in a continuum in which verrucous carcinoma is more aggressive, although barely histologically distinguishable. The approach to anal warts should be similar to that of colonic polyps; that is, they should all be excised rather than biopsied and should be carefully examined for dysplasia and invasion.

19.3 TUMOURS OF THE ANAL CANAL

Carcinoma arising in the anal canal appears clinically indistinguishable from a low rectal adenocarcinoma, despite a different histogenesis. These tumours arise from either the transitional zone (ATZ)

or the pecten in a proportion of between two and three to one. Origin from the ATZ is commoner in women than men and the reverse is true of tumours arising in the pecten. The ATZ (Section 19.1) is normally lined by a stratified cuboidal mucosa (Fig. 19.2) and tumours of this zone show features unique to this site. So-called basaloid differentiation is that most frequently encountered (Pang and Morson, 1967; Singh *et al.*, 1981), particularly in tumours arising in the ATZ. Despite the term 'basaloid' these tumours are histogenetically unrelated to basal cell carcinoma of skin and metastasize to regional lymph nodes (Dougherty and Evans, 1985). It is likely that they arise in epithelium which first passes through a phase of dysplasia (Fenger and Nielsen, 1985). Pre-invasive squamous carcinoma of this region is known as anal intra-epithelial neoplasia (AIN). Malignant melanomas and tumours apparently arising in anal glands are relative rarities.

19.3.1 Anal intra-epithelial neoplasia

Pre-invasive squamous anal neoplasia has formerly been referred to as severe dysplasia and is also known as carcinoma *in situ* or anal squamous intra-epithelial lesion (ASIL). This can be an incidental finding in, for example, haemorrhoids, tags or warts but may present clinically as eczematous or papular plaques. It is usually related to HPV infection and occurs particularly in homosexual men (Palefsky, 1995) and in immunodeficiency states, either human immunodeficiency virus (HIV)-induced or as a result of immunosuppressive therapy. It is otherwise rare. Anal intra-epithelial neoplasia can be present in the ATZ, the pecten or the perianal skin, although in the last site it is commonly referred to as Bowen's disease. In biopsies (Fig. 19.15), AIN is seen as varying degrees of loss of epithelial cell stratification and nuclear polarity, nuclear pleomorphism and increased mitotic activity with mitoses high in the epithelium. Koilocytosis is frequently present and there may or may not be surface keratinization. Anal intra-epithelial neoplasia is conventionally graded into AIN I, II or III but a two-grade system, low grade and high grade, is more consistently reproducible and may be preferable.

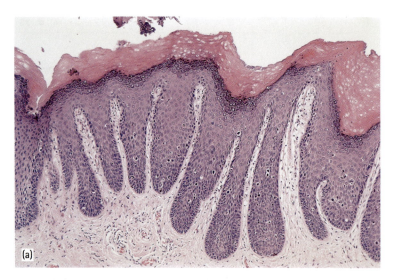

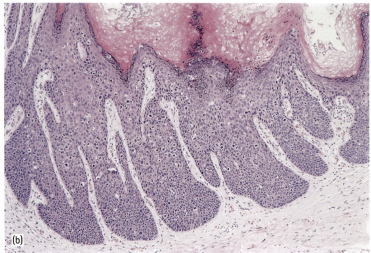

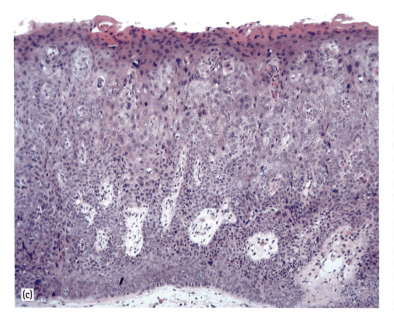

Figure 19.15 Anal intraepithelial neoplasia (AIN) is the failure of maturation of the squamous epithelium with or without cellular atypia (dysplasia) and is graded according to the level in the epithelium the dysplasia reaches. Keratinization of the surface is frequently present but is not obligatory. (a) AIN I: only the lower third of the epithelium is abnormal. (b) AIN II: the lower two-thirds are affected. (c) AIN III: the full thickness of the epithelium is immature and, in this case, highly atypical, with nuclear pleomorphism and mitotic figures.

19.3.2 Carcinoma of anal canal

Carcinoma of the anal canal is most commonly of squamous type (SCC), often with heterogeneous features. Tumours arising in the anal canal usually have a basaloid component of varying prominence and are associated with the sexually transmitted HPV 16 or 18 in 92 per cent (Frisch *et al.*, 1998b). This compares with 64 per cent in carcinoma of the perianal skin, which tends to be more purely squamous in type and associated with smoking, particularly in women. As with AIN, SCC of the anal canal has highest prevalence in homosexual men, especially with HIV infection (Fenger *et al.*, 2000). Despite these epidemiological differences, there is no difference in the behaviour or treatment between anal canal and perianal skin SCC and it is convenient to group them together for biopsy diagnostic purposes.

Biopsies of squamous carcinoma, sometimes taken in the belief that the tumour is a low-lying rectal adenocarcinoma, consist of irregular fragments of crumbly grey tissue. Histologically, there is a spectrum of appearances, some tumours being predominantly of classical squamous type but others showing an almost exclusively basaloid morphology, with solid sheets and nodules of small oval cells with dark-staining oval nuclei (Fig. 19.16a), resembling the cells of the basal or parabasal layers of the anal canal (Pang and Morson, 1967). Some tumours are heterogeneous, with basaloid, squamoid and even glandular areas. There is a variably well-formed pallisade at the periphery of the tumour cell islands. These tumours differ histologically from basal cell carcinoma of the skin in the frequent presence of squamoid differentiation with prickle cells and often keratin production (Fig. 19.16b). The stroma is desmoplastic rather than myxoid. An undifferentiated variant also occurs (Fig. 19.16c). There are often large areas of confluent necrosis in the centre of tumour islands.

Just as the epithelium of the transitional zone is variable in its cell population and includes 'aberrant' glandular structures, so are the carcinomas which arise from it. In addition to squamoid differentiation, mucin-secreting areas, occasionally with frank glandular differentiation, are sometimes observed (Fig 19.16d). There is some evidence that the presence of mucin and ductular structures is associated with a worse prognosis (Williams and Talbot, 1994). Occasional case reports of 'muco-epidermoid' carcinomas in this region may be variants of squamous cancers with unusually prominent tubules and mucin production (Fogler *et al.*, 1977).

Because of upward infiltration into the rectum, there may be an intact overlying colorectal-type mucosa, but there is usually central ulceration.

These tumours are analogous to the small cell variety of squamous carcinoma of cervix and

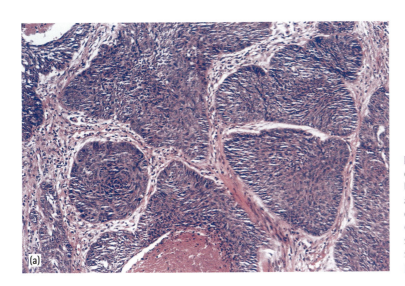

(a)

Figure 19.16 (a) Squamous cell carcinoma (SCC) of anal canal, basaloid features. Although classed as a subgroup of squamous carcinoma, these tumours can be composed entirely of small darkly staining oval cells arranged in sheets and nodules with peripheral pallisading.

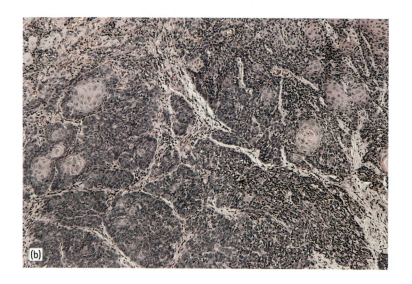

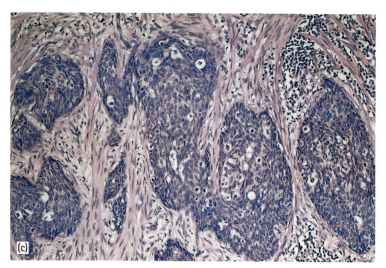

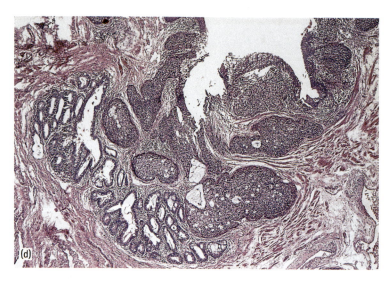

Figure 19.16 (b) Squamous cell carcinoma of anal canal. Many of these tumours of anal canal and anus contain classical squamous carcinomatous foci, including keratinization, within areas of 'basaloid' morphology. (c) Undifferentiated ('basaloid') SCC of anal canal. This tumour retains only rudimentary basaloid epithelial features, with a nodular pattern and relatively uniform, darkly stained cells. (d) Basaloid SCC with glandular differentiation. Acinar structures are frequently present in anal canal SCC and when prominent, as in this case, the tumour can resemble a mucoepidermoid carcinoma.

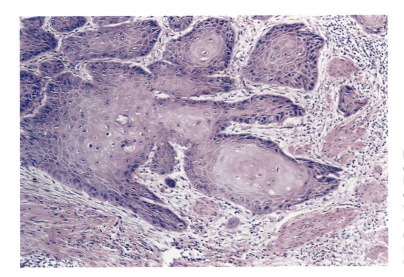

Figure 19.17 Squamous cell carcinoma (SCC) with keratinization. Tumours of anal canal or anus can show classical features of squamous carcinoma, with little sign of basaloid differentiation. Tumours of perianal skin are more frequently of this type.

behave in a similar way, metastasizing to lymph nodes, in preference to more extensive local and distant spread (Day *et al.*, 2003b). They are generally less aggressive than adenocarcinomas of the lower rectum with 5-year survival figures in excess of 60 per cent having been reported (Pang and Morson, 1967).

Tumours arising in the lower anal canal (the pecten) and the perianal skin tend to be more classical squamous carcinoma in type. Association with fistulae and other chronic inflammatory conditions (Sawyers, 1972) remains uncertain (Daling *et al.*, 1987; Frisch *et al.*, 1994, 1998a). These tumours are more common in men than women, in contrast to the sex incidence observed for carcinomas with basaloid morphology (Morson, 1959).

Histologically, these tumours are predominantly composed of prickle cells, without peripheral pallisading. Keratin nests are usually well developed (Fig. 19.17). Unequivocal infiltration of underlying connective tissue can be difficult to determine in biopsy fragments of low anal tumours of this type. Although, histologically, squamous carcinoma of perianal skin closely resembles squamous carcinoma of the lower anal canal, it should be appreciated that, because their lymphatic drainages differ, node involvement from perianal tumours tends to be in the inguinal region, rather than in the iliac nodes, to which anal canal tumours spread.

19.3.3 Verrucous carcinoma

This tumour is indistinguishable from giant condyloma and is regarded by most authorities as the same condition (Prioleau *et al.*, 1980; Fenger *et al.*, 2000). The histological features are considered in more detail in an earlier section (19.2.9a). The name 'verrucous carcinoma' betrays the invasive property of this lesion, which can invade and cause extensive destruction of local pelvic tissues, reaching enormous size. It resembles lesions of the same name, which are more frequently encountered at other muco-cutaneous junctions (Ackerman, 1948). In excised lesions, a papillomatous pattern and prominent keratin-filled, vertically orientated clefts can be appreciated (Fig. 19.18). However, in biopsies, the features can rarely be distinguished from a simple condyloma. If giant condyloma/verrucous carcinoma is suspected, complete excision is imperative. This is in contrast to the generality of anal squamous carcinomas, which are now usually treated effectively by chemoradiotherapy after biopsy diagnosis. Because of this difference in clinical practice when approaching the two lesions, we have no experience of the use of chemoradiotherapy for verrucous carcinoma/giant condyloma. It has been suggested that giant condyloma does not respond to radiotherapy. However, at case report level, chemoradiotherapy has been demonstrated

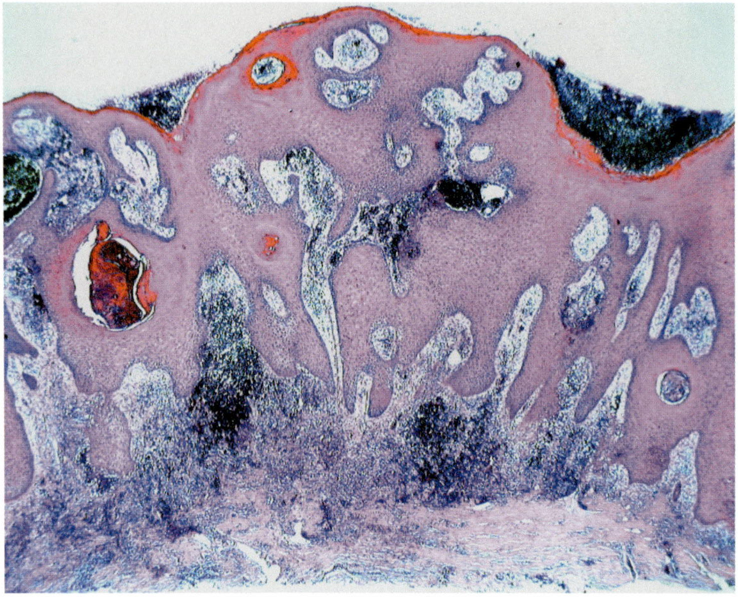

Figure 19.18 Verrucous carcinoma of anus. These tumours closely resemble large warts and, indeed, are often classified as giant condylomas. There is wart-like papillary acanthosis with keratin-filled clefts. The latter tend to be orientated vertically, a feature obscured in this section by tangential orientation. There is no cellular pleomorphism. There is typically a dense lymphocytic infiltrate at the base. Deep invasion, seen here, can be very difficult to identify.

to ablate a verrucous carcinoma (Hyacinthe *et al.*, 1998). So-called verrucous carcinoma should not exhibit epithelial atypia (dysplasia) and, if atypia is present, the diagnosis should be that of a well-differentiated squamous carcinoma of conventional type. The connective tissue underlying the tumour is characteristically heavily infiltrated by lympho-cytes and plasma cells. Human papilloma virus has been demonstrated in these lesions (Cuesta *et al.*, 1998), with implication of HPV 6 and 11 (Boshart and zur Hausen, 1986). It has been suggested that aberrant subtypes of HPV 6 may be responsible for more rapid growth of giant codyloma (Rando *et al.*, 1986). By analogy with the vulva, rare cases of giant condyloma behave in a more aggressive way with a tendency to metastasize, and this transform-ation is possibly caused by HPV 16 or 18 infection (Day *et al.*, 2003b).

19.3.4 Malignant melanoma

These rare tumours arise from the ATZ and grow upwards, sometimes becoming very large and resem-bling large thrombosed piles. Biopsies of malignant melanoma tend to be large fleshy fragments. Histologically, there are loosely arranged sheets of

pleomorphic cells, either epithelioid (Fig. 19.19a) or spindle shaped with prominent nucleoli (Fig. 19.19b,c). Bizarre giant cells are frequently present. Melanin is only detectable in about half of all cases (Day *et al.* 2003b). Often there is an ulcerated rectal mucosa on the surface and this obscures any junc-tional activity there may have been (Wanebo *et al.*, 1981). The tumour immediately beneath the surface may be modified by necrosis, inflammatory reaction and granulation tissue production.

There is a real possibility of confusing the biopsy appearances with undifferentiated carcinoma, basaloid squamous carcinoma, carcinoid tumour or stromal tumour (GIST). Positive features in favour of malignant melanoma are melanin pig-ment and tumour giant cells. Other tumours on rare occasions also show the same degree of sur-face oedema and inflammation related to ulcera-tion. The cells of undifferentiated carcinoma of both small cell (Fig. 18.3) and large cell varieties (Fig. 18.2) are more uniform, do not have large nucleoli and are arranged in more cohesive sheets. Basaloid carcinoma also has a more cohesive arrangement (Fig. 19.16a), often with intercellular bridges, and malignant melanoma does not have a peripheral pallisaded arrangement. Carcinoid tumours are composed of more uniform cells with

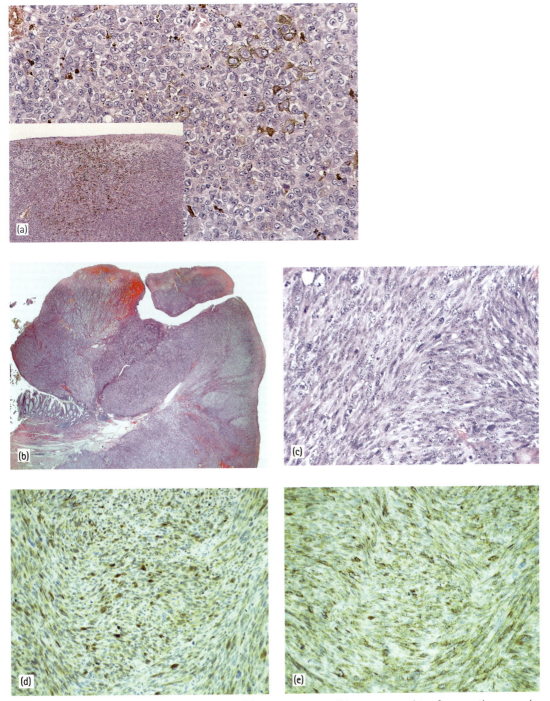

Figure 19.19 (a–f) Malignant melanoma of anus. (a) Epithelioid type. This tumour consists of compactly arranged sheets of large epithelioid cells with eosinophilic cytoplasm and prominent nucleoli. Melanin pigment is variable. There is a sprinkling of lymphocytes beneath the ulcerated surface. (b,c) Spindle cell type. This polypoid tumour is composed of large spindle cells with a whorled pattern, not to be mistaken for a stromal tumour. This tumour is amelanotic. Immunocytochemistry is helpful in achieving a diagnosis. (d) The spindle cells are positive for S-100 and (e) for HMB45.

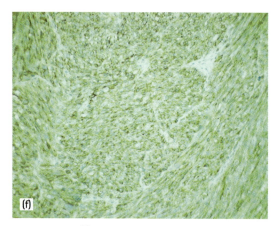

Figure 19.19 (f) Weak cell membrane positivity is displayed for CD117.

a trabecular or packetted (insular) arrangement (Figs 18.7 and 18.6), which malignant melanoma lacks. Immunohistochemical markers may be of value (Table 18.1), S-100 protein being positive in melanomas (Gatter *et al.*, 1985) (Fig 19.19d) although HMB45 (Fig 19.19e) is more specific. Confusingly, melanoma cells can express CD117 (Fig. 19.19f) and it is unwise to rely on this antibody alone when a GIST has to be excluded.

19.3.5 Adenocarcinoma of anal ducts

Although it is likely that some carcinomas of basaloid type arise in the ducts of anal glands, differentiated adenocarcinoma arising in this way is extremely rare (Wellman, 1962; Winkelman *et al.*, 1964). Only seven cases were present in a review of anal tumours seen in two North American centres over 30 years (Hobbs *et al.*, 2001). Such tumours infiltrate deeply beneath an intact anal canal or lower rectal mucosa and are well advanced by the time of biopsy. They show a columnar cell morphology, with well-formed glands, resembling those of the anal gland ducts, in a desmoplastic stroma. Distinction from an ordinary colorectal adenocarcinoma may not be possible from morphology alone, although carcinoma of anal duct is said to express CK7 (Hobbs *et al.*, 2001), unlike rectal adenocarcinoma.

19.3.6 Leukaemic infiltration

Occasionally, leukaemia patients develop lesions in the anal canal, or in relation to the cutaneous margin, which clinically resemble skin tags or haemorrhoids, but which prove on histological examination to be the result of infiltration by leukaemic cells; lymphocytic, myeloid or monocytic. This possibility should be considered when there is a monomorphic infiltrate of leucocytes which show cytological abnormalities with enlarged, hyperchromatic nuclei.

19.3.7 Granular cell tumour

Granular cell tumours may, rarely, present as nodules or masses in the anal canal or be mistaken for fibrous polyps or haemorrhoids (Johnston and Helwig, 1981). They show histological features in common with similar tumours at other, cutaneous sites, consisting of solid masses of large cells with finely granular cytoplasm, beneath a hyperplastic stratified squamous epithelium. The granules are periodic acid–Schiff (PAS)-positive after diastase treatment. Immunohistochemical staining for S-100 protein suggests a Schwann cell origin (Eng and Bigbee, 1978).

19.4 LESIONS OF PERIANAL SKIN

The same diseases which affect the external genitalia are also found around the anus.

19.4.1 Hidradenitis suppurativa

This is a clinical diagnosis and is not always biopsied. In many cases, biopsies show no more than chronic dermal inflammation with or without fibrosis. Less commonly, there are classical features, with a florid chronic inflammatory reaction around sweat glands, which are cystically dilated and often destroyed with the formation of dermal abscesses (McKee, 1989a; Elder *et al.*, 1997a). Stratified squamous epithelium extends down sweat ducts to form multiple sinuses and these may run parallel to the

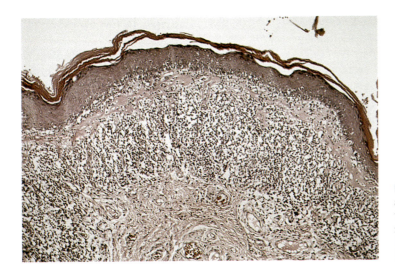

Figure 19.20 Lichen sclerosus et atrophicus. A dense hyaline zone in the upper dermis lies between a sharply defined dermal infiltrate of lymphocytes and the atrophic, hyperkeratotic epidermis.

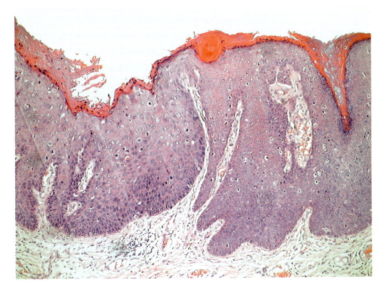

Figure 19.21 Bowen's disease of perianal skin. The epidermis is hyperkeratotic with parakeratosis. There is irregular acanthosis with incomplete maturation. Mitotic figures are numerous and sometimes abnormal. Vacuolated cells can be conspicuous.

anal canal, superficial to the internal sphincter, to form fistulae (Culp, 1983). There is oedema and fibrosis of the perianal connective tissue.

19.4.2 Lichen sclerosus et atrophicus

This condition occasionally occurs outside the vulval area in women (McKee, 1989b; Elder *et al.*, 1997b). Biopsy (Fig. 19.20) shows a well-defined band of lymphocytic infiltration in the dermis, separated from the overlying flat, thinned epidermis by a hyaline zone, proportional in thickness to the chronicity of the disease. In early cases the hyaline band may be lacking and the picture resembles leukaemic or lymphomatous infiltration.

19.4.3 Bowen's disease

This form of squamous carcinoma *in situ* presents as red scaly or warty patches which occasionally affect the perianal skin. It may or may not be in continuity with AIN of the anal canal. Biopsies show acanthosis, with atypia of the cells in all levels of the epidermis (Fig. 19.21). There is a lack of maturation towards the surface, although hyperkeratosis and parakeratosis are frequently present. It resembles AIN III, often with surface keratinization. Its diagnostic importance when examining haematoxylin and eosin (H and E) stained sections of biopsies is that sometimes atypical keratinocytes in Bowen's disease are vacuolated and can resemble Paget cells. However, they are negative when stained for mucin (e.g. with Alcian blue) and low molecular weight cytokeratins. Another differential diagnosis is from melanoma. If in doubt, immunocytochemistry for S-100 or HMB45 is helpful.

When hair follicles are present these are generally involved in the dysplastic process, together with sebaceous glands, although sweat gland duct epithelium is spared. This contrasts with the distribution of abnormal epithelium in Bowenoid papulosis, from which Bowen's disease should be distinguished.

In common with Bowen's disease elsewhere, despite its pre-invasive nature, local excision tends to be curative (Ramos et al., 1983), but an internal malignancy is frequently present – in 40 per cent of cases, according to Scoma and Levy (1975).

19.4.4 Epidermodysplasia verruciformis (Bowenoid papulosis)

This is a condition in which multiple small genital and perianal papules and warty lesions appear in young adults, often with itching (Wade et al., 1979).

Biopsy is rarely performed but the histological appearances are striking and specific (Patterson et al., 1986). There is circumscribed flat acanthosis of epidermis, resembling a verruca plana (Fig. 19.22). The acanthotic epidermis shows normal maturation but scattered through all layers are numerous large, atypical keratinocytes, often in mitosis and sometimes individually keratinized. These cells stand out against the background regularity of maturing epidermis. The abnormal cells are found also in the ducts of sweat glands but not in hair follicle epithelium.

The main feature distinguishing this condition from Bowen's disease is the normal maturation and orientation of the bulk of the epidermis.

Bowenoid papulosis is associated with a large variety of papilloma virus types (Day et al., 2003b). Regression occurs, either owing to topical therapy or spontaneously. Although recurrence has been described following excision, there is no evidence of a direct association with malignancy.

19.4.5 Basal cell carcinoma

Basal cell carcinoma can occasionally develop in the perianal skin, close to the anal orifice, in common with hair-bearing skin at other sites (Wittoesch et al., 1957).

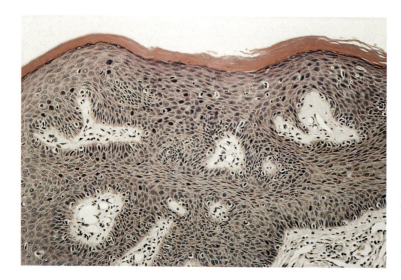

Figure 19.22 Bowenoid papulosis. The epidermis is acanthotic and hyperkeratotic. Bizarre keratinocytes with large hyperchromatic nuclei are scattered through the epidermis but overall maturation is normal.

19.4.6 Squamous carcinoma

See Section 19.3.2.

19.4.7 Keratoacanthoma

This is rare in the anal region and, when present, lies at the junction of anus with perianal skin. Rapid growth is a notable feature (Jensen and Sjolin, 1985). As with such lesions elsewhere, the diagnosis is made from examination of the overall architecture of a completely excised lesion.

A low-power appearance resembling an acorn in its cup, with 'beaking' of the edge of the overlying normal epidermis is characteristic and distinguishes keratoacanthoma from invasive squamous carcinoma (Fig. 19.23).

19.4.8 Paget's disease

This is a rare. but clinically problematical condition of perianal skin.

Characteristically, biopsy shows large vacuolated cells, often with signet ring forms, singly and in clusters in the basal and suprabasal layers of the epidermis (Fig. 19.24). Mention has been made of the histological distinction from Bowen's disease. The Paget's cells contain mucin which is stainable by

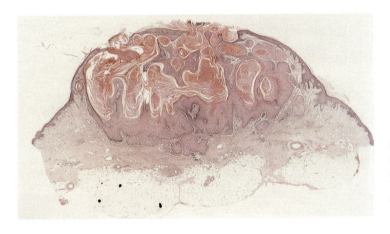

Figure 19.23 Keratoacanthoma of anus. This rapidly growing lesion has a configuration resembling an acorn in its cup, with 'beaking' of the adjacent uninvolved epidermis. There is partial 'glassy' keratinization.

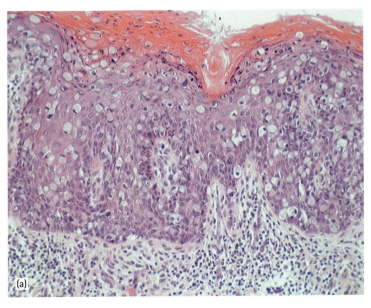

Figure 19.24 Paget's disease of anal skin. (a) This biopsy shows infiltration of the epidermis by large vacuolated cells, singly and in clusters.

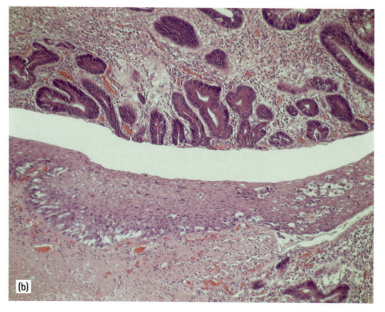

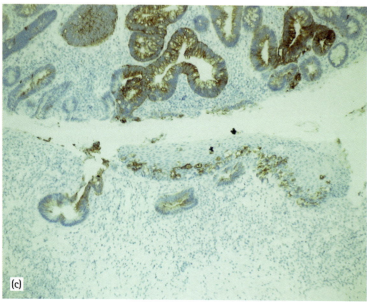

Figure 19.24 (b) Pagetoid spread into perianal skin of adenocarcinoma cells from a malignant polyp in the low rectum (partly shown in the upper half of this field). Immunocytochemistry shows the cytokeratin profile of colorectal cancer (the reverse of primary Paget's disease): (c) expression of CK20.

Alcian blue or the PAS method after diastase digestion. In common with sweat gland epithelium but unlike any other adnexal or epidermal cells Paget's cells express carcinoembryonic antigen (Nadji *et al.*, 1982).

It should be remembered that a similar appearance may be the result of downward lymphatic spread from a carcinoma of rectum (Fig 19.24b–e). Wood and Culling (1975) proposed that this eventuality could be detected by finding *O*-acetylated mucin in the abnormal cells, using the PB–KOH–PAS stain. However, the advent of cytokeratin immunohistochemistry has enabled the diagnosis to be made more conveniently (Table 18.1). Cells derived from sweat gland epithelium are usually CK7-positive and CK20-negative, whereas cells of colorectal

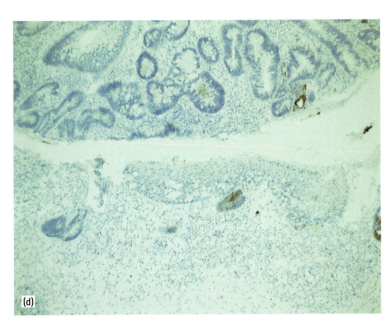

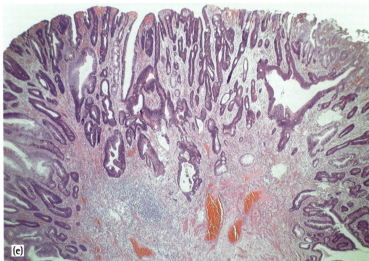

Figure 19.24 (d) no expression of CK7. (e) Examination of the locally excised rectal tubular adenoma reveals a focus of early adenocarcinoma.

adenocarcinomas are typically CK7-negative and CK20-positive (Fig 19.24c,d). It is of interest that the cells of some adenocarcinomas of the low rectum and upper anal canal are both CK7-positive and CK20-positive.

We have seen examples of perianal 'Paget's disease' presenting before the subsequent discovery of a low rectal adenomatous polyp containing a small focus of early adenocarcinoma (Fig 19.24b–e).

Although there is more usually an association with an underlying sweat gland carcinoma it may be many years before such a tumour becomes evident. In any case, extensive local excision of the perianal skin must be recommended.

19.4.9 Adenoma of apocrine gland

This is a small rounded mobile dermal nodule arising in anogenital sweat glands of middle-aged women. Histologically it shows the characteristic

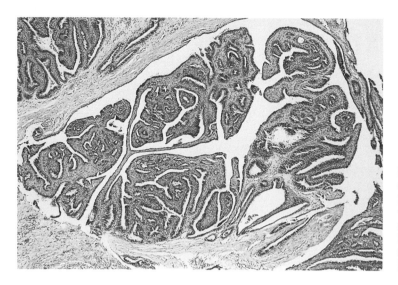

Figure 19.25 Adenoma of apocrine gland. This biopsy of a lesion at the anal margin, shows the nodular and papillary architecture of this circumscribed lesion. The tubules are branched and arborized and lined by a double layer of epithelium.

circumscribed papillary and glandular structure of a hidradenoma papilliferum (Meeker *et al.*, 1962), often with prominent apocrine type epithelium (Fig. 19.25). The cells stain with mucin stains.

REFERENCES

Ackerman, L.V. (1948) Verrucous carcinoma of the oral cavity. *Surgery*, 23, 670–8.

Bogomoletz, W.V., Potet, F., Molas, G. (1985) Condyloma acuminata, giant condyloma acuminatum (Buschke–Loewenstein tumour) and verrucous squamous carcinoma of the perianal and anorectal region: a continuous pre-cancerous spectrum? *Histopathology*, 9, 1115–69.

Bataille, F., Klebl, F., Rummele, P. *et al.* (2004) Morphological characterisation of Crohn's disease fistulae. *Gut*, 53, 1314–21.

Boshart, M., zur Hausen, H. (1986) Human papillomaviruses in Buschke–Lowenstein tumors: physical state of the DNA and identification of a tandem duplication in the noncoding region of a human papillomavirus 6 subtype. *J. Virol.*, 58, 963–6.

Cuesta, K.H., Palazzo, J.P., Mittal, K.R. (1998) Detection of human papillomavirus in verrucous carcinoma from HIV-seropositive patients. *J. Cutan. Pathol.*, 25, 165–70.

Culp, C.E. (1983) Chronic hidradenitis suppurativa of the anal canal. A surgical skin disease. *Dis. Col. Rectum*, 26, 669–76.

Daling, J.R., Weiss, N.S., Hislop, T.G. *et al.* (1987) Sexual practices, sexually transmitted diseases, and the incidence of anal cancer. *N. Engl. J. Med.*, 317, 973–7.

Day, D.W., Jass, J.R., Price, A.B. *et al.* (2003a) Lymphogranuloma venereum. In: *Morson and Dawson's gastrointestinal pathology*, 4th edn. Oxford: Blackwell Science, p. 480.

Day, D.W., Jass, J.R., Price, A.B. *et al.* (2003b) Tumours and tumour-like lesions of the anal region. In: *Morson and Dawson's gastrointestinal pathology*, 4th edn. Oxford: Blackwell Science, pp. 653–71.

Dougherty, B.G., Evans, H.L. (1985) Carcinoma of the anal canal: a study of 79 cases. *Am. J. Clin. Pathol.*, 83, 159–64.

Dyson, J.L., Walker, P.G., Singer, A. (1984) Human papillomavirus infection of the uterine cervix: histological appearances in 28 cases identified by immuno-histochemical techniques. *J. Clin. Pathol.*, 37, 126–30.

Elder, D., Elenitsas, R., Jaworsky, C., Johnson, B. Jr. (1997a) Follicular occlusion triad. In: *Lever's histopathology of the skin*, 8th edn.

Philadelphia and New York: Lippincott–Raven, pp. 461–2.

Elder, D., Elenitsas, R., Jaworsky, C., Johnson, B. Jr. (1997b) Lichen sclerosus et atrophicus. In: *Lever's histopathology of the skin*, 8th edn. Philadelphia and New York: Lippincott–Raven, pp. 280–3.

Eng, L.F., Bigbee, J.W. (1978) Immunohistochemistry of nervous system – specific antigens. *Adv. Neurochem.*, 3, 43.

Fenger, C. (1997) Anal canal. In: Sternberg, S.S. (ed.) *Histology for pathologists*, 4th edn. Philadelphia: Lippincott–Raven, pp. 551–71.

Fenger, C., Nielsen, V.T. (1985) Systematic histological investigation for squamous dysplasia in the anal canal. *Br. J. Surg.*, 72 (Suppl.), S134 (Abstract).

Fenger, C., Frisch, M., Marti, M.C., Parc, R. (2000) Verrucous carcinoma. In: Hamilton, S.R., Aaltonen, L.A. (eds) *Pathology and genetics of tumours of the digestive system.* Lyon: IARC Press, p. 149.

Fetissof, F., Dubois, M.P., Assan, R., Arbeille-Brassart, B., Baroudi, A., Tharanne, M.J., Jobard, P. (1984) Endocrine cells in the anal canal. *Virchows Arch. A.*, 404, 39–47.

Fogler, R., Lanter, B., Stern, G., Weiner, E. (1977) Mucoepidermoid carcinoma in an anal fistula with associated carcinoma in a villous adenoma of the descending colon: report of a case. *Dis. Col. Rectum*, 20, 428–35.

Frisch, M., Olsen, J.H., Bautz, A., Melbye, M. (1994) Benign anal lesions and the risk of anal cancer. *N. Engl. J. Med.*, 331, 300–2.

Frisch, M., Glimelius, B., van den Brule, A.J. *et al.* (1998a) Benign anal lesions, inflammatory bowel disease and risk for high-risk human papillomavirus-positive and -negative anal carcinoma. *Br. J. Cancer*, 78, 1534–8.

Frisch, M., Fenger, C., Glimelius, B. *et al.* (1998b) Variants of squamous cell carcinoma and perianal skin and their relation to human papillomaviruses. *Cancer Res.*, 59, 753–7.

Gatter, K.C., Ralfkiaer, E., Skinner, J. *et al.* (1985) An immunocytochemical study of malignant melanoma and its differential diagnosis from other malignant tumours. *J. Clin. Pathol.*, 38, 1353–7.

Helwig, E.B. (1983) Neoplasms of the anus. In: Norris, H.T. (ed.) *Pathology of the colon, small intestine and anus.* New York, Edinburgh, London, Melbourne: Churchill Livingstone, pp. 303–27.

Hill, S.A., Coghill, S.B. (1986) Human papillomavirus in squamous carcinoma of anus. *Lancet*, ii, 1333.

Hobbs, C.M., Lowry, M.A., Owen, D., Sobin, L.H. (2001) Anal gland carcinoma. *Cancer*, 92, 2045–9.

Hyacinthe, M., Karl, R., Coppola, D. *et al.* (1998) Squamous-cell carcinoma of the pelvis in a giant condyloma acuminatum: use of neo-adjuvant chemoradiation and surgical resection: report of a case. *Dis. Col. Rectum*, 41, 1450–3.

Jensen, S.L., Sjolin, K-E. (1985) Keratoacanthoma of the anus. Report of three cases. *Dis. Col. Rectum*, 28, 743–5.

Johnston, J., Helwig, E.B. (1981) Granular cell tumors of the gastrointestinal tract and perianal region. A study of 74 cases. *Dig. Dis. Sci.*, 26, 807–16.

Lobert, P.F., Appelman, H.D. (1981) Inflammatory cloacogenic polyp. A unique inflammatory lesion of the anal transitional zone. *Am. J. Surg. Pathol.*, 5, 761–6.

McCance, D.J., Lowe, D., Simmons, P., Thomson, P.S. (1986) Human papilloma virus in condyloma accuminata of the anus. *J. Clin. Pathol.*, 39, 927.

McKee, P.H. (1989a) Hidradenitis suppurativa. In: *Pathology of the skin.* Philadelphia: J.B. Lippincott Co., pp. 423–5.

McKee, P.H. (1989b). Lichen sclerosus et atrophicus. In: *Pathology of the skin.* Philadelphia: J.B. Lippincott Co., pp. 1127–30.

Meeker, J.H., Neubecker, R.D., Helwig, E.B. (1962) Hidradenoma papilliferum. *Am. J. Clin. Pathol.*, 37, 182–95.

Morson, B.C. (1959) The pathology and results of treatment of cancer of the anal region. *Proc. R. Soc. Med.*, 52 (Suppl.), 117–18.

Nadji, M., Morales, A.R., Cirtanner, R.E., Ziegels-Weissman, J., Penneys, N.S. (1982) Paget's disease of skin: a unifying concept of histogenesis. *Cancer*, 50, 2203–6.

Palefsky, J. (1995) Human papillomavirus-associated malignancies in HIV-positive men and women. *Curr. Opin. Oncol.*, 7, 437–41.

Pang, L.S.C., Morson, B.C. (1967) Basaloid carcinoma of the anal canal. *J. Clin. Pathol.*, 20, 128–35.

Patterson, J.W., Kao, G.F., Graham, J.H., Helwig, E.B. (1986) Bowenoid papulosis. A clinico-pathologic study with ultrastructural observations. *Cancer*, 57, 823–36.

Prioleau, P.G., Santa Cruz, D.J., Meyer, J.S. (1980) Verrucous carcinoma. A light and electron microscopic, autoradiographic and immunofluorescence study. *Cancer*, 45, 2849–57.

Ramos, R., Salinas, H., Tucker, L. (1983) Conservative approach to the treatment of Bowen's disease of the anus. *Dis. Col. Rectum*, 26, 712–15.

Rando, R.F., Sedlacek, T.V., Hunt, J., Jenson, A.B., Kurman, R.J., Lancaster, W.D. (1986) Verrucous carcinoma of the vulva associated with an unusual type 6 human papillomavirus. *Obstet. Gynecol.*, 67, 70S–5S.

Richens, J. (1992) The diagnosis and treatment of Donovanosis (granuloma inguinale). *Genitourin. Med.*, 32, 441–52.

Sawyers, J.L. (1972) Squamous cell carcinoma of the perianus and anus. *Surg. Clin. N. Am.*, 52, 935–41.

Scoma, J.A., Levy, E.I. (1975) Bowen's disease of the anus. *Dis. Col. Rectum*, 18, 137–40.

Singh, R., Nime, F., Mittelman, A. (1981) Malignant epithelial tumors of the anal canal. *Cancer*, 48, 411–15.

Wade, T.R., Kopf, A.W., Ackerman, A.B. (1979) Bowenoid papulosis of the genitalia. *Arch. Derm.*, 115, 306–8.

Wafai, M., Mohit, P. (1983) Granuloma of the anal canal due to *Enterobius vermicularis*. Report of a case. *Dis. Col. Rectum*, 26, 349–50.

Wanebo, H.J., Woodruff, J.M., Farr, G.H., Quan, S.H. (1981) Anorectal melanoma. *Cancer*, 47, 1891–1900.

Wellman, K.F. (1962) Adenocarcinoma of anal duct origin. *Can. J. Surg.*, 5, 311–18.

Williams, G.R., Talbot, I.C. (1994) Anal carcinoma – a histological review. *Histopathology*, 25, 507–16.

Winkelman, J., Grosfeld, J., Bigelow, B. (1964) Colloid carcinoma of anal gland origin. Report of a case and review of the literature. *Am. J. Clin. Pathol.*, 42, 395–401.

Wittoesch, J.H., Woolner, L.S., Jackson, R.J. (1957) Basal cell epithelioma and basaloid lesions of the anus. *Surg. Gynecol. Obstet.*, 104, 75–80.

Wood, W.S., Culling, W.G. (1975) Perianal Paget disease. *Arch. Pathol. Lab. Med.*, 99, 442–5.

CHAPTER 20

MISCELLANEOUS CONDITIONS

20.1	Angiodysplasia and other primary vascular lesions	377
	20.1.1 Angiodysplasia	377
	20.1.2 Connective tissue diseases	379
	20.1.3 Behçet's syndrome	379
20.2	Cystic pneumatosis (pneumatosis cystoides intestinalis, pneumatosis coli)	380
20.3	Malakoplakia	380
20.4	Chronic granulomatous disease of childhood	381
20.5	Whipple's disease	382
20.6	Sarcoidosis	382
20.7	Ceroid lipofuscinosis (including Batten's disease)	383
20.8	Amyloidosis	383
20.9	Cronkhite–Canada syndrome	385
20.10	Mucoviscidosis (cystic fibrosis)	386
20.11	Colitis cystica profunda	386
20.12	Endometriosis	387
20.13	Primary immunodeficiency syndromes	387
20.14	Irritable bowel syndrome	388
20.15	Brown bowel syndrome	389
References		389

20.1 ANGIODYSPLASIA AND OTHER PRIMARY VASCULAR LESIONS

20.1.1 Angiodysplasia

Angiodysplasia is alleged to be the commonest vascular malformation in the gastrointestinal tract (Gordon et al., 2001). It is usually regarded as a disease of the elderly (Boley et al., 1977), although this view has been challenged (Danesh et al., 1987), and of the right colon. It rivals diverticular disease as a major cause of bleeding. Its aetiology is unknown but the most acceptable theory to date is that it is a degenerative lesion resulting from chronic low-grade obstruction of submucosal veins due to continued high tension in the wall of the caecum and proximal right colon (Boley et al., 1977). The tension in the bowel wall is greatest in the segment with the greatest diameter. Lesions are almost invariably found directly opposite the ileo-caecal valve (Hemingway and Allison, 1986). However, angiodysplasias can also be scattered along the colon (Ottenjann et al., 1984) and, indeed, elsewhere in the gastrointestinal tract (Price, 1986), or even just confined to the appendix (Kyokane et al., 2001). They sometimes occur in younger patients (Allison and Hemingway, 1981) and may be asymptomatic and found incidentally at colonoscopy (Richter et al., 1984). There is a puzzling association with aortic stenosis (Galloway et al., 1974).

The term angiodysplasia may be defined as ectasia of the normal pre-existing colonic submucosal

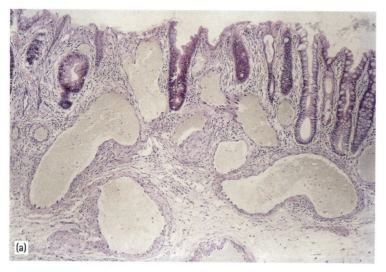

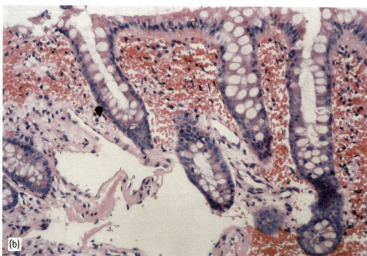

Figure 20.1 Angiodysplasia. (a) Colectomy specimen. Examination of the colon after injection of aqueous barium suspension into the veins revealed this lesion, showing the enormously dilated blood capillaries in the mucosa, displacing crypts and tortuous venous channels in the submucosa. (b) Endoscopic biopsy of a mucosal vascular ectasia from the right colon. The delicate sinusoidal vascular channels in the mucosa rarely survive biopsy and tissue processing as well as this.

veins with or without ectasia of overlying mucosal capillaries (Boley *et al.*, 1977). It is this variability in the presence of a mucosal abnormality that presents the problem in biopsy diagnosis.

The biopsy may show a cluster of large mucosal capillaries distorting the crypt architecture (Stamm *et al.*, 1985). If submucosa is included, classically, a thin-walled vein should be seen feeding the mucosal capillaries (Fig. 20.1).

There are two problems. First, the difficulty in obtaining a satisfactory biopsy from sponge-like mucosa and second, the distinction between congested and truly ectatic vessels. No easy distinguishing criteria exist. Furthermore, there may not be a cluster of mucosal vessels (Pounder *et al.*, 1982), but simply one or two and, indeed, the definition as given earlier does not require a mucosal element at all. On biopsy evidence alone, the mucosal lesion of angiodysplasia cannot be distinguished from a capillary haemangioma or the vascular lesion of the solitary ulcer syndrome (Fig. 3.54 on page 48). Interpretation of large submucosal vessels is, again, fraught with difficulty because of the wide normal range (Price, 1986).

Many of the problems are resolved by considering radiological and endoscopic findings. The diagnostic sequence of events usually begins with a characteristic picture on angiography, followed by the finding at endoscopy of a cherry-red lesion with a raised central vessel and peripheral flare (Danesh et al., 1987). When the colonoscopist is confident that the appearances are typical, it is common practice to coagulate the lesion without the need for biopsy (Boley and Brandt, 1986). Biopsy may only substantiate the diagnosis in up to 50 per cent of cases, presumably owing to sampling difficulties (Howard et al., 1982).

20.1.2 Connective tissue diseases

In diseases such as rheumatoid arthritis (RA), systemic sclerosis, ankylosing spondylitis, dermatomyositis, systemic lupus erythematosus (SLE), Wegener's granulomatosis and polyarteritis nodosa (PAN), a vasculitis may cause ischaemic colitis (Section 10.8) and occasionally, ischaemic proctitis. With systemic sclerosis there is a mucoid intimal thickening of arteries and the circular muscle of the bowel wall appears to be selectively affected by fibrosis and elastosis (Day et al., 2003a). In the rare instances in which there is colonic involvement due to PAN, the histology reveals the characteristic thickening of the arterioles in the submucosal layer (Day et al., 2003b); perforation secondary to PAN has been described (Burke et al., 1995). The involvement of the colon by Wegener's granulomatosis affects the mucosa in 50 per cent of the cases (Storesund et al., 1998). Ankylosing spondylitis can cause a lymphocytic infiltration in the lamina propria and intraepithelial infiltration (Lamarque et al., 2003). An association between Crohn's disease and SLE has also been described (Nishida et al., 1998).

The inflammatory changes occur in the terminal ileum and colon in patients with RA (Bjarnason et al., 1984), and are demonstrable in ileo-caecal biopsies at colonoscopy (Mielants et al., 1985; Cuvelier et al., 1987). The biopsy features are non-specific, including variously shaped ulcerative lesions, centred around the left hemicolon, with luminal narrowing (Nagahama et al., 2000), and may in part result from the non-steroidal anti-inflammatory drugs (NSAIDs) invariably given to these patients (Section 11.4.5). However, in the series of Cuvelier et al. (1987) the ileo-caecitis was restricted to patients with reactive arthritis rather than rheumatoid arthritis and not believed to be drug related. In some, granulomas were found and the features were indistinguishable from Crohn's disease.

20.1.3 Behçet's syndrome

This multisystem disorder is characterized by buccal and genital ulceration, eye lesions and skin lesions. These basic abnormalities may be accompanied by a host of others which include gastrointestinal problems, with the ileo-caecum and colon the most frequent extra-oral sites of gastrointestinal involvement (Bayraktar et al., 2000). Because of the variability in presentation it is considered a syndrome rather than a disease (Walport, 1984). In the gut, the commonest pattern, described particularly in Japan, is of localized penetrating ulcers in the ileo-caecal region, which frequently perforate (Shimizu et al., 1979; Kasahara et al., 1981; Lakhanpal et al., 1985). Using colonoscopy, three types of ulceration are recognized: geographic, aphthous and volcano-like. The last of these is associated with a less favourable response to medical treatment, a more frequent requirement for surgery, and more frequent recurrences (Kim et al. 2000). A tendency for development at sites of surgical anastomosis is also reported (Lee et al., 2001). When the whole of the colon and rectum is involved (Smith et al., 1973), a pattern more frequently described in the West, the problem then becomes one of distinction from ulcerative colitis and Crohn's disease (O'Duffy et al., 1971). This will not be possible by biopsy alone, as the histological features can include normal mucosa, actively inflamed mucosa, granulation tissue (from the ulcer floor) (Leonard et al., 1998) and even granulomas (Baba et al., 1976). In view of the last feature, and the tendency for there to be small intestinal involvement, transmural lesions and skip areas, it is unlikely that the intestinal manifestation of Behçet's syndrome is a variant of ulcerative colitis (O'Connell et al., 1980), although this rare association has been reported (Kobashigawa et al., 2004). The precise relationship with Crohn's disease remains a dilemma: Behçet's syndrome can simulate Crohn's disease macroscopically (Masugi *et al.*, 1994) or, it is claimed, even be associated with it (Tolia *et al.*, 1989). Such claims hinge on questions of definition and semantics. This overlap of histological features emphasizes, yet again, the need for the integration of all clinical data for the accurate classification of inflammatory bowel disease. Vasculitis is a feature of the cutaneous manifestations of Behçet's syndrome and infiltration of venules by lymphocytes ('lymphocytic venulitis'), a useful sign, has been described throughout the colon, even away from sites of ulceration (Lee, 1986).

20.2 CYSTIC PNEUMATOSIS (PNEUMATOSIS CYSTOIDES INTESTINALIS, PNEUMATOSIS COLI)

This is a condition in which large gas-filled cysts accumulate in the large intestine. The cysts contain air and may occupy any layer of the bowel wall, although the submucosa is most frequently involved (Gagliardi *et al.*, 1996). A large mass may develop, but intestinal obstruction is rare (Soutter *et al.*, 1985). Patients may complain of abdominal pain or mucous diarrhoea, but the condition is frequently symptomless and found only on barium enema or endoscopy for another obstructive or inflammatory disease (Koss, 1952). The endoscopic appearance may resemble clusters of pale, smooth-surfaced polyps, often with red, inflamed overlying mucosa. When clinically suspected, radiography and computed tomography are the best diagnostic tests (St Peter *et al.*, 2003). Any part of the small bowel or colon can be affected, in children or adults (Galandiuk and Fazio, 1986). The rectum is rarely involved (Gagliardi *et al.*, 1996). When acute complications appear, such as perforation and peritonitis, surgery is indicated (St Peter *et al.*, 2003). Cystic pneumatosis carries a bad prognosis when associated with gynaecological malignancies (Horowitz *et al.*, 2002).

Histologically, the cysts are often incomplete and collapsed, having been cut into and ruptured at the biopsy procedure. This can be accompanied by a popping noise. The cysts are usually lined by a rim of pale foamy histiocytes and foreign-body-type giant cells (Fig. 3.58) which tend to protrude into the lumen. This is in contrast to the flattened macrophages lining the fluid-filled cysts in oleogranulomas (Fig. 11.5). Cysts without a histiocytic lining are sometimes found and Whitehead (1985) suggests that these are early lesions. From observations on our own cases, the crypts overlying submucosal cysts can show irregularity. This could be a misleading sign unless the biopsy includes adequate submucosa.

Although there is evidence that cystic pneumatosis can develop as a result of air passing into the mediastinum following rupture of an emphysematous bulla and dissecting down into the retroperitoneal soft tissues (Keyting *et al.*, 1961), it is likely that the gas is more usually the result of local bacterial action (Yale *et al.*, 1974; Read *et al.*, 1984). Experimentally, intestinal *Clostridium perfringens* produces cystic pneumatosis in the germ-free rat. Yale and Balish (1985) postulate that the same mechanism applies in humans and cystic pneumatosis has been reported as a complication of pseudomembranous colitis (Kreiss *et al.*, 1999). Pieterse *et al.* (1985) have proposed a sequence of events beginning with crypt rupture and giant cell formation (Fig. 3.40 on page 40), followed by local gas production, with vesicle formation, as in pseudolipomatosis (Section 3.8.12), and eventual coalescence of cysts to produce the fully developed picture of pneumatosis. The process can presumably be subclinical. Cystic pneumatosis is known to develop in children following overt enterocolitis (Gruenberg *et al.*, 1979).

The cysts seem to appear and disappear spontaneously and can be made to shrink when the patient breathes 70 per cent oxygen for a prolonged period (Forgacs *et al.*, 1973).

20.3 MALAKOPLAKIA

Malakoplakia is characterized by the presence of sheets of loosely arranged large, pale-staining macrophages, often containing sharply defined spherical haematoxyphilic cytoplasmic granules

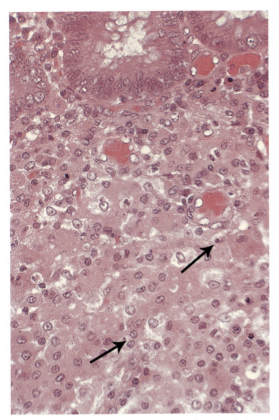

Figure 20.2 Malakoplakia. The mucosa is expanded by a sheet of large pale macrophages, many of which contain calcific Michaelis–Guttmann bodies (arrowed). From a patient with ulcerative colitis.

(Michaelis–Gutmann bodies) (Fig. 20.2). This is a rare finding, but is occasionally seen locally in relation to adenocarcinomas (Finlay-Jones et al., 1968; Moran et al., 1989; Sandmeier and Guillou, 1993; Bates et al., 1997; Pillay and Chetty, 2002) or diffusely, in chronic debilitating diseases including ulcerative colitis (Ng and Ng, 1993). This is in association with abnormal macrophages and impaired T-lymphocyte function (MacKay, 1978). An association with Hodgkin's disease has also been reported (Yang et al., 1983). The infiltrate can involve any layer of the bowel and may be the cause of bulky irregular thickening of the mucosa or of the whole bowel wall. The Michaelis–Guttmann bodies are periodic acid–Schiff (PAS)-positive and have been shown to contain calcium, phosphate and

sometimes iron (Underwood et al., 1982). They appear to form in lysosomes in relation to disintegrating bacilli, possibly Escherichia coli (Chaudhry et al., 1980). Malakoplakia appears to be the result of bacterial infection in circumstances of defective lysosomal function (Stevens and McClure, 1982).

The histological diagnosis in biopsy material is important, as clinically the lesion can mimic other diseases. Radiologically, malakoplakia shows features of polyps, bulky tumour-like masses, mucosal ulceration and fistulae (Radin et al., 1984).

20.4 CHRONIC GRANULOMATOUS DISEASE OF CHILDHOOD

Chronic granulomatous disease of childhood (CGDC) is one of the primary phagocytic disorders of childhood, caused by an X-linked genetic disorder (Segal and Holland, 2000). It results from a defect in any of the four subunits of NADPH oxidase and is characterized by recurrent life-threatening bacterial and fungal infections and abnormal tissue granuloma formation (Segal et al., 2000). Owing to a defect in electron transport resulting in lack of lysosomal production of hydrogen peroxide, neutrophil polymorphs are unable to destroy pyogenic bacteria (Segal, 1985). Secondary accumulation of vacuolated and pigmented histiocytes occurs in many tissues. Children with this condition often develop steatorrhoea, with or without diarrhoea.

Rectal biopsy (Ament and Ochs, 1973) shows large histiocytes in the lamina propria, with ample, finely vacuolated cytoplasm (Fig. 20.3). These cells contain brownish-yellow pigment which, on frozen section, stains positively with PAS, fat stains and Luxol fast blue, suggestive of lipochrome (glycolipid or phospholipid). Inflammatory cells may be present in increased numbers and multinucleate giant cells are sometimes found, giving a truly granulomatous appearance. The numbers of vacuolated histiocytes are said to be fewer than in Whipple's disease.

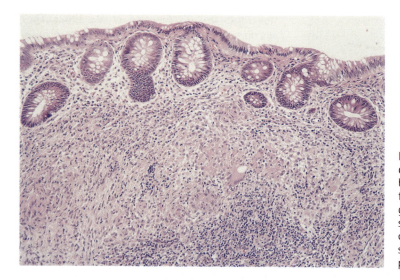

Figure 20.3 Chronic granulomatous disease of childhood. In this rectal biopsy there are collections of pale foamy histiocytes from confluent granulomas in the mucosa and submucosa. Multinucleate giant cells are present. There is a sprinkling of lymphocytes and plasma cells.

20.5 WHIPPLE'S DISEASE

This rare bacterial infection may lead to rectal biopsy for investigation of a patient with persistent diarrhoea. Although the disease predominantly affects the small intestine and lymph nodes, there may be clinical proctitis, with variable histological features (Yardley and Donowitz, 1977), and even concomitant oesophageal involvement (Marcial and Villafana, 1997).

The diagnosis should be suspected if foamy macrophages, resembling muciphages, are unusually prominent in the superficial part of the lamina propria. Staining with Alcian blue/PAS shows large numbers of intact and fragmented PAS-positive bacilliform organisms, concentrated within these cells. They are also present in other cells of the lamina propria and scattered extracellularly. The ultrastructural features of the macrophages have been documented by Watson and Haubrich (1969) and the ultrastructural features of the bacilli documented by Dobbins and Kawanishi (1981). The organism has been identified by polymerase chain reaction (PCR) as an actinomycete-like bacillus and has been named *Tropheryma whippeli* (Relman *et al.*, 1992). It is now known that the diagnosis of Whipple's disease is a multifaceted one, and can be supported by culture, immunohistochemistry and PCR analysis (Ratnaike, 2000; Fenollar and Raoult, 2001).

It is important to realize that limited numbers of intramucosal muciphages, resembling Whipple's cells, are seen both in normal mucosa and incidentally, during the course of other inflammatory conditions (Section 3.8.9). Very similar cells are seen in acquired immune-deficiency syndrome (AIDS) patients infected by *Mycobacterium avium* (Hamrock *et al.*, 1999) (Section 4.4.4). Occasionally in Whipple's disease, the muciphages may be sparse and there is a pattern of gut involvement that includes fibrosis, arteritis and vascular intimal proliferation (James *et al.*, 1984). From a purely histological viewpoint, a firm diagnosis depends on the examination of a small intestinal biopsy.

20.6 SARCOIDOSIS

In patients with sarcoidosis it has been shown that the gastrointestinal tract in general (Sprague *et al.*, 1984) and the rectal mucosa in particular may be the site of small non-caseating granulomas resembling those seen in Crohn's disease (Tobi *et al.*, 1982; Dumot *et al.*, 1998). These lesions are non-progressive and are usually incidental findings in an otherwise normal mucosa, not giving rise to symptoms; however, instances of rectal mass formation (Zech *et al.*, 1993) and obstruction (Hilzenrat *et al.*, 1995) have been reported. An example of colonic sarcoidosis mimicking polyposis has been recorded by Veitch and Badger (2004). An association of gastrointestinal sarcoidosis with malignant lymphoma and protein-losing enteropathy has been described by Godeau *et al.* (1992).

As well as reviewing six case reports and describing one further example, Tobi *et al.* (1982), recommend the use of rectal biopsy as a possible alternative to the Kveim test to confirm a suspected diagnosis of sarcoidosis.

Finally, it must be said that sarcoid-like granulomas may be present due to a different aetiology, for example, in reaction to diverticulitis (Naschitz *et al.*, 1990).

20.7 CEROID LIPOFUSCINOSIS (INCLUDING BATTEN'S DISEASE)

This is an ill-defined group of rapidly progressive congenital diseases, affecting mental and neurological function, characterized by accumulation of ceroid lipofuscin in nerve cells, Schwann cells and smooth muscle. The material is most readily found in the myenteric ganglia of Auerbach's plexus and full-thickness rectal biopsy is therefore required

(Brett and Lake, 1975). Frozen sections are preferable if fat stains (Fig. 20.4a) or autofluorescence are to be used, but the coarse granular material does resist processing into paraffin wax and can be identified with PAS and long Ziehl–Neelsen (ZN) as well as Sudan black (Lake, 1976). Electron-dense curvilinear cytoplasmic bodies seen on electron microscopy are diagnostic (Fig. 20.4b).

Different variants of the disease present in early infancy, late infancy, pre-adolescent juveniles and young adults. Their biopsy features are indistinguishable. The late-infantile (Batten–Bielschowsky–Jansky) form is the most common (Adams and Lyon, 1982). An adult form (Kufs disease) is reported to have been diagnosed by the finding of vascular and perivascular lipofuscin deposits and the ultrastructural curvilinear bodies in rectal biopsies (Gelot *et al.*, 1998; Pasquinelli *et al.*, 2004).

20.8 AMYLOIDOSIS

Amyloid, a fibrillar protein folded as a characteristic β-pleated sheet (Pepys, 2001), is found on the basement membrane of small submucosal blood vessels in rectal biopsies in 84 per cent of all patients with amyloidosis (Kyle, 1975). Histologically, no

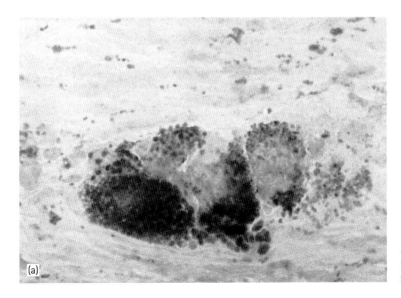

(a)

Figure 20.4 Lipofuscinosis (Batten's disease). (a) Submucosal ganglion cells packed with granular storage material (unfixed cryostat section, Sudan black ×1165).

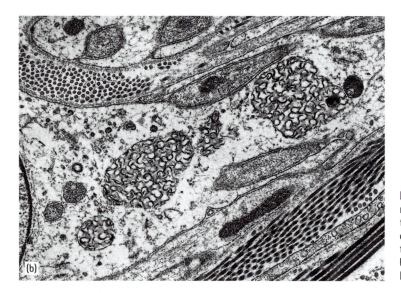

Figure 20.4 (b) Electron micrograph of Schwann cells from the submucosal plexus showing the curvilinear bodies characteristic of this group of diseases. (Photographs by courtesy of Professor Brian Lake, Institute of Child Health, London.)

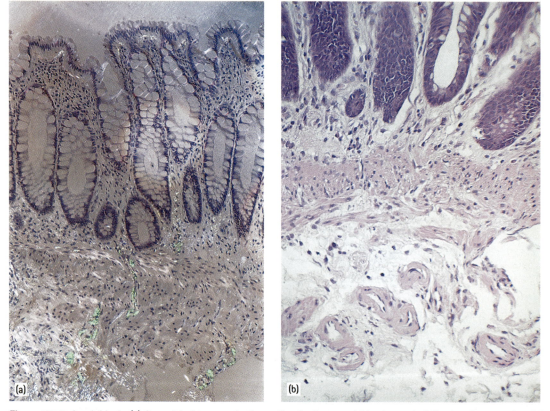

Figure 20.5 Amyloidosis. (a) Green birefringence in the walls of submucosal blood vessels following Congo red staining can sometimes be seen in the absence of a detectable abnormality in routine sections. (b) Thickening of submucosal arteriolar walls caused by amyloid deposition (haematoxylin and eosin).

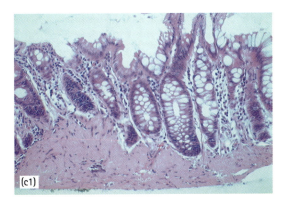

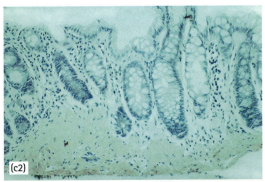

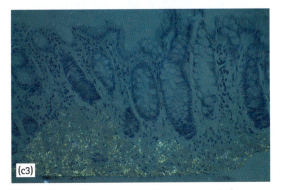

Figure 20.5 (c) Amyloid deposition in muscularis mucosae: (c1) haematoxylin and eosin; (c2) Congo red; (c3) polarized Congo red.

amyloid deposition there may be overt thickening of the walls of the blood vessels (Fig. 20.5b), of crypt basement membrane and even of the muscularis mucosae (Fig. 20.5c). Deposition beneath the surface epithelium may cause confusion with collagenous colitis.

In general, different types of amyloid lead to different patterns of deposition. The systemic reactive type of amyloidosis (AA) is more likely to show deposition in the mucosa and submucosa, while AL and AH amyloid deposition, associated with immunocytic dyscrasias, is more often found in the muscle layers, and thus is less likely to be detected by endoscopic biopsy (Tada *et al.*, 1993). Any AA amyloid can be identified by its lability when Congo red-stained sections are treated with potassium permanganate (Wright *et al.*, 1977). Senile amyloidosis tends to be found in the superficial vessels and the submucosa (Rocken *et al.*, 1994); dialysis-associated amyloid deposition occurs more in the submucosa and muscularis propria. On rare occasions, the excessive deposition leads to amyloid tumours (Deans *et al.*, 1995).

Amyloidosis may be responsible for impaired motility (Kumar *et al.*, 1983) and for ischaemia. However, it is important to remember that in many patients with amyloidosis no deposits are detectable in the mucosa. It is therefore essential that rectal biopsies taken for the diagnosis of amyloid disease should include an adequate amount of submucosa (Wegelius and Pasternack, 1976). Rectal biopsy tissue is often unsuitable for electron microscopic examination for amyloid material, owing to the difficulty of sampling the sparsely arranged submucosal blood vessels in small resin blocks.

abnormality may be visible in haematoxylin and eosin (H and E) sections, but typically, there is staining of the walls of submucosal blood vessels by Congo red, which is dichroic and shows green birefringence when examined with crossed polarizing filters (Fig. 20.5a), or is positive for the serum amyloid P component (a member of the non-fibrillar pentraxin plasma protein family) (Hirschfield, 2004) antibody by immunohistochemistry. In heavy

20.9 CRONKHITE–CANADA SYNDROME

This is a rare disease of the gastrointestinal tract, skin, hair and nails, occurring in middle-aged and elderly subjects (Manousos and Webster, 1966). Diarrhoea tends to be the major symptom, although the stomach and small intestine are also involved.

The large intestinal mucosa is characteristically diffusely thickened and nodular, owing to oedema of the lamina propria and cystic dilatation of glands (Fig. 15.34). There is also a variable infiltrate of plasma cells and eosinophils. Polymorphs may be present in the lumina of the glands. Sometimes the nodular thickening is polypoid and the condition must then be distinguished from multiple juvenile polyposis or the Peutz–Jeghers syndrome (Sections 15.7 and 15.8). The glandular epithelium is atrophic rather than hyperplastic (Jenkins *et al.*, 1985) and shows no dysplastic features. A total of 31 cases of colorectal carcinoma in patients with Cronkhite–Canada syndrome have been reported (Yashiro *et al.*, 2004). The latter authors postulate that there is a serrated adenoma-carcinoma sequence in such patients.

Cronkhite–Canada syndrome is an acquired condition, of obscure aetiology, possibly resulting from failure of normal crypt cell proliferation (Freeman *et al.*, 1985). It is possible that the atrophic but polypoid mucosa represents disordered epithelial cell proliferation mediated by damage to the pericrypt sheath, which has features in common with dermal perifollicular damage, and damage to the nail beds. It may be the result of an autoimmune state.

20.10 MUCOVISCIDOSIS (CYSTIC FIBROSIS)

The viscous mucus in this condition accumulates in the crypts of the large intestinal mucosa, resulting in a characteristic picture of multiple distended glands filled with lamellated eosinophilic material. Goblet cells are unusually prominent, apparently 'crowding out' the columnar cells (Parkins *et al.*, 1963). There is a scanty and variable polymorph infiltrate, but crypt abscesses are not seen. It is of interest that the glycoprotein content of the mucus and its export from the cell are normal (Neutra *et al.*, 1977) and the fault presumably lies in the protein core of the mucins.

Affected children may present with meconium ileus equivalent, intussusception, volvulus or rectal prolapse (Eggermont, 1996). Fibrosing colonopathy can develop in the right colon, but is not amenable to biopsy and is rare now that high dose pancreatic supplements are not given (Pawel *et al.*, 1997).

Although not the usual method for primary diagnosis in this condition, the features are sufficiently specific for rectal biopsy to be useful, particularly in patients presenting at an older age (Matseshe *et al.*, 1977). Multiple sequential biopsies may have to be examined, however, before the typical features are found.

20.11 COLITIS CYSTICA PROFUNDA

Colitis cystica profunda is the term applied to the presence of glands lined by columnar and goblet cells below the muscularis mucosae (Fig. 20.6). The glands are characteristically accompanied by lamina propria and show no dysplastic features. However, since they are often distended by mucus and may lie quite deeply, only small portions of epithelium may be included in a biopsy. Care may then be needed to distinguish the condition from cystic pneumatosis (Section 20.2). Three patterns of clinical presentation are described (Bentley *et al.*, 1985): (1) a rectal mass, which may mimic an obstructing carcinoma (Nielson *et al.*, 1984); (2) segmental lesions at various sites; and (3) diffuse involvement of lengths of bowel.

The misplaced glands form either from downgrowth of epithelium during regeneration in the healing of deeply penetrating ulceration or from deep-lying crypts in lymphoid-glandular complexes (Section 3.11.4).

The diagnosis is important clinically because it can mimic a malignant process (Guest and Reznick, 1989), particularly mucinous carcinoma (Valenzuela *et al.*, 1996). The aetiology is unknown, and associations have been described with both self-inflicted rectal trauma (Lifshitz *et al.*, 1994) or following post-radiation therapy (Ng and Chan, 1995). The pathogenesis is also variable, and includes repeated ulceration/regeneration or chronic colonic ischaemia (Ng and Chan, 1995).

Colitis cystica profunda may occur as a result of mucosal prolapse, localized to the anterior rectum in the solitary rectal ulcer syndrome (Levine, 1987) (Section 15.10). Focal segmental colitis cystica profunda may develop in Crohn's disease and in

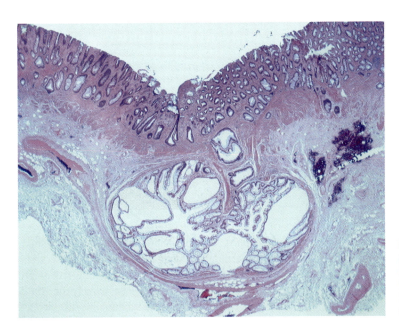

Figure 20.6 Colitis cystica profunda. Mucosal glands and lamina propria are misplaced below the thickened muscularis mucosae. Some of the glands are cystically dilated.

areas of healed radiation damage, sometimes in association with fibrous stricturing (Gardiner *et al.*, 1984).

Diffuse colitis cystica profunda occasionally results from healed ulceration following bacillary dysentery (Goodall and Sinclair, 1957) or ulcerative colitis (Magidson and Lewin, 1981).

20.12 ENDOMETRIOSIS

The sigmoid colon or rectum is affected in 18–25 per cent of cases of pelvic endometriosis (Spjut and Perkins, 1969), presenting with pain, constipation, tenesmus and occasionally cyclical rectal bleeding. There is irregular stricturing of the bowel. The mucosal surface is usually intact but the mucosa can show features that mimic inflammatory bowel disease (Langlois *et al.*, 1994; Gupta and Shepherd, 2003). The lesions are mostly situated on the serosal aspect or deep in the wall and biopsy is best performed at laparoscopy (Rowland and Langman, 1989). However, occasionally, endometriosis extends through the bowel wall to involve the submucosa and even the mucosa; sigmoidoscopic biopsy will

yield diagnostic tissue (Fig. 20.7). The typical stroma, together with a variable number of glands, is then seen. Haemorrhage and haemosiderin are not constant features. Confusion with colitis cystica profunda (Section 20.11) is unlikely, especially if the possibility is remembered in a woman of child-bearing age.

20.13 PRIMARY IMMUNODEFICIENCY SYNDROMES

A primary defect in antibody-mediated immunity or, less commonly, cell-mediated immunity may produce gastrointestinal disease (Eidelman, 1976). This usually takes the form of infection by opportunistic organisms. Adult common variable hypogammaglobulinaemia is the condition pathologists are most likely to see (Kalha and Sellin, 2004). A rectal biopsy in this condition will show reduced or absent plasma cells and a picture suggesting muted low-grade infection. That is, there will be a small number of neutrophils clearly invading the crypts and surface epithelium. Attention should focus on identifying any organisms such as cryptosporidia or cytomegalovirus (Chapter 4). Chronic *Campylobacter* infection may be present (Lever *et al.*, 1984).

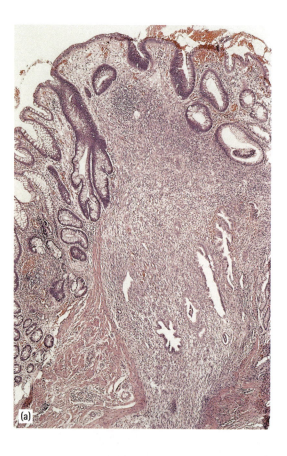

(a)

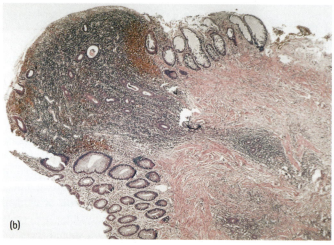

(b)

20.14 IRRITABLE BOWEL SYNDROME

Close to half of the patients with recurrent abdominal pain or bowel disturbance show no pathological abnormality, and are sufferers of the irritable bowel syndrome (Chaudhary and Truelove, 1962). The term is reserved for patients who have symptoms for at least 12 weeks during a 12-month period (Thompson *et al.*, 1999). This may affect up to 20 per cent of the general population according to some estimates (Schuster, 2001). The spectrum of colonic symptoms includes abdominal bloating, constipation, diarrhoea and pain (the so-called Rome criteria; Thompson *et al.*, 1999). It is becoming recognized that four groups of patients exist, namely those with spastic colon, diarrhoea-predominant spastic colon, functional diarrhoea and mid-gut dysmotility (Cole *et al.*, 2002). In general, the aetiology is poorly understood and has been associated with depression and anxiety (Ford *et al.*, 1987), food intolerance (Bentley *et al.*, 1983) and post-infective gastroenteritis (Chaudhary and Truelove, 1962; Spiller, 2003). The biopsy pathology is, as indicated above, characteristically negative. Therapy may include psychological support, biofeedback or drugs in the serotonin receptor modulator group (Thielecke *et al.*, 2004).

Figure 20.7 Rectal endometriosis. (a) There is a submucosal mass of endometrial glands and stroma. Although these extend slightly into the mucosa, the surface is largely intact. (b) Endometrial stroma, containing glands, displaces the mucosal crypts and extends through to an ulcerated surface.

20.15 BROWN BOWEL SYNDROME

Brown bowel syndrome is a particularly florid form of melanosis involving the smooth muscle cells of the muscularis propria, which are loaded with lipofuscin pigment. The muscularis mucosae is spared. Although the small bowel is predominantly affected, an occasional case of total enterocolonic involvement with clinical megacolon has been described (Robinson *et al.*, 1989). The pigment is located in lysosomes but the mitochondria show degenerative changes (Foster, 1979; Horn *et al.*, 1985). The condition may be a result of severe and prolonged malabsorption (Robinson *et al.*, 1989). There is some evidence that vitamin E deficiency is responsible (Foster, 1979). There is no causative association with chronic megacolon. This condition is not encountered in biopsy practice as the changes are deep to the mucosa. This topic is further considered in Chapter 13.

REFERENCES

Adams, R.D., Lyon, G. (1982) *Neurology of hereditary metabolic diseases of children.* New York, London: McGraw–Hill, pp. 149–52.

Allison, D.J., Hemingway, A.P. (1981) Angiodysplasia – does old age begin at 19? *Lancet*, ii, 979–80.

Ament, M.E., Ochs, H. (1973) Gastrointestinal manifestations of chronic granulomatous disease. *N. Engl. J. Med.*, 288, 382–7.

Baba, S., Maruta, M., Ando, K., Teramoto, T., Endo, I. (1976) Intestinal Behçet's disease: report of five cases. *Dis. Col. Rectum*, 19, 428.

Bates, A.W., Dev, S., Baithun, S.I. (1997) Malakoplakia and colorectal adenocarcinoma. *Postgrad. Med. J.*, 73, 171–3.

Bayraktar, Y., Ozaslan, E., van Thiel, D.H. (2000) Gastrointestinal manifestations of Behçet's disease. *J. Clin. Gastroenterol.*, 30, 144–54.

Bentley, E., Chandrasoma, P., Cohen, H., Radin, R., Ray, M. (1985) Colitis cystica profunda: Presenting with complete intestinal obstruction. *Gastroenterology*, 89, 1157–61.

Bentley, S.J., Pearson, D.J., Rix, K.J. (1983) Food hypersensitivity in irritable bowel syndrome. *Lancet*, ii, 295–7

Bjarnason, I., Williams, P., So, A. *et al.* (1984) Intestinal permeability and inflammation in rheumatoid arthritis: effects of non-steroidal anti-inflammatory drugs. *Lancet*, ii, 1171–4.

Boley, S.J., Brandt, L.J. (1986) Vascular ectasias. *Dig. Dis. Sci.*, 31 (Suppl. 9), 26–425.

Boley, S.J., Sammartano, R., Adams, A., DiBiase, A., Kleinhaus, S., Sprayregen, S. (1977) On the nature and etiology of vascular ectasias of the colon. Degenerative lesions of ageing. *Gastroenterology*, 72, 650–60.

Brett, E.M., Lake, B.D. (1975) Reassessment of rectal approach to neuropathology in childhood. Review of 307 biopsies over 11 years. *Arch. Dis. Child.*, 50, 753–62.

Burke, A.P., Sobin, L.H., Virmani, R. (1995) Localized vasculitis of the gastrointestinal tract. *Am. J. Surg. Pathol.*, 19, 338–49.

Chaudhary, N.A., Truelove, S.C. (1962) The irritable colon syndrome. A study of the clinical features, predisposing causes, and prognosis in 130 cases. *Q. J. Med.*, 31, 307–22.

Chaudhry, A.P., Satchidanand, S.K., Anthone, R., Baumler, R.A., Gaeta, J.F. (1980) An unusual case of supraclavicular and colonic malakoplakia – a light and ultrastructural study. *Pathology*, 131, 193–208.

Cole, S.J., Duncan, H.D., Claydon, A.H., Austin, D., Bowling, T.E., Silk, D.B. (2002) Distal colonic motor activity in four subgroups of patients with irritable bowel syndrome. *Dig. Dis. Sci.*, 47, 345–55.

Cuvelier, C., Barbatis, C., Mielants, H., De Vos, M., Roels, H., Veys, E. (1987) Histopathology of intestinal inflammation related to reactive arthritis. *Gut*, 28, 394–401.

Danesh, B.J., Spiliadis, C., Williams, C.B., Zambartas, C.M. (1987) Angiodysplasia – an uncommon cause of colonic bleeding: colonoscopic evaluation of 1,050 patients with rectal bleeding and anaemia. *Int. J. Colorectal Dis.*, 2, 218–22.

Day, D.W., Jass, J.R., Price, A.B., Shepherd, N.A., Talbot, I.C., Warren, B.F., Williams, G.T. (2003a) *Morson and Dawson's gastrointestinal pathology*. 4th edn. Oxford: Blackwell, p. 461.

Day, D.W., Jass, J.R., Price, A.B., Shepherd, N.A., Talbot, I.C., Warren, B.F., Williams, G.T. (2003b) *Morson and Dawson's gastrointestinal pathology*. 4th edn. Oxford: Blackwell, p. 548.

Deans, G.T., Hale, R.J., McMahon, R.F., Brough, W.A. (1995) Amyloid tumour of the colon. *J. Clin. Pathol.*, 48, 592–3.

Dobbins, W.O., Kawanishi, H. (1981) Bacillary characteristics in Whipple's disease: an electron microscopic study. *Gastroenterology*, 80, 1468–75.

Dumot, J.A., Adal, K., Petras, R.E., Lashner, B.A. (1998) Sarcoidosis presenting as granulomatous colitis. *Am. J. Gastroenterol.*, 93, 1949–51.

Eggermont, E. (1996) Gastrointestinal manifestations in cystic fibrosis. *Eur. J. Gastroenterol. Hepatol.*, 8, 731–8.

Eidelman, S. (1976) Intestinal lesions in immune deficiency. *Hum. Pathol.*, 7, 427–34.

Fenollar, F., Raoult, D. (2001) Molecular techniques in Whipple's disease. *Expert Rev. Mol. Diagn.*, 1, 299–309

Finlay-Jones, L.R., Blackwell, J.B., Papadimitriou, J.M. (1968) Malakoplakia of the colon. *Am. J. Clin. Pathol.*, 50, 320–9.

Ford, M.J., Miller, P.M., Eastwood, J., Eastwood, M.A. (1987) Life events, psychiatric illness and the irritable bowel syndrome. *Gut*, 28, 160–5.

Forgacs, P., Wright, P.H., Wyatt, A.P. (1973) Treatment of intestinal gas cysts by oxygen breathing. *Lancet*, i, 579.

Foster, C.S. (1979) The brown bowel syndrome: a possible smooth muscle mitochondrial myopathy? *Histopathology*, 3, 1–17.

Freeman, K., Anthony, P.P., Miller, D.S., Warin, A.P. (1985) Cronkhite–Canada syndrome: a new hypothesis. *Gut*, 26, 531–6.

Gagliardi, G., Thompson, I.W., Hershman, M.J., Forbes, A., Hawley, P.R., Talbot, I.C. (1996) Pneumatosis coli: a proposed pathogenesis based on study of 25 cases and review of the literature. *Int. J. Colorectal Dis.*, 11, 111–18.

Galandiuk, S., Fazio, V.W. (1986) Pneumatosis cystoides intestinalis. A review of the literature. *Dis. Colon Rectum*, 29, 358–63.

Galloway, S.J., Casarella, W.J., Shimkin, P.M. (1974) Vascular malformations of the right colon as a cause of bleeding in patients with aortic stenosis. *Radiology*, 113, 11–15.

Gardiner, G.W., McAuliffe, W., Murray, D. (1984) Colitis cystica profunda occurring in radiation induced colonic stricture. *Hum. Pathol.*, 15, 295–7.

Gelot, A., Maurage, C.A., Rodriguez, D., Perrier-Pallisson, D., Larmande, P., Ruchoux, M.M. (1998) *In vivo* diagnosis of Kufs' disease by extracerebral biopsies. *Acta Neuropathol. (Berl.)*, 96, 102–8.

Godeau, B., Farcet, J.P., Delchier, J.C., Xuan, D.H., Chaumette, M.T., Gaulard, P. (1992) Protein-losing enteropathy in gastrointestinal sarcoidosis associated with malignant lymphoma. *J. Clin. Gastroenterol.*, 14, 78–80.

Goodall, M.B., Sinclair, S.R. (1957) Colitis cystica profunda. *J. Pathol. Bacteriol.*, 73, 33–42.

Gordon, F.H., Watkinson, A., Hodgson, H. (2001) Vascular malformations of the gastrointestinal tract. *Best Pract. Res. Clin. Gastroenterol.*, 15, 41–58.

Gruenberg, J.C., Grodsinsky, C., Ponka, J.L. (1979) Pneumatosis intestinalis: a clinical classification. *Dis. Col. Rectum*, 22, 5–9.

Guest, C.B., Reznick, R.K. (1989) Colitis cystica profunda. Review of the literature. *Dis. Colon Rectum*, 32, 983–8.

Gupta, J., Shepherd, N.A. (2003) Colorectal mass lesions masquerading as chronic inflammatory bowel disease on mucosal biopsy. *Histopathology*, 42, 476-81.

Hamrock, D., Azmi, F.H., O'Donnell, E., Gunning, W.T., Philips, E.R., Zaher, A. (1999) Infection by *Rhodococcus equi* in a patient with AIDS: histological appearance mimicking Whipple's disease and *Mycobacterium avium-intracellulare* infection. *J. Clin. Pathol.*, 52, 68–71.

Hemingway, A.P., Allison, D.J. (1986) Angiodysplasia: a new concept in the localisation and aetiology of colonic angiodysplasia. *Gut*, 27, A619 (Abstract).

Hilzenrat, N., Spanier, A., Lamoureux, E., Bloom, C., Sherker, A. (1995) Colonic obstruction secondary to sarcoidosis: nonsurgical diagnosis and management. *Gastroenterology*, 108, 1556–9.

Hirschfield, G.M. (2004) Amyloidosis: a clinico-pathophysiological synopsis. *Semin. Cell Dev. Biol.*, 15, 39–44.

Horn, T., Svendsen, L.B., Johansen, A., Backer, O. (1985) Brown bowel syndrome. *Ultrastruct. Pathol.*, 8, 357–61.

Horowitz, N.S., Cohn, D.E., Herzog, T.J., Mutch, D.G., Rader, J.S., Bhalla, S., Gibb, R.K. (2002) The significance of pneumatosis intestinalis or bowel perforation in patients with gynecologic malignancies. *Gynecol. Oncol.*, 86, 79–84.

Howard, O.M., Buchanan, J.D., Hunt, R.H. (1982) Angiodysplasia of the colon. *Lancet*, ii, 16–19.

James, T.N., Bulkley, B.H., Kent, S.P. (1984) Vascular lesions of the gastrointestinal system in Whipple's disease. *Am. J. Med. Sci.*, 288, 125–9.

Jenkins, D., Stephensen, P.M., Scott, B.B. (1985) The Cronkhite–Canada syndrome: an ultrastructural study of pathogenesis. *J. Clin. Pathol.*, 38, 271–6.

Kalha, I., Sellin, J.H. (2004) Common variable immunodeficiency and the gastrointestinal tract. *Curr. Gastroenterol. Rep.*, 6, 377–83.

Kasahara, Y., Tanaka, S., Nishino, M., Umemura, H., Shiraha, S., Kuyama, T. (1981) Intestinal involvement in Behçet's disease: review of 136 surgical cases in the Japanese literature. *Dis. Col. Rectum*, 24, 103–6.

Keyting, W.S., McCarver, R.R., Kovarik, J.L., Daywitt, A.I. (1961) Pneumatosis intestinalis: a new concept. *Radiology*, 76, 733–41.

Kim, J.S., Lim, S.H., Choi, I.J., Moon, H., Jung, H.C., Song, I.S., Kim, C.Y. (2000) Prediction of the clinical course of Behçet's colitis according to macroscopic classification by colonoscopy. *Endoscopy*, 32, 635–40.

Kobashigawa, T., Okamoto, H., Kato, J. *et al.* (2004) Ulcerative colitis followed by the development of Behçet's disease. *Intern. Med.*, 43, 243–7.

Koss, L.G (1952) Abdominal gas cysts (pneumatosis cystoides intestinorum hominis): analysis with report of case and critical review of literature. *Arch. Pathol.*, 53, 523–49.

Kreiss, C., Forohar, F., Smithline, A.E., Brandt, L.J. (1999) Pneumatosis intestinalis complicating *C. difficile* pseudomembranous colitis. *Am. J. Gastroenterol.*, 94, 2560–1.

Kumar, S.S., Appavu, S.S., Abearin, H., Barreta, T.B. (1983) Amyloidosis of the colon. Report of a case and review of the literature. *Dis. Col. Rectum*, 26, 541–4.

Kyle, R.A. (1975) Amyloidosis: review of 236 cases. *Medicine*, 54, 271–99.

Kyokane, T., Akita, Y., Katayama, M., Kitagawa, Y., Sato, T., Shichino, S., Nimura, Y. (2001) Angiodysplasia of the appendix. *Am. J. Gastroenterol.*, 96, 242–4.

Lake, B.D. (1976) The differential diagnosis of the various forms of Batten disease by rectal biopsy. *Birth Defects*, XII (3), 455–62.

Lakhanpal, S., Tani, K., Lie, J.T., Katoh, K., Ishigatsubo, V., Ohokubo, T. (1985) Pathologic features of Behçet's syndrome. A review of Japanese Autopsy Registry Data. *Hum. Pathol.*, 16, 790–5.

Lamarque, D., Nhieu, J.T., Breban, M. *et al.* (2003) Lymphocytic infiltration and expression of inducible nitric oxide synthase in human duodenal and colonic mucosa is a characteristic feature of ankylosing spondylitis. *J. Rheumatol.*, 30, 2428–36.

Langlois, N.E., Park, K.G., Keenan, R.A. (1994) Mucosal changes in the large bowel with endometriosis: a possible cause of misdiagnosis of colitis? *Hum. Pathol.*, 25, 1030–4.

Lee, C.R., Kim, W.H., Cho, Y.S., Kim, M.H., Kim, J.H., Park, I.S., Bang, D. (2001) Colonoscopic findings in intestinal Behçet's disease. *Inflamm. Bowel Dis.*, 7, 243–9.

Lee, R.G. (1986) The colitis of Behçet's syndrome. *Am. J. Surg. Pathol.*, 10, 888–93.

Leonard, N., Palazzo, J., Jameson, J., Denman, A.M., Talbot, I.C., Price, A.B. (1998) Behçet's colitis has distinctive pathological features. *Int. J. Surg. Pathol.*, 6, 1–4.

Lever, A.M.L., Dolby, J.M., Webster, A.D.M., Price, A.B. (1984) Chronic *Campylobacter* colitis and uveitis in patient with hypogammoglobulinaemia. *Br. Med. J.*, 288, 531.

Levine, D.S. (1987) 'Solitary' rectal ulcer syndrome. Are 'solitary' rectal ulcer syndrome and 'localized' colitis cystica profunda analogous syndromes caused by rectal prolapse? *Gastroenterology*, 92, 243–53.

Lifshitz, D., Cytron, S., Yossiphov, J., Lelcuk, S., Rabau, M. (1994) Colitis cystica profunda: self-inflicted by rectal trauma? Report of a case. *Dig. Dis.*, 12, 318–20.

MacKay, E.H. (1978) Malakoplakia in ulcerative colitis. *Arch. Pathol. Lab. Med.*, 102, 140–5.

Magidson, J.G., Lewin, K.J. (1981) Diffuse colitis cystica profunda. *Am. Surg. Pathol.*, 5, 393–9.

Manousos, O., Webster, C.V. (1966) Diffuse gastrointestinal polyposis with ectodermal changes. *Gut*, 7, 375–9.

Marcial, M.A., Villafana, M. (1997) Whipple's disease with esophageal and colonic involvement: endoscopic and histopathologic findings. *Gastrointest. Endosc.*, 46, 263–6.

Masugi, J., Matsui, T., Fujimori, T., Maeda, S.A. (1994) A case of Behçet's disease with multiple longitudinal ulcers all over the colon. *Am. J. Gastroenterol.*, 89, 778–80.

Matseshe, J.W., Go, V.L.W., Dimagno, E.P. (1977) Meconium ileus equivalent complicating cystic fibrosis in postneonatal children and young adults. Report of 12 cases. *Gastroenterology*, 72, 732–6.

Mielants, H., Veys, E.M., Cuvelier, C., De Vos, M., Botelberghe, L. (1985) HLA-B27 related arthritis and bowel inflammation. Part 2. Ileocolonoscopy and bowel histology in patients with HLA-B27 related arthritis. *J. Rheumatol.*, 12, 294–8.

Moran, C.A., West, B., Schwartz, I.S. (1989) Malakoplakia of the colon in association with colonic adenocarcinoma. *Am. J. Gastroenterol.*, 84, 1580–2.

Nagahama, T., Matsui, T., Matsumura, M. *et al.* (2000) Rheumatoid arthritis accompanied by colonic lesions. *Intern. Med.*, 39, 235–8.

Naschitz, J.E., Yeshurun, D., Horovitz, I.L., Misselevitch, I., Boss, J.H. (1990) Colonic diverticulitis-related exuberant granulomatous reaction in a patient with sarcoidosis. *Dig. Dis. Sci.*, 35, 533–8.

Neutra, M.R., Grand, R.J., Trier, J.S. (1977) Glycoprotein synthesis, transport and secretion by epithelial cells of human rectal mucosa. Normal and cystic fibrosis. *Lab. Invest.*, 36, 535–46.

Ng, I.O., Ng, M. (1993) Colonic malakoplakia: unusual association with ulcerative colitis. *J. Gastroenterol. Hepatol.*, 8, 110–15.

Ng, W.K., Chan, K.W. (1995) Postirradiation colitis cystica profunda. Case report and literature review. *Arch. Pathol. Lab. Med.*, 119, 1170–3.

Nielsen, O.S., Sondergaard, J.O., Aru, A. (1984) Colitis cystica profunda lokalisata. *Acta Chir. Scand.*, 150, 191–2.

Nishida, Y., Murase, K., Ashida, R. *et al.* (1998) Familial Crohn's disease with systemic lupus erythematosus. *Am. J. Gastroenterol.*, 93, 2599–601.

O'Conell, D., Courtney, J.V., Riddell, R.H. (1980) Colitis of Behçet's syndrome radiologic and pathologic features. *Gastrointest. Radiol.*, 5, 173–9.

O'Duffy, J.D., Carney, J.A., Deodhar, S. (1971) Behçet's disease: report of 10 cases, 3 with new manifestations. *Ann. Intern. Med.*, 75, 561–70.

Ottenjann, R., Weingart, J., Kiihner, W., Frimberger, E. (1984) Colorectal angiodysplasias (vascular ectasias): endoscopic morphology, localization and frequency. *Dtsch. Med. Wochr.*, 109, 1549–52.

Parkins, R.A., Eidelman, S., Rubin, C.E., Dobbins, W.O., Phelps, P.C. (1963) The diagnosis of cystic fibrosis by rectal suction biopsy. *Lancet*, ii, 851–6.

Pasquinelli, G., Cenacchi, G., Piane, E.L., Russo, C., Aguglia, U. (2004) The problematic issue of Kufs disease diagnosis as performed on rectal biopsies: a case report. *Ultrastruct. Pathol.*, 28, 43–8.

Pawel, B.R., de Chadarevian, J.P., Franco, M.E. (1997) The pathology of fibrosing colonopathy of cystic fibrosis: a study of 12 cases and review of the literature. *Hum. Pathol.*, 28, 395–9.

Pepys, M.B. (2001) Pathogenesis, diagnosis and treatment of systemic amyloidosis. *Phil. Trans. R. Soc. Lond. B Biol. Sci.*, 356(1406), 203–10.

Pieterse, A.S., Leong, A.S-Y., Rowland, R. (1985) The mucosal changes and pathogenesis of pneumatosis cystoides intestinalis. *Hum. Pathol.*, 16, 683–8.

Pillay, K., Chetty, R. (2002) Malakoplakia in association with colorectal carcinoma: a series of four cases. *Pathology*, 34, 332–5.

Pounder, D.J., Rowland, R., Pieterse, A.S., Freeman, R., Hunter, R. (1982) Angiodysplasias of the colon. *J. Clin. Pathol.*, 35, 824–9.

Price, A.B. (1986) Angiodysplasia of the colon. *Int. J. Colorectal Dis.*, 1, 121–8.

Radin, D.R., Chandrasoma, P., Halls, J.M. (1984) Colonic malacoplakia. *Gastrointest. Radiol.*, 9, 359–61.

Ratnaike, R.N. (2000) Whipple's disease. *Postgrad. Med. J.* 76, 760–6.

Read, N.W., Al-Janabi, M.N., Cann, P.A. (1984) Is raised breath hydrogen related to the pathogenesis of pneumatosis coli? *Gut*, 839–45.

Relman, D.A., Schmidt, T.M., MacDermott, R.P., Falkow, S. (1992) Identification of the uncultured bacillus of Whipple's disease. *N. Engl. J. Med.*, 327, 293–301.

Richter, J.M., Hedberg, S.T., Athanasoulis, C.A., Schapiro, R.H. (1984) Angiodysplasia: clinical presentation and colonoscopic diagnosis. *Dig. Dis. Sci.*, 29, 481–5.

Robinson, M.H., Dowling, B.L., Clark, J.V., and Mason, C.H. (1989). Brown bowel syndrome: an unusual cause of massive dilatation of the colon. *Gut*, 30, 882–4.

Rocken, C., Saeger, W., Linke, R.P. (1994) Gastrointestinal amyloid deposits in old age. Report on 110 consecutive autopsical patients and 98 retrospective bioptic specimens. *Pathol. Res. Pract.*, 190, 641–9.

Rowland, R., Langman, J.M. (1989) Endometriosis of the large bowel: a report of 11 cases. *Pathology*, 21, 259–65.

Sandmeier, D., Guillou, L. (1993) Malakoplakia and adenocarcinoma of the caecum: a rare association. *J. Clin. Pathol.*, 46, 959–60.

Schuster, M.M. (2001) Defining and diagnosing irritable bowel syndrome. *Am. J. Manag. Care*, 7(8 Suppl), S246–51.

Segal, A.W. (1985) Variations on the theme of chronic granulomatous disease. *Lancet*, i, 137–82.

Segal, B.H., Holland, S.M. (2000) Primary phagocytic disorders of childhood. *Pediatr. Clin. N. Am.*, 47, 1311–38.

Segal, B.H., Leto, T.L., Gallin, J.I., Malech, H.L., Holland, S.M. (2000) Genetic, biochemical, and clinical features of chronic granulomatous disease. *Medicine (Baltimore)*, 79, 170–200.

Shimizu, T., Ehrlich, G.E., Inaba, K., Hayashi, K. (1979) Behçet's disease (Behçet's syndrome). *Semin. Arthritis Rheum.*, 8, 223–60.

Smith, G.E., Kime, L.R., Pitcher, J.L. (1973) The colitis of Behçet's Disease: A separate entity? Colonoscopic findings and literature review. *Am. J. Dig, Dis.*, 18, 987–99.

Soutter, D.I., Paloschi, G.B., Prentice, R.S. (1985) Pneumatosis cystoides intestinalis simulating malignant colonic obstruction. *Can. J. Surg.*, 28, 272–3.

Spjut, H.J., Perkins, D.E. (1969) Endometriosis of the sigmoid colon and rectum. *Am. J. Roentgenol.*, 82, 1070–5.

Spiller, R.C. (2003) Postinfectious irritable bowel syndrome. *Gastroenterology*, 124, 1662–71.

Sprague, R., Harper, P., McClain, S., Trainer, T., Beeken, W. (1984) Disseminated gastrointestinal sarcoidosis. Case report and review of the literature. *Gastroenterology*, 87, 421–5.

Stamm, B., Heer, M., Buhler, H., Ammann, R. (1985) Mucosal biopsy of vascular ectasia (angiodysplasia) of the large bowel detected during routine colonoscopic examination. *Histopathology*, 9, 639–46.

St Peter, S.D., Abbas, M.A., Kelly, K.A. (2003) The spectrum of pneumatosis intestinalis. *Arch. Surg.*, 138, 68–75.

Stevens, S., McClure, J. (1982) The histochemical features of the Michaelis–Gutmann body and a consideration of the pathophysiological mechanisms of its formation. *J. Pathol.*, 137, 119–27.

Storesund, B., Gran, J.T., Koldingsnes, W. (1998) Severe intestinal involvement in Wegener's granulomatosis: report of two cases and review of the literature. *Br. J. Rheumatol.*, 37, 387–90.

Tada, S., Iida, M., Yao, T., Kitamoto, T., Fujishima, M. (1993) Intestinal pseudo-obstruction in patients with amyloidosis: clinicopathologic differences between chemical types of amyloid protein. *Gut*, 34, 1412–17.

Thielecke, F., Maxion-Bergemann, S., Abel, F., Gonschior, A.K. (2004) Update in the pharmaceutical therapy of the irritable bowel syndrome. *Int. J. Clin. Pract.*, 58, 374–81.

Thompson, W.G., Longstreth, G.F., Drossman, D.A., Heaton, K.W., Irvine, E.J., Muller-Lissner, S.A. (1999) Functional bowel disorders and functional abdominal pain. *Gut*, 45 (Suppl 2), II43–7.

Tobi, M., Kobrin, I., Ariel, 1. (1982) Rectal involvement in sarcoidosis. *Dis. Col. Rectum*, 25, 491–3.

Tolia, V., Abdullah, A., Thirumoorthi, M.C., Chang, C.H. (1989) A case of Behçet's disease with intestinal involvement due to Crohn's disease. *Am. J. Gastroenterol.*, 84, 322–5.

Underwood, J.C., Durrant, T.E., Coup, A.J. (1982) X-ray microanalysis of the Michaelis–Gutmann bodies of malakoplakia. *J. Pathol.*, 138, 41–7.

Valenzuela, M., Martin-Ruiz, J.L,. Alvarez-Cienfuegos, E., Caballero, A.M., Gallego, F., Carmona, I., Rodriguez-Tellez, M. (1996) Colitis cystica profunda: imaging diagnosis and conservative treatment: report of two cases. *Dis. Colon Rectum*, 39, 587–90.

Veitch, A.M., Badger, I. (2004) Sarcoidosis presenting as colonic polyposis: report of a case. *Dis. Colon Rectum*, 47, 937–9.

Walport, M. (1984) Behçet's syndrome. In: Bouchier, I.A.D., Allan, R.N., Hodgson, H.J.F., Keighley, M.R.B. (eds) *Textbook of Gastroenterology*. London: Bailliere Tindall, pp. 657–66.

Watson, J.H.L., Haubrich, W.S. (1969) Bacilli bodies in the lumen and epithelium of the jejunum in Whipple's disease. *Lab. Invest.*, 21, 347–57.

Wegelius, O., Pasternack, A. (1976) Amyloidosis. In: *Proceedings of the fifth Sigrid Juselius Foundation Symposium*. London: Academic Press, p. 408.

Whitehead, R. (1985) *Mucosal biopsy of the gastrointestinal tract*. Philadelphia, London, Toronto, Mexico City, Rio de Janeiro, Sydney and Tokyo: W.B. Saunders, pp. 276–8.

Wright, J.R., Calkins, E., Humphrey, R.L. (1977) Potassium permanganate reaction in amyloidosis. A histologic method to assist in differentiating forms of this disease. *Lab. Invest.*, 36, 274–81.

Yale, C.E., Balish, E. (1985) Evidence for Clostridial involvement in pneumatosis cystoides intestinalis. In: Borriello, S.P. (ed.), *Clostridia in gastrointestinal disease*. Boca Raton: CRC Press, pp. 60–6.

Yale, C.E., Balish, E., Wu, J.P. (1974) The bacterial etiology of pneumatotis coli intestinalis. *Arch. Surg.*, 109, 89–94.

Yamano, T., Shimada, M., Okada, S., Yutaka, T., Kato, T., Yabuuchi, H. (1982) Ultrastructural study of biopsy specimens of rectal mucosa. Its use in neuronal storage diseases. *Arch. Pathol. Lab. Med.*, 106, 673–7.

Yang, C.C., Huang, T.Y., Tsung, S.H., Han, D.C. (1983) Rectal malacoplakia in a patient with Hodgkin's disease. Report of a case and review of the literature. *Dis. Colon Rectum*, 26, 129–32.

Yardley, J.H., Donowitz, M. (1977) Colo-rectal biopsy in inflammatory bowel disease. In: Yardley, J.H., Morson, B.C., Abell, M.R. (eds) *The gastrointestinal tract. International Academy of Pathology monograph*. Baltimore: Williams and Wilkins, pp. 77–8.

Yashiro, M., Kobayashi, H., Kubo, N., Nishiguchi, Y., Wakasa, K., Hirakawa, K. (2004) Cronkhite–Canada syndrome containing colon cancer and serrated adenoma lesions. *Digestion*, 69, 57–62.

Zech, J.R., Kroger, E., Bonnin, A.J., Richmond, G.W. (1993) Sarcoidosis: unusual cause of a rectal mass. *South. Med. J.*, 86, 1054–5.

INDEX

Figures are comprehensively referred to from the text. Therefore, significant material in figures has only been given a page reference in the absence of their concommitant mention in the text referring to that figure. Note that 'vs' indicates the differentiation of two or more conditions. Abbreviations: IBD, inflammatory bowel disease.

abscess, crypt 27–8, 34
    in collagenous colitis 152–3
    in Crohn's disease 117
    incipient see cryptitis
    in ulcerative colitis 94, 96
acanthotic epidermis 370
O-acetyltransferase (OAT) gene 7
acquired immunodeficiency
        syndrome see HIV
        disease/AIDS
acetycholinesterase staining
        233–42
adenocarcinoma 293–5, 332–4,
        334–7, 368
    adenoma progression to see
        adenoma–carcinoma
        sequence
    in adenomatous polyps, focal
        295–8
    anal ducts 368
    definition/grading/features
        related to small biopsy
        interpretation 330–2
    diagnosis 292–300, 334–7
        vs adenoma 275–6, 299
    histological subtypes 332–3
    local excision 337
    Peutz–Jeghers syndrome 267
    secondary 345–6
    stroma 293–5
adenoma(s) (non-polypoid or in
        general) 254
    apocrine gland 373–4
    carcinoma arising from

glandular see adenoma–
        carcinoma (adenocarcinoma)
        sequence
    squamous 334
dysplasia 31, 254–5, 257, 258,
        259, 263, 293
    flat 254, 258–60
    malignancy vs 275–6, 299
    stromal fibrosis 275, 294
    in ulcerative colitis, sporadic
        319–23
adenoma(s) (polypoid; adenomatous
        polyps) 253–60
    colonoscopic excision 284
        repeat 285
    focal carcinoma in 295–8
    ileoanal pouch, in FAP patients
        130
    juvenile polyps vs 276
    misplaced glands 52, 293
    multiple see polyposis
    pseudocarcinomatous invasion
        52, 275, 293
    serrated 263–4
        sessile 262
    tubular 253, 256
    tubulovillous 253, 256–7
    villous 253, 257–8
adenoma–carcinoma
        (adenocarcinoma) sequence
        254
    Peutz–Jeghers syndrome and
        267
    sessile serrated adenoma 262

adenoma-like dysplasia-associated
        lesion or mass/DALM 305,
        320–1
adenomatous polyposis see APC;
        familial adenomatous
        polyposis
adenosquamous carcinoma 334
adenovirus 73–4
adhesion molecules in ulcerative
        colitis 100
adjuvant radiotherapy,
        preoperative, mucosal
        effects 183–4
Aeromonas 61
aganglionosis see Hirschsprung's
        disease
AIDS see HIV disease
AIN (anal intra-epithelial neoplasia)
        361
allergic (eosinophilic) colitis 50,
        217–18
5-aminosalicylic acid influence on
        biopsy in ulcerative colitis
        104
amoebiasis 15–16, 44, 74–6
    differential diagnosis 76
amyloid deposits/amyloidosis 52,
        158, 243, 383–5
anal biopsy 351–76
    inflammatory lesions
        352–61
    normal morphology 351–2
    perianal skin 368–74
    tumours see tumours

anaplastic carcinoma *see* undifferentiated carcinoma
anastomotic ulceration   195
aneuploidy detection, dysplasia   316
angiodysplasia   377–80
ankylosing spondylitis   379
antibiotic-associated colitis   138–9, 189–90
  crypt dilatation   25
  differential diagnosis   140
    IBD   140, 213
  terminology/definition   134
antibiotic-associated diarrhoea (AAD)   133, 139–40
  terminology/definition   134
antibodies in serology   212
anus *see* anal biopsy
APC
  adenoma-like dysplasia-associated lesion or mass and   321
  ulcerative colitis-associated cancer and   317
aphthoid ulcers
  in Crohn's disease   113, 117–18
  NSAID-associated   189
  terminal ileum   221
apocrine gland adenoma   373–4
apoptosis/apoptotic bodies
  crypt cells   23–4
    drug-associated colitis   186
    graft-vs-host disease   192, 193
  flat/depressed adenoma   259–60
  surface epithelium   16–17
appendix, ulcerative colitis   103
argentaffin cells   8
argyrophilic cells   8
arterial supply   168–9
  occlusion   168
arthritis
  reactive   223–4
  rheumatoid   379
atrophy
  crypt   21, 98
  ulcerative colitis   98, 100
  villous *see* villous atrophy
atypia, definition   303
Auerbach's plexus *see* myenteric plexus
autistic spectrum disorder and ileal lymphoid nodular hyperplasia   226
autoimmunity and microscopic colitis   161

B cell, IBD and   211
B cell lymphomas   340–1, 342
backwash ileitis   224–5
bacterial infections, anus   357–8
bacterial infections, large bowel (incl. diarrhoea and dysentery)   57–70
  acute forms   57–65
    causes/specific pathogens   57
    inflammatory/invasive   57
    less typical/other biopsy patterns   57–8
    non-inflammatory/non-invasive   57, 63
    typical biopsy   57–60
    see also colitis, acute self-limiting
  cryptitis   28
  lamina propria   42
bacterial infections, terminal ileum   220–1
Balantidium   77
barium granulomas   184
basal cell carcinoma, anal   370
basal lamina   5
  abnormalities   18
  see also basement membrane
basaloid anal carcinoma   361, 363
  melanoma vs   366
basement membrane   9
  see also basal lamina
Batten's disease   383
bcl2 and adenoma-like dysplasia-associated lesion or mass   321
Behçet's syndrome   379–80
biopsy tissue handling   2
bile acids and microscopic colitis   152
bladder carcinoma, colorectal metastases   346
bleeding *see* haemorrhage
blood, free   48
blood vessels *see* vascular supply
bowel preparation-induced colitis   194
Bowen disease   369–70
bowenoid papulosis   370
BRAF   262
Brainerd diarrhoea   153, 159
breast carcinoma, colorectal metastases   347
brown bowel syndrome   196, 389
brown pigment   37, 53, 195–6, 389

budding, of adenocarcinoma cells   297–8
Burkitt lymphoma   340, 341

cadherin (E-) immunostaining, benign vs malignant signet ring cells   136
caecum, ulcerative colitis   103
Cam   5.2 333
Campylobacter jejuni   25, 61
Canada–Cronkhite syndrome   275, 385–6
cancer (malignant tumours)
  anal   361, 363–8, 370–1
  diagnosis   292–300
    overdiagnosis   275, 293
    underdiagnosis   275–6
  familial syndromes with predisposition to *see* hereditary cancer syndromes
  in IBD patients (=carcinoma)   301
    risk factors   303–5
    surveillance, reliability of dysplasia   305–6
  schistosomiasis and   79
  see also metastases; precancerous conditions; precancerous lesions *and specific histological types*
'cap' polyps, inflammatory   270, 274, 276
capillaries, lamina propria   10
  abnormalities   48
  endothelial cell inclusions in CMV infection   71
carcinoids
  anus   366–8
  large bowel   337–8
carcinoma   330–7, 363–6
  adenoma progression to *see* adenoma–carcinoma sequence
  in adenomatous polyps, focal   295–8
  anal canal   361, 363–6, 373
  definition/grading/features related to small biopsy interpretation   330–2
  diagnosis   292–300, 334–7
    vs adenoma   275–6, 299
    overdiagnosis   275, 293
    underdiagnosis   275–6
  histological subtypes   332–4

intramucosal, definition/
categorization 249, 302
schistosomiasis 79
secondary 345-6
signet ring cell 137, 332
submucosal *see* submucosa
carcinoma *in situ*
anal *see* Bowen's disease; intraepithelial neoplasia, anal
colonic, definition 302
β-catenin and adenoma-like
dysplasia-associated lesion
or mass 321
cathartic colon 196, 217
cavernous haemangioma 279
CD antigens and lymphoma 342
cellulose nitrate filter 1-2
ceroid lipofuscinosis 383
cervical carcinoma, colorectal
metastases 347
cestodes 78
Chagas' disease 242
chemoradiotherapy, anal verrucous
carcinoma 365-6
children
chronic granulomatous disease
381
constipation 233
biopsy policy 241-2
IBD, indefinite for dysplasia
312-14
idiopathic megacolon 242
see also infants; juvenile polyps
Chlamydia trachomatis 67
lymphogranuloma venereum
67, 357-8
cholinesterase staining, lamina
propria 10
chromogranin 8
chronic granulomatous disease of
childhood 381
cleansing agents, instrumentation
194-5
clinicians' role 1-2
cloacogenic polyp, inflammatory
271, 358
Clostridium difficile 62, 133,
140-2, 189
diarrhoea 134, 140
pseudomembranous collagenous
colitis and 153
toxigenic 140-2
positive toxin test 142
see also pseudomembranous
colitis

Clostridium perfringens 65
CMV *see* cytomegalovirus
cobblestoning 113
cocaine 190
coccidia 77
coccidioidomycosis 82
coeliac disease and microscopic
colitis 156
colectomy, ileal pathology 224-5
colitis
acute, use of term 90
acute fulminant 106-7
see also toxic dilatation
acute self-limiting (ASLC) 60,
216
vs IBD 62-3, 216
in AIDS 67-8, 218
antibiotic-associated *see*
antibiotic-associated colitis
bowel preparation and
instrumentation-induced
194-5
collagenous *see* collagenous
colitis
drug-associated *see* drug-
associated colitis
duration (in ulcerative colitis) as
risk factor for dysplasia and
cancer 303-4
eosinophilic/allergic 50, 217-18
evanescent 171
extent (anatomical) as risk factor
for dysplasia and cancer
304
focal and focal active *see* focal
colitis
IBD vs 210-19
indeterminate 106-7, 128,
208-9
infective *see* infective colitis
ischaemic *see* ischaemic colitis
lymphocytic *see* lymphocytic
colitis
microscopic *see* microscopic
colitis
minimal change 216
necrotizing, syndromes of 177
neutropenic 194
non-specific 205, 205-6
obstructive 170-1, 244-6
pseudomembranous *see*
pseudomembranous colitis
radiation *see* radiation damage
ulcerative *see* ulcerative colitis
see also proctocolitis

colitis cystica profunda 29, 52,
386-7
radiation-related 183
colitus cystica superficialis 25, 62
colitis polyposa 271
collagen
lamina propria 9
subepithelial, thickening 19
submucosa 11
collagen band/plate, thickened
147, 157, 160
detection 148-51
differential diagnosis in presence
or absence 157-8
in terminal ileum 155-6
collagenous colitis 147, 216
diagnostic biopsy 148-53
differential diagnosis 157, 158
IBD 216
epidemiology 162
lymphocytic colitis and, overlap
147, 155
small bowel 156
terminology/definition 147
variant patterns 152-3
yersiniosis and, association
between 64
colloid (mucinous) carcinoma 332
colonoscopic biopsy
Crohn's disease 119, 120-1
ulcerative colitis 102-4
colonoscopic polypectomy
284-5
repeat 285
colonoscopy
cleansing agents 194-5
in follow-up of adenoma
excision 285
ischaemic colitis 171-2
see also sigmoidoscopy
columnar cells 5, 7
polarity loss 30-1
common variable
immunodeficiency
(hypogammaglobulinaemia)
35, 218-19, 387
computed tomography, ischaemic
colitis 172
condyloma, giant 359-61, 365,
366
condyloma accuminatum 358-9,
361
connective tissue
polyps, classification 243
rectal, normal 9

connective tissue disorders 219, 379
constipation 233
childhood *see* children
Cowden's syndrome 282
ganglioneuroma 280
Crohn's disease 113–23
activity 119–20
anal fistula 355
C. difficile-associated exacerbations 141
complications 121
differential diagnosis 118–19, 202–32
antibiotic-associated and pseudomembranous colitis 140, 213
Behçet's syndrome 379–80
infective colitis 76, 209–12
lymphocytic colitis 157–8, 216
tuberculosis 64–5, 118–19
ulcerative colitis 91, 209–12
dysplasia *see* dysplasia
histopathology 114–18, 209–10
giant cells 37–8, 38
granulomas 37–8, 39, 115–17, 118, 119, 210, 223, 355
microgranulomas 41, 65, 117, 210, 223
submucosa 50, 118
ileoanal pouch in 124, 130
lymphoid aggregates 35
making the diagnosis 113–14
mucin depletion 29
natural history 211
prognostic indicators 120
terminal ileum in 223
see also inflammatory bowel disease
Cronkhite–Canada syndrome 275, 385–6
crushing artefact 31
crypt(s) (intestinal glands)
abnormalities 19–33
aberrant crypt foci 252–3
abscess *see* abscess
atrophy *see* atrophy
branching *see* *subheading below*
in Crohn's disease 114–15, 117
damage/destruction/degenera- tion *see* *subheading below*

dilatation and enlargement 25–7
dysplasia *see* dysplasia
infective colitis 23, 25, 28–9, 57–60, 61
misplacement *see* *subheading below*
in pseudomembranous colitis 135
in radiation colitis 183, 184
serration 24–5
in ulcerative colitis *see* ulcerative colitis
apoptosis *see* apoptosis
branching 19–20
in IBD 314
damage/destruction/degeneration 21–4, 37–8, 39
graft-vs-host disease 23, 192, 193
ischaemic colitis *see* ischaemic colitis
epithelium between, abnormalities 16, 18
in flat adenoma 259
misplaced 29, 51–2, 293
in colitis cystica profunda 29, 386
normal 5, 6, 7, 8, 9–10
submucosal extension *see* lymphoid–glandular complex
crypt cell carcinoma 334
cryptitis (incipient crypt abscess) 28–9
collagenous colitis 152–3
infective colitis 28–9, 58
cryptosporidiosis 77
surface epithelium 18
crypt withering 58, 59, 60
cutaneous lesions, perianal 368–74
cyst(s)
Peutz–Jeghers polyps 267
in submucosal lymphoid follicles 42
cystic fibrosis (mucoviscidosis) 26, 386
cystic pneumatosis 50, 380
cytokeratin (CK) staining
malignant tumours 332, 333
Paget's disease of anal skin 372–3
cytomegalovirus (CMV) 70–2
anal fissures 352

graft-vs-host disease-related changes mimicked by 193
DCC and ulcerative colitis- associated cancer 317
debris, mucosal surface 15
degeneration
crypt *see* crypt
hyaline 46
mucosa, in ulcerative colitis 311–12
surface epithelium 16
dermatological lesions, perianal 368–74
desmoplastic stroma of adenocarcinoma 294–5
diarrhoea
adenovirus-associated 73
antibiotic-associated *see* antibiotic-associated diarrhoea
bacterial *see* bacterial infections
C. difficile-associated 134, 140
chronic secretory watery, causes 156
infective (in general), lymphocytic colitis and rare form of 153, 159
of microscopic colitis 152
travellers' 57, 61, 77
diffuse distension of crypts 26
diffuse inflammatory cell distribution 36
disseminated intravascular coagulation 174
diversion proctocolitis 191–2
diverticular disease, crypt dilatation 25
diverticulitis vs IBD 215–16
DNA aneuploidy, dysplasia 316
donovanosis 357
DPC4 and juvenile polyps 266
drug-associated colitis 185–91, 219
biopsy clues 186
general features 186
ischaemic colitis 169–70, 188
microscopic colitis 161, 188
drug therapy
microscopic colitis 162
ulcerative colitis, influence on biopsy 104
duodenum in microscopic colitis 156
dysentery, bacterial *see* bacterial infections

dysplasia, epithelial (precancerous) 248–9
  adenomas 31, 254–5, 257, 258, 259, 263, 293
  anal 361
  classification/grading 248–9, 302
    in IBD patients 311
  controversies in diagnosis 248–9
  crypt 30–2
    flat adenoma 259
    in IBD 31, 306, 308–9, 310, 314
  definitions 248–9, 302
  in IBD (predominantly ulcerative colitis over Crohn's disease) 301–29
    architectural abnormalities 309–10
    in cancer surveillance, reliability 305–6
    crypt 31, 306, 308–9, 310, 314
    cytological abnormalities 308–9
    failure to find a lesion following resection 323
    high-grade 308, 309, 314, 319
    histological recognition and classification 307–15
    indefinite for 312–14, 318
    low-grade 314, 318–19
    macroscopic features 306–7
    molecular studies 312, 321
    observer variation in diagnosis and grading 316
    other stains and methodologies 316–17
    pathologist's report, implications 317–18
    risk factors 303–5
    screening 302
  juvenile polyps 265
  post-inflammatory polyps 269
  pouch mucosa 131
  preoperative adjuvant radiation mucosal pathology resembling 183–4
  in schistosomiasis 79
dysplasia, neuronal 235–41
dysplasia-associated lesion or mass (DALM) 305, 319–23
  adenoma-like 305, 320–1

E-cadherin immunostaining, benign vs malignant signet ring cells 136
ectasia, capillary 48
ectopic gastric mucosa 282–4
elastic fibres
  muscularis mucosa 10–11
  submucosa 11
endocrine (neuroendocrine) cells 5, 7–8
  abnormal 33
  tumours see carcinoids
endometriosis 387
endoscopy see colonoscopy; sigmoidoscopy
endothelial cell inclusions in CMV infection 71
enemas, preparing 194
Entamoeba histolytica infection see amoebiasis
enteroadherent E. coli 61
enteroaggregative E. coli 61
Enterobius vermicularis 81
enterochromaffin cells 8
enterocolitic syndromes 65–8
enterohaemorrhagic E. coli 61
enteroinvasive E. coli 61
enteropathogenic C. difficile 141
enteropathogenic E. coli 61
enterotoxigenic E. coli 61
enterotoxin, C. difficile 140–2
eosinophil(s) 35–6
  in collagenous colitis 151
  in drug-associated colitis 186
  in eosinophilic colitis 217, 218
  in ulcerative colitis 94–5
eosinophilic colitis 50, 217–18
eosinophilic cytoplasm in ulcerative colitis 310
epidermodysplasia verruciformis 370
epithelial tumours/neoplasms
  anus 353, 361–8
  large bowel
    definitions and classification 248–50
    malignant 330–7
epithelialization of fistula track 353
epithelioid histiocytes 38–9, 39
  see also microgranulomas
epithelium
  abnormal 16–33
    atrophy see atrophy
    in Crohn's disease 114–15
    crypt see subheading below

misplacement 29, 51–2, 293
surface epithelium see surface epithelium abnormalities
in ulcerative colitis 91–3, 98
crypt, abnormal 29–33
dysplasia see dysplasia
in pseudomembranous colitis 136
lymphocytes see lymphocytes
normal
  anus 351–2
  large bowel 5–9
eroded polypoid hyperplasia 269
erosion, intercryptal epithelium 18
Escherichia coli 61
extracellular matrix abnormalities, lamina propria 44–9
exudate, inflammatory 34

familial adenomatous polyposis (FAP) 256
  ileoanal pouch in patients with adenomas 130
  pouchitis 128
  lymphoid polyps in 277
  see also APC
familial cancer syndromes see hereditary cancer syndromes
fat, submucosal 51
fat (and fat-like) vacuoles see vacuoles
fibroblasts, pericryptal 39
  microscopic colitis and 161
fibroepithelial polyps 357
fibrosis
  ileoanal pouch 129–30
  lamina propria 44–6, 157
    in ischaemic colitis 175
    in mucosal prolapse syndrome 46, 274
    in ulcerative colitis 93–5, 98–9
  stromal, in adenoma 275, 294
  submucosal, with pancreatic enzyme supplements 191
fibrous polyp, anal canal 358
fissures
  anal 352, 355
  in IBD 118, 355
fistulae, anal 353–4
flow cytometry, dysplasia 316
flukes (trematodes) 78, 79
foamy histiocytes 33, 50

focal carcinoma in adenomatous
    polyps   295–8
focal colitis/mucosal inflammation
    37
    active   28, 205, 207–8
        in ischaemic colitis   173
follicular lymphoma   341, 342
follicular proctitis   35, 107
foreign body giant cells   38
    anal fistulae   355
fungal infections   82

ganglia (nerve), submucosa   53
    normal deficiency
        (hypoganglionic zone)
        233–4
    pathology   235–46
ganglioneuroma   279–80
gangrenous ischaemia   172
gastric mucosa, heterotopic   282–4
gastroenteritis, eosinophilic
    218–19
gastrointestinal stromal tumours
    342–4
genetic cancer syndromes see
    hereditary cancer
    syndromes
giant cells   37–8
    in collagenous colitis   153
    foreign body see foreign body
        giant cells
    in IBD   210
        ulcerative colitis   96
    in lymphocytic colitis   154
giant condyloma   359–61, 365,
    366
giardiasis   76
glands, intestinal see crypts
glandular differentiation   293
glutaraldehyde   194–5
gluten enteropathy (coeliac disease)
    and microscopic colitis
    156
goblet cells   5, 6–7
    discharge and exhaustion   29
    loss/reduced numbers   29
    polarity loss with dysplastic
        epithelium   31
    in ulcerative colitis   96
        dystrophy   309
gold salts   190
gonorrhoea   66
graft-vs-host disease   192–4, 219
    crypt degeneration and apoptosis
        23, 192

endocrine cells   33
granular cell tumours
    anus   368
    large bowel   282
granularity, mucosal, ulcerative
    colitis   95
granulation tissue   48–9
    adenocarcinoma   294
    anal fistula   354, 355
    inflammatory cap polyps   260
granuloma(s)
    anal fistula   355, 357
    barium   184
    Crohn's disease   37–8, 39,
        115–17, 118, 119, 210, 223,
        355
    ileoanal pouch   129
    lamina propria   37–8, 38–9
    microscopic colitis   158
        collagenous colitis   153
        lymphocytic colitis   154–5
    submucosa   50–1
    tuberculosis   39–41, 64–5
    ulcerative colitis, crypt-
        associated   96
    see also microgranulomas;
        oleogranulomas
granuloma inguinale   357
granulomatosis, Wegener's   379
granulomatous disease of
    childhood, chronic   381
Griffith's point, blood supply
    susceptibility   169
gut-associated lymphoid tissue   9

haemangiomatous malformations
    279
haemorrhage   48
haemorrhagic antibiotic-associated
    colitis   139
haemorrhoids   358
haemosiderin   37, 53
hamartomas and hamartomatous
    polyps
    connective tissue   253, 279–82
    mucosa   253, 276
helminths   77–81
hereditary cancer syndromes
    Cowden's syndrome   282
    hereditary mixed polyposis
        syndrome   276
    hereditary non-polyposis colon
        cancer   256
    juvenile polyposis   265
herpes simplex   73

heterotopic gastric mucosa
    282–4
hidradenitis suppurativa   368–9
hidradenoma papilliferum   374
Hirschsprung's disease
    (aganglionosis)   2, 236–9
    diagnostic biopsy   236
    hypoganglionosis associated with
        239
    nerve bundles   53
histiocytes   37
    barium-laden   184
    epithelioid see epithelioid
        histiocytes;
        microgranulomas
    foamy   33, 50
    submucosal   51
histoplasmosis   82
HIV disease/AIDS 218
    adenovirus-associated diarrhoea
        73–4
    colitis   67–8, 218
    cryptosporidiosis   77
    Kaposi sarcoma   344
    lymphoma   341
hMLH1/hMSH2/hMSH6 see MLH1;
    MSH2; MSH6
HPV see human papilloma virus
HSV (herpes simplex virus)   73
human immunodeficiency virus see
    HIV disease
human papilloma virus (HPV), anal
    lesions
    condyloma accuminatum   361
    giant condyloma   361, 366
    intraepithelial neoplasia   361
    verrucous carcinoma   366
hyalinization   46
hydrogen peroxide   194, 195
hyperganglionosis (intestinal
    neuronal dysplasia)   235,
    239–41, 241, 242
    diagnostic biopsy   236
    transition zone with mixed
        picture of hypoganglionosis
        and   238
hyperplasia
    eroded polypoid   269
    lymphoid follicles (colon)   35
        in ulcerative colitis   35, 107
    lymphoid follicles (ileum)
        225–6
    regenerative, crypt epithelium
        29–30
    see also lipohyperplasia

hyperplastic polyps *see*
    metaplastic/hyperplastic
    polyp; metaplastic/
    hyperplastic polyposis
hypertonic enemas   194
hypertrophy, myocyte   47–8
hypogammaglobulinaemia   35,
    218–19, 387
hypoganglionic zone   233–4
hypoganglionosis   235, 239
    transition zone with mixed
        picture of hyperganglionosis
        and   238

iatrogenic disease   182–201
ileitis   220–1
    acute   220–1
    backwash   224–5
    chronic   221
    pre-pouch   119, 128
ileoanal pouch   124–32
    complications   119, 125–31
    indications/contraindications
        124
    normal adaptive changes
        124–5
ileocaecal valve, lipohyperplasia
        278
ileum
    colectomy-related pathology
        224–5
    nodular lymphoid hyperplasia
        225–6
    terminal   219–24
        in microscopic colitis   155–6,
            223
        normal biopsy   219–20
    in ulcerative colitis   224–5
iliac arteries   169
immunodeficiency states   218–19,
        387–8
    IBD vs   218–19
immunoglobulins, mucosal, IBD
        100, 211
immunology, mucosal, and IBD
        100, 210–11
immunostaining/immunochemistry
    CMV infection   71–3
    collagen band   151
    signet ring cells *see* signet ring
        cell
    tumours and precancerous
        lesions or conditions   333,
            334
        adenocarcinoma   333, 337

Bowen's disease   370
carcinoids   338
granular cell tumour   282,
    368
melanoma   368
Paget's disease   372–3
inclusions, intranuclear, in CMV
    infection   71
infants
    innervation abnormalities
        causing constipation   223
    newborn, necrotizing
        enterocolitis   65–6
infections, venereal *see* sexually-
        transmitted diseases
infective colitis and/or proctitis
        54–89
    acute bacterial forms *see*
        bacterial infections
    histopathology   209–12
        crypt   23, 25, 28–9, 57–60, 61
        neutrophil exudate   34
        surface epithelium   17–18
    IBD vs   62–3, 209–12
    lumen in   15–16
    microscopic colitis vs   158
    natural history   211
    see also specific
        pathogens/diseases
infective ileitis   220–1
infective plexitis   242
inflammation, large bowel
    acute non-specific   205–6
    chronic
        in diarrhoeal illness   60–1
        non-specific   206
        in collagenous colitis   151–2
        in Crohn's disease   50, 115, 118
        in ileoanal pouch   125–6
inflammation, terminal ileum
        220–4
    interpretation of biopsy   222–4
inflammatory bowel disease,
        chronic   90–123
    anal fistula and fissure   355
    differential diagnosis   202–32
        amoebiasis   76
        Behçet's syndrome   379–80
        general principles   203
        infective colitis   62–3,
            209–12
        microscopic colitis *see*
            subheading below
        minor abnormalities and
            204–9

normal biopsy and   203–4
inflammatory polyps   269–70
microscopic colitis vs   216
    collagenous colitis   216
    lymphocytic colitis   157–8,
        216
natural history   211
reliability of diagnosis   211–12
see also Crohn's disease;
    ulcerative colitis
inflammatory cells
    in collagenous colitis   151–2
    in Crohn's disease   210
    lamina propria   33–7
        distributions   36–7
        proportions   36
        in ulcerative colitis   93–5,
            209
    submucosa   50–1
inflammatory lesions of anus
        352–61
inflammatory polyps
        (pseudopolyps)   253,
            268–70
    'cap' polyps   270, 274, 276
    cloacogenic polyp   271, 358
    in Crohn's disease   121
    juvenile polyps vs   264, 268,
        276
    myoglandular polyp   269, 274,
        276
    in ulcerative colitis   106
innervation *see* nerve supply
innominate grooves   19
instrumentation cleansing agents
        194–5
insular carcinoids   337, 368
intercryptal epithelium
        abnormalities   16, 18
intra-epithelial lymphocytes *see*
        lymphocytes
intra-epithelial neoplasia, anal
        361
intramucosal carcinoma,
        definition/categorization
            249, 302
intranuclear inclusions in CMV
        infection   71
irradiation *see* radiation
irritable bowel syndrome   217, 388
    IBD vs   217
ischaemia
    gangrenous   172
    radiation-related   176, 182,
        183

ischaemic colitis 168–81, 213–14
aetiology and precipitating
factors 168, 169–71
drugs 169–71, 188
anatomical considerations
168–9
appearance on biopsy 172–5
crypt degeneration 21, 23,
172–3, 213
end result 175
differential diagnosis 171–2
difficulties 175–6
IBD 213–14
microscopic colitis 157
pseudomembranous colitis
140
endoscopic features 171–2
natural history 171
reparative phase 174–5
submucosa 51, 172, 174, 175
surface epithelium degeneration
16, 172

juvenile polyps 204–6
adenomas vs 276
inflammatory polyps vs 264,
268, 276

Kaposi sarcoma 344–5
keratoacanthoma, anal 371
Ki67 immunostaining, benign vs
malignant signet ring cells
136
Klebsiella granulomatis 357
koilocytosis
condyloma accuminatum 359
giant condyloma 361
Kufs disease 383

lamina propria 9–10
abnormalities 33–49
cellular 33–44
in Crohn's disease 115
in ischaemic colitis 173
matrix 44–9
in ulcerative colitis 93–5,
98–9
empty 33
in mucosal prolapse syndrome
46, 274
normal features
large bowel 9–10
terminal ileum 219–20
large cell high-grade B cell
lymphomas 342

laxative abuse (cathartic colon)
196, 217
lectins, ulcerative colitis 100
leiomyoma, polypoid 277
leiomyosarcoma 342
leucoplakia 358
leukaemic infiltration
anus 368
large bowel 340
lichen sclerosis et atrophicus 369
lipid and lipid-like vacuoles *see*
vacuoles
lipofuscin 53, 196
lipofuscinosis, ceroid 383
lipohyperplasia 51
ileocaecal valve 278
lipomatous polyps 278
LKB1 and Peutz–Jeghers syndrome
266
lumen 15–16
toxins, and microscopic colitis
161
lupus erythematosus, systemic
379
lymph node metastases
from anal carcinoma 365
from colon
adenocarcinoma 337
malignant polyps 297
lymphocytes 35
epithelial, normal counts 147,
153–4
epithelial, raised counts
(lymphocytosis) 147, 153,
154, 155, 156, 157, 160–1,
163
in collagenous colitis 151,
155
in drug-associated colitis 186
mildly raised 154, 155, 157,
158
see also B cell; T cell
lymphocytic colitis 153–5, 216
atypical 157, 160
differential diagnosis 157–8,
158, 159
IDB 157–8, 216
epidemiology 162
overdiagnosis 161
overlap with collagenous colitis
147, 155
small bowel 156
terminology/definition 147
lymphogranuloma venereum 67,
357–8

lymphoid follicles
large bowel 9
epithelium associated with 8
hyperplasia *see* hyperplasia
submucosal *see* lymphoid–
glandular complex
in ulcerative colitis *see*
ulcerative colitis
terminal ileum (Peyer's patches)
220
hyperplasia 225–6
lymphoid–glandular complex
(submucosal lymphoid
follicles) 10, 29, 51–2
cysts in 42
lymphoid polyps 276–7
lymphoid tissue, gut-associated 9
lymphomas 340–2
lymphocytic colitis vs 157

M cells 220
macrophages
brown pigment 37, 53, 195–6
intranuclear inclusions in CMV
infection 71
malakoplakia 380–1
malignant tumours *see* cancer
MALT lymphoma 340
mantle cell lymphoma vs
341–2
mantle cell lymphoma (malignant
lymphomatous polyposis)
340
MALT lymphoma vs 341–2
marginal artery 168–9
mast cells 36
ulcerative colitis 94–5
mechanical stress, polyps
associated with 253
medullary carcinoma 332
megacolon 235–46
acquired 242–3
congenital 235–42
features associated with 244–6
idiopathic, childhood 242
toxic *see* toxic dilatation
Meissner's plexus 11
melanoma, malignant 366–8
melanosis coli 37, 53, 195–6, 244,
389
mesenchymal tumours
benign 277–80
malignant 342–5
mesenteric arteries
anatomy 168–9

occlusive disease   169
metaplasia, Paneth cell *see* Paneth
    cells
metaplastic/hyperplastic polyp(s)
    260–3
  crypt abnormalities   24
metaplastic/hyperplastic polyposis
    256, 262–3
metastases
  from anus to lymph node   365
  from large bowel
    to lymph node *see* lymph node
      metastases
    malignant polyps   296–7
  to large bowel   345–6
microadenomas   256
microgranulomas in Crohn's disease
    41, 65, 117, 210, 223
micro-organisms, lamina propria
    42–4
microsatellite instability (MSI)
  adenocarcinoma   332, 334–7
  metaplastic/hyperplastic polyps
    262
  serrated adenomas   264
microscopic colitis   146–67
  aetiology/pathogenesis   161–2
    drugs   161, 188
  course and therapy   162
  diagnostic biopsy   148–61
  diagnostic pitfalls   160–1
  differential diagnosis   156–9
    IBD   156–7, 158, 216
  epidemiology   162
  non-collagenous non-
      lymphocytic   147–8,
      159–60, 216
  overlap forms   147, 155
  pathophysiology   162
  small bowel and   155–6
  terminal ileum in   155–6, 223
  terminology/definition   147
microvilli
  columnar cell   7
  goblet cell   7
minimal change colitis   216
mismatch repair proteins and
    adenocarcinoma   337
MLH1 (hMLH1)
  adenocarcinoma and   337
  serrated adenomas and   264
MMR vaccine and ileal lymphoid
    nodular hyperplasia   226
molecular studies, dysplasia   312,
    321

motility disorders   2, 233–47
MSH2 and adenocarcinoma   337
MSH6 and adenocarcinoma   337
MSI-H, concept of   334–7
mucin
  adenovirus infection and   74
  columnar cell   7
  goblet cell   6–7
    depletion   29
  Peutz–Jeghers polyps   267
  tumours
    anus   363
    colon   333
  in ulcerative colitis   100
    in dysplastic cells   309
mucinous carcinoma   332
muciphages   9
mucoepidermoid carcinoma, anus
    363
mucosa
  anal   351
  carcinoma, definition/
      categorization   249
  debris covering   15
  dissection and coiling to detect
      dysplasia in ulcerative
      colitis   323
  epithelium *see* epithelium
  gastric, heterotopic   282–4
  giant cells   37–8
  of ileoanal pouch   124–5,
      128–30
    dysplasia   131
  immunology, and IBD 100, 210–11
  in ischaemic colitis   172–4
  normal architecture
    large bowel   5
    terminal ileum   219
  polyps
    classification   243
    diagnostic problems   275–6
  preoperative adjuvant
      radiotherapy affecting
      183–4
  prolapse *see* prolapse; ulcers,
      solitary rectal
  tags   269–70
  transitional   26–7
  in ulcerative colitis
    degenerative features   311–12
    regenerative   321
    thickening   309–10
mucosa-associated lymphoid tissue
    lymphoma *see* MALT
    lymphoma

mucosectomy   284
mucoviscidosis   26, 386
multinucleate giant cells of foreign
    body type *see* foreign body
    giant cells
multiple endocrine neoplasia (MEN)
    syndrome, ganglioneuroma
    280
mumps/measles/rubella vaccine and
    ileal lymphoid nodular
    hyperplasia   226
muscle fibres *see* smooth muscle
    fibres
muscularis mucosa   10–11
  abnormalities   49–50
    strictures *see* strictures
    ulcerative colitis   95
  smooth muscle fibres *see* smooth
      muscle fibres
*Mycobacterium avium-
    intracellulare* complex   68
Mycobacterium tuberculosis see
    tuberculosis
myenteric (Auerbach's) plexus
    234–5
  infection   242
myoblastoma, granular cell   282
myocyte hypertrophy   47–8
myoglandular polyps, inflammatory
    269, 274, 276
myopathy, visceral   242–3

necrosis
  pseudomembranous colitis   136
  schistosomiasis   79, 80
necrotizing colitis syndromes
    177
necrotizing enterocolitis   65–6
Neisseria gonorrhoea   66
nematodes   78, 79–81
neoadjuvant (preoperative
    adjuvant) radiotherapy,
    mucosal effects   183–4
neonates, necrotizing enterocolitis
    65–6
neoplasms *see* tumours
nerve supply (innervation)
  lamina propria   10
  muscularis mucosa   11
  submucosa   11, 233–4
    abnormalities (in general)   53
    in Crohn's disease   118
neural supply *see* nerve supply
neuroendocrine cells *see* endocrine
    cells

neurofibroma 279
neurofibromatosis type I (von
        Recklinghausen's disease)
    ganglioneuroma 279–80
    neurofibromas 279
neuronal dysplasia 235–41
neurone-specific enolase 8
neutropenic colitis 194
neutrophils 34
    collagenous colitis 151
    ulcerative colitis 93, 94
newborns (neonates), necrotizing
        enterocolitis 65–6
nodular lymphoid hyperplasia, ileal
        225–6
non-steroidal anti-inflammatory
        drugs 187–9
nuclei
    of crypt epithelium, in dysplasia
        30–1
    inclusions in CMV infection 71
    of surface epithelial cells
        degeneration into nuclear dust
            16
        displaced upwards 18–19

obstruction, large intestinal
    colitis due to 170–1, 244–6
    ischaemic effects 170–1
    see also pseudo-obstruction
occlusive disease (intestinal vessels)
        169
    natural history 171
oedema
    mucosal 46–7
        in infective colitis 57, 60
    submucosal 50
oleogranulomas 184–5
ovarian carcinoma, colorectal
        metastases 345
oxyuriasis 81

p53
    adenoma-like dysplasia-
        associated lesion or mass
        and 321
    in benign vs malignant signet
        ring cells, immunostaining
        for protein product
        136
    ulcerative colitis-associated
        cancer and 317
paediatrics see children; infants
Paget's disease, perianal 371–3

pancreatic enzyme supplements
        190–1
Paneth cells 5, 32–3
    metaplasia 32–3
        in lymphocytic colitis 152–3
        in ulcerative colitis 98
papilloma virus see human
        papilloma virus
papulosis, Bowenoid 370
PAR and Peutz–Jeghers syndrome
        266
paracoccidioidomycosis 82
parasites see helminths; protozoa
patchy distribution/disease
    Crohn's disease 115, 119
    ulcerative colitis 103
pathologist
    pseudomembranous colitis
        diagnosis 142
    report see report
pecten, anal 352, 353
    carcinoma arising from 361
pedunculated polyps 275
    fixation for polypectomy 284
    metaplastic/hyperplastic polyps
        260
    tubular adenoma 256
perianal skin lesions 368–74
pericryptal eosinophilic
        gastroenteritis 218
pericryptal fibroblasts see
        fibroblasts
perinuclear anti-neutrophilic
        cytoplasmic antibody 212
Peutz–Jeghers syndrome and
        polyps 266–7
    hamartoma vs 276
    smooth muscle fibres 48
Peyer's patches see lymphoid
        follicles, terminal ileum
phagocytes, mononuclear 37
pigbel 65–6
pigment deposition 37, 53
    brown 37, 53, 195–6, 389
piles (haemorrhoids) 358
pinworm 81
plasma cells 34–5
    in collagenous colitis 151
    in IBD 210–11
        ulcerative colitis 209
pleomorphic carcinoma 334
plexitis, infective 242
ploidy studies, dysplasia 316
pneumatosis, cystic 50, 380

polymorphonuclear neutrophils see
        neutrophils
polyp(s) 251–91
    adenomatous see adenomas
        (polypoid); familial
        adenomatous polyposis
    anal 357, 358
    classification 252, 253
    crypt abnormalities 19, 24
    definition 251
    diagnostic difficulties 275–6
    excision see polypectomy
    hamartomatous see
        hamartomas
    handling 251–2
    inflammatory see inflammatory
        polyps
    juvenile see juvenile polyps
    leimyomatous 277
    lipomatous 278
    lymphoid 276–7
    malignant 295–8
    metaplastic 24
    mucosal see mucosa
    pedunculated see pedunculated
        polyps
    Peutz–Jeghers see Peutz–Jeghers
        syndrome
    reporting 285–6
    serrated 260–4
    sessile 252, 261
    smooth muscle fibres 48
polypectomy 2
    colonoscopic see colonoscopic
        polypectomy
polyposis (multiple/many polyps)
        253, 256
    benign lymphoid 277
    'cap' 270
    familial adenomatous see familial
        adenomatous polyposis
    hereditary mixed polyposis
        syndrome 276
    inflammatory (colitis polyposa)
        271
    juvenile 265
    lipomatous 278
    malignant lymphomatous see
        mantle cell lymphoma
    metaplastic/hyperplastic 256,
        262–3
    serrated adenomatous 264
post-inflammatory polyps 269–70
pouch, ileoanal see ileoanal pouch

pouchitis
  differential diagnosis   128–30
  risk factors   126–8
precancerous conditions (disorders),
      definition   302
precancerous lesions
  crypt epithelium   31
  definition   302
  see also adenoma–carcinoma
      sequence
premalignancy see precancerous
      conditions; precancerous
      lesions
preparing enemas   194
proctitis
  follicular see follicular proctitis
  infective see infective colitis
      and/or proctitis
  mild acute non-specific   60
  non-specific, use of term   91
proctocolitis
  diversion   191–2
  ulcerative see ulcerative colitis
prolapse, anorectal mucosal   358
  see also ulcers, solitary rectal
prostatic carcinoma, colorectal
      metastases   346
protozoa   42, 74–7
pseudocarcinomatous invasion of
      adenoma   52, 254, 293
pseudolipomatosis   41–2
pseudomembranous colitis   133,
      134–7, 177
  crypts   135, 136
      degeneration   21
      dilatation   25, 136
  diagnostic biopsy   134–7
  differential diagnosis   140
      ischaemic colitis   176
  intercryptal erosion   18
  lumen   15
  pathologist's role in diagnosis
      142
  terminology/definition   134
  type I lesion   135–6, 140
  type II lesion   136
  type III lesion   136–7, 140
pseudomembranous collagenous
      colitis   153
pseudo-obstruction   242
pseudopolyps see inflammatory
      polyps
PTEN and Cowden's syndrome   282
pus, luminal   15

radiation damage, chronic (radiation
      colitis)   182–4, 218
  hyalinization   46
  IBD vs   218
  ischaemic colitis vs   176
radiotherapy
  anal verrucous carcinoma   365–6
  preoperative adjuvant, mucosal
      effects   183–4
reactive arthritis   223–4
regenerative hyperplasia, crypt
      epithelium   29–30
regenerative mucosa in IBD 312
report
  colonoscopist's
      Crohn's disease   120
      ulcerative colitis   102–3
  neoplastic tissue, decisions
      298–9
  pathologist's   2–3
      dysplasia   317–18
  polyps   285–6
research and development   3
resolution of acute diarrhoea   61
rheumatoid arthritis   379
roundworms (nematodes)   78, 79–81

Salmonella   62
sarcoidosis   382–3
sarcoma
  Kaposi   344–5
  smooth muscle (leiomyosarcoma)
      342
schistosomiasis   79
  granulomas   41
  inflammatory polyps   268
schwannosis   243
serology, IBD   212
sessile polyps   252, 261
sexually-transmitted (venereal)
      diseases
  anal lesions   357–8
  large bowel lesions   66–8
Shigella   61–2
sialylated mucin   6–7
sigmoid colon, ulcerative colitis
      102, 104, 105
sigmoidoscopy, ulcerative colitis
      91, 95
signet ring cell (and their
      immunostaining)
  benign change, in
      pseudomembranous colitis
      136, 137

carcinoma   137, 332
skin lesions, perianal   368–74
skin tags, anal   357
skip lesion
  Crohn's disease   114, 115
  ulcerative colitis   103
SMAD4 and juvenile polyps   266
small bowel and microscopic colitis
      155–6
  see also ileum
small cell undifferentiated
      carcinoma   334, 366
small vessel disease   169
smooth muscle fibres of muscularis
      mucosa extending into
      lamina propria   9, 10–11
  hyperextension/splaying upwards
      47–8, 49–50
snare polypectomy   284
spindle cell tumours   342
spirochaetosis   69–70
  lamina propria   42
  surface epithelium   17
splenic flexure, blood supply
      susceptibility   169
spondylitis, ankylosing   379
squamous carcinoma
  anal   363
  colon   334
      secondary (from cervix)   347
squamous carcinoma in situ see
      Bowen disease; intra-
      epithelial neoplasia, anal
squamous epithelial differentiation,
      adenomas   255
Staphylococcus aureus   62
stem cell(s) (epithelial)   5, 8
  carcinoma   334
stercoral ulceration   245
stomach mucosa, heterotopic
      282–4
strictures (of muscularis mucosa),
      non-malignant   50
  ischaemic colitis   175
  NSAIDs   187–8
string of pearls' sign   58, 60
strip biopsy   2
stroma
  adenoma, fibrosis   275, 294
  invasive adenocarcinoma
      293–5
stromal tumours, gastrointestinal
      342–4
strongyloidiasis   79

subepithelial zone abnormalities
      18–19
submucosa   11, 50–2
   abnormalities   50–2
      ischaemic colitis   51, 172,
         174, 175
      ulcerative colitis   95
   carcinoma
      definition/categorization
         249
      focal (in adenomatous polyps)
         296–8
   crypts/lymphoid follicles
         extending into see
         lymphoid–glandular
         complex
   fibrosis, with pancreatic enzyme
      supplements   191
   giant cells   38
   innervation see nerve supply
   lymphoid follicles, cysts in   42
   resection with tumours   2
surface epithelium abnormalities
      16–18
   in collagenous colitis   152
   in ischaemic colitis   16, 172
surgery   2
   adenocarcinoma   337
   in ulcerative colitis following
      biopsy diagnosis of
      dysplasia, failure to find
      lesion after   323
   see also specific techniques
sweat gland carcinoma   373
syphilis
   anus   357
   large bowel   66
systemic lupus erythematosus   379
systemic sclerosis   243, 379

T cell, IBD and   211
T cell lymphomas   340
tags
   anal skin   357
   mucosal   269–70
tapeworms   78
tenascin stain, collagen band   151
threadworm   81
thrombosis (causing ischaemia)
      169, 214
   small vessel   174, 176
toxic dilatation/megacolon
   Crohn's disease   121
   ulcerative colitis   106–7

toxins
   C. difficile see Clostridium
      difficile
   luminal, and microscopic colitis
      161
trabecular carcinoids   337–8, 368
transitional cell carcinoma of
      bladder   346
transitional mucosa   26–7
transitional zone, anal (ATZ)
      351–2
   carcinoma arising from   361
trematodes   78, 79
Treponema pallidum infection see
      syphilis
trichuriasis   79–81
Tropheryma whippeli   382
trophozoites, Balantidium   77
Trypanosoma cruzi   242
tuberculosis   64–5
   Crohn's disease vs   64–5,
      118–19
   granulomas   39–41, 64–5
tubular adenoma   253, 256
tubulovillous adenoma   253,
      256–7
tufts, surface epithelial cell   17
tumours (neoplasms)   248–50,
      361–8, 370–4
   anus
      anal canal   361–8
      perianal skin   370–4
   decisions when reporting
      298–9
   epithelial see epithelial tumours
   ileoanal pouch   130–1
   local excision   2
   malignant see cancer; metastases
typhoid fever   62

ulcer(s)
   amoebiasis   75
   anastomotic   195
   aphthoid see aphthoid ulcers
   ileoanal pouch   126
   NSAID-associated   188, 189
   solitary rectal (mucosal prolapse
      syndrome)   214–15, 271–4
      colitis cystica profunda with
         386
      IBD vs   214–15
      intercryptal erosion   18
      lamina propria in   46, 274
      misplaced crypts   29

pseudomembranous colitis
      type I lesion vs   135
stercoral   245
terminal ileum   221
ulcerative colitis/proctocolitis
      90–112, 301–29
   active phase   91–6
   C. difficile-associated
      exacerbations   141
   colonoscopic biopsy   102–4
   complications   106–7
      follicular proctitis   35, 107
   crypt abnormalities   20, 21, 25,
      28, 91–3, 96, 100, 101
      abscesses   94
      atrophy   21, 98
      dysplasia   31, 306, 308–9,
         310, 314
   diagnostic biopsy   91–101
   diagnostic difficulties   95–6, 96,
      99–100
   differential diagnosis   202–32
      Behçet's syndrome   379
      Crohn's disease   91, 209–12
      infective colitis   76, 209–12
      microscopic colitis   158, 216
      radiation colitis   183
   dysplasia see dysplasia;
      dysplasia-associated lesion
      or mass
   equivocal   101
   histopathology   209–12
      crypts see subheading above
      endocrine cell abnormalities
         33
      granulation tissue   49
      inflammatory polyps   269
      lymphoid follicles, see
         subheading below
   lymphoid follicles in   93–4,
      107
      hyperplasia   35, 107
   natural history/resolving phase
      96, 211
   remission/quiescent phase
      98–100
   sequential/follow-up biopsy
      101–2
   sporadic adenoma   319–23
   terminal ileum in   223
   treatment influence on biopsy
      104–6
   see also inflammatory bowel
      disease

undifferentiated/anaplastic
carcinomas
anus 363
vs melanoma 366
colon 334
urinary bladder carcinoma,
colorectal metastases 346

vacuoles
adenovirus-infected cells 74
koilocytic 359, 361
lipid 184
lipid-like/fat-like, lamina propria
33, 41
vascular lesions 377–80
hamartoma 279
vascular supply (blood vessels)
anatomy (relevant to ischaemic
colitis) 168–9
inflammatory disease see
vasculitis
lamina propria 10
abnormalities 48
occlusive disease see occlusive
disease

radiation damage 182, 183
submucosa, abnormalities 52
see also capillaries
vasculitis 175–6
in Behçet's syndrome 380
venereal infections see sexually-
transmitted diseases
venous occlusion 168
verrucous carcinoma, anal 361,
365–6
Vienna classification of
gastrointestinal epithelial
neoplasia 248, 249
villiform pattern, ulcerative colitis
93
villous adenoma 253, 257–8
mixed tubular and (tubulovillous
adenoma) 253, 256–7
villous atrophy
ileoanal pouch 124, 126
ileum, in microscopic colitis
156, 223
vimentin, tumours 333
viral infections 42, 70–4
visceral myopathy 242–3

von Recklinghausen's disease see
neurofibromatosis type I

wart(s)/condyloma accuminatum
358–9, 361
Warthin–Starry stain,
spirochaetosis 17, 69
Wegener's granulomatosis 379
Whipple's disease 382
AIDS-related colitis resembling
68
whipworm 79–81
World Health Organization (WHO)
classification of
gastrointestinal epithelial
neoplasia 248, 249, 250,
330
metaplastic polyposis 262–3
worms (helminths) 77–81

xanthoma 37

yersiniosis 63–4

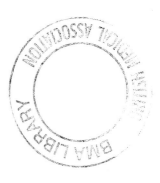